Delmar's

Respiratory Care

Drug Reference

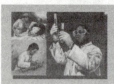

Delmar's Respiratory Care Drug Reference

Fred Hill, MA, RRT
Director of Clinical Education and
Assistant Professor
Department of Cardiorespiratory Care
College of Allied Health Professions
University of South Alabama
Mobile, Alabama

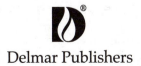

Delmar Publishers

an International Thomson Publishing company I(T)P®

Albany • Bonn • Boston • Cincinnati • Detroit • London • Madrid
Melbourne • Mexico City • New York • Pacific Grove • Paris • San Francisco
Singapore • Tokyo • Toronto • Washington

NOTICE TO THE READER

Publisher does not warrant or guarantee any of the products described herein or perform any independent analysis in connection with any of the product information contained herein. Publisher does not assume, and expressly disclaims, any obligation to obtain and include information other than that provided to it by the manufacturer.

The reader is expressly warned to consider and adopt all safety precautions that might be indicated by the activities herein and to avoid all potential hazards. By following the instructions contained herein, the reader willingly assumes all risks in connections with such instructions.

The publisher makes no representation or warranties of any kind, including but not limited to, the warranties of fitness for particular purpose or merchantability, nor are any such representations implied with respect to the material set forth herein, and the publisher takes no responsibility with respect to such material. The publisher shall not be liable for any special, consequential, or exemplary damages resulting, in whole or in part, from the readers' use of, or reliance upon, this material.

Delmar Staff:

Publisher: Susan Simpfenderfer
Acquisitions Editor: Dawn Gerrain
Developmental Editor: Debra Flis
Project Editor: William Trudell
Production Manager: Linda Helfrich
Marketing Manager: Darryl Caron
Editorial Assistant: Donna Leto

COPYRIGHT © 1999
By Delmar Publishers
an International Thomson Publishing company I(T)P®

The ITP logo is a trademark under license
Printed in Canada

For more information contact:

Delmar Publishers
3 Columbia Circle, Box 15015
Albany, New York 12212-5015

International Thomson Publishing Europe
Berkshire House
168-173 High Holborn
London, WC1V7AA
United Kingdom

Nelson ITP, Australia
102 Dodds Street
South Melbourne,
Victoria, 3205 Australia

Nelson Canada
1120 Birchmont Road
Scarborough, Ontario
M1K5G4, Canada

International Thomson Publishing France
Tour Maine-Montparnasse
33 Avenue du Maine
75755 Paris Cedex 15, France

International Thomson Editores
Seneca 53
Colonia Polanco
11560 Mexico D.F. Mexico

International Thomson Publishing GmbH
Königswinterer Strasße 418
53227 Bonn
Germany

International Thomson Publishing Asia
60 Albert Street
#15-01 Albert Complex
Singapore 189969

International Thomson Publishing Japan
Hirakawa-cho Kyowa Building, 3F
2-2-1 Hirakawa-cho, Chiyoda-ku,
Tokyo 102, Japan

ITE Spain/Paraninfo
Calle Magallanes, 25
28015-Madrid, Espana

ISBN: 0-8273-9066-1

Notice to the Reader

Preface

Delmar's Respiratory Care Drug Reference provides up-to-date information on drugs of particular interest to the respiratory care practitioner. These drugs are presented alphabetically in Chapter 3.

Chapter 1 and the "Quick Guide to the Use of *Delmar's Respiratory Care Drug Reference* should be consulted first because they outline how to use the text. General information on drug classes, including respiratory care considerations, is found in Chapter 2. This information is easy to locate and use and prevents lengthy repetitions throughout the text. A list of drugs that are in that drug class appears at the beginning of each class discussed.

Trade names of drugs marketed in the United States and Canada are listed; trade names of drugs marketed only in Canada are designated by a maple leaf ✹. For ease of location, the FDA pregnancy category immediately follows the pronunciation of the drug at the beginning of the information for each drug in Chapter 3.

One of the important features of *Delmar's Respiratory Care Drug Reference* is the format whereby dosage information is presented. The dosage form and/or route of administration are clearly delineated and are often correlated with the disease state(s) for which the dosage is used. This makes finding dosage information easy. Another important feature is the designation in boldface italics of life-threatening side effects. Immediately following the listing of side effects is a section entitled *Overdose Management,* OD that lists the symptoms and treatment for drug overdose. The use of an icon for overdose helps to locate this section quickly. The section entitled *Special Concerns* provides information of special note to the practitioner, including safety and efficacy considerations for use of the drug in certain disease states, in children, during lactation, during pregnancy, and in the geriatric client.

The presentation of *Respiratory Care Considerations* is one of the most important features of the text. Such information provides the practitioner with a mechanism to assess the client before and after prescribed drug therapy, to obtain and review specific items (assessments, labs) related to the drug being administered, to initiate appropriate interventions, to incorporate appropriate client/family teaching to ensure proper drug therapy, and to evaluate the effectiveness and outcomes of drug therapy. The expected outcome(s) of the drug therapy are addressed and identified under the *Evaluate* section. Chapter 1 should be consulted for a more thorough discussion of how respiratory care considerations are presented.

Appendices include a definition and listing of drugs controlled either by the United States Controlled Substances Act of the Canadian Controlled Substances Law (Appendix 1); information on the elements and interpretation of a prescription (Appendix 2); definitions of FDA pregnancy categories (Appendix 3); commonly used laboratory test values (Appendix 4); nomogram for estimating the body surface area (Appendix 5); easy formulas for IV rate calculations (Appendix 6); commonly accepted therapeutic drug levels (Appendix 7); and table of weights and measures (Appendix 8). The index is extensively cross-referenced and facilitates locating drugs by pairing generic and trade names.

I believe that the information provided and the format used for *Delmar's Respiratory Care Drug Reference* makes the book an easy-to-use and valuable text and reference for the latest information on drugs and the proper monitoring of drug therapy by the practitioner.

Acknowledgments

I would like to extend my thanks to the Delmar team that work so diligently to ensure that the manuscript process flows smoothly and to try to keep us on track. Team members include Debra Flis, Lisa Santy, Dawn Gerrain, Bill Trudell, and Linda Helfrich.

Special thanks are extended to Deanna Winn for her assistance in the technical preparation of the manuscript.

Delmar and the author would like to recognize the following individuals who reviewed the manuscript and made valuable suggestions:

Allen W. Barbaro, MS, RRT
Program Director, Respiratory Care Program
Collin County Community College
McKinney, Texas

Melanie A. Ciesielski, BS, RRT
Faculty, Respiratory Care Program
Forsyth Technical Community College
Winston-Salem, North Carolina

Leanna Konechne, Med, RRT
Respiratory Therapy Program Director
Pima Medical Institute
Tucson, Arizona

Kathy Miller, MA, RRT
Director, Respiratory Care Program
Marygrove College
Detroit, Michigan

Quick Guide to the Use of *Delmar's Respiratory Care Drug Reference*

An understanding of the format of *Delmar's Respiratory Care Drug Reference* will help you reference information quickly.

- There are three chapters:
  1. Detailed information on "How to Use *Delmar's Respiratory Care Drug Reference*"
  2. Alphabetical listing of therapeutic/chemical drug classes with general information for the class, plus a listing of drugs in the class covered in Chapter 3.
  3. Alphabetical listing of drugs by generic name.

- Each entry in Chapter 3 consists of two parts: general drug information and respiratory care considerations

General drug information (similar in format to Chapter 2) includes the following categories (not all categories may be provided for each drug):

- **Combination Drug** heading indicates two or more drugs are combined in the same product.
- **Generic name** of drug with simplified **phonetic pronunciation**
- **FDA pregnancy category**
- **Trade name(s)** by which drug is marketed; a maple leaf (✤) indicates trade names available only in Canada
- **Drug schedule** if drug is controlled by U.S. Federal Controlled Substances Act (such as C-II, C-III)
- **Rx** = prescription drug; **OTC** = nonprescription, over-the-counter drug
- See also reference to classification in Chapter 2, if applicable
- **Classification** is the chemical or pharmacologic class to which the drug has been assigned.
- **Content** (for combination drugs) is the generic name and amount of each drug in the combination product.
- **General Statement:** General information and/or specific aspects of drugs in a class; also diseases for which drugs may be used
- **Action/Kinetics:** Mechanism(s) by which drug achieves therapeutic effect, rate of absorption, distribution, minimum effective serum or plasma level, half-life (time for half the drug to be removed from blood), duration of action, metabolism, excretion routes, and other pertinent information
- **Uses:** Therapeutic indications, including investigational uses for the drug
- **Contraindications:** Diseases or conditions for which drug should not be used
- **Special Concerns:** Considerations for use in pediatric, geriatric, pregnant, or lactating clients. Also situations or disease states when the drug should be used with caution.

- **Side Effects:** Undesired or bothersome effects in some clients, listed by body organ or system affected. Life-threatening side effects are designated in boldface italics
- **Overdose Management:** Lists the symptoms of drug overdose, as well as treatment approaches and/or antidotes to treat the symptoms of the drug overdose. Designated by a special `OD` icon.
- **Drug Interactions:** Drugs that may interact with one another resulting in an increase or decrease in effect of drug; when listed for a class of drugs, are likely to apply to all drugs in the class
- **Laboratory Test Interferences:** Effect on laboratory test values; may also appear in *Respiratory Care Considerations* section
- **Dosage:** Recommended adult and pediatric dosages for designated disease states, dosing intervals, and available dosage forms

  Respiratory Care Considerations: Guides the practitioner in applying the nursing process to pharmacotherapeutics to ensure safe practice.
- **Administration/Storage:** Guidelines for preparing and administering medications, as well as proper storage
- **Assessment:** Guidelines to assist the practitioner in what to obtain, identify, and assess before, during, and after drug therapy
- **Interventions:** Guidelines for specific appropriate nursing actions related to the drug being administered
- **Client/Family Teaching:** Guidelines to promote education, active participation, understanding, precautions, and compliance with drug therapy
- **Evaluate:** Identifies measurable outcome criteria to determine effectiveness of drug therapy and the anticipated client response

- **Additional Contraindications, Additional Side Effects,** or **Additional Respiratory Care Considerations:** Information relevant to a specific drug but not necessarily to the class overall. More complete data can be found in the discussion of the drug class (Chapter 2).

- **Index:** Extensively cross-referenced; **boldface** = generic drug name; *italics* = therapeutic drug class; regular type = trade name; CAPITALS = combination drug names; trade name is paired with generic name to facilitate ease of locating

Table of Contents

Commonly Used Abbreviations and Symbols

aa, A	of each
ABG	arterial blood gas
a.c.	before meals
ACE	angiotensin-converting enzyme
ACLS	advanced cardiac life support
ACTH	adrenocorticotropic hormone
ad	to, up to
a.d.	right ear
ad lib	as desired, at pleasure
ADA	adenosine deaminase
ADH	antidiuretic hormone
ADL	activities of daily living
AFB	acid fast bacillus
AHF	antihemophilic factor
AIDS	acquired immunodeficiency syndrome
a.l.	left ear
ALT	alanine aminotransferase
a.m., A.M.	morning
AMI	acute myocardial infarction
AML	acute myeloid leukemia
AMP	adenosine monophosphate
ANA	antinuclear antibody
ANC	active neutrophil count
ANS	autonomic nervous system
aq	water
aq dest.	distilled water
ARC	AIDS-related complex
ARDS	adult respiratory distress syndrome
ASA	aspirin
ASAP	as soon as possible
ASHD	arteriosclerotic heart disease
AST	aspartate aminotransferase
ATC	around the clock
ATP	adenosine triphosphate
a.u.	each ear, both ears
AV	atrioventricular
AZT	zidovudine
b.i.d.	two times per day
b.i.n.	two times per night
BMR	basal metabolic rate
BP	blood pressure
BPH	benign prostatic hypertrophy
BSA	body surface area

BSE	breast self-exam
BSP	Bromsulphalein
BUN	blood urea nitrogen
C	Centigrade/Celsius
CABG	coronary artery bypass graft
CAD	coronary artery disease
caps, Caps	capsule(s)
CBC	complete blood count
CD_4	helper T_4 lymphocyte cells
C&DB	cough and deep breathe
CHF	congestive heart failure
CLL	chronic lymphocytic leukemia
cm	centimeter
CML	chronic myelocytic leukemia
CMV	cytomegalovirus
CN	cranial nerve
CNS	central nervous system
CO	cardiac output
COPD	chronic obstructive pulmonary disease
CPAP	continuous positive airway pressure
CPB	cardiopulmonary bypass
CPK	creatine phosphokinase
CPR	cardiopulmonary resuscitation
C&S	culture and sensitivity
CSF	cerebrospinal fluid
CT	computerized tomography
CTZ	chemoreceptor trigger zone
CV	cardiovascular
CVA	cerebrovascular accident
CVP	central venous pressure
CXR	chest X ray
dATP	deoxy ATP
DBP	diastolic BP
dc	discontinue
DI	diabetes insipidus
DIC	disseminated intravascular coagulation
dil.	dilute
dL	deciliter (one-tenth of a liter)
DNA	deoxyribonucleic acid
DOE	dyspnea on exertion
dr.	dram (0.0625 ounce)
DTR	deep tendon reflex
EC	enteric-coated
ECB	extracorporeal cardiopulmonary bypass
ECG, EKG	electrocardiogram, electrocardiograph
EDTA	ethylenediaminetetraacetic acid
EENT	eye, ear, nose, and throat
e.g.	for example
elix	elixir
emuls.	emulsion
ER	extended release
ESR	erythrocyte sedimentation rate
ET	endotracheal
ext.	extract
F	Fahrenheit, fluoride
FBS	fasting blood sugar

FDA	Food and Drug Administration
FFP	fresh frozen plasma
FSH	follicle-stimulating hormone
F/U	follow-up
g, gm	gram (1,000 mg)
GABA	gamma-aminobutyric acid
GERD	gastroesophageal reflux disease
GFR	glomerular filtration rate
gi, GI	gastrointestinal
GnRH	gonadotropin-releasing hormone
G6PD	glucose-6-phosphate dehydrogenase
gr	grain
gtt	a drop, drops
GU	genitourinary
h, hr	hour
HA, HAL	hyperalimentation
Hb	hemoglobin
HcG	human chorionic gonadotropin
HCP	health-care provider
HDL	high density lipoprotein
HFN	high flow nebulizer
H&H	hematocrit and hemoglobin
HIV	human immunodeficiency virus
HMG-CoA	3-hydroxy-3-methyl-glutaryl-coenzyme A
HR	heart rate
h.s.	at bedtime
HSV	herpes simplex virus
5-HT	5-hydroxytryptamine
IA	intra-arterial
ICP	intracranial pressure
Ig	immunoglobulin
im, IM	intramuscular
IMV	intermittent mandatory ventilation
INR	international normalized ratio
I&O	intake and output
IPPB	intermittent positive pressure breathing
ITP	idiopathic thrombocytopenia purpura
IU	international units
iv, IV	intravenous
IVPB	IV piggyback, a secondary IV line
JVD	jugular vein distension
kg	kilogram (2.2 lb)
KVO	keep vein open
l, L	liter (1,000 mL)
L	left
LDH	lactic dehydrogenase
LDL	low density lipoprotein
LFTs	liver function tests
LH	luteinizing hormone
LHRH	luteinizing hormone–releasing hormone
LOC	loss of consciousness
LV	left ventricular
M	mix
m^2, M^2	square meter

m., min.	minimum
MAO	monoamine oxidase
MAP	mean arterial pressure
max	maximum
mcg	microgram
mCi	millicurie
MDI	metered-dose inhaler
mEq	milliequivalent
mg	milligram
MI	myocardial infarction
MIC	minimum inhibitory concentration
min	minute
mist, mixt	mixture
mL	milliliter
MRI	magnetic resonance imaging
NaCl	sodium chloride
ng	nanogram
NG	nasogastric
NGT	nasogastric tube
NKA	no known allergies
NKDA	no known drug allergies
noct	at night, during the night
non rep	do not repeat
NPN	nonprotein nitrogen
NPO	nothing by mouth
NR	do not refill (e.g., a prescription)
NSAID	nonsteroidal anti-inflammatory drug
NSR	normal sinus rhythm
NSS	normal saline solution
N&V	nausea and vomiting
O_2	oxygen
o.d.	once a day
O.D.	right eye
OOB	out of bed
OR	operating room
os	mouth
O.S.	left eye
O_2 sat	oxygen saturation
OTC	over the counter
O.U.	each eye, both eyes
oz	ounce
PA	pulmonary artery
PABA	para-aminobenzoic acid
PAWP	pulmonary artery wedge pressure
PBI	protein-bound iodine
p.c.	after meals
PCA	patient-controlled analgesia
PCN	penicillin
PCP	*Pneumocystis carinii* pneumonia
PE	pulmonary embolus
PEEP	positive end expiratory pressure
per	by, through
PFTs	pulmonary function tests
pH	negative logarithm of hydrogen ion concentration
PMH	past medical history
PMI	point of maximum impulse

PMS	premenstrual syndrome
PND	paroxysmal nocturnal dyspnea
po, p.o., PO	by mouth
PPD	purified protein derivative
PR	by rectum
p.r.n., PRN	when needed or necessary
PSA	prostatic specific antigen
PSVT	paroxysmal supraventricular tachycardia
PT	prothrombin time
PTT	partial thromboplastin time
PUD	peptic ulcer disease
PVC	premature ventricular contraction, polyvinyl chloride
PVD	peripheral vascular disease
q.d.	every day
q.h.	every hour
q2h	every two hours
q3h	every three hours
q4h	every four hours
q6h	every six hours
q8h	every eight hours
qhs	every night
q.i.d.	four times per day
q.o.d.	every other day
q.s.	as much as is needed, quantity sufficient
RA	right atrium
RBC	red blood cell
RDA	recommended daily allowance
REM	rapid eye movement
Rept.	let it be repeated
RNA	ribonucleic acid
ROM	range of motion
R/T	related to
RTC	round the clock
RV	right ventricular
Rx	symbol for a prescription
SA	sinoatrial or sustained-action
SAH	subarachnoid hemorrhage
SBE	subacute bacterial endocarditis
SBP	systolic BP
sc, SC, SQ	subcutaneous
SCID	severe combined immunodeficiency disease
SGOT	serum glutamic-oxaloacetic transaminase
SGPT	serum glutamic-pyruvic transaminase
S., Sig.	mark on the label
SIMV	synchronized intermittent mandatory ventilation
SL	sublingual
SLE	systemic lupus erythematosus
SOB	shortness of breath
sol	solution
sp	spirits
SR	sustained-release
ss	one-half
S&S	signs and symptoms
stat	immediately, first dose
STD	sexually transmitted disease

SV	stroke volume
SVT	supraventricular tachycardia
syr	syrup
tab	tablet
TB	tuberculosis
TENS	transcutaneous electric nerve stimulation
t.i.d.	three times per day
t.i.n.	three times per night
T.O.	telephone order
TPN	total parenteral nutrition
TSH	thyroid stimulating hormone
U	unit
μ	micron
μCi	microcurie
μg	microgram
ung	ointment
URI, URTI	upper respiratory infection
USP	U.S. Pharmacopeia
ut dict	as directed
UTI	urinary tract infection
vin	wine
VLDL	very low density lipoprotein
V.O.	verbal order
VS	vital signs
WBC	white blood cell
&	and
>	greater than
<	less than
↑	increased, higher
↓	decreased, lower
-	negative
/	per
%	percent
+	positive
×	times, frequency

CHAPTER 1
How To Use Respiratory Care Drug Reference

Respiratory Care Drug Reference is intended to be a quick reference to obtain useful information on drugs. An important objective is to provide information on the proper monitoring of drug therapy. Information is provided to assist practitioners in teaching clients and family members about important aspects of most traditional respiratory care drugs.

Chapter 2 includes general information on important therapeutic or chemical classes of drugs. The classes of drugs are listed alphabetically. Specific drugs in therapeutic or chemical classes are found in Chapter 3 (alphabetical listing of drugs). The information on each therapeutic or chemical class in Chapter 2 begins with a list of the drugs addressed in the drug class. Information on the specific drugs is provided under that drug in Chapter 3. Information on many other drugs also is provided in Chapter 3.

The format for information on individual drugs (and for drug classes when appropriate) is presented as follows:

Drug Names: The generic name for the drug is presented first; this is followed by the correct pronunciation of the generic name. The FDA pregnancy category A, B, C, D, or X (see Appendix 3 for definitions) to which the drug has been assigned is also listed in this section. All trade names follow this; if the trade name is available only in Canada, the name is followed by a maple leaf (✦). Also, if the drug is controlled by the U.S. Federal Controlled Substances Act, the schedule in which the drug has been placed follows the trade name

(e.g., C-II, C-III, C-IV or I, II, III, IV, V). See Appendix 1 for a listing of controlled substances in both the United States and Canada.

Classification: This section defines the type of drug or the class under which the drug has been listed. This information is most useful in learning to categorize drugs. To minimize the need to repeat general information, a cross reference to Chapter 2 is often made for drugs listed in Chapter 3. This information should also be consulted.

General Statement: Information about the class of drug and/or what might be specific or unusual about a particular group of drugs is presented. In addition, brief information may be presented about the disease(s) for which the drugs are indicated.

Action/Kinetics: The action portion of this entry describes the proposed mechanism(s) by which a drug achieves its therapeutic effect (e.g., certain antibiotics interfere with the growth of bacteria). Not all mechanisms of action are known, and some are self-evident. The kinetics entry lists pertinent pharmacologic properties, if known, about rate of drug absorption, distribution, minimum effective serum or plasma level, biologic half-life (t½), duration of action, metabolism, and excretion. Metabolism and excretion routes may be important for clients with systemic liver disease, kidney disease, or both. Again, information is not available for all therapeutic agents.

The time it takes for half the drug to be excreted or removed from the blood, t½ (half-life), is important in determining how often a drug is to be administered and how long to assess for side effects. Therapeutic serum or plasma levels indicate the desired concentration, in serum or plasma, for the drug to exert its beneficial effect and is helpful in predicting the possible onset of side effects or the lack of effect. More and more drug therapy is being monitored in this fashion (e.g., antibiotics, theophylline, dilantin, amiodarone). An additional feature is a listing of commonly accepted therapeutic drug levels on the inside front cover.

Uses: Approved therapeutic application(s) for the particular drug are presented. Investigational uses are also listed for selected drugs.

Contraindications: Disease states or conditions in which the drug should not be used are noted. The safe use of many of the newer pharmacologic agents during pregnancy, lactation, or childhood has not been established. As a general rule, the use of drugs during pregnancy is contraindicated unless specified by the provider where the benefits of drug therapy outweigh the potential risks.

Special Concerns: This section lists information of special concern to the practitioner. For example, whether the drug is considered safe and effective for use in children, during lactation, during pregnancy, and in the geriatric client may be listed. Situations and disease states when the drugs should be used with caution also are listed.

Side Effects: Undesired or bothersome effects the client *may* experience while taking a particular agent are described. Side effects are listed by the body organ or system affected. This feature allows easy access to information on potential side effects of each drug. It is important to note that nearly all of the potential side effects are listed; in any given clinical situation, however, a client may show no side effects, one or two side effects, or multiple side effects. If the side effect may be life threatening,

the effect is highlighted in boldface italics. Thus, it is mandatory to monitor the client carefully.

OD **Overdose Management:** When appropriate, this section provides a list of the symptoms observed following an overdose (*symptoms*) of the drug as well as the approaches for the treatment of the overdose (*treatment*).

Drug Interactions: An alphabetical listing of drugs that may interact with one another are listed under this heading. The study of drug interactions is an important area of pharmacology and drug therapy and is changing constantly with the influx of new drugs, clinical feedback, and increased client usage. The compilation of such interactions is far from complete; therefore, listings in this manual are to be considered *only* as general cautionary guidelines.

Drug interactions may result from a number of different mechanisms (e.g., additive or inhibitory effects, interference with degradation of drug, increased speed of elimination, decreased absorption from the GI tract, and receptor site competition or displacement from plasma protein binding sites). Such interferences may manifest themselves in a variety of ways; however, an attempt has been made throughout the text to describe these interactions whenever possible as an increase ($\uparrow$) or a decrease ($\downarrow$) in the effect of the drug, followed by a brief description of the reason for the change.

It is important to realize that any side effects that accompany the administration of a particular agent also may be increased as a result of a drug interaction.

The reader should be aware that the drug interactions are often listed for classes of drugs. Thus, the drug interaction would be likely to occur for all drugs in that particular class. Thus, information in Chapter 2 should be consulted.

Laboratory Test Interferences: The manner in which a drug may affect the laboratory test values of the client is presented. Some of these interferences are caused by the therapeutic or toxic effects of the drugs; others result from interference with the testing method itself. Interferences are described as false positive (+), or increased (↑), values and as false negative (–), or decreased (↓), values. Many of the laboratory test interferences are also noted under the *Respiratory Care Considerations* for each drug.

Dosage: The adult and pediatric doses, as well as the dosage form(s) for which the drug is available, are presented when possible. The dosage form and route of administration is clearly delineated and is followed by the disease state or condition (in italics) for which the dosage is recommended. The listed dosage is to be considered as a general guideline; the exact amount of the drug to be given is determined by the provider. However, one should question orders when dosages differ markedly from the accepted norm. We have tried to give complete data for drugs that are frequently prescribed.

Respiratory Care Considerations: These were developed to assist the practitioner to apply the assessment process to pharmacotherapeutics. The Administration/Storage section assists the practitioner in preparing the medications for administration, how best to administer the drug, and proper storage. Guidelines assessing the client before, during, and after prescribed drug therapy are identified, as are interventions appropriate for the prescribed drug therapy. Important client/family teaching issues related to the particular drug therapy are addressed for most respiratory care drugs, and specific therapeutic outcome criteria are listed to help the practitioner evaluate the effectiveness of the prescribed drug therapy. Respiratory Care considerations that include assessments and interventions may contain specifics such as:

1. Gathering of physical data and client history.
2. Assessment of specific physiologic functions that may be affected by the drug.
3. Specific laboratory tests to monitor during drug therapy.
4. Identification of sensitivities/interactions and conditions that may preclude a particular drug therapy.
5. Documenting specific indications for therapy and describing related symptom characteristics related to this condition.
6. Physiologic, pharmacologic, and psychologic effects of the drug and how these may affect the client and impact on therapeutic results.
7. Emergency situations or adverse reactions that can arise as a result of drug therapy and appropriate interventions for these situations.
8. Specific interventions that help relieve a client's discomfort, which may have been precipitated by a particular drug.
9. Interventions that help ensure the safety of the client when receiving drug therapy.

The practitioner must also assess the client for the *Side Effects* listed for that drug. Side effects must be documented and reported to the provider. Severe side effects generally are cause for dosage modification or discontinuation of the drug.

Specific information on client education is provided in the *Respiratory Care Considerations* for respiratory care drugs. *Respiratory Care Considerations,* related to client/family teaching, emphasizes the practitioner's role as he/she provides client education and promotes drug compliance. Emphasis is placed on helping the client/family recognize side effects, avoiding potentially dangerous situations, and alleviating anxiety that may result from taking a particular drug. Details on administration, including methods and return demonstrations, have been included to enhance client understanding and compliance. Side effects that require medical intervention are included as well as specifics on how to minimize side effects for certain medications (i.e., take medication with food to decrease GI upset or take at bedtime to minimize daytime sedative effects).

The proper education of clients is a challenging aspect of respiratory care, but the instructions must be tailored to the needs, awareness, and sophistication of each client. Some drugs and drug therapy require the active participation of clients and/or family. For example, clients who take bronchodilators should assume responsibility for taking their own pulse or identifying someone who can or is willing to learn how to take their pulse. Clients should be taught to carry identification listing the drugs currently prescribed, to know what they are taking and why, to develop a mechanism to remind themselves to take their medication, and to avoid counting pills, wondering if they have taken their dose(s) in a given day. A daily or weekly slotted pill box, a blocked check-off sheet, calendar, or a written record may assist clients to minimize errors when taking prescribed drug therapy. Clients should be instructed to bring these records with them whenever they go for a check-up or seek medical care. The drug list may also be shared with the pharmacist if there is a question concerning drugs prescribed, if the client is considering taking an over-the-counter medication, or if the client has to change pharmacies. The records should be shared with the health care provider to ensure accurate evaluation of the response to the prescribed drug therapy. This may also alert the provider to any medication consumption by the client that was not prescribed, or that may interfere with (i.e., potentiate, antagonize) the current pharmacologic regimen. The practitioner should use a return demonstration teaching format to ensure understanding and compliance, and to identify early any problems or lack of client ability to comply with the prescribed therapy. They may also provide the client with a phone number and encourage them to call with any questions or concerns about their therapy.

Finally, when taking the history, emphasis should be placed on the client's ability to read and to follow directions. The ability to comprehend what is written or said should not be assumed based on the client's level of education or command of language. Given the current rate of illiteracy, it is possible that clients may not be able to comprehend what is taught concerning their drug therapy. Clients with language barriers should be identified, and appropriate written translations should be provided. In addition, client life-style, cultural factors, and income as well as the availability of health insurance and transportation are important factors that may affect compliance with prescribed drug therapy. The potential for a client being/becoming pregnant, and whether a mother is breast feeding her infant should be included in assessments as appropriate. The age of clients and their state of mental acuity, whether learned from personal observation or from discussion with close friends or family members, can be critical in determining potential relationships between drug therapy and/or drug interactions. Including these factors in the assessment will assist all on the health care team to determine the type of therapy and drug delivery system best suited to a particular client and will promote the highest level of compliance.

An evaluation section has been included to assist the practitioner in determining the effectiveness and positive therapeutic outcome of the prescribed drug therapy. Specific outcome criteria related to each drug have been delineated to help evaluate the effectiveness of the drug therapy and to assess the client's response (some of which may include a decrease in BP, subjective reports of symptomatic improvement in the disease state, and relief of pain).

The previous points are covered for all drugs or drug classes. When drugs are presented as a group (as in Chapter 2) rather than individually, the points may be covered only once for each group. In this case the practitioner should look for the appropriate entry in the drug class.

Information that requires emphasizing or is relevant to a particular drug is listed under appropriate headings, such as *Additional Contraindications, Additional Side Effects,* or *Additional Respiratory Care Considerations.* Such entries are *in addition to* and not *instead of* the regular entry, which is referenced and must also be consulted.

Additional information to assist the practitioner in administering drugs and monitoring drug therapy appropriately is also found in the text. For example, commonly used laboratory test values are found in Appendix 4. Nomograms for computing the BSA (for children) are provided in Appendix 5. Also helpful are A Table of Weights and Measures (Appendix 8) and Commonly Used Abbreviations and Symbols (front portion of book).

The scope of drugs covered in this reference includes traditional respiratory care drugs used in the treatment of asthma and other respiratory diseases that are often administered by respiratory care practitioners, usually via the inhalation route. Also, coverage is provided for other respiratory related drugs that are given systemically for the treatment of respiratory disorders which includes asthma drugs and antimicrobial agents. Coverage also includes cardiovascular drugs, narcotic analgesics, narcotic antagonists, paralyzing agents, drugs used for smoking cessation programs, and certain other drugs of special interest to respiratory care practitioners.

You are now ready to use Respiratory Care Drug Reference. We hope that the text will be useful and assist you in your education, profession, and practice. Even though the material presented might, at first, appear overwhelming, remember that the effective drugs currently at the disposal of the health care team are the key to today's better, more effective, and efficient medical care. Certainly, the safe administration of drugs, assessment of potential interactions and adverse effects, as well as the evaluation of their outcome on the client are crucial parts of the health care process.

CHAPTER 2
Therapeutic Drug Classifications

ALPHA-1-ADRENERGIC BLOCKING AGENTS

See also the following individual entries:

Doxazosin mesylate
Prazosin hydrochloride
Terazosin

General Statement: As their name implies, the adrenergic blocking agents (sympatholytics) reduce or prevent the action of the sympathomimetic agents. They do this by competing with norepinephrine or epinephrine (the neurotransmitters) for the various subtypes of either alpha-adrenergic or beta-adrenergic receptor sites. For example, alpha-adrenergic blocking agents prevent the smooth muscles surrounding the arterioles from contracting, whereas beta-adrenergic blocking agents prevent the excitatory effect of the neurotransmitters on the heart. It should also be noted that several antihypertensive agents act by blocking alpha (especially in the CNS) or beta receptors.

Some of the adrenergic blocking agents also have a direct systemic cardiac effect in addition to their peripheral vasodilating effect. The fall in BP accompanying their administration may trigger a compensatory tachycardia (reflex stimulation). The cardiac blood vessels of a client with arteriosclerosis may be unable to dilate rapidly enough to accommodate these changes in blood volume, and the client may experience an acute attack of angina pectoris or even cardiac failure.

Adrenergic blocking agents have many undesirable effects which, although not toxic, limit their use. Treatment should always be started at low doses and increased gradually.

ALPHA-ADRENERGIC BLOCKING AGENTS: These drugs reduce the tone of muscles surrounding peripheral blood vessels and consequently increase peripheral blood circulation and decrease BP.

Action/Kinetics: The drugs in this group selectively block postsynaptic alpha-1-adrenergic receptors. This results in dilation of both arterioles and veins leading to a decrease in supine and standing BP. Diastolic BP is affected the most. Prazosin and terazosin do not produce reflex tachycardia. Terazosin also relaxes smooth muscle in the bladder neck and prostate, making it useful to treat benign prostatic hypertrophy.

Uses: Alone or in combination with diuretics or beta-adrenergic blocking agents to treat hypertension. Doxazocin and terazosin are used to treat benign prostatic hypertrophy. *Investigational:* Prazosin is used for refractory CHF, for management of Raynaud's vasospasm, and to treat benign prostatic hyperplasia. Doxazosin, along with digoxin and diuretics, is used to treat CHF.

Contraindications: Hypersensitivity to these drugs (i.e., quinazolines).

Special Concerns: The first few doses may cause postural hypotension and syncope with sudden loss of consciousness. Use with caution in those with impaired hepatic function or in clients receiving drugs known to influence hepatic metabolism. Use with caution during lactation. Safety and efficacy have not been established in children.

Side Effects: The following side effects are common to alpha-1-adrenergic blockers. Please see individual drugs as well. *CV:* Palpitations, postural hypotension, hypotension, tachycardia, chest pain, arrhythmia. *GI:* N&V, dry mouth, diarrhea, constipation, abdominal discomfort or pain, flatulence. *CNS:* Dizziness, depression, decreased libido, sexual dysfunction, nervousness, paresthesia, somnolence, anxiety, insomnia, asthenia, drowsiness. *Musculoskeletal:* Pain in the shoulder, neck, or back; gout, arthritis, joint pain, arthralgia. *Respiratory:* Dyspnea, nasal congestion, sinusitis, bronchitis, **bronchospasm,** cold symptoms, epistaxis, increased cough, flu symptoms, pharyngitis, rhinitis. *Ophthalmic:* Blurred vision, abnormal vision, reddened sclera, conjunctivitis. *GU:* Impotence, urinary frequency, incontinence. *Miscellaneous:* Tinnitus, vertigo, pruritus, sweating, alopecia, lichen planus, headache, edema, weight gain, facial edema, fever.

OD **Overdose Management:** *Symptoms:* Extension of the side effects, especially on BP. *Treatment:* Keep the client supine to restore BP and normalize heart rate. Shock may be treated with volume expanders or vasopressors; support renal function.

Drug Interactions: Alpha-1 blockers ↓ the antihypertensive effect of clonidine.

Laboratory Test Interferences: ↑ Urinary VMA.

Dosage ───────────────
See individual agents.

RESPIRATORY CARE CONSIDERATIONS

Administration/Storage: The first dose of prazosin and terazosin should be taken at bedtime.

Assessment
1. Obtain a thorough history noting any evidence or history of PUD as

drugs should be used cautiously in this setting.
2. Document indications for therapy, and type and onset of symptoms.
3. Determine baseline electrolytes, ECG, BP, and pulse; monitor throughout drug therapy.
4. Document any evidence of heart or lung disease and note currently prescribed therapy. Some agents may cause vasospasm with Prinzmetal or vasospastic angina.

Interventions
1. Use cautiously in older clients due to possibility of orthostatic hypotension. They may tolerate a slower, more gradual increase in dosage (i.e., terazosin 1 mg/day for 7 days followed by 2 mg/day for 7 days, etc., until desired response).
2. Initiate therapy with a low dose and at bedtime to prevent syncope and postural hypotensive effects.
3. Titration generally should be based on standing BP due to postural effects.
4. Drug does not affect glucose levels and may be useful in clients with diabetes.

Evaluate
• Control of hypertension
• Improvement in symptoms of nocturia, urgency, and frequency with BPH

AMINOGLYCOSIDES

See also the following individual entries:

General Statement: The aminoglycosides are broad-spectrum antibiotics, primarily used for the treatment of serious gram-negative infections caused by *Pseudomonas, Escherichia coli, Proteus, Klebsiella,* and *Enterobacter.* Aminoglycoside antibiotics are distributed in the extracellular fluid and cross the placental barrier, but not the blood-brain barrier. Penetration of the CSF is increased when the meninges are inflamed.

The aminoglycosides are excreted, largely unchanged, in the urine. This makes the drugs suitable for UTIs. Concomitant administration of bicarbonate (alkalinization of urine) improves the treatment of such infections. Considerable cross-allergenicity occurs among the aminoglycosides. These drugs are powerful antibiotics and can induce serious side effects. They should not be used for minor infections. Except for streptomycin, resistance of the organisms to aminoglycosides develops slowly. Whenever possible, the sensitivity of the infectious agent should be determined before instituting therapy.

Action/Kinetics: Believed to inhibit protein synthesis by binding irreversibly to ribosomes (30S subunit), thereby interfering with an initiation complex between messenger RNA and the 30S subunit. This leads to production of nonfunctional proteins; polyribosomes are split apart and are unable to synthesize protein. The aminoglycosides are usually bactericidal as a result of disruption of the bacterial cytoplasmic membrane.

The aminoglycosides are poorly absorbed from the GI tract and are therefore usually administered parenterally, the only occasional exceptions being some enteric infections of the GI tract and prior to surgery. They are also absorbed from the peritoneum, bronchial tree, wounds, denuded skin, and joints.

The aminoglycosides are rapidly absorbed after IM injection. **Peak plasma levels:** Usually attained –2 hr after IM administration. Measurable levels persist for 8–12 hr after a single administration. **t½:** 2–3 hr. This value increases sharply in clients with impaired kidney function. Ranges of t½ from 24 to 110 hr have

been observed. Excreted mainly unchanged in urine.

Uses: Gram-negative bacteria causing bone and joint infections, septicemia (including neonatal sepsis), skin and soft tissue infections (including those from burns), respiratory tract infections, postoperative infections, intra-abdominal infections (including peritonitis), UTIs. In combination with clindamycin for mixed aerobic-anaerobic infections. Also, see individual drugs.

They should be used for gram-positive bacteria only when other less toxic drugs are either ineffective or contraindicated. Their use in CNS *Pseudomonas* infections such as meningitis or ventriculitis is questionable.

Contraindications: Hypersensitivity to aminoglycosides, long-term therapy (except streptomycin for tuberculosis). Use with extreme caution in clients with impaired renal function or preexisting hearing impairment. Safe use in pregnancy and during lactation not established.

Special Concerns: Premature infants, neonates, and older clients receiving aminoglycosides should be assessed closely as they are particularly sensitive to their toxic effects.

Side Effects: *Ototoxicity:* Both auditory and vestibular damage have been noted. The risk of ototoxicity and vestibular impairment is increased in clients with poor renal function and in the elderly. Auditory symptoms include tinnitus and hearing impairment, while vestibular symptoms include dizziness, nystagmus, vertigo, and ataxia.

Renal Impairment: This may be characterized by cylindruria, oliguria, proteinuria, azotemia, hematuria, increase or decrease in frequency of urination; increased BUN, NPN, or creatinine; and increased thirst. *Neurotoxicity:* Neuromuscular blockade, headache, tremor, lethargy, paresthesia, peripheral neuritis (numbness, tingling, or burning of face/mouth), arachnoiditis, encephalopathy, acute organic brain syndrome. CNS depression, characterized by stupor, flaccidity, and rarely, *coma, and respiratory depression in infants.* Optic neuritis with blurred vision or loss of vision. *GI:* N&V, diarrhea, increased salivation, anorexia, weight loss. *Allergic:* Rash, urticaria, pruritus, burning, fever, stomatitis, eosinophilia. Rarely, *agranulocytosis and anaphylaxis.* Cross-allergy among aminoglycosides has been observed. *Miscellaneous:* Joint pain, *laryngeal edema, pulmonary fibrosis,* superinfection.

OD **Overdose Management:** *Symptoms:* Extension of side effects. *Treatment:* Undertake hemodialysis (preferred) or peritoneal dialysis.

Drug Interactions
Bumetanide / ↑ Risk of ototoxicity
Capreomycin / ↑ Muscle relaxation
Cephalosporins / ↑ Risk of renal toxicity
Ciprofloxacin HCl / Additive anti-bacterial activity
Cisplatin / Additive renal toxicity
Colistimethate / ↑ Muscle relaxation
Digoxin / Possible ↑ or ↓ effect of digoxin
Ethacrynic acid / ↑ Risk of ototoxicity
Furosemide / ↑ Risk of ototoxicity
Methoxyflurane / ↑ Risk of renal toxicity
Penicillins / ↓ Effect of aminoglycosides
Polymyxins / ↑ Muscle relaxation
Skeletal muscle relaxants (surgical) / ↑ Muscle relaxation
Vancomycin / Additive ototoxicity and renal toxicity
Vitamin A / ↓ Effect of vitamin A due to ↓ absorption from GI tract

Laboratory Test Interferences: ↑ BUN, BSP retention, creatinine, AST, ALT, bilirubin. ↓ Cholesterol values.

RESPIRATORY CARE CONSIDERATIONS

See also *General Respiratory Care Considerations for All Anti-Infectives.*

Administration/Storage
1. Check expiration date.
2. Warn client if the particular drug being administered stings or causes a burning sensation.
3. During IM administration
• Inject drug deep into muscle mass to minimize transient pain.
• Use a Z track method for thin, elderly clients.
• Rotate and document injection sites.
4. With IV administration
• Dilute with the appropriate compatible solution.
• Infuse at the rate ordered to prevent excessive serum concentrations.
5. Administer for only 7–10 days and avoid repeating course of therapy unless a serious infection is present that does not respond to other antibiotics.
6. Administer around the clock to maintain therapeutic drug levels.

Assessment:
1. Assess for allergic reactions; note any history of adverse reactions and hypersensitivity to anti-infective medications.
2. Weigh client prior to administering medication to ensure correct calculation of dosage.
3. Determine baseline liver, renal, auditory, and vestibular function. Assess regularly during drug administration for any symptoms of nephrotoxicity.
4. Assess client for the presence and possibly source(s) of infection. Document VS (evidence of fever), culture and lab reports, and wound appearance (i.e., color, odor, drainage) when applicable.
5. Ensure that appropriate culture studies have been performed before initiating drug therapy.

Interventions
1. Monitor VS and I&O and ensure adequate fluid intake to prevent renal tubule irritation.
2. During therapy, monitor serum drug levels and if levels are elevated, withhold drug and report (e.g., blood levels exceeding 30 mcg/mL of amikacin are considered toxic.)
3. Protect client with vestibular dysfunction by supervising ambulation and providing side rails if necessary.

Flag chart and bedside with (potential for) fall hazard.

4. Monitor for signs of ototoxicity; pretreatment audiograms may be helpful, as hearing loss is a dose-related side effect of drug therapy most commonly associated with amikacin, kanamycin, neomycin, or paromomycin. Also, assess for tinnitus, dizziness, and loss of balance, as these are signs of vestibular injury and are more commonly seen with gentamicin and streptomycin. Continue to monitor for ototoxicity, because the onset of deafness may occur several weeks after the aminoglycoside has been discontinued.

5. Do not administer concurrently or sequentially with a topical or systemic nephrotoxic or ototoxic drug (e.g., potent diuretics such as ethacrynic acid or furosemide) unless provider determines that the benefits outweigh the risks.

6. Observe for neuromuscular blockade with muscular weakness leading to apnea, when an aminoglycoside is administered with a muscle relaxant or after anesthesia. Have calcium gluconate or neostigmine available to reverse blockade.

7. Note the presence of cells or casts in the urine, oliguria, proteinuria, lowered specific gravity, or increasing BUN, or creatinine, all of which are indicators of altered renal function.

Evaluate

• A positive clinical response as evidenced by negative follow-up lab culture reports

• Clinical evidence of resolution of infection such as ↓ WBCs, ↓ fever, ↓ drainage and reports of symptomatic improvement

• Laboratory confirmation that serum drug levels are within desired therapeutic range

ANGIOTENSIN-CONVERTING ENZYME (ACE) INHIBITORS

See also the following individual entries:

Benazepril hydrochloride
Captopril
Enalapril maleate
Fosinopril sodium
Lisinopril
Moexipril hydrochloride
Quinapril hydrochloride
Ramipril

Action/Kinetics: The ACE inhibitors are believed to act by suppressing the renin-angiotensin-aldosterone system. Renin, which is synthesized by the kidneys, is released into the general circulation where it produces angiotensin I, an inactive decapeptide derived from plasma globulin substrate. Angiotensin I is converted to angiotensin II by ACE. Angiotensin II is a potent vasoconstrictor that also stimulates secretion of aldosterone from the adrenal cortex, resulting in sodium and fluid retention. The ACE inhibitors prevent the conversion of angiotensin I to angiotensin II. This results in a decrease in plasma angiotensin II and subsequently a decrease in peripheral resistance and decreased aldosterone secretion (leading to sodium and fluid loss) and therefore a decrease in BP. There may be either no change or an increase in CO. Several weeks of therapy may be required to achieve the maximum effect to reduce BP. Standing and supine BPs are lowered to about the same extent. The drugs are also antihypertensive in low renin hypertensive clients. ACE Inhibitors are additive with thiazide diuretics in lowering blood pressure; however, β-blockers and captopril have less than additive effects when used with ACE inhibitors.

Uses: Alone or in combination with other antihypertensive agents (especially thiazide diuretics) for the treatment of hypertension. Captopril may be used initially in clients with normal renal function where risk is low. Captopril, enalapril, fosinopril, lisinopril, quinapril, and ramipril are used, usually with other drugs, for CHF. Captopril and enalapril are used for left ventricular dysfunction. Lisinopril is used to treat hemodynamically stable clients within 24 hr of an acute MI in order to improve survival. See also individual drug entries.

Contraindications: History of angioedema due to previous treatment with an ACE inhibitor.

Special Concerns: Use of ACE inhibitors during the second and third trimesters of pregnancy can result in injury and even death to the developing fetus. ACE inhibitors may cause a profound drop in BP following the first dose; therapy should be initiated under close medical supervision. Use with caution in renal disease (especially renal artery stenosis) as increases in BUN and serum creatinine have occurred; thus, monitor carefully in clients with impaired renal function. Use with caution in clients with aortic stenosis due to possible decreased coronary perfusion following vasodilator use. With the exception of fosinopril (contraindicated), use with caution during lactation. Geriatric clients may show a greater sensitivity to the hypotensive effects of ACE inhibitors although these drugs may preserve or improve renal function and reverse LV hypertrophy. For most ACE inhibitors, safety and effectiveness have not been determined in children.

Side Effects: See individual entries. Side effects common to most ACE inhibitors include the following. *GI:* Abdominal pain, N&V, diarrhea, constipation, dry mouth. *CNS:* Sleep disturbances, insomnia, headache, dizziness, fatigue, nervousness, paresthesias. *CV:* Hypotension (especially following the first dose), palpitations, angina pectoris, *MI,* orthostatic hypotension, chest pain. *Hepatic:* Rarely, cholestatic jaundice progressing to *hepatic necrosis and death.* *Miscellaneous:* Chronic cough, dyspnea, increased sweating, diaphoresis, pruritus, rash, impotence, syncope, asthenia, arthralgia, myalgia. *Angioedema* of the face, lips, tongue, glottis, larynx, extremities, and mucous membranes. *Anaphylaxis.*

OD **Overdose Management:** *Symptoms:* Hypotension is the most common. *Treatment:* Supportive measures. The treatment of choice to restore BP is volume expansion with an IV infusion of NSS. Certain of the ACE inhibitors (captopril, enalaprilat, lisinopril) may be removed by hemodialysis.

Drug Interactions

Allopurinol / ↑ Risk of hypersensitivity reactions

Anesthetics / ↑ Risk of hypotension if used with anesthetics that also cause hypotension

Antacids / Possible ↓ bioavailability of ACE inhibitors

Capsaicin / Capsaicin may cause or worsen cough associated with ACE inhibitor use

Digoxin / ↑ Plasma digoxin levels

Indomethacin / ↓ Hypotensive effects of ACE inhibitors, especially in low renin or volume-dependent hypertensive clients

Lithium / ↑ Serum lithium levels → ↑ risk of toxicity

Phenothiazines / ↑ Effect of ACE inhibitors

Potassium-sparing diuretics / ↑ Serum potassium levels

Potassium supplements / ↑ Serum potassium levels

Thiazide diuretics / Additive effect to ↓ BP

Laboratory Test Interferences: ↑ BUN and creatinine (both are transient and reversible). ↑ Liver enzymes, serum bilirubin, uric acid, blood glucose. Small ↑ in serum potassium.

Dosage ———————————
See individual drugs.

RESPIRATORY CARE CONSIDERATIONS

Administration/Storage: ACE inhibitor therapy should not be interrupted or discontinued without consulting provider.

Assessment

1. Note any previous therapy with ACE inhibitors and antihypertensive agents and the results.

2. Obtain baseline VS (BP—both arms while lying, standing, and sitting). Assess electrolytes, CBC, and renal function studies, and check urine for proteins during therapy.

3. List other medications client currently prescribed noting any that may interact unfavorably.

4. Document any history of hereditary angioedema (especially if caused by a deficiency of C1 esterase inhibitor).

5. Assess mental status and evaluate extent of client's understanding of the disease of hypertension (or CHF) and the therapy as prescribed.

6. Determine client's ability to take own BP measurement and maintain a record as requested.

7. Document weight, risk factors, and any other medical problems.

8. Ascertain life-style changes clients may need to make to achieve and maintain the goal of lowered BP. Assess motivation and, if not already performed and condition permits, offer client a trial of "good behavior" with dietary modifications and a regular exercise program for 3–6 months and note the outcome.

Interventions

1. Observe clients closely for evidence of neutropenia (especially in those receiving captopril), as this is an indication to discontinue drug therapy.

2. Monitor for and instruct client to report any evidence of angioedema (swelling of face, lips, extremities, tongue, mucous membranes, glottis, or larynx) especially after first dose of drug (but this may also be a delayed response). Symptoms may be relieved with antihistamines. If angioedema involves laryngeal edema, client warrants astute observation for airway obstruction. *Discontinue* drug therapy and have epinephrine (1:1000 SC) readily available.

3. Monitor VS, I&O, weight, serum potassium, and renal function studies. Clients who are hypovolemic due to diuretics, GI fluid loss, or salt restric-

tion may exhibit severe hypotension after initial doses of ACE inhibitors.

4. Monitor BP closely during initiation of therapy, assessing for the development of severe hypotension. Observe and supervise ambulation until drug response is evident.

5. For clients undergoing surgery or general anesthesia with drugs that cause hypotension, ACE inhibitors will block angiotensin II formation; thus, hypotension can be corrected by volume expansion.

Evaluate

- ↓ BP with control of hypertension
- Improvement in S&S of CHF
- Reduction of proteinuria and renal damage with diabetes
- ↓ Morbidity post-AMI

ANTIANGINAL DRUGS– NITRATES/NITRITES

See also the following individual entries:

> Amyl nitrite
> Isosorbide dinitrate
> Isosorbide mononitrate, oral
> Nitroglycerin IV
> Nitroglycerin sublingual
> Nitroglycerin sustained release
> Nitroglycerin topical ointment
> Nitroglycerin transdermal system
> Nitroglycerin translingual spray
> Nitroglycerin transmucosal
> Pentaerythritol tetranitrate

General Statement: Angina pectoris may occur as a result of coronary atherosclerotic disease where there is an imbalance between the demand for oxygen by the myocardium and the oxygen supply (called secondary angina). The oxygen supply is compromised due to the inability of coronary blood flow to increase proportionally to increases in myocardial oxygen requirements. Angina pectoris may also result from vasospasm of large, surface coronary vessels or one of their major branches (called primary angina). In some clients, angina is due to a combination of constriction of coronary vessels and an insufficient oxygen supply.

Three groups of drugs are currently used for the treatment of angina. These agents include the nitrates/nitrites, beta-adrenergic blocking agents, and calcium channel blocking drugs. These drugs reduce the frequency and/or severity of angina by either increasing myocardial oxygen supply and/or decreasing the oxygen demand of the myocardium.

Action/Kinetics: The main mechanism of action of nitrates is to relax vascular smooth muscle by stimulating production of intracellular cyclic guanosine monophosphate. Dilation of postcapillary vessels decreases venous return to the heart due to pooling of blood; thus, LV end-diastolic pressure (preload) is reduced. Relaxation of arterioles results in a decreased systemic vascular resistance and arterial pressure (afterload). The oxygen requirements of the myocardium are also reduced. There is also a more efficient redistribution of blood flow through collateral channels in myocardial tissue. Diastolic, systolic, and mean BP are decreased. Also, elevated central venous and pulmonary capillary wedge pressures, pulmonary vascular resistance, and systemic vascular resistance are reduced. Reflex tachycardia may occur due to the overall decrease in BP. Cardiac index may increase, decrease, or remain the same; those with elevated left ventricular filling pressure and systemic vascular resistance values with a depressed cardiac index are likely to see improvement of the cardiac index. For nitrates, several dosage forms are available, including sublingual, topical, transdermal, parenteral, oral, and buccal. The onset and duration depend on the product and route of administration. Onset ranges from less than 1 min for amyl nitrite to 1 to 3 min for IV, sublingual, translingual, and transmucosal nitroglycerin or sublingual isosorbide dinitrate; 20 to 60 min for sustained-release, topical, and transdermal nitroglycerin or oral isosorbide dinitrate or mononi-

trate; and up to 4 hr for sustained-release isosorbide dinitrate. Duration of action also varies over a wide range including 3 to 5 min for amyl nitrite and IV nitroglycerin; 30 to 60 min for sublingual or translingual nitroglycerin; several hours for transmucosal, sustained-release, or topical nitroglycerin and all isosorbide dinitrate products; and up to 24 hr for transdermal nitroglycerin.

Uses: Treatment and prophylaxis of acute angina pectoris (use sublingual, transmucosal, or translingual nitroglycerin; amyl nitrite). Nitrates are first-line therapy for unstable angina. Prophylaxis of chronic angina pectoris (topical, transdermal, translingual, transmucosal, or oral sustained-release nitroglycerin; isosorbide dinitrate and mononitrate; erythrityl tetranitrate; pentaerythritol tetranitrate). IV nitroglycerin is used to decrease BP in surgical procedures resulting in hypertension, as well as an adjunct in treating hypertension or CHF associated with MI. *Investigational:* Nitroglycerin ointment has been used as an adjunct in treating Raynaud's disease. Also, isosorbide dinitrate with prostaglandin E_1 for peripheral vascular disease. Sublingual and topical nitroglycerin and oral nitrates have been used to decrease cardiac workload in clients with acute MI and in CHF.

Contraindications: Sensitivity to nitrites, which may result in severe hypotensive reactions, MI, or tolerance to nitrites. Severe anemia, cerebral hemorrhage, recent head trauma, postural hypotension, closed angle glaucoma, impaired hepatic function, hypertrophic cardiomyopathy, hypotension, recent MI. PO dosage forms should not be used in clients with GI hypermotility or with malabsorption syndrome. IV nitroglycerin should not be used in clients with hypotension, uncorrected hypovolemia, inadequate cerebral circulation, constrictive pericarditis, increased ICP, or pericardial tamponade.

Special Concerns: Use with caution during lactation and in glaucoma. Tolerance to the antianginal and vascular effects may occur. Safety and efficacy have not been determined during lactation and in children.

Side Effects: *CNS:* Headaches (most common) which may be severe and persistent, restlessness, dizziness, weakness, apprehension, vertigo, anxiety, insomnia, confusion, nightmares, hypoesthesia, hypokinesia, dyscoordination. *CV:* Postural hypotension (common) with or without paradoxical bradycardia and increased angina, tachycardia, palpitations, syncope, rebound hypertension, crescendo angina, retrosternal discomfort, *CV collapse,* atrial fibrillation, PVCs, *arrhythmias.* *GI:* N&V, dyspepsia, diarrhea, dry mouth, abdominal pain, involuntary passing of feces and urine, tenesmus, tooth disorder. *Dermatologic:* Crusty skin lesions, pruritus, rash, exfoliative dermatitis, cutaneous vasodilation with flushing. *GU:* Urinary frequency, impotence, dysuria. *Respiratory:* Upper respiratory tract infection, bronchitis, pneumonia. *Allergic:* Itching, wheezing, tracheobronchitis. *Miscellaneous:* Perspiration, muscle twitching, methemoglobinemia, cold sweating, blurred vision, diplopia, *hemolytic anemia,* arthralgia, edema, malaise, neck stiffness, increased appetite, rigors. **Topical use:** Peripheral edema, contact dermatitis.

Tolerance can occur following chronic use. Nitrites convert hemoglobin to methemoglobin, which impairs the oxygen-carrying capacity of the blood, resulting in *anemic hypoxia.* This interaction is dangerous in clients with preexisting anemia.

OD **Overdose Management:** *Symptoms (Toxicity):* Severe toxicity is rarely encountered with therapeutic use. Symptoms include hypotension, flushing, tachycardia, headache, palpitations, vertigo, perspiring skin followed by cold and cyanotic skin, visual disturbances, syncope, nausea, dizziness, diaphoresis, initial hyperpnea, dyspnea and slow breathing, slow pulse, *heart block,* vomiting

with the possibility of bloody diarrhea and colic, anorexia, and increased ICP with symptoms of confusion, moderate fever, and paralysis. Tissue hypoxia (due to methemoglobinemia) may result in *cyanosis, metabolic acidosis, coma, seizures, and death due to CV collapse.* *Treatment (Toxicity):*

• Induction of emesis or gastric lavage followed by activated charcoal (nitrates are usually rapidly absorbed from the stomach). Gastric lavage may be used if the drug has been recently ingested.

• Maintain client in a recumbent shock position and keep warm. Give oxygen and assisted ventilation if required.

• Methemoglobin levels should be monitored.

• Elevate the legs and administer IV fluids to treat severe hypotension and reflex tachycardia. Phenylephrine or methoxamine may also be helpful.

• Epinephrine and similar drugs are ineffective in reversing severe hypotension and should not be used to treat overdosage.

Drug Interactions
Acetylcholine / Effects ↓ when used with nitrates
Alcohol, ethyl / Hypotension and CV collapse due to vasodilator effect of both agents
Antihypertensive drugs / Additive hypotension
Aspirin / ↑ Serum levels and effects of nitrates
Beta-adrenergic blocking drugs / Additive hypotension
Calcium channel blocking drugs / Additive hypotension, including significant orthostatic hypotension
Dihydroergotamine / ↑ Effect of dihydroergotamine due to increased bioavailability or antagonism resulting in ↓ antianginal effects
Heparin / Possible ↓ effect of heparin
Narcotics / Additive hypotensive effect
Phenothiazines / Additive hypotension

✦ = Available in Canada   ***bold italic*** = life threatening side effect

Sympathomimetics / ↓ Effect of nitrates; also, nitrates may ↓ effect of sympathomimetics resulting in hypotension

Laboratory Test Interferences: ↑ Urinary catecholamines. False negative ↓ in serum cholesterol.

Dosage
See individual agents.

RESPIRATORY CARE CONSIDERATIONS
Administration/Storage
1. Nitrites and nitrates are available in a variety of dosage forms including sublingual, chewable, topical, transdermal, PO, inhalation, and parenteral. It is important to understand the appropriate use of each of these dosage forms. Changing from one brand to another should not be undertaken without consulting the provider or pharmacist as products manufactured by different companies may not be equivalent.
2. Tablets and capsules should be stored tightly closed in their original container. Avoid exposure to air, heat, and moisture.
3. Oral nitrates should be taken on an empty stomach with a glass of water.
4. Inhalation products should be used with the client either lying or sitting down.
5. Inhalation products are flammable and should not be used under situations where they might ignite.

Assessment
1. Note any history of sensitivity to nitrites.
2. Document indications for therapy, type and onset of symptoms, and other agents prescribed and the outcome.
3. Assess and document location, intensity, duration, extension, and any precipitating factors (i.e., activity, stress) surrounding client's anginal pain. Use a pain-rating scale to enable the client to report pain levels more reliably and consistently.
4. If client has a history of anemia, document and administer this category of drugs with extreme caution.

5. Nitrates are contraindicated with elevated intracranial pressure.
6. Determine client experience with self-administered medications and note if sublingual tablets were ordered for the bedside.
7. Note any changes in ECG or elevated cardiac panel. Document results of echocardiogram, stress test, and/or catheterization.

Interventions
1. If hospitalized clients are instructed to keep sublingual tablets at the bedside, instruct them so that accurate records of attacks, amounts and frequency of drug use, and the extent of medication relief are noted.
2. While caring for the client in the hospital, mutually record how much drug the client requires to keep angina under control. Record:
- How frequently the drug is given
- The intensity of pain (use a rating scale 1–10 to ensure consistent reporting; have client rate pain initially and 5 min after drug administration)
- The duration of the attacks
- Whether the relief is partial or complete
- How long it takes for relief to occur
- Whether or not there are any side effects
3. Remind client to notify someone when the medication is consumed so that effectiveness can be determined and usage monitored.
4. Monitor BP and pulse. Assess for symptoms of sensitivity to the hypotensive effects of nitrites. These may include the presence of N&V, pallor, restlessness, and CV collapse.
5. Monitor for the presence of hypotension when clients are receiving additional drugs that may cause hypotension. Adjustment of drug dosage may be necessary. Supervise activities and ambulation until drug effects are realized.
6. Be alert for signs of tolerance, which generally occur following chronic use but may begin several days after treatment is started. This is manifested by absence of response to the usual dose. (Nitrites may be discontinued temporarily until such tol-

erance is lost, and then reinstituted. During the interim, other vasodilators may be ordered.)

7. Observe clients for nausea, vomiting, complaints of drowsiness, headache, or visual disturbances during long-term prophylaxis. These are prolonged effects and may require a change in medication.

8. Note change in client activity and response to the drug therapy. Determine if client experiences less discomfort when performing regular activity.

Evaluate

• Clinical evidence of ↓ myocardial oxygen requirements; ↑ activity tolerance

• Improved perfusion to ischemic myocardium

• Relief of coronary artery spasm

ANTIARRHYTHMIC DRUGS

See also the following individual entries:

Adenosine
Amiodarone hydrochloride
Bretylium tosylate
Calcium Channel Blocking Drugs
Digitoxin
Digoxin
Diltiazem hydrochloride
Disopyramide phosphate
Flecainide acetate
Ibutilide fumarate
Lidocaine hydrochloride
Moricizine hydrochloride
Phenytoin
Phenytoin sodium
Procainamide hydrochloride
Propafenone hydrochloride
Propranolol hydrochloride
Quinidine bisulfate
Quinidine gluconate
Quinidine polygalacturonate
Quinidine sulfate
Tocainide hydrochloride
Verapamil

General Statement: The orderly sequence of contraction of the heart chambers, at an efficient rate, is necessary so that the heart can pump enough blood to the body organs. Normally the atria contract first, then the ventricles. Altered patterns of contraction, or marked increases or decreases in the rate of the heart, reduce the ability of the heart to pump blood. Such altered patterns are called *cardiac arrhythmias.* Some examples of cardiac arrhythmias are:

1. *Premature ventricular beats* or beats that occasionally originate in the ventricles instead of in the sinus node region of the atrium. This causes the ventricles to contract before the atria and ultimately results in a decrease in the volume of blood pumped into the aorta.

2. *Ventricular tachycardia.* A rapid heartbeat with a succession of beats originating in the ventricles.

3. *Atrial flutter.* Rapid contraction of the atria at a rate too fast to enable it to force blood into the ventricles efficiently.

4. *Atrial fibrillation.* The rate of atrial contraction is even faster than that noted during atrial flutter and more disorganized.

5. *Ventricular fibrillation.* Rapid, irregular, and uncoordinated ventricular contractions that are unable to pump any blood to the body. This condition will cause death if not corrected immediately.

6. *Atrioventricular heart block.* Slowing or failure of the transmission of the cardiac impulse from atria to ventricles, in the AV junction. This can result in atrial contraction *not* followed by ventricular contraction.

The effective treatment of arrhythmias depends on accurate diagnosis, changing the causative factors, and, if appropriate, selecting an antiarrhythmic drug. The various antiarrhythmic drugs are classified according to both their mechanism of action and their effects on the action potential of cardiac cells. Importantly, one drug in a particular class may be more effective and safer in an individual client. The antiarrhythmic drugs are classified as follows:

1. Group I. These drugs decrease the rate of entry of sodium during cardiac membrane depolarization, decrease the rate of rise of phase O of the cardiac membrane action potential, prolong the effective refractory period of fast-response fibers, and require that a more negative membrane potential be reached before the membrane becomes excitable (and thus can propagate to other membranes). Drugs classified as group I are further listed in subgroups (according to their effects on action potential duration) as follows:

• Group IA: Depress phase O and prolong the duration of the action potential. The drugs are disopyramide, procainamide, and quinidine.

• Group IB: Slightly depress phase O and are thought to shorten the action potential. The drugs include lidocaine, mexiletine (no longer marketed), phenytoin, and tocainide.

• Group IC: Slight effect on repolarization but marked depression of phase O of the action potential. Significant slowing of conduction. The drugs in this group are flecainide, indecainide, and propafenone.

NOTE: Moricizine is classified as a group I agent but it has characteristics of agents in groups IA, B, and C.

2. Group II. The drugs of this group competitively block beta-adrenergic receptors and depress phase 4 depolarization. Acebutolol, esmolol, and propranolol are group II antiarrhythmics.

3. Group III. The drugs in this group prolong the duration of the membrane action potential (relative refractory period) without changing the phase of depolarization or the resting membrane potential. Drugs in this group include amiodarone, bretylium, and sotalol.

4. Group IV. The drug in this group (verapamil) is a calcium channel blocker, slows conduction velocity, and increases the refractoriness of the AV node.

Although not in one of the preceding groups, adenosine and digoxin are used to treat arrhythmias. Adenosine slows conduction time through the AV node and can interrupt the reentry pathways through the AV node. Digoxin causes a decrease in maximal diastolic potential and duration of the action potential; it also increases the slope of phase 4 depolarization.

Special Concerns: It is important to monitor serum levels of antiarrhythmic drugs since some drugs can cause toxic side effects which can be confused with the purpose for which the drug is used. For example, toxicity from quinidine can result in cardiac arrhythmias. Antiarrhythmic drugs may cause new or worsening of arrhythmias, ranging from an increase in frequency of PVCs to severe ventricular tachycardia, ventricular fibrillation, or tachycardia that is more sustained and rapid. Such situations (called proarrhythmic effect) may make it difficult to distinguish the proarrhythmic effect from the underlying rhythm disorder.

RESPIRATORY CARE CONSIDERATIONS
Assessment

1. Obtain a thorough history and note any reports of drug sensitivity and previous experiences with this class of drugs.

2. Assess the extent of the client's palpitations, fluttering sensations, or missed beats prior to initiating the therapy and obtain a pretreatment ECG with arrhythmia documentation.

3. Note client complaints of chest pains or fainting episodes.

4. Obtain BP, pulse, and apical HR; listen to heart sounds. Record findings as these should serve as baseline data against which to measure the outcome of the prescribed therapy.

5. Ensure that lab tests for liver and renal function and electrolytes and blood glucose levels have been completed.

6. Assess lab values to ensure that serum pH and electrolytes are within

normal limits and that pO$_2$ and/or O$_2$ saturations are within desired range.

7. Determine if electrophysiologic studies will be conducted to assess the drug efficacy (i.e., amiodarone with ventricular tachycardia).

8. Review client life-style related to cigarettes and caffeine use, alcohol consumption, and a lack of regular exercise. Certain foods, emotional stress, and other environmental factors may trigger arrhythmias in certain individuals. These should be identified and if possible eliminated before instituting pharmacologic agents.

9. Obtain periodic evaluations to determine the need for continued therapy.

Interventions

1. Attach client to a cardiac monitor if administering antiarrhythmic drugs by IV route and use an electronic infusion device for safety.

2. Obtain specific written guidelines concerning what to do should the client develop unusual changes in HR or rhythm.

3. Monitor BP and pulse. A HR of less than 50 beats/min or greater than 120 should generally be avoided, depending on the client's baseline level. Request written parameters for BP and pulse.

4. Monitor for changes in cardiac rhythm. Document with rhythm strips and report as the drug therapy may need to be altered.

• Report any new onset of bradycardia, as this may be an early indicator of approaching cardiac collapse.

• Note any depression of cardiac activity, such as the prolongation of the PR interval, widening of the QRS complex, increased AV block, or aggravation of the arrhythmia.

• Have emergency drugs and equipment available in the event of an adverse reaction to therapy. Be prepared to help withdraw the medication, administer emergency drugs, and use resuscitative techniques.

5. Monitor serum concentrations of the antiarrhythmic agent to ensure therapeutic concentration ranges.

6. Monitor serum electrolyte levels, diet, and drug regimens to determine if the serum potassium levels are sufficient to enhance drug effectiveness.

Evaluate

• Knowledge and understanding of cardiac arrhythmias and level of compliance with prescribed therapy

• ECG evidence of control of arrhythmias and restoration of stable cardiac rhythm

• Laboratory confirmation that serum drug concentrations are within therapeutic range

• ↓ Drug-related side effects

ANTIHISTAMINES (H$_1$ BLOCKERS)

See also the following individual entries:

> Astemizole
> Brompheniramine maleate
> Cetirizine hydrochloride
> Chlorpheniramine maleate
> Cyproheptadine hydrochloride
> Dexchlorpheniramine maleate
> Diphenhydramine hydrochloride
> Fexofenadine hydrochloride
> Loratidine
> Promethazine hydrochloride
> Terfenadine
> Tripelennamine hydrochloride

Action/Kinetics: The effects of histamine may be reversed either by drugs that block H$_1$-histamine receptors (antihistamines) or by drugs that have effects opposite to those of histamine (e.g., epinephrine). Antihistamines used for the treatment of allergic conditions are referred to as *H$_1$-receptor blockers* while antihistamines used for the treatment of GI disorders (e.g., peptic ulcer) are referred to as *H$_2$-receptor blockers* (see *Cimetidine, Famotidine, Nizatidine,* and *Ranitidine*).

Antihistamines do not prevent the release of histamine, antibody production, or antigen-antibody interactions. Rather, they compete with histamine for histamine receptors (competitive inhibition), thus preventing or reversing the effects of histamine. Antihistamines prevent or reduce increased capillary permeability (i.e., decrease edema, itching) and bronchospasms. Allergic reactions unrelated to histamine release are not affected by antihistamines.

The H_1 blockers manifest varying degrees of sedation, as well as anticholinergic, antiemetic, antipruritic, and antiserotonin effects. Although antihistamines may relieve symptoms of the common cold, they neither prevent or cure colds nor do they shorten the course of a cold. Clients unresponsive to a certain antihistamine may regain sensitivity by switching to a different antihistamine.

From a chemical point of view, the antihistamines can be divided into the following classes.

1. **Ethylenediamine Derivatives.** This group manifests low to moderate sedative effects and almost no anticholinergic or antiemetic activity. They frequently cause GI distress. Available agents: pyrilamine, tripelennamine.

2. **Ethanolamine Derivatives.** This group is most likely to cause CNS depression (drowsiness). There is a low incidence of GI side effects. There are significant anticholinergic and antiemetic effects. Available agents: carbinoxamine, clemastine, diphenhydramine.

3. **Alkylamines.** Members of this group are among the most potent antihistamines. They are effective at relatively low dosage and are most suitable agents for daytime use. This group manifests minimal sedation, moderate anticholinergic effects, and no antiemetic effects. Paradoxical excitation may also occur. Individual response to agents is variable. Available agents: brompheniramine, chlorpheniramine, dexchlorpheniramine, triprolidine.

4. **Phenothiazines.** These agents possess significant antihistaminic action, varying degrees of sedation, and a high degree of both anticholinergic and antiemetic effects. Available agents: methdilazine, promethazine, trimeprazine.

5. **Piperidines.** Members of this group have prolonged antihistaminic activity, with a comparatively low incidence of drowsiness, moderate anticholinergic activity, and no antiemetic effects. Available agents: azatadine, cyproheptadine, diphenylpyraline, phenindamine.

6. **Miscellaneous.** The drugs in this group are specific in that they bind to peripheral rather than central H_1-histamine receptors. They have no sedative, anticholinergic, or antiemetic effects. Available agents: astemizole, azelastine, fexofenadine, loratadine, terfenadine.

The kinetics of most antihistamines are similar. **Onset:** 15–30 min; **peak:** 1–2 hr; **duration:** 4–6 hr (piperidines have a longer duration). Many antihistamines are available as timed-release preparations. Most antihistamines are metabolized by the liver and excreted in the urine.

Uses: PO: Treatment of vasomotor, perennial, or seasonal allergic rhinitis and allergic conjunctivitis. Treatment of angioedema, urticarial transfusion reactions, urticaria, pruritus. Atopic dermatitis, contact dermatitis, pruritus ani, pruritus vulvae, insect bites. Sneezing and rhinorrhea due to the common cold. Treatment of anaphylaxis, parkinsonism, drug-induced extrapyramidal reactions, vertigo. Prophylaxis and treatment of motion sickness, including N&V. Nighttime sleep aid.

Parenteral: Relief of allergic reactions due to blood or plasma. As an adjunct to epinephrine in treating anaphylaxis. Uncomplication allergic conditions when PO therapy is not possible.

See also the individual drugs.

Contraindications: Hypersensitivity to the drug, narrow-angle glaucoma, prostatic hypertrophy, stenosing peptic ulcer, and pyloroduodenal or bladder neck obstruction. Use with MAO inhibitors. Pregnancy or possibility thereof (some agents), lactation, premature and newborn infants. The phenothiazine-type antihistamines are contraindicated in CNS depression from any cause, bone marrow depression, jaundice, dehydrated or acutely ill children, and in comatose clients. Use to treat lower respiratory tract symptoms such as asthma.

Special Concerns: Administer with caution to clients with convulsive disorders and in respiratory disease. Excess dosage may cause hallucinations, convulsions, and death in infants and children. Use in geriatric clients may result in dizziness, excessive sedation, syncope, toxic confusional states, and hypotension. Rare cases of serious CV side effects (including torsades de pointes, prolongation of the QT interval, other ventricular arrhythmias, cardiac arrest, and death) can occur with astemizole and terfenadine (see individual drugs). These effects do not appear to occur with loratadine.

Side Effects: *CNS:* Sedation ranging from mild drowsiness to deep sleep. Dizziness, incoordination, faintness, fatigue, confusion, lassitude, restlessness, excitation, nervousness, tremor, *tonic-clonic seizures,* headache, irritability, insomnia, euphoria, paresthesias, oculogyric crisis, torticollis, catatonic-like states, hallucinations, disorientation, tongue protrusion (usually with IV use or overdosage), disturbing dreams, nightmares, pseudoschizophrenia, weakness, diplopia, vertigo, hysteria, neuritis, paradoxical excitation, epileptiform seizures in clients with focal lesions. Extrapyramidal reactions include opisthotonus, dystonia, akathisia, dyskinesia, and parkinsonism. *CV:* Postural hypotension, palpitations, bradycardia, tachycardia, reflex tachycardia, extrasystoles, increased or decreased BP, ECG changes (including blunting of T waves and prolongation of the Q-T interval),

cardiac arrest. GI: Epigastric distress, anorexia, increased appetite and weight gain, N&V, diarrhea, constipation, change in bowel habits, stomatitis. *GU:* Urinary frequency, dysuria, urinary retention, gynecomastia, inhibition of ejaculation, decreased libido, impotence, early menses, induction of lactation. *Hematologic:* Hypoplastic anemia, *aplastic anemia, hemolytic anemia,* thrombocytopenia, leukopenia, pancytopenia, *agranulocytosis,* thrombocytopenic purpura. *Respiratory:* Thickening of bronchial secretions, wheezing, nasal stuffiness, chest tightness, sore throat, *respiratory depression;* dry mouth, nose, and throat. *Ophthalmic:* Blurred vision, diplopia. *Miscellaneous:* Tinnitus, acute labyrinthitis, obstructive jaundice, erythema, high or prolonged glucose tolerance curves, glycosuria, elevated spinal fluid proteins, increased plasma cholesterol, increased perspiration, chills; tingling, heaviness, and weakness of the hands.

Topical use: Prolonged use may result in local irritation and allergic contact dermatitis.

OD **Overdose Management:** *Symptoms (Acute Toxicity):* Although antihistamines have a wide therapeutic range, overdosage can nevertheless be fatal. Children are particularly susceptible. Early toxic effects may be seen within 30–120 min and include drowsiness, dizziness, blurred vision, tinnitus, ataxia, and hypotension. Symptoms range from CNS depression (sedation, *coma,* decreased mental alertness) to *CV collapse* and CNS stimulation (insomnia, hallucinations, tremors, or *seizures*). Also, *profound hypotension, respiratory depression, coma, and death* may occur. Anticholinergic effects include flushing, dry mouth, hypotension, fever, *hyperthermia* (especially in children), and fixed, dilated pupils. Body temperature may be as high as 107°F. In children, symptoms include hallucinations, toxic psychosis, delirum tremens,

---

ataxia, incoordination, muscle twitching, excitement, athetosis, *hyperthermia, seizures,* and hyperreflexia followed by postictal depression and *cardiorespiratory arrest. Treatment:*

• Treat symptoms and provide supportive care.

• Vomiting is induced with syrup of ipecac (do not use for phenothiazine overdosage) followed by activated charcoal and a cathartic. If vomiting has not been induced within 3 hr of ingestion, gastric lavage can be undertaken.

• Hypotension can be treated with a vasopressor such as norepinephrine, dopamine, or phenylephrine (do not use epinephrine).

• For convulsions, use only short-acting depressants (e.g., diazepam). IV physostigmine can be used to treat centrally mediated convulsions.

• Ice packs and a cool sponge bath are effective in reducing fever in children.

• Severe cases of overdose can be treated by hemoperfusion.

Drug Interactions
Alcohol, ethyl / See *CNS depressants*
Anticoagulants / Antihistamines may ↓ the anticoagulant effects
Antidepressants, tricyclic / Additive anticholinergic side effects
CNS depressants, antianxiety agents, barbiturates, narcotics, phenothiazines, procarbazine, sedative-hypnotics / Potentiation or addition of CNS depressant effects. Concomitant use may lead to drowsiness, lethargy, stupor, respiratory depression, coma, and possibly death
Heparin / Antihistamines may ↓ the anticoagulant effects
MAO inhibitors / Intensification and prolongation of anticholinergic side effects; use with phenothiazine antihistamine → hypotension and extrapyramidal reactions

NOTE: Also see *Drug Interactions* for *Phenothiazines.*

Laboratory Test Interferences: Discontinue antihistamines 4 days before skin testing to avoid false – result.

Dosage ─────────────
Usually PO. Parenteral administration is seldom used because of irritating nature of drugs. Topical usage is also limited because antihistamines often cause hypersensitivity reactions. When given for motion sickness, antihistamines are usually given 30–60 min before anticipated travel. See individual drugs.

RESPIRATORY CARE CONSIDERATIONS
Administration/Storage
1. Inject IM preparations deep into the muscle. Preparations tend to be irritating to the tissues.
2. Sustained-release preparations should be swallowed whole. Scored tablets may be broken before swallowing. If the client has difficulty swallowing capsules, they can be opened and the contents put into soft food for ingestion.
3. Topical preparations should not be applied to raw, blistered, or oozing areas of the skin.
4. Do not apply to the eyes, around the genitalia, or to mucous membranes.
5. PO preparations may cause gastric irritation. Therefore, administer the medication with meals, milk, or a snack.

Assessment
1. Note any history of drug sensitivity to antihistamines and document known allergens.
2. Note if the client has any medical history of ulcers or glaucoma or if the client is pregnant. Antihistamines are contraindicated under these circumstances.
3. Document indications for therapy and the onset of symptoms. Assess the extent of the allergic response for which the antihistamine is being ordered.
4. Review medications currently prescribed, noting those which may interact unfavorably.
5. Determine if skin testing is to be conducted. Antihistamines generally should be *discontinued* 2–4 days

prior to skin testing to avoid false negative results.

6. Obtain baseline BP, pulse, and respirations; assess CV status and document.

7. Assess lung sounds and note characteristics of secretions produced.

8. Assess skin condition. Note extent and characteristics of any rash, if present.

Interventions

1. Note client complaints of severe CNS depression. This is a symptom of overdosage and may require the administration of syrup of ipecac. See Treatment of Overdose.

2. Monitor VS; document if the client develops hypotension or palpitations.

3. Monitor I&O and ensure adequate hydration. If clients experience difficulty in voiding, have them void prior to receiving the medication.

4. If the client complains of constipation, encourage at least 2 L/day of fluids unless restriction of fluids is necessary. Instruct client to increase the amount of exercise performed (if condition permits), and to consume more fruits, fruit juices, and dietary fiber. A stool softener may also be indicated if these measures are not successful.

5. Monitor lung sounds and secretion production. If bronchial secretions are thick, increase fluid intake to decrease the viscosity of secretions and advise to avoid milk temporarily.

6. If the client is hospitalized and sedated with antihistamines, put up the side rails, supervise ambulation and activities, and incorporate safety precautions.

7. If the client complains of dizziness, weakness, or lassitude, provide assisted ambulation and report.

8. Report any complaints of local irritation as client may have developed an adverse reaction to the drug.·

9. Recurrent reactions of a chronic nature should be referred to an allergist. Clients should be taught how to protect themselves from undue exposure and how to create an allergen-free living area.

Client/Family Teaching

1. Explain that the medication should be taken before or at the onset of symptoms as antihistamines cannot reverse reactions but they may prevent them.

2. Review the appropriate steps to follow during an *acute* allergic reaction and how to differentiate, such as with a bee sting, and ensure the client has epinephrine available for self-administration.

3. Report all adverse effects immediately. Include onset of the side effects and duration, describing exactly what occurred. Another drug with fewer side effects may be indicated.

4. Provide a printed list of drugs to avoid. Report any depressants that may be ordered since antihistamines tend to potentiate the effects of other CNS depressants.

5. Caution the client not to drive a car or operate other machinery until response to the medication (drowsiness) has worn off. Sedative effects may disappear spontaneously after several days of therapy or may not occur at all.

6. If daytime sedation is a problem there are nondrowsy antihistamines available such as terfenadine and astemizole.

7. Report the development of sore throat, fever, unexplained bruising, bleeding, or petechiae. Laboratory studies (CBC and platelets) may be indicated to rule out a blood dyscrasia.

8. Advise that there is potential for developing a sensitivity to sun or ultraviolet light. Avoid any undue exposure to the sun, use a sunscreen, and wear a hat, sunglasses, and protective clothing when in the sun.

9. If the drug is being used for motion sickness, it should be taken 30 min before it is time to use the vehicle or board a plane.

10. Advise that symptoms of dry mouth may be reduced by frequent rinsing with water, good oral hy-

---

giene, and the use of sugarless gum or hard candies.

11. Explain that these products raise BP and should only be used for hypertensive clients under strict medical supervision.

12. Avoid alcohol and any OTC products unless prescribed or approved.

13. Advise parents that children may manifest excitation rather than sedation at ordinary dosages.

14. The clinical effectiveness of one class may diminish with continued usage; switching to another class may restore drug effectiveness.

15. Encourage family/significant other to learn CPR and explain that survival is greatly increased when CPR is initiated immediately.

Evaluate
- ↓ Frequency and intensity of allergic manifestations
- Control of severe itching and associated swelling
- Prevention of motion sickness
- Effective nighttime sedation

ANTIHYPERTENSIVE AGENTS

See also the following drug classes and individual drugs:

Agents Acting Directly on Vascular Smooth Muscle

Diazoxide IV
Hydralazine hydrochloride
Nitroprusside sodium

Alpha-1-Adrenergic Blocking Agents

Doxazosin mesylate
Prazosin hydrochloride
Terazosin

Angiotensin-Converting Enzyme Inhibitors

Benazepril hydrochloride
Captopril
Enalapril maleate
Fosinopril sodium
Lisinopril
Quinapril hydrochloride
Ramipril

Beta-Adrenergic Blocking Agents

Calcium Channel Blocking Agents

Amlodipine
Bepridil hydrochloride
Diltiazem hydrochloride
Felodipine
Isradipine
Nicardipine hydrochloride
Nifedipine
Verapamil

Centrally-Acting Agents

Clonidine hydrochloride
Guanabenz acetate
Guanfacine hydrochloride
Methyldopa
Methyldopate hydrochloride

Combination Drugs Used for Hypertension

Amiloride and
    Hydrochlorothiazide
Amlodipine and Benazepril
    hydrochloride
Bisoprolol fumarate and
    Hydrochlorothiazide
Enalapril maleate and
    Hydrochlorothiazide
Fosinopril sodium
Lisinopril and
    Hydrochlorothiazide
Losartan potassium and
    Hydrochlorothiazide
Methyldopa and
    Hydrochlorothiazide
Propranolol and
    Hydrochlorothiazide
Spironolactone and
    Hydrochlorothiazide
Triamterene and
    Hydrochlorothiazide

Miscellaneous Agents

Carvedilol
Epoprostenol sodium
Labetalol hydrochloride
Losartan potassium
Mecamylamine hydrochloride
Minoxidil, oral

Peripherally-Acting Agents

Guanadrel Sulfate
Guanethidine sulfate
Phenoxybenzamine
    hydrochloride
Phentolamine mesylate

General Statement: Hypertension is a condition in which the mean arterial BP is elevated. It is one of the most widespread chronic conditions for which medication is prescribed and taken on a regular basis. Most cases of hypertension are of unknown etiology and result from a generalized increase in resistance to flow in the peripheral vessels (arterioles). Such cases are known as primary or essential hypertension. Treatment of essential hypertension is aimed at reducing BP to normal or near-normal levels, because this is believed to prevent or halt the slow, albeit permanent, damage caused by constant excess pressure.

Essential hypertension is commonly classified according to its severity as stage 1 (mild: systolic BP, 140–159 mm Hg; diastolic BP: 90–99 mm Hg), stage 2 (moderate: systolic BP, 160–179 mm Hg; diastolic BP: 100–109 mm Hg), stage 3 (severe: systolic BP, 180–209 mm Hg; diastolic BP: 110–119 mm Hg), or stage 4 (very severe: systolic BP, over 210 mm Hg; diastolic BP: over 120 mm Hg). Moderate or severe (malignant) hypertension can result in degenerative changes in the brain, heart, and kidneys and can be fatal.

Other types of hypertension (secondary hypertension) have a known etiology and can result from a complication of pregnancy (toxemic hypertension) or certain other diseases that cause impairment of kidney function. It can also be caused by a tumor of the adrenal gland (pheochromocytoma) or by blockage of certain arteries leading into the kidney (renal hypertension). The latter two cases can be corrected by surgery.

Most pharmacologic agents used to treat hypertension lower BP by relaxing the constricted arterioles leading to a decrease in the resistance to peripheral blood flow. These drugs exert this effect by decreasing the influence of the sympathetic nervous system on smooth muscle of arterioles, by directly relaxing arteriolar smooth muscle, or by acting on the centers in the brain that control BP.

Antihypertensive drug therapy is usually initiated when diastolic BP is greater than 90 mm Hg. Treatment of hypertension involves a stepped-care approach. The first step is life-style modifications that include weight reduction, reduction of sodium intake, regular exercise, cessation of smoking, and moderate alcohol intake. If these steps are not effective, step II approaches may be initiated that include continuation of life-style modifications, and initiation of a diuretic or beta-adrenergic blocking agent (drugs from either group are preferred due to a decrease in morbidity and mortality). Other drugs that may be used include ACE inhibitors, calcium channel blockers, alpha-1 blockers, and an alpha-beta blocker. Step III therapy is initiated when there is inadequate response to step II approaches and includes increasing the drug dose, substituting another drug, or adding a second agent from a different drug class. Step IV therapy is initiated when step III therapy is inadequate; step IV therapy includes adding a second or third agent or diuretic (if not already prescribed). Supplemental antihypertensive drugs include clonidine, guanabenz, guanfacine, methyldopa, guanadrel, guanethidine, rauwolfia alkaloids, hydralazine, minoxidil.

Attempts should be made to decrease the dosage or number of antihypertensive drugs (step-down therapy) while maintaining life-style modifications. Step-down therapy may be tried if the client has been controlled effectively for 1 year or at least four visits to the physician. It should be noted that an antihypertensive drug withdrawal syndrome may occur after discontinuation of antihypertensives. The syndrome is due to catecholamine excess and may or may not include a rapid rise in BP; symptoms include nervousness, agitation, tremors, palpitations, insomnia,

---

sweating, flushing, headache, N&V. Rarely, malignant hypertension, MI, angina, and cardiac arrhythmias may be seen. To prevent such problems, client compliance should be stressed and excessive doses and combining beta blockers with sympatholytics avoided. If the medication is to be discontinued, the dose should be tapered slowly, one drug at a time, with special caution taken in clients with coronary artery or cerebrovascular disease.

RESPIRATORY CARE CONSIDERATIONS
Assessment
1. Obtain a complete history and include any family history of hypertension, stroke, CVD, CHD, dyslipidemia, and diabetes.
2. Determine baseline BP before starting any antihypertensive therapy. To ensure accuracy of baseline readings, take BP in both arms (lying, standing, and sitting) 2 min apart (30 min after last cigarette) at least three times during one visit and on two subsequent visits.
3. Evaluate the extent of client's understanding of the disease of hypertension and the therapy as prescribed. Document weight and risk factors.
4. Ascertain life-style modifications (in the area of weight reduction, moderation of alcohol intake, obtaining regular physical activity, reduction of sodium intake, and smoking cessation) clients may have to make in order to achieve the goal of lowered BP. Offer client a trial of "good behavior" following these modifications and reassess in 3–6 months.
5. Assess the probability of the client's willingness to adhere to prescribed therapy.
6. List all OTC agents consumed.
7. Determine client's ability to take own BP measurements.
8. Ensure that baseline ECG, electrolytes, fasting blood sugar, CBC, uric acid, urinalysis, and liver and renal function studies have been performed.
9. During complete PE include funduscopic and neurologic exam and note findings.
10. Assess for any thyroid enlargement and the presence of target organ damage. With difficult-to-control or complex clients, assess for 24-hr ambulatory BP monitoring.
11. Note if essential or secondary hypertension.
Evaluate
• Knowledge and understanding of illness and evidence of compliance with prescribed therapy
• Evidence of a consistent ↓ in BP to within desired range (SBP < 140 and DBP < 90 mm Hg)
• Evidence of ↓ weight, if on a reducing diet
• Freedom from complications/side effects of drug therapy

ANTI-INFECTIVE DRUGS

See also the following individual drugs and drug classes:

Aminoglycosides
Aztreonam for injection
Bacitracin
Cephalosporins
Chloramphenicol
Clindamycin
Erythromycins
Fluoroquinolones
Imipenem-Cilastatin sodium
Levofloxacin
Lincomycin hydrochloride
Loracarbef
Penicillins
Pentamidine isethionate
Tetracyclines
Trimetrexate glucuronate
Vancomycin hydrochloride

General Statement: The beginning of modern medicine is generally related to two events: the proof by Pasteur that many diseases are caused by microorganisms and the discovery of effective anti-infective drugs. The first of these drugs were the sulfonamides (1938), followed by penicillin during the early 1940s. Since then, dozens of anti-infectives have been added to the list. Moreover, significant progress has been made in the development of antiviral drugs.

Unfortunately, the advent of the anti-infectives has not been a pure panacea. Some of the bacteria and other microorganisms have adapted to the anti-infectives, and there has been a gradual emergence of bacteria resistant to certain anti-infectives, especially the antibiotics. Fortunately, most resistant strains can be eradicated by new and/or different antibiotics, antibiotic combinations, or higher dosages. Nevertheless, awareness of the problem has prompted somewhat greater scrutiny by the provider as to when and how to prescribe antibiotics.

The following general guidelines apply to the use of most anti-infective drugs:

1. Anti-infective drugs can be divided into those that are *bacteriostatic;* that is, arrest the multiplication and further development of the infectious agent, or *bactericidal;* that is, eradicate all living microorganisms. Both time of administration and length of therapy may be affected by this difference.

2. Some anti-infectives halt the growth of or eradicate many different microorganisms and are termed *broad-spectrum antibiotics.* Others affect only certain specific organisms and are termed *narrow-spectrum antibiotics.*

3. Some of the anti-infectives elicit a hypersensitivity reaction in some persons. Penicillins cause more severe and more frequent hypersensitivity reactions than any other drug.

4. Because of differences in susceptibility of infectious agents to anti-infectives, the sensitivity of the microorganism to the drug ordered should be determined before treatment is initiated. Several sensitivity tests are commonly used for this purpose. The most widely used test—the Kirby-Bauer or disk-diffusion test—gives qualitative results; there are also various quantitative tests aimed at determining the minimal inhibitory concentration (MIC).

5. Certain anti-infective agents have marked side effects, some of the more serious of which are neurotoxicity, including ototoxicity, and nephrotoxicity. Care must be taken not to administer two anti-infectives with similar side effects concomitantly, or to administer these drugs to clients in whom the side effects might be damaging (e.g., a nephrotoxic drug to a client suffering from kidney disease). The choice of anti-infective also depends on its distribution in the body (i.e., whether it passes the blood-brain barrier).

6. Another difficulty associated with anti-infective therapy is that these drugs can eradicate the normal intestinal flora necessary for proper digestion, synthesis of vitamin K, and control of fungi that may gain access to the GI tract (superinfection).

Action/Kinetics: The mechanism of action of the anti-infectives varies. The following modes of action have been identified.* Note the considerable overlap among these mechanisms:

1. Inhibition of synthesis of or activation of enzymes that disrupt bacterial cell walls leading to loss of viability and possibly cell lysis (e.g., penicillins, cephalosporins, cycloserine, bacitracin, vancomycin, miconazole, ketoconazole, clotrimazole).

2. Direct effect on the microbial cell membrane to affect permeability and leading to leakage of intracellular components (e.g., polymyxin, colistimethate, nystatin, amphotericin).

3. Effect on the function of bacterial ribosomes to cause a reversible inhibition of protein synthesis (e.g., chloramphenicol, tetracyclines, erythromycin, clindamycin).

4. Bind to the 30S ribosomal subunit

---

*Sande, M.A., Kapusnik-Uner, J.E., Mandel, G.L.: Antimicrobial agents. In *Goodman and Gilman's The Pharmacological Basis of Therapeutics,* 8th ed. Edited by Gilman, A.G., Rall, T.W., Nies, A.S., Taylor, P. New York, Pergamon Press, 1990, p. 1019.

that alters protein synthesis and leads to cell death (e.g., aminoglycosides).

5. Effect on nucleic acid metabolism, inhibits DNA-dependent RNA polymerase (e.g., rifampin), or inhibition of DNA supercoiling and DNA synthesis (e.g., quinolones).

6. Antimetabolites that block specific metabolic steps essential to the life of the microorganism (e.g., trimethoprim, sulfonamides).

7. Bind to viral enzymes that are essential for DNA synthesis leading to a halt of viral replication (e.g., acyclovir, ganciclovir, vidarabine, zidovudine).

Uses: Antibiotics as a group are effective against most bacterial pathogens, as well as against some of the rickettsias and a few of the larger viruses. They are ineffective against viruses that cause influenza, hepatitis, and the common cold. Other anti-infectives are effective against a number of parasites including helminths, the malarial parasite, fungi, trichomonas, and others.

The choice of the anti-infective depends on the nature of the illness to be treated, the sensitivity of the infecting agent, and the client's previous experience with the drug. Hypersensitivity and allergic reactions may preclude the use of the agent of choice.

In addition to their use in acute infections, anti-infectives may be given prophylactically in the following instances:

1. To protect persons exposed to a known specific organism

2. To prevent secondary bacterial infections in acutely ill clients suffering from infections unresponsive to antibiotics

3. To reduce risk of infection in clients suffering from various chronic illnesses

4. To inhibit spread of infection from a clearly defined focus, as after accidents or surgery

5. To "sterilize" the bowel or other areas of the body in preparation for extensive surgery

Instead of using a single agent, the provider may sometimes prefer to prescribe a combination of anti-infective agents.

Contraindications: Hypersensitivity or allergic reaction to certain anti-infectives is common and may preclude the use of a particular agent.

Side Effects: The antibiotics and anti-infective agents have few direct toxic effects. Kidney and liver damage, deafness, and blood dyscrasias are occasionally observed.

The following undesirable manifestations, however, occur frequently:

1. Antibiotic therapy often suppresses the normal flora of the body, which in turn keeps certain pathogenic microorganisms, such as *Candida albicans, Proteus,* or *Pseudomonas,* from causing infections. If the flora is altered, *superinfections* (monilial vaginitis, enteritis, UTIs), which necessitate the discontinuation of therapy or the use of other antibiotics, can result.

2. Incomplete eradication of an infectious organism. Casual use of anti-infectives favors the emergence of *resistant* strains insensitive to a particular drug. Resistant strains often are either mutants of the original infectious agents that have developed a slightly different metabolic pathway and can exist despite the antibiotic, or are variants that have developed the ability to release a chemical substance—for instance, the enzyme penicillinase—which can destroy the antibiotic.

To minimize the chances for the development of resistant strains, anti-infectives are usually given for a prescribed length of time after acute symptoms have subsided. Casual use of antibiotics is discouraged for the same reasons.

OD **Overdose Management:** *Treatment:* Discontinue the drug and treat symptomatically. Supportive measures should be instituted as needed. Hemodialysis may be used although its effectiveness is questionable, depending on the drug and the status of the client (i.e., more effective in impaired renal function).

Laboratory Tests: The bacteriologic sensitivity of the infectious organism to the anti-infective (especially the antibiotic) should be tested by the lab before initiation of therapy and during treatment.

GENERAL RESPIRATORY CARE CONSIDERATIONS FOR ALL ANTI-INFECTIVES
Administration/Storage
1. Check expiration date on container.
2. Check for recommended method of storage for the drug and store accordingly.
3. Clearly mark the date and time of reconstitution, your initials, and the strength of solutions of all drugs. Note the length of time that the drug may be stored after dilution and store under appropriate conditions.
4. Complete the administration of anti-infective agents by IVPB (or as ordered) before the drug loses potency.
Assessment
1. Document indications for therapy, type and onset of symptoms, and location and source of infection (if known).
2. Determine if client has experienced any unusual reaction or problems associated with any anti-infectives (usually penicillin) or related drug therapy and note.
3. Ensure that diagnostic cultures have been done before administering empiric therapy. Use correct procedure for obtaining, storing, and transporting specimen to the lab.
4. Obtain baseline liver and renal function studies and CBC with long-term therapy.
Interventions
1. Conspicuously mark in red on the client's chart, medication record, care plan, pharmacy record, and bed the fact that the client has an allergy and to what. Inform client not to take that drug again unless the provider gives approval after reviewing the history of past allergic reactions to this medication.
2. Once drug therapy is initiated, ask the client about any unusual reactions or problems with the medication. Review with the client possible side effects such as hives, rashes, difficulty breathing, etc. If any of these occur, they may indicate a hypersensitivity or allergic response and the drug should be discontinued and the provider notified immediately.
3. Monitor VS and I&O and ensure adequate hydration.
4. If the anti-infective is mainly excreted by the kidneys, anticipate reduced dosage in clients with renal dysfunction. Nephrotoxic drugs are usually contraindicated in persons with renal dysfunction because toxic levels of the drugs are rapidly attained when renal function is impaired.
5. Verify orders when two or more anti-infectives are ordered for the same client, especially if the drugs have similar side effects, such as nephrotoxicity and/or neurotoxicity.
6. Assess client for therapeutic response, such as reduction of fever, increased appetite, and increased sense of well-being.
7. Assess client for superinfections, particularly of fungal origin, characterized by black furred tongue, nausea, and/or diarrhea.
8. *Prevent superinfections by*
• Limiting client's exposure to persons suffering from an active infectious process
• Rotating the site of IV administration q 72 hr and by changing IV tubing q 24–48 hr
• Providing and emphasizing need for good hygiene
• Instructing care provider to wash own hands carefully before and after contact with the client
9. Have the order for an anti-infective (administered in the hospital) evaluated at least q 5–7 days for renewal, revision, or cancellation.
10. Schedule drug administration throughout 24-hr period to maintain appropriate drug levels. A drug administration schedule is determined by

the half-life ($t\frac{1}{2}$) of the drug, the severity of the infection, evidence of organ dysfunction, and the client's need for sleep.

11. Obtain and monitor serum drug levels (peak and trough) throughout therapy to ensure that client is receiving the appropriate dose.

Evaluate

• Prevention or resolution of infection

• ↓ Fever

• ↓ WBCs

• Negative follow-up culture results

• ↑ Appetite

• Reports of symptomatic improvement

• Laboratory evidence of therapeutic serum drug levels

• Freedom from complications of drug therapy

BETA-ADRENERGIC BLOCKING AGENTS

See also Alpha-1-Adrenergic Blocking Agents and the following individual agents:

Acebutolol hydrochloride
Atenolol
Betaxolol hydrochloride
Bisoprolol fumarate
Carteolol hydrochloride
Esmolol hydrochloride
Metoprolol succinate
Metoprolol tartrate
Nadolol
Penbutolol sulfate
Pindolol
Propranolol hydrochloride
Sotalol hydrochloride
Timolol maleate

Action/Kinetics: Beta-adrenergic blocking agents combine reversibly with beta-adrenergic receptors to block the response to sympathetic nerve impulses, circulating catecholamines, or adrenergic drugs. Beta-adrenergic receptors have been classified as beta-1 (predominantly in the cardiac muscle) and beta-2 (mainly in the bronchi and vascular musculature). Blockade of beta-1 receptors decreases HR, myocardial contractility, and CO; in addition, AV conduction is slowed. These effects lead to a decrease in BP, as well as a reversal of cardiac arrhythmias. Blockade of beta-2 receptors increases airway resistance in the bronchioles and inhibits the vasodilating effects of catecholamines on peripheral blood vessels. The various beta-blocking agents differ in their ability to block beta-1 and beta-2 receptors (see individual drugs); also, certain of these agents have intrinsic sympathomimetic action.

Certain of these drugs (betaxolol, carteolol, levobunolol, metipranolol, and timolol) are used for glaucoma. The drugs appear to act by reducing production of aqueous humor; metipranolol and timolol may also increase outflow of aqueous humor. These drugs have little or no effect on the pupil size or on accommodation.

Uses: Depending on the drug, these agents may be used to treat one or more of the following conditions: hypertension, angina pectoris (first-line agents for unstable angina), cardiac arrhythmias, MI, prophylaxis of migraine, tremors (essential, lithium-induced, parkinsonism), situational anxiety, aggressive behavior, antipsychotic-induced   akathisia, esophageal varices rebleeding, and alcohol withdrawal syndrome. Propranolol is indicated for a number of other conditions (see information on propranolol).

Decrease intraocular pressure in chronic open-angle glaucoma. If intraocular pressure is not adequately controlled with a beta blocker, concomitant therapy with pilocarpine, other miotics, dipivefrin, or systemic carbonic anhydrase inhibitors may be instituted.

Contraindications: Sinus bradycardia, second- and third-degree AV block, cardiogenic shock, CHF unless secondary to tachyarrhythmia treatable with beta blockers, overt cardiac failure. Most are contraindicated in chronic bronchitis, bronchial asthma or history thereof, bronchospasm, emphysema, severe COPD.

Special Concerns: Use with caution in diabetes, thyrotoxicosis, cerebrovascular insufficiency, and impaired hepatic and renal function. Withdrawing beta blockers before major surgery is controversial. Safe use during pregnancy and lactation and in children has not been established. The drugs may be absorbed systemically when used for glaucoma; thus, there is the potential for an additive effect with beta blockers used systemically. Certain of the products for use in glaucoma contain sulfites, which may result in an allergic reaction. Also, see individual agents.

Side Effects: *CV:* Bradycardia, hypotension (especially following IV use), CHF, cold extremities, claudication, worsening of angina, strokes, edema, syncope, arrhythmias, chest pain, peripheral ischemia, flushing, SOB, sinoatrial block, pulmonary edema, vasodilation, increased HR, palpitations, conduction disturbances, *first- and third-degree heart block,* worsening of AV block, thrombosis of renal or mesenteric arteries, precipitation or worsening of Raynaud's phenomenon. Sudden withdrawal of large doses may cause angina, ventricular tachycardia, *fatal MI, sudden death,* or *circulatory collapse. GI:* N&V, diarrhea, flatulence, dry mouth, constipation, anorexia, cramps, bloating, gastric pain, dyspepsia, distortion of taste, weight gain or loss, retroperitoneal fibrosis, ischemic colitis. *Hepatic:* Hepatomegaly, acute pancreatitis, elevated liver enzymes, liver damage (especially with chronic use of phenobarbital). *Respiratory:* Asthma-like symptoms, *bronchospasms, bronchial obstruction, laryngospasm with respiratory distress,* wheeziness, worsening of chronic obstructive lung disease, dyspnea, cough, nasal stuffiness, rhinitis, pharyngitis, rales. *CNS:* Dizziness, fatigue, lethargy, vivid dreams, depression, hallucinations, delirium, psychoses, paresthesias, insomnia, nervousness, nightmares, headache, vertigo, disorientation of time and

place, hypoesthesia or hyperesthesia, decreased concentration, short-term memory loss, change in behavior, emotional lability, slurred speech, lightheadedness. In the elderly, paranoia, disorientation, and combativeness have occurred. *Hematologic: Agranulocytosis,* thrombocytopenia. *Allergic:* Fever, sore throat, respiratory distress, rash, pharyngitis, *laryngospasm, anaphylaxis. Skin:* Pruritus, rashes, increased skin pigmentation, sweating, dry skin, alopecia, skin irritation, psoriasis (reversible). *Musculoskeletal:* Joint and muscle pain, arthritis, arthralgia, back pain, muscle cramps, muscle weakness when used in clients with myasthenic symptoms. *GU:* Impotence, decreased libido, dysuria, UTI, nocturia, urinary retention or frequency, pollakiuria. *Ophthalmic:* Visual disturbances, eye irritation, dry or burning eyes, blurred vision, conjunctivitis. When used ophthalmically: keratitis, blepharoptosis, diplopia, ptosis, and visual disturbances including refractive changes. *Other:* Hyperglycemia or hypoglycemia, lupus-like syndrome, Peyronie's disease, tinnitus, increase in symptoms of myasthenia gravis, facial swelling, decreased exercise tolerance, rigors, speech disorders. *Systemic effects due to ophthalmic beta-1 and beta-2 blockers:* Headache, depression, arrhythmia, heart block, CVA, syncope, CHF, palpitation, cerebral ischemia, nausea, localized and generalized rash, bronchospasm (especially in those with pre-existing bronchospastic disease), respiratory failure, masked symptoms of hypoglycemia in insulin-dependent diabetics, keratitis, visual disturbances (including refractive changes), blepharoptosis, ptosis, diplopia.

OD **Overdose Management:**
Symptoms: CV symptoms include bradycardia, hypotension, CHF, *cardiogenic shock,* intraventricular conduction disturbances, *AV block, pulmonary edema, asystole,* and tachycardia.

Also, overdosage of pindolol may cause hypertension and overdosage of propranolol may result in systemic vascular resistance. CNS symptoms include respiratory depression, decreased consciousness, **coma, and seizures.** Miscellaneous symptoms include **bronchospasm** (especially in clients with obstructive pulmonary disease), hyperkalemia, and hypoglycemia. *Treatment:*

• To improve blood supply to the brain, place client in a supine position and raise the legs.

• Measure blood glucose and serum potassium. Monitor BP and ECG continuously.

• Provide general supportive treatment such as inducing emesis or gastric lavage and assisted ventilation.

• *Seizures:* Give IV diazepam or phenytoin.

• *Excessive bradycardia:* If hypotensive, give atropine, 0.6 mg; if no response, give q 3 min for a total of 2–3 mg. Cautious administration of isoproterenol may be tried. Also, glucagon, 5–10 mg rapidly over 30 sec, followed by continuous IV infusion of 5 mg/hr may reverse bradycardia. Transvenous cardiac pacing may be needed for refractory cases.

• *Cardiac failure:* Digitalis, diuretic, and oxygen; if failure is refractory, IV aminophylline or glucagon may be helpful.

• *Hypotension:* Place client in Trendelenburg position. IV fluids unless pulmonary edema is present; also vasopressors such as norepinephrine (may be drug of choice), dobutamine, dopamine with monitoring of BP. If refractory, glucagon may be helpful. In intractable cardiogenic shock, intra-aortic balloon insertion may be required.

• *Premature ventricular contractions:* Lidocaine or phenytoin. Disopyramide, quinidine, and procainamide should be avoided as they depress myocardial function further.

• *Bronchospasms:* Give a beta-2-adrenergic agonist, epinephrine, or theophylline.

• *Heart block, second or third degree:* Isoproterenol or transvenous cardiac pacing.

Drug Interactions

Anesthetics, general / Additive depression of myocardium

Anticholinergic agents / Counteract bradycardia produced by beta-adrenergic blockers

Antihypertensives / Additive hypotensive effect

Ophthalmic beta blockers / Additive systemic beta-blocking effects if used with oral beta blockers

Chlorpromazine / Additive beta-adrenergic blocking action

Cimetidine / ↑ Effect of beta blockers due to ↓ breakdown by liver

Clonidine / Paradoxical hypertension; also, ↑ severity of rebound hypertension

Disopyramide / ↑ Effect of both drugs

Epinephrine / Beta blockers prevent beta-adrenergic action of epinephrine but not alpha-adrenergic action → ↑ systolic and diastolic BP and ↓ HR

Furosemide / ↑ Beta-adrenergic blockade

Hydralazine / ↑ Beta-adrenergic blockade

Indomethacin / ↓ Effect of beta blockers possibly due to inhibition of prostaglandin synthesis

Insulin / Beta blockers ↑ hypoglycemic effect of insulin

Lidocaine / ↑ Effect of lidocaine due to ↓ breakdown by liver

Methyldopa / Possible ↑ BP to alpha-adrenergic effect

NSAIDs / ↓ Effect of beta blockers, possibly due to inhibition of prostaglandin synthesis

Oral contraceptives / ↑ Effect of beta blockers due to ↓ breakdown by liver

Phenformin / ↑ Hypoglycemia

Phenobarbital / ↓ Effect of beta blockers due to ↑ breakdown by liver

Phenothiazines / ↑ Effect of both drugs

Phenytoin / Additive depression of myocardium; also phenytoin ↓ effect of beta blockers due to ↑ breakdown by liver

Prazosin / ↑ First-dose effect of prazosin (acute postural hypotension)

Reserpine / Additive hypotensive effect

Rifampin / ↓ Effect of beta blockers due to ↑ breakdown by liver

Ritodrine / Beta blockers ↓ effect of ritodrine

Salicylates / ↓ Effect of beta blockers, possibly due to inhibition of prostaglandin synthesis

Succinylcholine / Beta blockers ↑ effects of succinylcholine

Sympathomimetics / Reverse effects of beta blockers

Theophylline / Beta blockers reverse the effect of theophylline; also, beta blockers ↓ renal clearance of theophylline

Tubocurarine / Beta blockers ↑ effects of tubocurarine

Verapamil / Possible side effects since both drugs ↓ myocardial contractility or AV conduction; bradycardia and asystole when beta blockers are used ophthalmically

Laboratory Test Interferences: ↓ Serum glucose.

Dosage —————————————
See individual drugs.

RESPIRATORY CARE CONSIDERATIONS

Administration/Storage

1. Sudden cessation of beta blockers may precipitate or worsen angina.
2. The lowering of intraocular pressure may take a few weeks to stabilize when using betaxolol or timolol.
3. Due to diurnal variations in intraocular pressure, the response to b.i.d. therapy is best assessed by measuring intraocular pressure at different times during the day.
4. If intraocular pressure is not controlled using beta blockers, additional drugs should be added to the regimen, including pilocarpine, dipivefrin, or systemic carbonic anhydrase inhibitors.

Assessment

1. Note indications for therapy and assess client's mental status. Document any symptoms or history of depression.
2. Determine pulse and BP in both arms with client lying, sitting, and standing, before beginning therapy.
3. Obtain baseline EKG, serum glucose level, CBC, electrolytes, and liver and renal function studies.
4. Note any history of asthma, diabetes, or impaired renal function.
5. With any history of asthma, avoid nonselective beta antagonists due to beta-2 receptor blockade which may lead to increased airway resistance.
6. Review drugs currently prescribed to ensure none interact unfavorably.

Interventions

1. Monitor pulse rate and BP; obtain written parameters for medication administration (e.g., hold for SBP < 90 or HR < 50).
2. When assessing the client's respirations note the rate and quality. Drugs in this category may cause dyspnea and bronchospasm.
3. Monitor I&O and daily weights. Observe for increasing dyspnea, coughing, client complaint of difficulty breathing or fatigue, or the presence of edema. These are symptoms of CHF and indicate that the client may require digitalization, diuretics, and/or discontinuation of drug therapy.
4. Assess any client complaints of "having a cold, easy fatigue, or feeling of lightheadedness." These side effects may indicate a need to have the medication changed.
5. If working with a client with diabetes be especially cognizant of symptoms of hypoglycemia, such as hypotension or tachycardia. Most beta-adrenergic blocking agents mask these signs.
6. During IV drug administration, monitor EKG (drug may slow AV conduction and increase PR interval) and activities closely until drug effects are realized.

Evaluate

- ↓ BP
- ↓ Intraocular pressure
- Reports of ↓ frequency and severity of anginal attacks and improved exercise tolerance
- ↓ Anxiety levels
- ↓ Tremors
- Effective migraine prophylaxis
- ECG confirmation of control of cardiac arrhythmias

CALCIUM CHANNEL BLOCKING AGENTS

See also the following individual entries:

Amlodipine
Bepridil hydrochloride
Diltiazem hydrochloride
Felodipine
Isradipine
Nicardipine hydrochloride
Nifedipine
Nisoldipine
Verapamil

Action/Kinetics: Calcium ions are important for generation of action potentials and for excitation/contraction of muscles. For contraction of cardiac and smooth muscle to occur, extracellular calcium must move into the cell through openings called *calcium channels*. The calcium channel blocking agents (also called *slow channel blockers* or *calcium antagonists*) inhibit the influx of calcium through the cell membrane, resulting in a depression of automaticity and conduction velocity in both smooth and cardiac muscle. This leads to a depression of contraction in these tissues. Although all drugs in this class act similarly, they have different degrees of selectivity on vascular smooth muscle, myocardium, and conduction and pacemaker tissues. In the myocardium, these drugs dilate coronary vessels in both normal and ischemic tissues and inhibit spasms of coronary arteries. They also decrease total peripheral resistance, thus reducing energy and oxygen requirements of the heart. These ef-

fects benefit various types of angina. These agents also are effective against certain cardiac arrhythmias by slowing AV conduction and prolonging repolarization. In addition, they depress the amplitude, rate of depolarization, and conduction in atria.

Uses: See individual drugs. Depending on the drug, calcium channel blockers are used for vasospastic angina, chronic stable angina, unstable angina, and essential hypertension. Selected drugs are used for atrial flutter or atrial fibrillation (oral verapamil, IV diltiazem), supraventricular tachyarrhythmias (IV verapamil), or subarachnoid hemorrhage (nimodipine).

Contraindications: Sick sinus syndrome, second- or third-degree AV block (except with a functioning pacemaker). Use of bepridil, diltiazem, or verapamil for hypotension (<90 mm Hg systolic pressure). Lactation.

Special Concerns: Abrupt withdrawal of calcium channel blockers may result in increased frequency and duration of chest pain. Hypertensive clients treated with calcium channel blockers have a higher risk of heart attack than clients treated with diuretics or beta-adrenergic blockers. Safety and effectiveness of bepridil, diltiazem, felodipine, and isradipine have not been established in children.

Side Effects: Side effects vary from one calcium channel blocker to another; refer to individual drugs.

OD **Overdose Management:** *Symptoms:* Nausea, weakness, drowsiness, dizziness, slurred speech, confusion, marked and prolonged hypotension, bradycardia, junctional rhythms, *second- or third-degree block. Treatment:*

- Treatment is supportive. Monitor cardiac and respiratory function.
- If client is seen soon after ingestion, emetics or gastric lavage should be considered followed by cathartics.
- *Hypotension:* IV calcium, dopamine, isoproterenol, metaraminol, norepinephrine. Also, provide IV

fluids. Place client in Trendelenburg position.

• *Ventricular tachycardia:* IV procainamide or lidocaine; also, cardioversion may be necessary. Also, provide slow-drip IV fluids.

• *Bradycardia, asystole, AV block:* IV atropine sulfate (0.6–1 mg), calcium gluconate (10% solution), isoproterenol, norepinephrine; also, cardiac pacing may be indicated. Provide slow-drip IV fluids.

Drug Interactions
Beta-adrenergic blocking agents / Beta blockers may cause depression of myocardial contractility and AV conduction
Cimetidine / ↑ Effect of calcium channel blockers due to ↓ first-pass metabolism
Fentanyl / Severe hypotension or increased fluid volume requirements
Ranitidine / ↑ Effect of calcium channel blockers due to ↓ first-pass metabolism

Dosage —————————
See individual drugs.

RESPIRATORY CARE CONSIDERATIONS
Assessment
1. Document indications for therapy and type and onset of symptoms.
2. Identify other agents used for these symptoms and the outcome.
3. Note if the client has had any experience with calcium channel blocking drugs in the past and the response.
4. Assess and document CV and mental status.
5. Determine that baseline VS, weight, and ECG have been performed.
6. Document pulse and BP in both arms with client lying, sitting, and standing.
7. Obtain baseline serum glucose, electrolytes, and liver and renal function studies.
Interventions
1. During IV drug administration, monitor activities and hemodynamics closely until drug effects are realized.
2. These drugs cause peripheral vasodilation. Therefore, clients should have their BP and pulse monitored during the initial administration of the drug. Any excessive hypotensive response and increased HR may precipitate angina. Request written parameters for safe drug administration.
3. Monitor I&O and daily weights. Assess for symptoms of CHF (weight gain, peripheral edema, dyspnea, rales, jugular vein distention).
Evaluate
• Control of hypertension
• ↓ HR
• Reports of ↓ frequency and intensity of anginal attacks
• ECG evidence of control of cardiac arrhythmias

CALCIUM SALTS

See also the following individual entries:

Calcium chloride
Action/Kinetics: Calcium is essential for maintaining normal function of nerves, muscles, the skeletal system, and permeability of cell membranes and capillaries. For example, calcium is necessary for activation of many enzyme reactions and is required for nerve impulses; contraction of cardiac, smooth, and skeletal muscle, renal function, respiration, and blood coagulation. It has a role in the release of neurotransmitters and hormones, in the uptake and binding of amino acids, in vitamin B_{12} absorption, and in gastrin secretion. The normal serum calcium concentration is 9–10.4 mg/dL (4.5–5.2 mEq/L). When the calcium level of the extracellular fluid falls below this level, calcium is first mobilized from bone. However, eventually blood calcium depletion may be significant. Hypocalcemia is characterized by muscular fibrillation, twitching, skeletal muscle spasms, leg cramps,

tetanic spasms, cardiac arrhythmias, smooth muscle hyperexcitability, mental depression, and anxiety states. Excessive, chronic hypocalcemia is characterized by brittle, defective nails, poor dentition, and brittle hair. The daily RDA for elemental calcium is 0.8 g/day for adults over 25 years of age and children 1–10 years of age, 1.2 g for pregnant or lactating women and both males and females 11–24 years of age, 0.6 g for children 6–12 months of age, and 0.4 g for infants less than 6 months of age. Calcium deficiency can be corrected by the administration of various calcium salts. Calcium is well absorbed from the upper GI tract. However, severe low-calcium tetany is best treated by IV administration of calcium gluconate. The presence of vitamin D is necessary for maximum calcium utilization. The hormone of the parathyroid gland is necessary for the regulation of the calcium level.

Uses: IV: Acute hypocalcemic tetany secondary to renal failure, hypoparathyroidism, premature delivery, maternal diabetes mellitus in infants, and poisoning due to magnesium, oxalic acid, radiophosphorus, carbon tetrachloride, fluoride, phosphate, strontium, and radium. To treat depletion of electrolytes. Also during cardiac resuscitation when epinephrine or isoproterenol has not improved myocardial contraction (may also be given into the ventricular cavity for this purpose). To reverse cardiotoxicity or hyperkalemia. **IM or IV:** Reduce spasms in renal, biliary, intestinal, or lead colic. To relieve muscle cramps due to insect bites and to decrease capillary permeability in various sensitivity reactions. **PO:** Osteoporosis, osteomalacia, chronic hypoparathyroidism, rickets, latent tetany, hypocalcemia secondary to use of anticonvulsant drugs. Myasthenia gravis, Eaton-Lambert syndrome, supplement for pregnant, postmenopausal, or nursing women. Also, prophylactically for primary osteoporosis. *Investigational:* As an infusion to diagnose Zollinger-Ellison syndrome and medullary thyroid carcinoma. To antagonize neuromuscular blockade due to aminoglycosides.

Contraindications: Digitalized clients, sarcoidosis, renal or cardiac disease, ventricular fibrillation. Cancer clients with bone metastases. Renal calculi, hypophosphatemia, hypercalcemia.

Special Concerns: Calcium requirements decrease in geriatric clients; thus, dose may have to be adjusted. Also, low levels of active vitamin D metabolites may impair calcium absorption in older clients. Use with caution in cor pulmonale, respiratory acidosis, renal disease or failure, ventricular fibrillation, hypercalcemia.

Side Effects: Following PO use: GI irritation, constipation. **Following IV use:** Venous irritation, tingling sensation, feeling of oppression or heat, chalky taste. Rapid IV administration may result in vasodilation, decreased BP and HR, *cardiac arrhythmias,* syncope, or *cardiac arrest.* **Following IM use:** Burning feeling, necrosis, tissue sloughing, cellulitis, soft tissue calcification. *NOTE:* If calcium is injected into the myocardium rather than into the ventricle, *laceration of coronary arteries, cardiac tamponade, pneumothorax, and ventricular fibrillation* may occur. *Symptoms due to excess calcium (hypercalcemia):* Lassitude, fatigue, GI symptoms (anorexia, N&V, abdominal pain, dry mouth, thirst), polyuria, depression of nervous and neuromuscular function (emotional disturbances, confusion, skeletal muscle weakness, and constipation), confusion, delirium, stupor, *coma,* impairment of renal function (polyuria, polydipsia, and azotemia), renal calculi, arrhythmias, and bradycardia.

OD **Overdose Management:** *Symptoms:* Systemic overloading from parenteral administration can result in an acute hypercalcemic syndrome with symptoms including markedly increased plasma calcium levels, lethargy, intractable N&V, weakness, *coma, and sudden death.* *Treatment:* Discontinue therapy and lower serum calcium levels by giving an IV infusion of sodium chloride plus a potent diuretic such as furosemide. Consider hemodialysis.

Drug Interactions

Atenolol / ↓ Effect of atenolol due to ↓ bioavailability and plasma levels

Cephalocin / Incompatible with calcium salts

Corticosteroids / Interfere with absorption of calcium from GI tract

Digitalis / ↑ Digitalis arrhythmias and toxicity. Death has resulted from combination of digitalis and IV calcium salts

Iron salts / ↓ Absorption of iron from the GI tract

Milk / Excess of either may cause hypercalcemia, renal insufficiency with azotemia, alkalosis, and ocular lesions

Norfloxacin / ↓ Bioavailability of norfloxacin

Sodium polystyrene sulfonate / Metabolic alkalosis and ↓ binding of resin to potassium in clients with renal impairment

Tetracyclines / ↓ Effect of tetracyclines due to ↓ absorption from GI tract

Thiazide diuretics / Hypercalcemia due to thiazide-induced renal tubular reabsorption of calcium and bone release of calcium

Verapamil / Calcium antagonizes the effect of verapamil

Vitamin D / Enhances intestinal absorption of dietary calcium

Dosage ───────────────
See individual agents.

RESPIRATORY CARE CONSIDERATIONS
Administration/Storage

ORAL

1. Administer 1–1.5 hr after meals. Alkalis and large amounts of fat decrease the absorption of calcium.
2. If the client has difficulty swallowing large tablets, obtain a calcium in water suspension. Because calcium goes into suspension six

times more readily in hot water than in cold water, the solution can be prepared by diluting the medication with *hot* water. Solution may then be cooled before administering to the client.

IV

1. Warm solutions to body temperature and give slowly (0.5–2 mL/min), stopping administration if client complains of discomfort.
2. Administer slowly, observing VS closely for evidence of bradycardia, hypotension, and cardiac arrhythmias.
3. Prevent leakage of medication into the tissues. These salts are extremely irritating.
4. Client should remain recumbent for a short time following the injection.
5. Calcium salts should not be mixed with carbonates, phosphates, sulfates, or tartrates in parenteral admixtures.

IM

1. Rotate the injection sites because this medication may cause sloughing of tissue.
2. Do not administer IM calcium gluconate to children.

Assessment

1. Perform a thorough nursing history, noting indications for therapy and any underlying causes.
2. Note if the client is receiving digitalis products as the drug is generally contraindicated.
3. Obtain baseline serum calcium level and renal function studies to determine if renal disease is present.

Interventions

1. Monitor serum calcium levels. Administer vitamin D as prescribed to facilitate absorption.
2. If the client goes into hypocalcemic tetany, provide appropriate safety precautions to protect the client from injury.
3. Observe for symptoms of hypercalcemia, such as fatigue and CNS depression.

Evaluate
- Resolution of clinical symptoms of hypocalcemia
- Reports of relief of muscle cramps
- Osteoporosis prophylaxis
- Laboratory confirmation that serum calcium level is within desired range (8.8–10.4 mg/dL)

CARDIAC GLYCOSIDES

See also the following individual entries:

Digitoxin
Digoxin

General Statement: Cardiac glycosides, such as digitoxin, are plant alkaloids. They are the oldest, yet still the most effective, drugs for treating CHF. By improving myocardial contraction, they improve blood supply to all organs, including the kidney, thereby improving function. This action results in diuresis, thereby correcting the edema often associated with cardiac insufficiency. Digitalis glycosides are also used for the treatment of cardiac arrhythmias, since they decrease pulse rate as well. The cardiac glycosides are cumulative in action. This effect is partially responsible for the difficulties associated with their use.

Action/Kinetics: Cardiac glycosides increase the force and velocity of myocardial contraction (positive inotropic effect) by increasing the refractory period of the AV node and increasing total peripheral resistance. This effect is due to inhibition of sodium/potassium–ATPase in the sarcolemmal membrane, which alters excitation–contraction coupling. Inhibiting sodium, potassium–ATPase, results in an increase of calcium influx and an increased release of free calcium ions within the myocardial cells, which then potentiate the contractility of cardiac muscle fibers. The digitalis glycosides also decrease the rate of conduction and increase the refractory period of the AV node. This effect is due to an increase in parasympathetic tone and a decrease in sympathetic tone. The cardiac glycosides are absorbed from the GI tract. Absorption varies from 40% to 90%, depending on the preparation and brand as well as the presence of food. These drugs are widely distributed in tissues, with the highest levels seen in the myocardium, skeletal muscle, liver, brain, and kidneys. With most preparations, peak plasma concentrations are reached within 2–3 hr. Half-life ranges from 1.7 days for digoxin to 7 days for digitoxin. The drugs are primarily excreted through the kidneys, either unchanged (digoxin) or metabolized (digitoxin). Due to the long half-lives, clinical effects are not seen until steady-state plasma levels are reached. The initial dose of digitalis glycosides is larger (loading dose) and is traditionally referred to as the *digitalizing dose;* subsequent doses are referred to as *maintenance doses.*

Uses: All types of CHF, including that due to venous congestion, edema, dyspnea, orthopnea, and cardiac arrhythmia. These drugs are most effective in low-output failure and less effective in high-output failure (e.g., bronchopulmonary insufficiency, arteriovenous fistula, anemia, infection, and hyperthyroidism). Control of rapid ventricular contraction rate in clients with atrial fibrillation or flutter. Slow HR in sinus tachycardia due to CHF. Supraventricular tachycardia. Prophylaxis and treatment of recurrent paroxysmal atrial tachycardia with paroxysmal AV junctional rhythm. Cardiogenic shock (value not established).

Contraindications: Ventricular fibrillation or tachycardia (unless congestive failure supervenes after protracted episode not due to digitalis), in presence of digitalis toxicity, hypersensitivity to cardiac glycosides, beriberi heart disease, certain cases of hypersensitive carotid sinus syndrome.

Special Concerns: Use with caution in clients with ischemic heart disease, acute myocarditis, hypertrophic subaortic stenosis, hypoxic or myxedemic states, Adams-Stokes or carotid sinus syndromes, cardiac amyloidosis, or cyanotic heart and lung disease, including emphysema and partial heart block. Those with carditis associated with rheumatic fever or viral myocarditis are especially sensitive to digoxin-induced disturbances in rhythm. Electric pacemakers may sensitize the myocardium to cardiac glycosides. The cardiac glycosides should also be given cautiously and at reduced dosage to elderly, debilitated clients, pregnant women and nursing mothers, and newborn, term, or premature infants who have immature renal and hepatic function. Similar precautions also should be observed for clients with reduced renal and/or hepatic function, since such impairment retards excretion of cardiac glycosides, and in those still experiencing effects from previous digitalis products. Digitalis toxicity may result in arrhythmias which are similar to those for which these drugs are utilized.

Side Effects: Cardiac glycosides are extremely toxic and have caused death even in clients who have received the drugs for long periods of time. There is a narrow margin of safety between an effective therapeutic dose and a toxic dose. Overdosage caused by the cumulative effects of the drug is a constant danger in therapy with cardiac glycosides. Digitalis toxicity is characterized by a wide variety of symptoms, which are hard to differentiate from those of the cardiac disease itself.

CV: Changes in the rate, rhythm, and irritability of the heart and the mechanism of the heartbeat. Extrasystoles, bigeminal pulse, coupled rhythm, ectopic beat, and other forms of arrhythmias have been noted. *Death most often results from ventricular fibrillation.* Cardiac glycosides should be discontinued in adults when pulse rate falls below 60 beats/min. All cardiac changes are best detected by the ECG, which is also most useful in clients suffering from intoxication. *Acute hemorrhage.*

GI: Anorexia, N&V, excessive salivation, epigastric distress, abdominal pain, diarrhea, bowel necrosis. Clients on digitalis therapy may experience two vomiting stages. The first is an early sign of toxicity and is a direct effect of digitalis on the GI tract. Late vomiting indicates stimulation of the vomiting center of the brain, which occurs after the heart muscle has been saturated with digitalis. *CNS:* Headaches, fatigue, lassitude, irritability, malaise, muscle weakness, insomnia, stupor. Psychotomimetic effects (especially in elderly or arteriosclerotic clients or neonates) including disorientation, confusion, depression, aphasia, delirium, hallucinations, and, rarely, *convulsions.* *Neuromuscular:* Neurologic pain involving the lower third of the face and lumbar areas, paresthesia. *Visual disturbances:* Blurred vision, flickering dots, white halos, borders around dark objects, diplopia, amblyopia, color perception changes. *Hypersensitivity (5–7 days after starting therapy):* Skin reactions (urticaria, fever, pruritus, facial and *angioneurotic edema*). *Other:* Chest pain, coldness of extremities.

OD Overdose Management: The relationship of cardiac glycoside levels to symptoms of toxicity varies significantly from client to client; thus, it is not possible to identify glycoside levels that would define toxicity accurately. *Symptoms (Toxicity):* *GI:* Anorexia, N&V, diarrhea, abdominal discomfort, or pain. *CNS:* Blurred, yellow, or green vision and halo effect; headache, weakness, drowsiness, mental depression, apathy, restlessness, disorientation, confusion, *seizures,* EEG abnormalities, delirium, hallucinations, neuralgia, psychosis. *CV:* Ventricular tachycardia, unifocal or multiform PVCs (especially in bigeminal or trigeminal patterns), paroxysmal and nonparoxysmal nodal rhythms, AV dissociation, accelerated junctional rhythm, excessive slowing of the pulse, *AV block (may proceed to complete block),*

✦ = Available in Canada   ***bold italic*** = life threatening side effect

atrial fibrillation, **_ventricular fibrillation (most common cause of death)._** Chil-dren: Visual disturbances, headache, weakness, apathy, and psychosis occur but may be difficult to recognize. *CV:* Conduction disturbances, supraventricular tachyarrhythmias (e.g., **_AV block_**), atrial tachycardia with or without block, nodal tachycardia, unifocal or multiform ventricular premature contractions, ventricular tachycardia, sinus bradycardia (especially in infants).*Treatment in Adults:*

• Discontinue drug and admit to the intensive care area for continuous monitoring of ECG.

• If serum potassium is below normal, potassium chloride should be administered in divided PO doses totaling 3–6 g (40–80 mEq). Potassium should not be used when severe or complete heart block is due to digitalis and not related to tachycardia.

• *Atropine:* A dose of 0.01 mg/kg IV to treat severe sinus bradycardia or slow ventricular rate due to secondary AV block.

• *Cholestyramine, colestipol, activated charcoal:* To bind digitalis in the intestine, thus preventing enterohepatic recirculation.

• *Digoxin immune FAB:* See drug entry. Given in approximate equimolar quantities as digoxin, it reverses S&S of toxicity, often with improvement seen within 30 min.

• *Lidocaine:* A dose of 1 mg/kg given over 5 min followed by an infusion of 15–50 mcg/kg/min to maintain normal cardiac rhythm.

• *Phenytoin:* For atrial or ventricular arrhythmias unresponsive to potassium, can give a dose of 0.5 mg/kg at a rate not exceeding 50 mg/min (given at 1–2 hr intervals). The maximum dose should not exceed 10 mg/kg/day.

• *Countershock:* A direct-current countershock can be used *only as a last resort.* If required, therapy should be initiated at low voltage levels.

Treatment in Children: Give potassium in divided doses totaling 1–1.5 mEq/kg (if correction of arrhythmia is urgent, a dose of 0.5 mEq/kg/hr can be used) with careful monitoring of the ECG. The potassium IV solution should be dilute to avoid local irritation although IV fluid overload must be avoided. Digoxin immune FAB may also be used.

Digoxin is not removed effectively by dialysis, by exchange transfusion, or during cardiopulmonary bypass as most of the drug is found in tissues rather than the circulating blood. Digitoxin is not effectively removed by either peritoneal or hemodialysis due to its high degree of plasma protein binding.

Drug Interactions: One of the most serious side effects of digitalis-type drugs is hypokalemia (lowering of serum potassium levels). This may lead to cardiac arrhythmias, muscle weakness, hypotension, and respiratory distress. Other agents causing hypokalemia reinforce this effect and increase the chance of digitalis toxicity. Such reactions may occur in clients who have been on digitalis maintenance for a long time.

Albuterol / ↑ Skeletal muscle binding of digoxin

Amiloride / ↓ Inotropic effects of digoxin

Aminoglycosides / ↓ Effect of digitalis glycosides due to ↓ absorption from GI tract

Aminosalicylic acid / ↓ Effect of digitalis glycosides due to ↓ absorption from GI tract

Amphotericin B / ↑ K depletion caused by digitalis; ↑ risk of digitalis toxicity

Antacids / ↓ Effect of digitalis glycosides due to ↓ absorption from GI tract

Beta blockers / Complete heart block possible

Calcium preparations / Cardiac arrhythmias if parenteral calcium given with digitalis

Chlorthalidone / ↑ K and Mg loss with ↑ chance of digitalis toxicity

Cholestyramine / Binds digitoxin in the intestine and ↓ its absorption

Colestipol / Binds digitoxin in the intestine and ↓ its absorption

Ephedrine / ↑ Chance of cardiac arrhythmias

Epinephrine / ↑ Chance of cardiac arrhythmias

Ethacrynic acid / ↑ K and Mg loss with ↑ chance of digitalis toxicity

Furosemide / ↑ K and Mg loss with ↑ chance of digitalis toxicity

Glucose infusions / Large infusions of glucose may cause ↓ in serum potassium and ↑ chance of digitalis toxicity

Hypoglycemic drugs / ↓ Effect of digitalis glycosides due to ↑ breakdown by liver

Methimazole / ↑ Chance of toxic effects of digitalis

Metoclopramide / ↓ Effect of digitalis glycosides by ↓ absorption from GI tract

Muscle relaxants, nondepolarizing / ↑ Risk of cardiac arrhythmias

Propranolol / Potentiates digitalis-induced bradycardia

Reserpine / ↑ Chance of cardiac arrhythmias

Spironolactone / Either ↑ or ↓ toxic effects of digitalis glycosides

Succinylcholine / ↑ Chance of cardiac arrhythmias

Sulfasalazine / ↓ Effect of digitalis glycosides by ↓ absorption from GI tract

Sympathomimetics / ↑ Chance of cardiac arrhythmias

Thiazides / ↑ K and Mg loss with ↑ chance of digitalis toxicity

Thioamines / ↑ Effect and toxicity of cardiac glycosides

Thyroid / ↓ Effectiveness of digitalis glycosides

Triamterene / ↑ Pharmacologic effects of digoxin

Laboratory Test Interferences: May ↓ PT. Alters tests for 17-ketosteroids and 17-hydroxycorticosteroids.

Dosage

PO, IM, or IV. *Highly individualized.* See individual drugs: digitoxin, digoxin. Initially, the drugs are usually given at higher ("digitalizing" or loading) doses. These are reduced as soon as the desired therapeutic effect is achieved or undesirable toxic reactions develop. The client's response to cardiac glycosides is gauged by clinical and ECG observations. The rates at which clients become digitalized vary considerably. Clients with mild signs of congestion can often be digitalized gradually over a period of several days. Clients suffering from more serious congestion, for example, those showing signs of acute LV failure, dyspnea, or lung edema, can be digitalized more rapidly by parenteral administration of a fast-acting cardiac glycoside. Once digitalization has been attained (pulse 68–80 beats/min) and symptoms of CHF have subsided, the client is put on maintenance dosage. Depending on the drug and the age of the client, the daily maintenance dose is often approximately 10% of the digitalizing dose.

RESPIRATORY CARE CONSIDERATIONS

Administration/Storage

1. Many cardiac glycosides have similar names. However, their dosage and duration of their effect differ markedly. Therefore, check the order, the medication administration record/card, and the bottle label of the medication to be administered. If a client questions the drug (size, color, etc.) recheck the drug order, bottle label, and the name of the client to whom the drug is to be given.

2. Measure all oral liquid cardiac medications precisely, using a calibrated dropper or a syringe.

3. The half-life of cardiac glycosides is prolonged in the elderly. When working with elderly clients, anticipate the doses of drug will be smaller than for those in other age groups.

4. Obtain written parameters indicating the pulse rates, both high and low, at which cardiac glycosides are to be withheld. Any change in rate or rhythm may indicate digitalis toxicity.

FOR CLIENTS STARTING ON A DIGITALIZING DOSE

Assessment

1. Document indications for therapy, type and onset of symptoms, and other agents prescribed. If administered for heart failure note causes and ensure that failure not solely related to diastolic dysfunction as drug's positive inotropic effect may increase cardiac outflow obstruction with hypertrophic cardiomyopathy.

2. Note any drugs the client may be taking that would adversely interact with digitalis glycosides. Diuretics may increase toxicity.

3. Obtain and review the following lab tests before administering the medication: CBC, serum electrolytes, calcium, magnesium, and liver and renal function tests.

4. Ascertain that an ECG has been completed and note rhythm and rate before administration.

5. Assess and document cardiopulmonary findings; note presence of S3, JVD, HJR, laterally displaced PMI, HR above 100 bpm, rales, peripheral edema, DOE, PND, and echo, MUGA, and/or cardiac cath findings. Note New York Heart Association Classification based on client symptoms.

FOR CLIENTS BEING DIGITALIZED AND FOR CLIENTS ON A MAINTENANCE DOSE OF A CARDIAC GLYCOSIDE

Interventions

1. During digitalization the client should be in a closely monitored environment where emergency equipment is readily available.

2. Observe cardiac monitor for evidence of bradycardia and/or arrhythmias, or count the apical pulse rate for at least 1 min before administering the drug. Obtain written parameters (e.g., HR > 50) for drug administration.

• Document if the adult pulse rate is below 50 beats/min or if an arrhythmia (irregular heart beat/pulse) not previously noted occurs and report.

• If a child's pulse rate is 90–110 beats/min or if an arrhythmia is present, withhold the drug and report.

3. Anticipate more than once daily dosing in most children (up to age 10) due to higher metabolic activity.

4. With co-worker simultaneously take the client's apical/radial pulse for 1 min, report if there is a pulse deficit (e.g., the wrist rate is less than the apical rate). A pulse deficit may indicate that the client is having an adverse reaction to the drug.

5. Monitor weights and place the client on I&O. Determine that the client is adequately hydrated and that elimination is in line with the intake. Weight gain may indicate edema. Adequate intake will help prevent cumulative toxic effects of the drug.

6. Anticipate that clients taking nonpotassium-sparing diuretics as well as a cardiac glycoside will require potassium supplements.

7. When a potassium supplement is needed, ask the pharmacist to provide the client with the most palatable preparation available. (Liquid potassium preparations are usually bitter.)

8. If the client complains of gastric distress, an antacid preparation may be ordered.

• Antacids containing aluminum or magnesium and kaolin/pectin mixtures should be given 6 hr before or 6 hr after dose of cardiac glycoside to prevent decreased therapeutic effect of glycoside.

9. When the drug is given to newborns, use a cardiac monitor to identify early evidence of toxicity. Any excessive slowing of sinus rate, sinoatrial arrest, or prolonged PR interval should be reported immediately and the drug withheld.

10. Monitor serum digoxin levels periodically (therapeutic range 0.5–2.0 ng/mL) and assess for symptoms of toxicity. For steady state draw specimen more than 6 hr after last dose.

11. Have digoxin antidote available (digoxin immune FAB) for management of clients with severe toxicity.

12. Use caution; digoxin withdrawal may worsen heart failure.

Evaluate

- A positive response to digitalization, as evidenced by a stable cardiac rate and rhythm, improved breathing patterns, ↓ severity of S&S of CHF, improved CO, improved activity tolerance, ↓ weight, and improved diuresis

- Laboratory confirmation that serum levels of drug are within therapeutic range (e.g., digoxin 0.5–2.0 ng/mL) and client does not manifest symptoms of toxicity

Special Concerns

1. Elderly clients must be observed for early S&S of toxicity, because their rate of drug elimination is slower than with other clients. N&V, anorexia, confusion, and visual disturbances may be signs of toxicity and should be reported immediately.

2. The half-life of cardiac glycosides is prolonged in the elderly. Anticipate small doses of drug for those in this age group.

3. Be especially alert to cardiac arrhythmias in children. This sign of toxicity occurs more frequently in children than in adults.

CEPHALOSPORINS

See also the following individual entries:

Cefaclor
Cefadroxil monohydrate
Cefamandole nafate
Cefazolin sodium
Cefepime hydrochloride
Cefixime oral
Cefmetazole sodium
Cefonicid sodium
Cefoperazone sodium
Cefotaxime sodium
Cefotetan disodium
Cefoxitin sodium
Cefpodoxime proxetil
Cefprozil
Ceftazidime
Ceftibuten
Ceftizoxime sodium
Ceftriaxone sodium
Cefuroxime axetil
Cefuroxime sodium
Cephalexin hydrochloride monohydrate
Cephalexin monohydrate
Cephalothin sodium
Cephapirin sodium
Cephradine
Loracarbef

General Statement: The cephalosporins are semisynthetic antibiotics resembling the penicillins both chemically and pharmacologically. Some cephalosporins are rapidly absorbed from the GI tract and quickly reach effective concentrations in the urinary, GI, and respiratory tracts except in clients with pernicious anemia or obstructive jaundice. The drugs are eliminated rapidly in clients with normal renal function.

The cephalosporins are broad-spectrum antibiotics classified as first-, second-, and third-generation drugs. The difference among generations is based on antibacterial spectra; third-generation cephalosporins have more activity against gram-negative organisms and resistant organisms and less activity against gram-positive organisms than first-generation drugs. Third-generation cephalosporins are also stable against beta-lactamases. Cephalosporins can be destroyed by cephalosporinase. Also, the cost increases from first- to third-generation cephalosporins.

Action/Kinetics: The cephalosporins interfere with a final step in the formation of the bacterial cell wall (inhibition of mucopeptide biosynthesis), resulting in unstable cell membranes that undergo lysis (same mechanism of actions as penicillins). Also, cell division and growth are inhibited. The cephalosporins are most effective against young, rapidly dividing organisms and are considered bactericidal. The **t½** ranges from 69 to 132 min, and serum protein binding ranges from 5% to 86%. Cephalosporins are widely distributed to most tissues and fluids. First- and second-generation drugs do not enter

---

the CSF well but third-generation drugs enter inflamed meninges readily. The cephalosporins are rapidly excreted by the kidneys.

Uses: Cephalosporins are effective against infections of the biliary tract, GI tract, GU system, bones, joints, upper and lower respiratory tract, skin, and skin structures. Also, gynecologic infections, meningitis, osteomyelitis, endocarditis, intra-abdominal infections, peritonitis, otitis media, gonorrhea, septicemia, and prophylaxis prior to surgery. A listing of the organisms against which cephalosporins are effective follows.

First-Generation Cephalosporins. Gram-positive cocci including *Staphylococcus aureus, S. epidermidis, S. pyogenes, Streptococcus pneumoniae, S. viridans,* group A and B streptococci, and anaerobic streptococci. Activity against gram-negative bacteria includes *Escherichia coli, Haemophilus influenzae, Klebsiella,* and *Proteus mirabilis.* Drugs include cefadroxil, cefazolin, cephalexin, cephalothin, cephapirin, cephradine.

Second-Generation Cephalosporins. Spectrum similar to that of first-generation cephalosporins. Also active against certain gram-negative bacteria and anaerobes including *Providencia rettgeri, Bacteroides* species, *Peptococcus,* and *Peptostreptococcus* species. Selected second-generation cephalosporins are effective against the following genera: *Citrobacter, Enterobacter, Providencia, Clostridium,* and *Fusobacterium,* as well as *Morganella morganii, Neisseria gonorrhoeae,* and *Proteus vulgaris.* Second-generation drugs include cefaclor, cefamandole, cefmetazole, cefonicid, cefotetan, cefoxitin, cefpodoxime, cefprozil, cefuroxime, and loracarbef.

Third-Generation Cephalosporins. Less active against gram-positive cocci. Spectrum similar to first- and second-generation cephalosporins. Most are also active against the following gram-negative and anaerobic species: *Acinetobacter, Citrobacter, Enterobacter, Providencia, Salmonella, Serratia, Shigella, Bacteroides,*

Clostridium, Fusobacterium, Peptococcus, and *Peptostreptococcus.* Most are effective against *M. morganii, N. gonorrhoeae, Neisseria meningitidis, P. vulgaris, Pseudomonas aeruginosa,* and *Bacteroides fragilis.* Selected third-generation cephalosporins are effective against *Haemophilus parainfluenzae, Moraxella catarrhalis, Salmonella thypi, Clostridium difficile,* and *Eubacterium* species. Third-generation drugs include cefixime, cefoperoxazone, cefotaxime, ceftazidime, ceftizoxime, ceftriaxone.

Contraindications: Hypersensitivity to cephalosporins.

Special Concerns: Safe use in pregnancy and lactation has not been established. Use with caution in the presence of impaired renal or hepatic function or together with other nephrotoxic drugs. Creatinine clearances should be performed on all clients with impaired renal function who receive cephalosporins. Use with caution in clients over 50 years of age. Clients hypersensitive to penicillin may occasionally cross-react to cephalosporins.

Side Effects: *GI:* N&V, diarrhea, abdominal cramps or pain, dyspepsia, glossitis, heartburn, sore mouth or tongue, dysgeusia, anorexia, flatulence, cholestasis. Pseudomembranous colitis. *Allergic:* Urticaria, rashes (maculopapular, morbilliform, or erythematous), pruritus (including anal and genital areas), fever, chills, erythema, **angioedema,** serum sickness, joint pain, exfoliative dermatitis, chest tightness, myalgia, erythema multiforme, edema, itching, numbness, chills, **Stevens-Johnson syndrome, anaphylaxis.** *NOTE:* Cross-allergy may be manifested between cephalosporins and penicillins. *Hematologic:* Leukopenia, leukocytosis, lymphocytosis, neutropenia (transient), eosinophilia, thrombocytopenia, thrombocythemia, **agranulocytosis,** granulocytopenia, bone marrow depression, **hemolytic anemia,** pancytopenia, decreased platelet function, **aplastic anemia,** hypoprothrombinemia (may lead to bleeding), thrombocytosis (transient). *CNS:* Headache, malaise, fatigue, vertigo, dizziness, lethargy, confusion, paresthesia, precipitation of **seizures** (especially in clients with impaired renal function). *Hepatic:* Hepatomegaly, hepatitis. Intrathecal use may result in hallucinations, nystagmus, or **seizures.** *Miscellaneous:* Superinfection including oral candidiasis and enterococcal infections, hypotension, sweating, flushing, dyspnea, interstitial pneumonitis.

IV or IM use may result in local swelling, inflammation, cellulitis, paresthesia, burning, phlebitis, thrombophlebitis. IM use may also cause pain and induration, tenderness, increased temperature. Sterile abscesses have been observed following SC use. Nephrotoxicity (↑ BUN with and without ↑ serum creatinine) may occur in clients over 50 and in young children.

OD **Overdose Management:** *Symptoms:* Parenteral use of large doses of cephalosporins may cause seizures, especially in clients with impaired renal function. *Treatment:* If seizures occur, discontinue the drug immediately and give anticonvulsant drugs. Hemodialysis may also be effective.

Drug Interactions
Aminoglycosides / ↑ Risk of renal toxicity with certain cephalosporins
Anticoagulants / Certain cephalosporins ↑ PT
Bacteriostatic agents / ↓ Effect of cephalosporins
Bumetanide / ↑ Risk of renal toxicity
Colistimethate / ↑ Risk of renal toxicity
Colistin / ↑ Risk of renal toxicity
Ethacrynic acid / ↑ Risk of renal toxicity
Furosemide / ↑ Risk of renal toxicity
Polymyxin B / ↑ Risk of renal toxicity
Probenecid / ↑ Effect of cephalosporins by ↓ excretion by kidneys

Vancomycin / ↑ Risk of renal toxicity

Laboratory Test Interferences: False + for urinary glucose with Benedict's solution, Fehling's solution, or Clinitest tablets. Enzyme tests (Clinistix, Tes-Tape) are unaffected. False + Coombs' test and urinary 17-ketosteroids.

↑ AST, ALT, total bilirubin, GGTP, LDH, alkaline phosphatase.

Dosage
See individual drugs.

RESPIRATORY CARE CONSIDERATIONS

See also *General Respiratory Care Considerations for All Anti-Infectives.*

Administration/Storage
1. Parenteral solutions infused too rapidly may cause pain and irritation; infuse over 30 min unless otherwise indicated and assess site frequently.
2. Therapy should be continued for at least 2–3 days after symptoms of infection have disappeared.
3. For group A beta-hemolytic streptococcal infections, therapy should be continued for at least 10 days to prevent the development of glomerulonephritis or rheumatic fever.

Assessment
1. Assess client with a history of hypersensitivity reaction to penicillin for cross-sensitivity to cephalosporins. Cephalosporins are sensitizing and may elicit a hypersensitivity reaction, so do not administer.
2. Assess client's financial status. Many in this group of antibiotics are quite expensive and clients on fixed incomes with limited health benefits may be unable to afford the prescription expense.
3. Document indications for therapy and symptoms of infection and ensure that appropriate cultures have been performed prior to initiating drug therapy.
4. Obtain baseline CBC, serum glucose, electrolytes, and liver and renal

function studies. Anticipate lower doses for clients with renal impairment; for dialysis clients, administer after treatment.

5. Drug may cause a false positive Coombs' test; document appropriately and instruct client.

Interventions

1. The cephalosporins all have similar sounding and similarly spelled names. Use care when transcribing orders for administration of these drugs and request clarification as needed.

2. Pseudomembranous colitis may occur in clients receiving cephalosporins. If diarrhea develops, note any fever and report immediately. Continue to monitor VS, I&O, stool C&S, and for lab evidence of electrolyte imbalance.

3. Persistent temperature elevations may be indicative of drug-induced fever.

Evaluate

• Evidence (presence/absence) of pretreatment symptoms and review of C&S results to determine effectiveness of treatment

• Clinical evidence of resolution of infection, such as ↓ WBCs, ↓ temperature, improved appetite

• Reports of symptomatic improvement

CHOLINERGIC BLOCKING AGENTS

Atropine sulfate
Glycopyrrolate
Ipratropium bromide
Scopolamine hydrobromide
Scopolamine transdermal
    therapeutic system

Action/Kinetics: The cholinergic blocking agents prevent the neurotransmitter acetylcholine from combining with receptors on the postganglionic parasympathetic nerve terminal (muscarinic site). In therapeutic doses, these drugs have little effect on transmission of nerve impulses across ganglia (nicotinic sites) or at the neuromuscular junction.

The main effects of cholinergic blocking agents are:

1. To reduce spasms of smooth muscles like those controlling the urinary bladder or spasms of bronchial and intestinal smooth muscle.

2. To block vagal impulses to the heart, resulting in an increase in the rate and speed of impulse conduction through the AV conducting system.

3. To suppress or decrease gastric secretions, perspiration, salivation, and secretion of bronchial mucus.

4. To relax the sphincter muscles of the iris and cause pupillary dilation (mydriasis) and loss of accommodation for near vision (cycloplegia).

5. To act in diverse ways on the CNS, producing such reactions as depression (scopolamine) or stimulation (toxic doses of atropine). Many of the anticholinergic drugs also have antiparkinsonism effects. They abolish or reduce the S&S of Parkinson's disease, such as tremors and rigidity, and result in some improvement in mobility, muscular coordination, and motor performance. These effects may be due to blockade of the effects of acetylcholine in the CNS. This section also discusses miscellaneous synthetic antispasmodics related to anticholinergic drugs.

The anticholinergics that are related to atropine are quickly absorbed following PO ingestion. These agents cross the blood-brain barrier and may exert significant CNS effects. Examples of these drugs are scopolamine, l-hyoscyamine, and belladonna alkaloids. The drugs classified as quaternary ammonium anticholinergic drugs are erratically absorbed from the GI tract and exert minimal CNS effects, since they do not cross the blood-brain barrier. Examples of these drugs are glycopyrrolate, methantheline, propantheline, tridihexethyl chloride, clidinium bromide, isopropamide, and others.

Uses: See individual drugs.

Contraindications: Glaucoma, adhesions between iris and lens of the eye, tachycardia, myocardial ischemia, unstable CV state in acute hemorrhage, partial obstruction of the GI and biliary tracts, prostatic hypertrophy, renal disease, myasthenia gravis, hepatic disease, paralytic ileus, pyloroduodenal stenosis, pyloric obstruction, intestinal atony, ulcerative colitis, obstructive uropathy. Cardiac clients, especially when there is danger of tachycardia; older persons suffering from atherosclerosis or mental impairment. Lactation.

Special Concerns: Use with caution in pregnancy. Infants and young children are more susceptible to the toxic side effects of anticholinergic drugs. Of particular importance is use of such drugs in children when the ambient temperature is high; due to suppression of sweat glands, the body temperature may increase rapidly. Geriatric clients are particularly likely to manifest anticholinergic side effects such as dry mouth, constipation, and urinary retention (especially in males). Geriatric clients are also more likely to experience agitation, confusion, drowsiness, excitement, glaucoma, and impaired memory. Use with caution in hyperthyroidism, CHF, cardiac arrhythmias, hypertension, Down syndrome, asthma, spastic paralysis, blonde individuals, allergies, and chronic lung disease.

Side Effects: These are desirable in some conditions and undesirable in others. Thus, the anticholinergics have an antisalivary effect that is useful in parkinsonism. This same effect is unpleasant when the drug is used for spastic conditions of the GI tract.

Most side effects are dose-related and decrease when dosage decreases. Sometimes it helps to discontinue the medication for several days. With this in mind, anticholinergic drugs have the following side effects. *GI:* N&V, dry mouth, dysphagia, constipation, heartburn, change in taste perception, bloated feeling, paralytic ileus. *CNS:* Dizziness, drowsiness, nervousness, disorientation, headache, weakness, insomnia,

fever (especially in children). Large doses may produce CNS stimulation including tremor and restlessness. Anticholinergic psychoses: ataxia, euphoria, confusion, disorientation, loss of short-term memory, decreased anxiety, fatigue, insomnia, hallucinations, dysarthria, agitation. *CV:* Palpitations. *GU:* Urinary retention or hesitancy, impotence. *Ophthalmologic:* Blurred vision, dilated pupils, photophobia, cycloplegia, precipitation of acute glaucoma. *Allergic:* Urticaria, skin rashes, **anaphylaxis.** *Other:* Flushing, decreased sweating, nasal congestion, suppression of glandular secretions including lactation. Heat prostration (fever and heat stroke) in presence of high environmental temperatures due to decreased sweating.

OD **Overdose Management:** *Symptoms ("Belladonna Poisoning"):* Infants and children are especially susceptible to the toxic effects of atropine and scopolamine. Poisoning (dose-dependent) is characterized by the following symptoms: dry mouth, burning sensation of the mouth, difficulty in swallowing and speaking, blurred vision, photophobia, rash, tachycardia, increased respiration, **increased body temperature** (up to 109°F, 42.7°C), restlessness, irritability, confusion, muscle incoordination, dilated pupils, hot dry skin, **respiratory depression and paralysis,** tremors, **seizures,** hallucinations, and **death.** *Treatment ("Belladonna Poisoning"):*

• Gastric lavage or induction of vomiting followed by activated charcoal. General supportive measures.

• Anticholinergic effects can be reversed by physostigmine (Eserine), 1–3 mg IV (effectiveness uncertain; thus use other agents if possible). Neostigmine methylsulfate, 0.5–2 mg IV, repeated as necessary.

• If there is excitation, diazepam, a short-acting barbiturate, IV sodium thiopental (2% solution), or chloral hydrate (100–200 mL of a 2% solution by rectal infusion) may be given.

• For fever, cool baths may be used. Keep client in a darkened room if photophobia is manifested.
• Assisted ventilation should be instituted if there is paralysis of respiratory muscles.

Drug Interactions

Amantadine / Additive anticholinergic side effects
Antacids / ↓ Absorption of anticholinergics from GI tract
Antidepressants, tricyclic / Additive anticholinergic side effects
Antihistamines / Additive anticholinergic side effects
Atenolol / Anticholinergics ↑ effects of atenolol
Benzodiazepines / Additive anticholinergic side effects
Corticosteroids / Additive ↑ intraocular pressure
Cyclopropane / ↑ Chance of ventricular arrhythmias
Digoxin / ↑ Effect of digoxin due to ↑ absorption from GI tract
Disopyramide / Potentiation of anticholinergic side effects
Guanethidine / Reversal of inhibition of gastric acid secretion caused by anticholinergics
Haloperidol / Additive ↑ intraocular pressure
Histamine / Reversal of inhibition of gastric acid secretion caused by anticholinergics
Levodopa / Possible ↓ effect of levodopa due to ↑ breakdown of levodopa in stomach (due to delayed gastric emptying time)
MAO inhibitors / ↑ Effect of anticholinergics due to ↓ breakdown by liver
Meperidine / Additive anticholinergic side effects
Methylphenidate / Potentiation of anticholinergic side effects
Metoclopramide / Anticholinergics block action of metoclopramide
Nitrates, nitrites / Potentiation of anticholinergic side effects
Nitrofurantoin / ↑ Bioavailability of nitrofurantoin
Orphenadrine / Additive anticholinergic side effects
Phenothiazines / Additive anticholinergic side effects; also, effects of phenothiazines may ↓
Primidone / Potentiation of anticholinergic side effects
Procainamide / Additive anticholinergic side effects
Quinidine / Additive anticholinergic side effects
Reserpine / Reversal of inhibition of gastric acid secretion caused by anticholinergics
Sympathomimetics / ↑ Bronchial relaxation
Thiazide diuretics / ↑ Bioavailability of thiazide diuretics
Thioxanthines / Potentiation of anticholinergic side effects

Dosage ─────────────
See individual drugs.

───────────────────────

RESPIRATORY CARE CONSIDERATIONS
Administration/Storage
1. Check dosage and measure the drug exactly. Some drugs in this category are given in small amounts. As a consequence, overdosage is quickly achieved and can lead to toxicity.
2. Review the list of drugs with which drugs in this category interact.

Assessment
1. Document indications for therapy and assess client for a history of asthma, glaucoma, or duodenal ulcer, all of which contraindicate the use of these drugs.
2. Note client history of renal disease, cardiac problems, or hepatic disease.
3. Determine the age of the client. Elderly clients, especially those with mental impairment or atherosclerosis, should not receive these drugs.
4. Assess for constipation and urinary retention and tolerance.

Interventions
1. If the client complains of a dry mouth, provide frequent mouth care and cold drinks, especially postoperatively. Sugarless hard candies and chewing gum may also be of some benefit.
2. Observe the client for evidence of drug interactions that may occur. A

reduction in dosage of one of the medications may be necessary.

3. Drugs such as atropine may suppress thermoregulatory sweating; counsel client concerning activity (especially in hot weather) and appropriate clothing. Also, children and infants may exhibit "atropine fever."

ADDITIONAL RESPIRATORY CARE CONSIDERATIONS RELATED TO PATHOLOGIC CONDITIONS FOR WHICH THE DRUG IS ADMINISTERED

CARDIOVASCULAR

Interventions

1. Monitor VS and ECG. Assess for any hemodynamic changes and intraventricular conduction blocks.

2. Note any client complaints of palpitations.

Evaluate

• ↑ HR

• Evidence of ↓ production of secretions

CORTICOSTEROIDS

See also the following individual entries:

Beclomethasone dipropionate
Betamethasone
Betamethasone dipropionate
Betamethasone sodium
    phosphate
Betamethasone sodium
    phosphate and Betamethasone
    acetate
Betamethasone valerate
Budesonide
Cortisone acetate
Dexamethasone
Dexamethasone acetate
Dexamethasone sodium
    phosphate
Flunisolide
Fluticasone propionate
Hydrocortisone
Hydrocortisone acetate
Hydrocortisone butyrate
Hydrocortisone cypionate
Hydrocortisone sodium
    phosphate

Hydrocortisone sodium succinate
Hydrocortisone valerate
Methylprednisolone
Methylprednisolone acetate
Methylprednisolone sodium
    succinate
Prednisolone
Prednisolone acetate
Prednisolone acetate and
    Prednisolone sodium
    phosphate
Prednisolone sodium phosphate
Prednisolone tebutate
Prednisone
Triamcinolone
Triamcinolone acetonide
Triamcinolone diacetate
Triamcinolone hexacetonide

Action/Kinetics: The hormones of the adrenal gland influence many metabolic pathways and all organ systems and are essential for survival.

The release of corticosteroids is controlled by hormones such as corticotropin-releasing factor, produced by the hypothalamus, and ACTH (corticotropin), produced by the anterior pituitary.

The natural corticosteroids play an important role in most major metabolic processes. They have the following effects:

1. **Carbohydrate metabolism.** Deposition of glucose as glycogen in the liver and the conversion of glycogen to glucose when needed. Gluconeogenesis (i.e., the transformation of protein into glucose).

2. **Protein metabolism.** The stimulation of protein loss from many organs (catabolism). This is characterized by a negative nitrogen balance.

3. **Fat metabolism.** The deposition of fatty tissue in facial, abdominal, and shoulder regions.

4. **Water and electrolyte balance.** Alteration of glomerular filtration rate; increased sodium and consequently fluid retention. Also affects the excretion rate of potassium, calcium, and phosphorus. Urinary excretion rate of creatine and uric acid increases.

According to their chemical structure

---

and chief physiologic effect, the corticosteroids fall into two subgroups, which have considerable functional overlap.

1. Those, like cortisone and hydrocortisone, that mainly regulate the metabolic pathways involving protein, carbohydrate, and fat. This group is often referred to as *glucocorticoids*. Glucocorticoids are qualitatively similar. Differences between these agents are due to duration of action and half-life (see individual agents).

2. Those, like aldosterone and desoxycorticosterone, that are more specifically involved in electrolyte and water balance. These are often referred to as *mineralocorticoids*. Hormones with mineralocorticoid activity result in reabsorption of sodium (and therefore water retention) and enhanced potassium and hydrogen excretion. Substances such as cortisone and hydrocortisone, although classified as glucocorticoids, possess significant mineralocorticoid activity.

Therapeutically, the corticosteroids are used for a variety of purposes; a distinction must be made between physiologic doses used for replacement therapy and pharmacologic doses used to treat inflammatory and other disease states. Many slightly modified synthetic variants are available today that possess glucocorticoid but minimal or no mineralocorticoid activity.

The hormones have a marked anti-inflammatory effect because of their ability to inhibit prostaglandin synthesis. These agents also inhibit accumulation of macrophages and leukocytes at sites of inflammation as well as inhibit phagocytosis and lysosomal enzyme release. They aid the organism in coping with various stressful situations (trauma, severe illness). The immunosuppressant effect is thought to be due to a reduction of the number of T lymphocytes, monocytes, and eosinophils. Corticosteroids also decrease binding of immunoglobulin to receptors on the cell surface and inhibit the

synthesis and/or release of interleukins which, in turn, decrease T-lymphocyte blastogenesis and reduce the primary immune response.

Uses: When used for anti-inflammatory or immunosuppressant therapy, the corticosteroid should possess minimal mineralocorticoid activity. Therapy with glucocorticoids is not curative and in many situations should be considered as adjunctive rather than primary therapy.

1. **Replacement therapy.** Acute and chronic adrenal insufficiency, including Addison's disease, congenital adrenal hyperplasia, adrenal insufficiency secondary to anterior pituitary insufficiency. However, not all drugs can be used for replacement therapy; some lack glucocorticoid effects, whereas others lack mineralocorticoid effects. For replacement therapy, drugs must possess both effects.

2. **Rheumatic disorders.** Rheumatoid arthritis (including juveniles), ankylosing spondylitis, acute and subacute bursitis, acute nonspecific tenosynovitis, acute gouty arthritis, psoriatic arthritis, posttraumatic osteoarthritis, synovitis of osteoarthritis, epicondylitis.

3. **Collagen diseases.** Including SLE, acute rheumatic carditis, polymyositis.

4. **Allergic diseases.** Control of severe allergic conditions refractory to conventional treatment as serum sickness, drug hypersensitivity reactions, anaphylaxis, urticarial transfusion reactions, acute noninfectious laryngeal edema.

5. **Respiratory diseases.** Including bronchial asthma (and status asthmaticus), symptomatic sarcoidosis, seasonal or perennial rhinitis, berylliosis, aspiration pneumonitis, fulminating or disseminated pulmonary tuberculosis (with appropriate antitubercular therapy), Loeffler's syndrome refractory to other treatment. Used for the maintenance treatment of asthma as prophylactic therapy. As supplemental therapy when systemic corticosteroids are required in order to

reduce the dose or eliminate the need for systemic steroids.

6. **Ocular diseases.** Severe acute and chronic allergic and inflammatory conditions including conjunctivitis, keratitis, herpes zoster ophthalmicus, iritis, iridocyclitis, chorioretinitis, diffuse posterior uveitis and choroiditis, optic neuritis, allergic corneal marginal ulcers, sympathetic ophthalmia, and anterior segment inflammation.

7. **Dermatologic diseases.** Including severe erythema multiforme (Stevens-Johnson syndrome), exfoliative dermatitis, mycosis fungoides, severe seborrheic dermatitis, bullous dermatitis herpetiformis, severe psoriasis, angioedema or urticaria, contact dermatitis, atopic dermatitis, pemphigus.

8. **Diseases of the intestinal tract.** To assist client through crises of chronic ulcerative colitis, regional enteritis, intractable sprue.

9. **Nervous system.** Acute exacerbations of multiple sclerosis. Short-term treatment with high doses of methylprednisolone and prednisone in clients with optic neuritis (often the first sign of multiple sclerosis) may prevent full-blown multiple sclerosis for 2 years.

10. **Malignancies.** Including leukemias and lymphomas in adults and acute leukemia in children.

11. **Nephrotic syndrome.** To induce diuresis or remission of proteinuria due to lupus erythematosus or of the idiopathic type.

12. **Hematologic diseases.** Including acquired hemolytic anemia, RBC anemia, idiopathic and secondary thrombocytopenic purpura in adults, congenital hypoplastic anemia.

13. **Intra-articular or soft tissue administration.** To treat acute episodes of synovitis of osteoarthritis, rheumatoid arthritis, acute gouty arthritis, epicondylitis, acute nonspecific tenosynovitis, posttraumatic osteoarthritis.

14. **Intralesional administration.** To treat keloids, psoriatic plaques, granuloma annulare, lichen simplex chronicus, discoid lupus erythematosus, cystic tumors of an aponeurosis or ganglia, lesions of lichen planus, necrobiosis lipoidica diabeticorum, alopecia areata.

15. **Miscellaneous.** Septic shock (use controversial), trichinosis with neurologic or myocardial involvement, tuberculosis meningitis with subarachnoid block or impending block (with appropriate antitubercular therapy).

Contraindications: Corticosteroids are contraindicated if infection is suspected because these drugs may mask infections. Also peptic ulcer, psychoses, acute glomerulonephritis, herpes simplex infections of the eye, vaccinia or varicella, the exanthematous diseases, Cushing's syndrome, active tuberculosis, myasthenia gravis. Recent intestinal anastomoses, CHF or other cardiac disease, hypertension, systemic fungal infections, open-angle glaucoma. Also, hyperlipidemia, hyperthyroidism or hypothyroidism, osteoporosis, myasthenia gravis, tuberculosis. Lactation (if high doses are used). Inhalation products to relieve acute bronchospasms.

Topical application in the treatment of eye disorders is contraindicated in dendritic keratitis, vaccinia, chickenpox, or other viral disease that may involve the conjunctiva or cornea. Also tuberculosis and fungal or acute purulent infections of the eye. Topical treatment of the ear is contraindicated in aural fungal infections and perforated eardrum. Topical use in dermatology is contraindicated in tuberculosis of the skin, herpes simplex, vaccinia, varicella, and infectious conditions in the absence of anti-infective agents.

Special Concerns: Glucocorticoids should be used with caution in the presence of diabetes mellitus, hypertension, chronic nephritis, thrombophlebitis, convulsive disorders, infectious diseases, renal or hepatic insufficiency, pregnancy. Chronic use of

---

corticosteroids may inhibit the growth and development of children or adolescents. Pediatric clients are also at greater risk for developing cataracts, osteoporosis, avascular necrosis of the femoral heads, and glaucoma. Geriatric clients are more likely to develop hypertension and osteoporosis (especially postmenopausal women).

Side Effects: Small physiologic doses given as replacement therapy or short-term high-dosage therapy during emergencies rarely cause side effects. Prolonged therapy may cause a Cushing-like syndrome with atrophy of the adrenal cortex and subsequent adrenocortical insufficiency. A steroid withdrawal syndrome may occur following prolonged use; symptoms include anorexia, N&V, lethargy, headache, fever, joint pain, desquamation, myalgia, weight loss, hypotension.

Fluid and electrolyte: Edema, hypokalemic alkalosis, hypokalemia, hypocalcemia, hypotension or shock-like reaction, hypertension, CHF. *Musculoskeletal:* Muscle wasting, muscle pain or weakness, osteoporosis, spontaneous fractures including vertebral compression fractures and fractures of long bones, tendon rupture, aseptic necrosis of femoral and humeral heads. *GI:* N&V, anorexia or increased appetite, diarrhea or constipation, abdominal distention, pancreatitis, gastric irritation, ulcerative esophagitis. *Development or exacerbation of peptic ulcers with the possibility of perforation and hemorrhage; perforation of the small and large bowel,* especially in inflammatory bowel disease. *Endocrine:* Cushing's syndrome (e.g., central obesity, moonface, buffalo hump, enlargement of supraclavicular fat pads), amenorrhea, postmenopausal bleeding, menstrual irregularities, decreased glucose tolerance, hyperglycemia, glycosuria, increased insulin or sulfonylurea requirement in diabetics, development of diabetes mellitus, negative nitrogen balance due to protein catabolism, suppression of growth in children, secondary adrenocortical and pituitary unresponsiveness (especially during periods of stress). *CNS/Neurologic:* Headache, vertigo, insomnia, restlessness, increased motor activity, ischemic neuropathy, EEG abnormalities, *seizures,* pseudotumor cerebri. Also, euphoria, mood swings, depression, anxiety, personality changes, psychoses. *CV:* Thromboembolism, thrombophlebitis, ECG changes (due to potassium deficiency), fat embolism, necrotizing angiitis, cardiac arrhythmias, *myocardial rupture following recent MI,* syncopal episodes. *Dermatologic:* Impaired wound healing, skin atrophy and thinning, petechiae, ecchymoses, erythema, purpura, striae, hirsutism, urticaria, *angioneurotic edema,* acneiform eruptions, allergic dermatitis, lupus erythematosus-like lesions, suppression of skin test reactions, perineal irritation. *Ophthalmic:* Glaucoma, posterior subcapsular cataracts, increased intraocular pressure, exophthalmos. *Miscellaneous:* Hypercholesterolemia, atherosclerosis, aggravation or masking of infections, leukocytosis, increased or decreased motility and number of spermatozoa.

In children: Suppression of linear growth; reversible pseudobrain tumor syndrome characterized by papilledema, oculomotor or abducens nerve paralysis, visual loss, or headache.

PARENTERAL USE: Sterile abscesses, Charcot-like arthropathy, subcutaneous and cutaneous atrophy, burning or tingling (especially in the perineal area following IV use), scarring, inflammation, paresthesia, induration, hyperpigmentation or hypopigmentation, blindness when used intralesionally around the face and head (rare), transient or delayed pain or soreness, nystagmus, ataxia, muscle twitching, hiccoughs, *anaphylaxis with or without circulatory collapse, cardiac arrest, bronchospasm,* arachnoiditis after intrathecal use, foreign body granulomatous reactions.

INTRA-ARTICULAR: Postinjection

flare, Charcot-like arthropathy, tendon rupture, skin atrophy, facial flushing, osteonecrosis. Due to reduction in inflammation and pain, clients may overuse the joint.

INTRASPINAL: Aseptic, bacterial, chemical, cryptococcal, or tubercular meningitis; adhesive arachnoiditis, conus medullaris syndrome.

INTRAOCULAR: Application of corticosteroid preparations to the eye may reduce aqueous outflow and increase ocular pressure, thereby inducing or aggravating simple glaucoma. Ocular pressure therefore should be checked frequently in the elderly or in clients with glaucoma. Stinging, burning, dendritic keratitis (herpes simplex), corneal perforation (especially when the drugs are used for diseases that cause corneal thinning). Posterior subcapsular cataracts, especially in children. Exophthalmos, secondary fungal or viral eye infections.

TOPICAL USE: Except when used over large areas, when the skin is broken, or with occlusive dressings, topically applied corticosteroids are not absorbed systemically in sufficiently large quantities to cause the side effects noted in the previous paragraphs. Topically applied corticosteroids, however, may cause atrophy of the epidermis, drying of the skin, or atrophy of the dermal collagen. When used on the face, the agents may cause diffuse thinning and homogenization of the collagen, epidermal thinning, and striae formation. Topical corticosteroids should be used cautiously, or not at all, for infected lesions, and in that case, the use of occlusive dressings is contraindicated. Occasionally, topical corticosteroids may cause a sensitization reaction, which necessitates discontinuation of the drug.

OD **Overdose Management:** *Symptoms (Continued Use of Large Doses)—Cushing's Syndrome:* Acne, hypertension, moonface, striae, hirsutism, central obesity, ecchymoses,

myopathy, sexual dysfunction, osteoporosis, diabetes, hyperlipidemia, increased susceptibility to infection, peptic ulcer, electrolyte and fluid imbalance. Acute toxicity or death is rare. *Treatment of Chronic Overdose:* Gradually taper the dose of the steroid and frequently monitor lab tests. During periods of stress, steroid supplementation is necessary. Dose should be reduced to the lowest one that will control the symptoms (or discontinue the steroid completely). Recovery of normal adrenal and pituitary function may take up to 9 months. Large, acute overdoses may be treated with gastric lavage, emesis, and general supportive measures.

Drug Interactions

Acetaminophen / ↑ Risk of hepatotoxicity due to ↑ rate of formation of hepatotoxic acetaminophen metabolite

Alcohol / ↑ Risk of GI ulceration or hemorrhage

Amphotericin B / Corticosteroids ↑ K depletion caused by amphotericin B

Aminoglutethimide / ↓ Adrenal response to corticotropin

Anabolic steroids / ↑ Risk of edema

Antacids / ↓ Effect of corticosteroids due to ↓ absorption from GI tract

Antibiotics, broad-spectrum / Concomitant use may result in emergence of resistant strains, leading to severe infection

Anticholinergics / Combination ↑ intraocular pressure; will aggravate glaucoma

Anticoagulants, oral / ↓ Effect of anticoagulants by ↓ hypoprothrombinemia; also ↑ risk of hemorrhage due to vascular effects of corticosteroids

Anticholinesterases / Corticosteroids may ↓ effect of anticholinesterases when used in myasthenia gravis

Antidiabetic agents / Hyperglycemic effect of corticosteroids may necessitate an ↑ dose of antidiabetic agent

---

Asparaginase / ↑ Hyperglycemic effect of asparaginase and the risk of neuropathy and disturbances in erythropoiesis

Barbiturates / ↓ Effect of corticosteroids due to ↑ breakdown by liver

Bumetanide / Enhanced potassium loss due to potassium-losing properties of both drugs

Carbonic anhydrase inhibitors / Corticosteroids ↑ K depletion caused by carbonic anhydrase inhibitors

Cholestyramine / ↓ Effect of corticosteroids due to ↓ absorption from GI tract

Colestipol / ↓ Effect of corticosteroids due to ↓ absorption from GI tract

Contraceptives, oral / Estrogen ↑ anti-inflammatory effect of hydrocortisone by ↓ breakdown by liver

Cyclophosphoramide / ↑ Effect of cyclophosphoramide due to ↓ breakdown by liver

Cyclosporine / ↑ Effect of both drugs due to ↓ breakdown by liver

Digitalis glycosides / ↑ Chance of digitalis toxicity (arrhythmias) due to hypokalemia

Ephedrine / ↓ Effect of corticosteroids due to ↑ breakdown by liver

Estrogens / ↑ Anti-inflammatory effect of hydrocortisone by ↓ breakdown by liver

Ethacrynic acid / Enhanced potassium loss due to potassium-losing properties of both drugs

Folic acid / Requirements may ↑

Furosemide / Enhanced potassium loss due to potassium-losing properties of both drugs

Heparin / Ulcerogenic effects of corticosteroids may ↑ risk of hemorrhage

Immunosuppressant drugs / ↑ Risk of infection

Indomethacin / ↑ Chance of GI ulceration

Insulin / Hyperglycemic effect of corticosteroids may necessitate ↑ dose of antidiabetic agent

Isoniazid / ↓ Effect of isoniazid due to ↑ breakdown by liver and ↑ excretion

Ketoconazole / ↓ Effect of corticosteroids due to ↑ rate of clearance

Mexiletine / ↓ Effect of mexiletine due to ↑ breakdown by liver

Mitotane / ↓ Response of adrenal gland to corticotropin

Muscle relaxants, nondepolarizing / ↓ Effect of muscle relaxants

Neuromuscular blocking agents / ↑ Risk of prolonged respiratory depression or paralysis

NSAIDs / ↑ Risk of GI hemorrhage or ulceration

Phenobarbital / ↓ Effect of corticosteroids due to ↑ breakdown by liver

Phenytoin / ↓ Effect of corticosteroids due to ↑ breakdown by liver

Potassium supplements / ↓ Plasma levels of potassium

Rifampin / ↓ Effect of corticosteroids due to ↑ breakdown by liver

Ritodrine / ↑ Risk of maternal edema

Salicylates / Both are ulcerogenic; also, corticosteroids may ↓ blood salicylate levels

Somatrem, Somatropin / Glucocorticoids may inhibit effect of somatrem

Streptozocin / ↑ Risk of hyperglycemia

Theophyllines / Corticosteroids ↑ effect of theophyllines

Thiazide diuretics / Enhanced potassium loss due to potassium-losing properties of both drugs

Tricyclic antidepressants / ↑ Risk of mental disturbances

Vitamin A / Topical vitamin A can reverse impaired wound healing in clients receiving corticosteroids

Laboratory Test Interferences: ↑ Urine glucose, serum cholesterol, serum amylase. ↓ Serum potassium, triiodothyronine, serum uric acid. Alteration of electrolyte balance.

Dosage

Dosage is highly individualized, according to both the condition being treated and the client's response. Although the various corticosteroids are similar in their actions, clients may respond better to one type of drug than to another. It is most important that therapy not be discontinued abruptly. Except for replacement therapy, treatment should always involve the minimum effective dose and the shortest period of time. Long-term use often causes severe side effects. If corticosteroids are used for replacement therapy or high doses are used for prolonged periods of time, the dose must be *increased* if surgery is required.

For topical use, ointment, cream, lotion, solution, plastic tape, aerosol suspension, and aerosol cream are selected, depending on dermatologic condition to be treated.

Lotions are considered best for weeping eruptions, especially in areas subject to chafing (axilla, feet, and groin). Creams are suitable for most inflammations; ointments are preferred for dry, scaly lesions.

RESPIRATORY CARE CONSIDERATIONS

Administration of Oral Corticosteroids

1. Administer PO forms of drug with food to minimize ulcerogenic effect.
2. When corticosteroids are given chronically, use the smallest dose possible that will achieve the desired effect.
3. At frequent intervals, the dose of medication should be gradually decreased to determine if symptoms of the disease can be effectively controlled by the smaller amount of drug.
4. When treating clients with conditions such as asthma, ulcerative colitis, and rheumatoid arthritis, corticosteroids, given every other day, may maintain therapeutic effects while reducing or eliminating undesirable side effects. When ordered every other day, administer in the morning to coincide with the normal body secretion of cortisol.
5. Local administration of corticosteroids is preferred over systemic therapy to minimize systemic side effects.
6. Corticosteroids should be discontinued gradually if used chronically.

7. Alternate day therapy may be beneficial in selected clients requiring chronic steroid therapy. With this therapy, twice the usual daily dose of an intermediate-acting steroid is given every other morning. This regimen provides the beneficial effect of the steroid while minimizing pituitary-adrenal suppression.

Administration of Topical Corticosteroids

1. Cleanse the area before applying the medication.
2. Wear gloves to apply the agent; apply sparingly and rub gently into the area.
3. When prescribed, apply an occlusive dressing to promote hydration of the stratum corneum and increase the absorption of the medication.
4. The following are two methods of applying an occlusive type dressing (do not apply an occlusive dressing if infection is present):
• Apply a large amount of medication to the cleansed area. Cover with a thin, pliable, nonflammable plastic film (film enhances absorption), which is then sealed to the surrounding tissue with skin tape or held in place with gauze. Change the dressing q 3–4 days.
• Apply a small amount of medication to the area and cover with a damp cloth. Then cover with a thin, pliable, nonflammable plastic film and seal to the surrounding tissue with tape, or hold in place with gauze. Change dressing b.i.d.

Assessment: (General)

1. Document indications for therapy, type and onset of symptoms, and underlying cause: adrenal or nonadrenal disorder.
2. Record baseline data concerning the client's mental status (i.e., mood, affect, aggression, behavioral changes, depression) and neurologic function.
3. Check medication history for evidence of allergic reactions to corticosteroids or tartrazine, a coloring agent used in certain preparations.
4. Obtain baseline ECG, electro-

---

bold italic = life threatening side effect

lytes, glucose, urinalysis, and liver and renal function studies.

5. Document baseline VS and weight. Obtain CXR and PPD if prolonged therapy is anticipated.

6. Note childhood illnesses and immunization status.

7. List any medication the client is taking and identify those that may interact with corticosteroids. These include antidiabetic agents, cardiac glycosides, oral contraceptives, anticoagulants, and drugs influenced by liver enzymes.

8. If the client is female, of childbearing age, and sexually active, discuss the possibility of pregnancy and notify the provider if pregnancy is determined.

9. With specific conditions, carefully assess and describe the affected area requiring treatment. This may be useful as a baseline against which to evaluate the effectiveness of prescribed therapy.

Interventions

TOPICAL CORTICOSTEROIDS

1. Assess for local sensitivity reaction at the site of application. Withhold the medication and report any sensitivity response.

2. Absorption varies regionally with the highest absorption in scrotal skin and the lowest on the foot. Inflamed skin enhances absorption several-fold.

3. Better action has been noted with the ointment bases than with the lotion or cream vehicles.

4. Observe the client closely for signs of infections since corticosteroids tend to mask the problem. Do not apply an occlusive dressing when an infection is present. Document the site of the infection, the nature of the infection, and characteristics (e.g., redness, swelling, odor, or drainage).

5. If the client has a large occlusive dressing, take temperatures q 4 hr. Report if the temperature is elevated and remove the dressing unless otherwise specified.

6. Routinely assess the client for evidence of systemic absorption of the medication. Protracted use of large quantities of potent topical corticosteroids to large BSAs may precipitate iatrogenic Cushing's syndrome. Symptoms may include edema and transient inhibition of pituitary-adrenal cortical function as manifested by muscular pain, lassitude, depression, hypotension, and weight loss.

7. If family members are to apply the topical ointment, advise them to wash their hands and to wear gloves or to apply the medication with a sterile applicator (e.g., tongue blade). Instruct them concerning what to expect in response to the prescribed therapy.

8. Review adverse side effects that should be reported such as erythema, telangiectases, purpura, bruising, pustules, and depressed shiny, wrinkled skin. Prolonged use of potent topical corticosteroids may increase incidence of systemic side effects.

Interventions

ORAL CORTICOSTEROIDS

1. When the client is first placed on corticosteroids, take the BP at least b.i.d. until a maintenance dose has been established. Document and report any significant increases in BP.

2. Short-term oral therapy (e.g., 60 mg PO for 5 days) does not require divided doses or titration. With long-term therapy, continuously monitor for symptoms of adrenal insufficiency, which include hypotension, confusion, restlessness, lethargy, weakness, N&V, anorexia, and weight loss and titrate dose to withdraw.

3. Repeatedly evaluate the client for increased sodium and fluid retention. Monitor the client's weight and observe for other evidences of edema. If fluid and salt retention are noted, adjust the client's diet to one that is low in sodium and high in potassium. Weigh daily under standard conditions. Anticipate a small weight gain due to increased appetite, but sudden increases are probably due to edema and must be reported. Edema occurs most frequently with cortisone or desoxycorticosterone

acetate and occurs less frequently with the new synthetic agents.

4. Assess for SOB, distended neck veins, edema, and easy fatigue. The client may be in CHF. Obtain a CXR and ECG and compare with the baseline studies.

5. Conduct periodic blood glucose determinations and monitor serum electrolytes and platelet counts with long-term therapy. Report any unusual bleeding, bruising, the presence of petechiae, symptoms of diabetes, and any other skin changes.

6. Assess muscles for weakness and wasting as these are signs of a negative nitrogen balance.

7. Report changes in appearance, especially those resembling Cushing's syndrome (such as rounding of the face, hirsutism, presence of acne, and thinning of the hair and nails) so that dosage can be adjusted.

8. With diabetes, monitor the blood glucose levels frequently while on corticosteroid therapy. The client may develop hyperglycemia and a change in diet and insulin dosage may be necessary.

9. Assess for signs of depression, lack of interest in personal appearance, complaints of insomnia and anorexia. Document on the client's record, compare with initial clinical presentation, and report findings.

10. Discuss with female clients the potential for menstrual difficulties and amenorrhea that may be caused by long-term therapy with corticosteroids.

11. Observe for S&S of other illnesses during therapy with corticosteroids as these drugs tend to mask the severity of most illnesses.

12. GI bleeding may occur. Therefore, with long-term therapy, periodically test the stools for the presence of occult blood and monitor hematologic profile.

Client/Family Teaching

1. Take the oral medication with food and report any symptoms of gastric distress. To prevent the problem of gastric irritation, discuss the use of antacids and special diets. Suggest eating frequent small meals. If the symptoms persist, diagnostic X rays may be indicated.

2. High doses of glucocorticoids stimulate the stomach to produce excess acid and pepsin and may cause peptic ulcers. Advise that antacids 3–4 times/day may relieve epigastric distress.

3. Review the appropriate method for administration or application and the prescribed dosing intervals.

4. Explain that these agents generally work by inhibiting or decreasing the inflammatory response.

5. Review the symptoms of adrenal insufficiency (see #2 under Interventions) and provide a printed list of adverse drug reactions that should be reported if they occur.

6. Caution clients and family members to report any changes in mood or affect immediately.

7. Instruct clients to monitor and record their weight, BP, temperature, and pulse for evidence of physiologic changes that should be further evaluated. Advise clients to weigh themselves daily at the same time, wearing clothing of approximately the same weight, and using the same scales. Consistent weight gain may be evidence of fluid retention but caloric management should be instituted to prevent obesity.

8. Assist in identifying foods high in potassium and low in sodium content to prevent electrolyte disturbances. Explain how to supplement the diet with potassium-rich foods such as citrus juices and bananas. Instruct in what to look for on labels of canned or processed foods and refer to dietician for assistance in shopping, meal planning, and preparation.

9. Encourage clients to eat a diet high in protein to compensate for the loss due to protein breakdown from gluconeogenesis.

10. To decrease the possibility of osteoporosis (due to catabolic bone effects), explain the need to exercise daily and review foods high in cal-

cium that should be included in the diet. Stress the importance of adequate intake of protein, calcium, and vitamin D to minimize bone loss and for short-term drug use. On-going bone resorption with depressed bone formation is the cause of osteoporosis.

11. Be especially careful to avoid falls and other accidents. Steroids may cause osteoporosis, which makes the bones more susceptible to fractures. To reduce the possibility of falling and subsequent injury, advise clients to use a night light and to have a hand rail or other device for support if they get up at night.

12. Women using oral contraceptives need to be warned that corticosteroids can cause a loss of contraceptive action. Teach the client how to keep an accurate record of her menstrual periods and to consider alternative methods of birth control, and advise to report immediately if pregnancy is suspected.

13. Warn males that corticosteroids may have an adverse effect on the sperm production and count.

14. Review the possible effects on body image (weight gain, acne, excess hair growth, etc.) and explore coping mechanisms and identify support persons and groups.

15. Explain that there is a need to gradually withdraw the medication when therapy has exceeded 7 consecutive days. The process should proceed slowly so that the client's own adrenal cortex will gradually be reactivated and take over the production of hormones. Sudden withdrawal may be life-threatening. If adverse side effects occur, remind the client not to discontinue therapy with the idea that the changes will be reversed. Any sudden change will provoke symptoms of adrenal insufficiency.

16. If dosage of drug is reduced, provide supportive measures and reassurance to clients who are having flare-ups. Explain that these symptoms are caused by the reduction of drug dosage.

17. Explain to clients with arthritis that they should not overuse the joint once it has become painless. Permanent joint damage may result from overuse, because underlying pathology is still present.

18. If the client has diabetes, discuss the need to monitor glucose levels frequently while taking steroids. Any changes should be reported as alterations in insulin dose and diet may be necessary.

19. Explain that wounds may heal slowly because steroid therapy causes a delay in development of granulation tissue. The potential for infection also increases. Therefore, clients should observe any healing process carefully for signs of infection and report any injury so that appropriate medical supervision can be implemented. Postoperative clients should report any separation of wound or suture line.

20. These drugs mask symptoms of infection and cause immunosuppression. Because antibody production is decreased by corticosteroids, clients are at risk for infection. Explain the need to maintain general hygiene and scrupulous cleanliness to avoid infection. Advise clients to report if they have a sore throat, cough, fever, malaise, or an injury that does not heal. Avoid contact with persons with known contagious diseases.

21. Advise the client to delay any vaccinations, immunizations, or skin testing while receiving corticosteroid therapy because there is limited immune response during therapy with steroids.

22. Clients on long-term ophthalmic therapy are prone to developing cataracts, exophthalmus, and increased intraocular pressure. Advise these clients to have routine visits to the ophthalmologist for eye examinations.

23. Assist the client in establishing a means of maintaining a supply of medication on hand to avoid running out of the drug.

24. Avoid any OTC medications, including aspirin and ibuprofen compounds, as well as alcohol, since

these may aggravate gastric irritation and bleeding.

25. Stress the need for regular medical supervision to have the dosage of medication checked and periodically adjusted.

26. Remind the client to wear a Medic Alert tag and/or to carry identification listing the drug being used, the dosage, the condition being treated, and who to contact in the event of an emergency.

Evaluate

• Clinical response to date and the need for modifications in diet, drug dosage, or length of therapy

• Effective wound healing

• Suppression of inflammatory and immune responses or disease manifestation in allergic reactions, autoimmune diseases, and organ transplant recipients

• Laboratory confirmation that serum cortisol levels are within desired range in adrenal deficiency states (8 a.m. level 110–520 nmol/L)

Special Concerns

1. Check the height and weight of children regularly and maintain a graph because growth suppression is a hazard of corticosteroid therapy and is not prevented by growth hormone administration.

2. Advise parents that large doses of glucocorticoids in children may increase intracranial pressure (pseudotumor cerebri). Symptoms of this disorder include vertigo, headache, and convulsions. This should be reported immediately and advise that these symptoms should disappear once the therapy is discontinued (under medical supervision).

DIURETICS, LOOP

See also the following individual entries:

Bumetanide
Ethacrynate sodium
Ethacrynic acid
Furosemide
Torsemide

See also *Diuretics, Thiazides.*

Action/Kinetics: Loop diuretics inhibit reabsorption of sodium and chloride in the proximal and distal tubules and the loop of Henle. These diuretics are metabolized in the liver and excreted primarily through the urine. They are significantly bound to plasma protein.

Uses: Are potent diuretics and are used when a significant diuretic effect is required. Edema associated with CHF, hepatic cirrhosis, and renal disease (including nephrotic syndrome). Furosemide and torsemide are used alone or in combination with antihypertensive drugs to treat hypertension. Ethacrynic acid is used for short-term management of ascites due to malignancy, idiopathic edema, and lymphedema; it is also used for nephrotic syndrome and congenital heart disease in hospitalized pediatric clients (but not infants). Ethacrynic acid is used as adjunctive therapy in acute, pulmonary edema.

Contraindications: Hypersensitivity to loop diruetics or to sulfonylureas. In hepatic coma or severe electrolyte depletion (until condition improves or is corrected). Use during lactation.

Special Concerns: Sudden alterations of electrolytes in hepatic cirrhosis and ascites may precipitate hepatic encephalopathy and coma. SLE may be activated or worsened. Ototoxicity is most common with rapid injection, in severe renal impairment, with doses several times the usual dose, and with concurrent use of other ototoxic drugs. Safety and efficacy of most loop diuretics have not been determined in children or infants.

Side Effects: See individual drugs. Excessive diuresis may cause dehydration with the possibility of *circulatory collapse and vascular thrombosis or embolism.* Ototoxicity including tinnitus, hearing impairment, deafness (usually reversible), and vertigo with a sense of fullness are possible.

★ = Available in Canada   *bold italic* = life threatening side effect

Electrolyte imbalance, especially in clients with restricted salt intake. Photosensitivity. Changes include hypokalemia, hypomagnesemia, and hypocalcemia.

OD **Overdose Management:** *Symptoms:* Acute profound water loss, volume and electrolyte depletion, dehydration, decreased blood volume, and **circulatory collapse with possibility of fascicular thrombosis and embolism.** *Treatment:* Replace fluid and electrolyte loss. Carefully monitor urine and plasma electrolyte levels. Emesis and gastric lavage may be useful. Supportive measures may include oxygen or assisted ventilation.

Drug Interactions
Aminoglycosides / ↑ Ototoxicity with hearing loss
Anticoagulants / ↑ Anticoagulant activity
Chloral hydrate / Transient diaphoresis, hot flashes, hypertension, tachycardia, weakness and nausea
Cisplatin / Additive ototoxicity
Digitalis glycosides / ↑ Risk of arrhythmias due to diuretic-induced electrolyte disturbances
Lithium / ↑ Plasma levels of lithium → toxicity
Muscle relaxants, nondepolarizing / Effect of muscle relaxants may be either ↑ or ↓ , depending on the dose of diuretic
Nonsteroidal anti-inflammatory drugs / ↓ Effect of loop diuretics
Probenecid / ↓ Effect of loop diuretics
Salicylates / Diuretic effect may be ↓ in clients with cirrhosis and ascites
Sulfonylureas/ Loop diuretics may ↓ glucose tolerance
Theophyllines / Action of theophyllines may be ↑ or ↓
Thiazide diuretics / Additive effects with loop diuretics → profound diuresis and serious electrolyte abnormalities

Dosage —————————
See individual drugs.

RESPIRATORY CARE CONSIDERATIONS

See also *Diuretics, Thiazides*.
Administration/Storage
1. Since these drugs increase urination, they should be taken early in the day.
2. Take with food or milk to decrease GI upset.

Assessment
1. Document indications for therapy and type and onset of symptoms. Note other agents prescribed and the outcome.
2. Obtain baseline CBC, electrolytes, Mg, Ca, glucose, uric acid, and liver and renal function studies.
3. List other agents prescribed to ensure that none interact unfavorably.
4. Note any history of sensitivity to sulfonamides. Furosemide is a derivative and client may exhibit cross-reactivity.
5. Determine any evidence or history of SLE, as drug may worsen condition.
6. Assess auditory function carefully especially when large doses are anticipated or when used concurrently with other ototoxic agents. Ototoxicity is dose related and generally reversible.

Evaluate
• ↓ Edema
• Reports of symptomatic relief (↓ weight, ↓ swelling, ↑ diuresis)
• Clinical improvement in S&S associated with CHF and renal failure

DIURETICS, THIAZIDES

See also the following individual entries:

Chlorothiazide
Chlorothiazide sodium
Chlorthalidone
Hydrochlorothiazide
Indapamide

General Statement: The kidney is a complex organ with three main functions:
1. Elimination of waste materials and return of useful metabolites to the blood.

2. Maintenance of the acid-base balance.

3. Maintenance of an adequate electrolyte balance, which in turn governs the amount of fluid retained in the body.

Malfunction of one or more of these regulatory processes may result in the retention of excessive fluid by various tissues (edema). The latter can be an important manifestation of many conditions (e.g., CHF, pregnancy, and premenstrual tension).

Action/Kinetics: Diuretic drugs increase the urinary output of water and sodium (prevention or correction of edema), mostly through one of the following mechanisms:

1. Increasing the glomerular filtration rate.

2. Decreasing the rate at which sodium is reabsorbed from the glomerular filtrate by the renal tubules; therefore, water is excreted along with sodium.

3. Promoting the excretion of sodium, and therefore water, by the kidney.

Some of the commonly used diuretics, especially the thiazides, also have an antihypertensive effect. Diuretic drugs can enhance the normal function of the kidney but cannot stimulate a failing kidney into functioning. According to their mode of action and chemical structure, the diuretics fall into the following classes: thiazides (benzothiadiazides which are related chemically to the sulfonamides); carbonic anhydrase inhibitors (used mainly for glaucoma); osmotic diuretics; loop diuretics; and potassium-sparing drugs.

The thiazide diuretics are related chemically to the sulfonamides. Although devoid of anti-infective activity, the thiazides can cause the same hypersensitivity reactions as the sulfonamides.

The thiazides and related diuretics promote diuresis by decreasing the rate at which sodium and chloride are reabsorbed by the distal renal tubules of the kidney. By increasing the excretion of sodium and chloride, they force excretion of additional water. They also increase the excretion of potassium and, to a lesser extent, bicarbonate, as well as decrease the excretion of calcium and uric acid. Sodium and chloride are excreted in approximately equal amounts. The thiazides do not affect the glomerular filtration rate.

The antihypertensive mechanism of action of the thiazides is attributed to direct dilation of the arterioles, as well as to a reduction in the total fluid volume of the body and altered sodium balance. *Diuretic effect:* Usual, **Onset:** 1–2 hr. **Peak:** 4–6 hr. **Duration:** 6–24 hr. *Antihypertensive effect:* **Onset:** several days. *Optimal therapeutic effect:* 3–4 weeks.

Most thiazides are absorbed from the GI tract; a large fraction is excreted unchanged in urine.

Uses: Edema, CHF, hypertension, pregnancy, and premenstrual tension. Thiazides are used for edema due to CHF, nephrosis, nephritis, renal failure, PMS, hepatic cirrhosis, corticosteroid or estrogen therapy. Hypertension. *Investigational:* Thiazides are used alone or in combination with allopurinol (or amiloride) for prophylaxis of calcium nephrolithiasis. Nephrogenic diabetes insipidus.

Contraindications: Hypersensitivity to drug, anuria, renal decompensation. Impaired renal function and advanced hepatic cirrhosis.

Drugs should not be used indiscriminately in clients with edema and toxemia of pregnancy, even though they may be therapeutically useful, because the thiazides may have adverse effects on the newborn (thrombocytopenia and jaundice).

Thiazides and related diuretics may precipitate MIs in elderly clients with advanced arteriosclerosis, especially if the client is also receiving therapy with other antihypertensive agents.

Clients with advanced heart failure, renal disease, or hepatic cirrho-

---

sis are most likely to develop hypokalemia.

Thiazides may activate or worsen SLE.

Special Concerns: Geriatric clients may manifest an increased risk of hypotension and changes in electrolyte levels. Administer with caution to debilitated clients or to those with a history of hepatic coma or precoma, gout, diabetes mellitus, or during pregnancy and lactation. Particular care must be exercised when thiazides are administered concomitantly with drugs that also cause potassium loss, such as digitalis, corticosteroids, and some estrogens.

Side Effects: The following side effects may be observed with most thiazides. See also individual drugs. *Electrolyte imbalance:* Hypokalemia (most frequent) characterized by cardiac arrhythmias. Hyponatremia characterized by weakness, lethargy, epigastric distress, and N&V. Hypokalemic alkalosis. *GI:* Anorexia, epigastric distress or irritation, N&V, cramping, bloating, abdominal pain, diarrhea, constipation, jaundice, pancreatitis. *CNS:* Dizziness, lightheadedness, headache, vertigo, xanthopsia, paresthesias, weakness, insomnia, restlessness. *CV:* Orthostatic hypotension. *Hematologic:* **Agranulocytosis, aplastic or hypoplastic anemia, hemolytic anemia,** leukopenia, thrombocytopenia. *Dermatologic:* Purpura, photosensitivity, photosensitivity dermatitis, rash, urticaria, necrotizing angiitis, vasculitis, cutaneous vasculitis. *Metabolic:* neutropenia, hemolytic anemia. *Endocrine:* Hyperglycemia, glycosuria, hyperuricemia. *Miscellaneous:* Blurred vision, impotence, reduced libido, fever, muscle cramps, muscle spasm, respiratory distress.

OD Overdose Management: *Symptoms:* Symptoms of plasma volume depletion, including orthostatic hypotension, dizziness, drowsiness, syncope, electrolyte abnormalities, hemoconcentration, hemodynamic changes. Signs of potassium depletion, including confusion, dizziness, muscle weakness, and GI disturbances.

Also, N&V, GI irritation, GI hypermotility, CNS effects, cardiac abnormalities, **seizures, hypotension, decreased respiration, and coma.** *Treatment:*
• Induce emesis or perform gastric lavage followed by activated charcoal. Undertake measures to prevent aspiration.
• Electrolyte balance, hydration, respiration, CV, and renal function must be maintained. Cathartics should be avoided, as use may enhance fluid loss.
• Although GI effects are usually of short duration, treatment may be required.

Drug Interactions
Allopurinol / ↑ Risk of hypersensitivity reactions to allopurinol
Amphotericin B / Enhanced loss of electrolytes, especially potassium
Anesthetics / Thiazides may ↑ effects of anesthetics
Anticholinergic agents / ↑ Effect of thiazides due to ↑ amount absorbed from GI tract
Anticoagulants, oral / Anticoagulant effects may be decreased
Antidiabetic agents / Thiazides antagonize hypoglycemic effect of antidiabetic agents
Antigout agents / Thiazides may ↑ uric acid levels; thus, ↑ dose of antigout drug may be necessary
Antihypertensive agents / Thiazides potentiate the effect of antihypertensive agents
Antineoplastic agents / Thiazides may prolong leukopenia induced by antineoplastic agents
Calcium salts / Hypercalcemia due to renal tubular reabsorption or bone release may be ↑ by exogenous calcium
Cholestyramine / ↓ Effect of thiazides due to ↓ absorption from GI tract
Colestipol / ↓ Effect of thiazides due to ↓ absorption from GI tract
Corticosteroids / Enhanced potassium loss due to potassium-losing properties of both drugs
Diazoxide / Enhanced hypotensive effect. Also, ↑ hyperglycemic response

Digitalis glycosides / Thiazides produce ↑ potassium and magnesium loss with ↑ chance of digitalis-induced arrhythmias
Ethanol / Additive orthostatic hypotension
Fenfluramine / ↑ Antihypertensive effect of thiazides
Furosemide / Profound diuresis and electrolyte loss
Guanethidine / Additive hypotensive effect
Indomethacin / ↓ Effect of thiazides, possibly by inhibition of prostaglandins
Insulin / ↓ Effect due to thiazide-induced hyperglycemia
Lithium / ↑ Risk of lithium toxicity due to ↓ renal excretion; may be used together but use should be carefully monitored
Loop diuretics / Additive effect to cause profound diuresis and serious electrolyte losses
Methenamine / ↓ Effect of thiazides due to alkalinization of urine by methenamine
Methyldopa / ↑ Risk of hemolytic anemia (rare)
Muscle relaxants, nondepolarizing / ↑ Effect of muscle relaxants due to hypokalemia
Norepinephrine / Thiazides ↓ arterial response to norepinephrine
Quinidine / ↑ Effect of quinidine due to ↑ renal tubular reabsorption
Reserpine / Additive hypotensive effect
Sulfonamides / ↑ Effect of thiazides due to ↓ plasma protein binding
Sulfonylureas / ↓ Effect due to thiazide-induced hyperglycemia
Tetracyclines / ↑ Risk of azotemia
Tubocurarine / ↑ Muscle relaxation and ↑ hypokalemia
Vasopressors (sympathomimetics) / Thiazides ↓ responsiveness of arterioles to vasopressors
Vitamin D / ↑ Effect of vitamin D due to thiazide-induced hypercalcemia
Laboratory Test Interferences: Hypokalemia, hypercalcemia, hyponatremia, hypomagnesemia, hypochlo-

remia, hypophosphatemia, hyperuricemia. ↑ BUN, creatinine, glucose in blood and urine. ↓ Serum PBI levels (no signs of thyroid disturbance). Initial ↑ total cholesterol, LDL cholesterol, and triglycerides.

Dosage

Drugs are preferentially given **PO**, but some preparations can be given parenterally. They are usually given in the morning, so the peak effect occurs during the day.

RESPIRATORY CARE CONSIDERATIONS
Administration/Storage
1. If a diuretic is to be taken daily, administer it in the morning so that the major diuretic effect will occur before bedtime.
2. Liquid potassium preparations are bitter. Therefore, when they are to be used, administer with fruit juice or milk to make them more palatable.
3. Thiazides may be taken with food or milk if GI upset occurs.
4. Clients resistant to one type of thiazide may respond to another.
5. Thiazides should not be taken with any other medication (including OTC drugs for asthma, cough and colds, hay fever, weight control) unless approved by the provider.
6. To minimize electrolyte imbalance, thiazides may be taken every other day or on a 3–5-day basis for treatment of edema.
7. To prevent excess hypotension, the dose of other antihypertensive agents should be reduced when beginning thiazide therapy.
Assessment
1. Note if the client has any history of hypersensitivity to the drug. Document indications for therapy and any previous experience with this class of drugs.
2. Obtain baseline CBC, glucose, electrolytes, Ca, Mg, and liver and renal function tests prior to initiating therapy.
3. Note any history of heart disease, an indication that the client will re-

---

quire close monitoring once the drug has been administered.

4. Determine if client has a history of gout and check baseline uric acid level.

5. Determine the extent of client's edema and assess skin turgor, mucous membranes, and lung fields.

6. Review drugs the client has been taking to identify those with which diuretics interact so that appropriate adjustments and/or changes can be made.

7. Note any history of hepatic cirrhosis and if evident, closely monitor serum K to avoid depletion and hepatic encephalopathy.

Interventions

1. Weigh each morning after the client has voided and before the client has eaten or taken fluids. Record the weight and report any sudden increase.

2. Monitor I&O and keep bedpan or urinal within reach. Report any absence of or decrease in diuresis and note any changes in lung sounds.

3. Check ambulatory clients for edema in the extremities. Check clients on bed rest for edema in the sacral area. Measure daily, document the extent of edema or ascites, and report.

4. Monitor for serum electrolyte levels, pH, and the following *signs of electrolyte imbalance:*

• *Hyponatremia* (low-salt syndrome)—characterized by muscle weakness, leg cramps, dryness of mouth, dizziness, and GI disturbances.

• *Hypernatremia* (excessive sodium retention in relation to body water)—characterized by CNS disturbances such as confusion, loss of sensorium, stupor, and coma. Poor skin turgor or postural hypotension are not as prominent as when there are combined deficits of sodium and water.

• *Water intoxication* (caused by defective water diuresis)—characterized by lethargy, confusion, stupor, and coma. Neuromuscular hyperexcitability with increased reflexes, muscular twitching, and convulsions if water intoxication is acute.

• *Metabolic acidosis*—characterized by weakness, headache, malaise, abdominal pain, and N&V. Hyperpnea occurs in severe metabolic acidosis. Signs of volume depletion, such as poor skin turgor, soft eyeballs, and a dry tongue may also be observed.

• Metabolic alkalosis—characterized by irritability, neuromuscular hyperexcitability, and, in severe cases, tetany.

• Hypokalemia (deficiency of potassium in the blood)—characterized by muscular weakness, failure of peristalsis, postural hypotension, respiratory embarrassment, and cardiac arrhythmias.

• *Hyperkalemia* (excess of potassium in the blood)—characterized by early signs of irritability, nausea, intestinal colic, and diarrhea; and by later signs of weakness, flaccid paralysis, dyspnea, difficulty in speaking, and arrhythmias.

5. All signs of electrolyte imbalance should be reported and documented in the chart. Electrolyte levels should be monitored and the physical safety of the client should be safeguarded.

6. With high doses monitor for hyperlipidemia and hyperuricemia. Increased serum uric acid levels may precipitate a gout attack.

7. If the client is receiving enteric-coated potassium tablets, monitor for the presence of abdominal pain, distention, or GI bleeding. These tablets can cause small bowel ulceration. If these symptoms occur, discontinue the tablets. Also, monitor the client's stool to ensure that the tablets have not passed through intact.

8. If the client is also receiving antihypertensive drugs, monitor for excessively low BP. Diuretics potentiate the effects of antihypertensive agents.

9. Diuretics may precipitate symptoms of diabetes mellitus in clients with latent or mild diabetes. Therefore, test the urine or perform finger sticks routinely in clients with diabetes and observe for signs of hyperglycemia.

10. If the client is taking digitalis,

check the apical pulse. Hyper- or hypokalemia associated with diuretic therapy may potentiate the toxic effects of digitalis and precipitate cardiac arrhythmias.

11. Assess the client for complaints of sore throat, the presence of a skin rash, and yellowing of the skin or sclera, and report. These may be signs of blood dyscrasias due to drug hypersensitivity.

12. If the client has a history of liver disease, be alert for electrolyte imbalances, which could cause stupor, coma, and death.

13. If the client has a history of gout, note any increase in the frequency of acute attacks that may be precipitated by diuretics and report.

Interventions (Thiazides)

1. If the client is to undergo surgery, anticipate that the drug will be stopped at least 48 hr before the procedure. Thiazide inhibits the pressor effects of epinephrine.

2. Evaluate dietary potassium intake. Potassium chloride supplements should be given only when dietary measures are inadequate.

3. If potassium supplements are required, use liquid preparations to avoid ulcerations that may be produced by potassium salts in the solid dosage form. Exceptions include slow-K forms (potassium salt imbedded in a wax matrix) and micro-K forms (microencapsulated potassium salt).

4. If the client has diabetes, monitor blood glucose levels more frequently after beginning thiazide therapy. It may be necessary to change the dose of insulin or oral hypoglycemic agent.

Evaluate

• Control of hypertension with ↓ BP to within desired range

• Reports of ↑ urine output

• Evidence of ↓ edema with resultant ↓ weight

• Adequate tissue perfusion as evidenced by warm dry skin and good pulses

• Freedom from complications of drug therapy

• Laboratory confirmation of normal electrolyte levels and fluid balance

ERYTHROMYCINS

See also the following individual entries:

Erythromycin base
Erythromycin estolate
Erythromycin ethylsuccinate
Erythromycin lactobionate
Erythromycin stearate

Action/Kinetics: The erythromycins are produced by strains of *Streptomyces erythraeus* and have bacteriostatic and bactericidal activity (at high concentrations or if microorganism is particularly susceptible). The erythromycins are considered to be macrolide antibiotics.

The erythromycins inhibit protein synthesis of microorganisms by binding reversibly to a ribosomal subunit (50S), thus interfering with the transmission of genetic information and inhibiting protein synthesis. The drugs are effective only against rapidly multiplying organisms. The erythromycins are absorbed from the upper part of the small intestine. Erythromycins for PO use are manufactured in enteric-coated or film-coated forms to prevent destruction by gastric acid. Erythromycin is approximately 70% bound to plasma proteins and achieves concentrations in body tissues about 40% of those in the plasma. Erythromycin diffuses into body tissues; peritoneal, pleural, ascitic, and amniotic fluids; saliva; through the placental circulation; and across the mucous membrane of the tracheobronchial tree. It diffuses poorly into spinal fluid, although penetration is increased in meningitis. Alkalinization of the urine (to pH 8.5) increases the gram-negative antibacterial action. **Peak serum levels:** PO, 1–4 hr. **t½:** 1.5–2 hr, *but prolonged in clients with renal im-*

pairment. The drug is partially metabolized by the liver and primarily excreted in bile. Erythromycins are also excreted in breast milk. The strength of erythromycin products is based on erythromycin base equivalents. Many erythromycins are available in ointments and solutions for ophthalmic, otic, and dermatologic use.

Uses

1. Upper respiratory tract infections due to *Streptococcus pyogenes* (group a beta-hemolytic streptococci), *Streptococcus pneumoniae,* and *Haemophilus influenzae* (combined with sulfonamides).

2. Mild to moderate lower respiratory tract infections due to *S. pyogenes* and *S. pneumoniae.* Respiratory tract infections due to *Mycoplasma pneumoniae.*

3. Pertussis (whooping cough) caused by *Bordetella pertussis;* may also be used as prophylaxis of pertussis in exposed individuals.

4. Mild to moderate skin and skin structure infections due to *S. pyogenes* and *Staphylococcus aureus.*

5. As an adjunct to antitoxin in diphtheria (caused by *Corynebacterium diphtheriae*), to prevent carriers, and to eradicate the organism in carriers.

6. Intestinal amebiasis due to *Entamoeba histolytica* (PO erythromycin only).

7. Acute pelvic inflammatory disease due to *Neisseria gonorrhoeae.*

8. Erythrasma due to *Corynebacterium minutissimum.*

9. *Chlamydia trachomatis* infections causing urogenital infections during pregnancy, conjunctivitis in the newborn, or pneumonia during infancy. Also, uncomplicated chlamydial infections of the urethra, endocervix, or rectum in adults (when tetracyclines are contraindicated or not tolerated).

10. Nongonococcal urethritis caused by *Ureaplasma urealyticum* when tetracyclines are contraindicated or not tolerated.

11. Legionnaires' disease due to *Legionella pneumophilia.*

12. As an alternative to penicillin (in penicillin-sensitive clients) to treat primary syphilis caused by *Treponema pallidum.*

13. Prophylaxis of initial or recurrent attacks of rheumatic fever in clients allergic to penicillin or sulfonamides.

14. Infections due to *Listeria monocytogenes.*

15. Bacterial endocarditis due to alpha-hemolytic streptococci, Viridans group, in clients allergic to penicillins.

Investigational: Infections due to *N. gonorrhoeae,* including uncomplicated urethral, rectal, or endocervical infections and disseminated gonococcal infections (including use in pregnancy). Severe or prolonged diarrhea due to *Campylobacter jejuni.* Genital, inguinal, or anorectal infections due to *Lymphogranuloma venereum.* Chancroid due to *Haemophilus ducreyi.* Primary, secondary, or early latent syphilis due to *T. pallidum.* Erythromycin base used with PO neomycin prior to elective colorectal surgery to reduce wound complications. As an alternative to penicillin to treat anthrax, Vincent's gingivitis, erysipeloid, actinomycosis, tetanus, with a sulfonamide to treat *Nocardia* infections, infections due to *Eikenella corrodens,* and *Borrelia* infections (including early Lyme disease).

Contraindications: Hypersensitivity to erythromycin; in utero syphilis.

Special Concerns: Use with caution in liver disease and during lactation. Use may result in bacterial and fungal overgrowth (i.e., superinfection).

Side Effects: Erythromycins have a low incidence of side effects (except for the estolate salt). *GI* (most common): N&V, diarrhea, cramping, abdominal pain, stomatitis, anorexia, melena, heartburn, pruritus ani, pseudomembranous colitis. *Allergic:* Skin rashes with or without pruritus, bullous fixed eruptions, urticaria, eczema, **anaphylaxis** (rare). *CNS:* Fear, confusion, altered thinking, uncontrollable crying or hysterical laughter, feeling of impending loss of consciousness. *CV:* Rarely, ventricular arrhythmias, including **ventricular tachycardia and torsades de pointes in clients with prolonged QT intervals.** *Miscellaneous:* Superinfection, hepatotoxicity, ototoxicity. *Following topical use:* Itching, burning, irritation, or stinging of skin. Dry, scaly skin.

IV use may result in venous irritation and thrombophlebitis; IM use produces pain at the injection site, with development of necrosis or sterile abscesses.

OD **Overdose Management:** *Symptoms:* N&V, diarrhea, epigastric distress, acute pancreatitis (mild), hearing loss (with or without tinnitus and vertigo). *Treatment:* Induce vomiting. General supportive measures. Allergic reactions should be controlled with conventional therapy.

Drug Interactions
Alfentanil / ↓ Excretion of alfentanil → ↑ effect
Anticoagulants / ↑ Anticoagulant effect → possible hemorrhage
Astemizole / Serious CV side effects, including torsades de pointes and other ventricular arrhythmias (including QT interval prolongation), cardiac arrest, and death
Bromocriptine / ↑ Serum levels of bromocriptine → ↑ pharmacologic and toxic effects
Carbamazepine / ↑ Effect (and toxicity requiring hospitalization and resuscitation) of carbamazepine due to ↓ breakdown by liver
Cyclosporine / ↑ Effect of cyclosporine due to ↓ excretion (possibly with renal toxicity)
Digoxin / Erythromycin ↑ bioavailability of digoxin
Disopyramide / ↑ Plasma levels of disopyramide → arrhythmias and ↑ QTc intervals
Ergot alkaloids / Acute ergotism manifested by peripheral ischemia
Lincosamides / Drugs antagonize each other

Methylprednisolone / ↑ Effect of methylprednisolone due to ↓ breakdown by liver
Penicillin / Erythromycins either ↓ or ↑ effect of penicillins
Sodium bicarbonate / ↑ Effect of erythromycin in urine due to alkalinization
Terfenadine / Serious CV side effects, including torsades de pointes and other ventricular arrhythmias (including QT interval prolongation), cardiac arrest, and death
Theophyllines / ↑ Effect of theophylline due to ↓ breakdown in liver; ↓ erythromycin levels may also occur
Triazolam / ↑ Bioavailability of triazolam → ↑ CNS depression
Laboratory Test Interferences: False + or ↑ values of urinary catecholamines, urinary steroids, and AST and ALT.

Dosage
PO and **IM** (painful); some preparations can be given **IV.** See individual drugs.

RESPIRATORY CARE CONSIDERATIONS

See also *General Respiratory Care Considerations for All Anti-Infectives.*
Administration/Storage: Inject deep into muscle mass. Injections are painful and irritating.
Assessment
1. Note if client is allergic to any other antibiotics or to other allergens.
2. Document indications for therapy, type and onset of symptoms, other agents used, and the outcome.
3. Ensure that appropriate cultures have been performed prior to initiating therapy.
4. Determine that baseline hematologic profile and liver and renal function studies have been performed, if prolonged therapy is anticipated.
5. Assess for skin reactions when using erythromycin ointment. Plan to discontinue therapy and report if reactions are evident.

6. When using ophthalmic solutions, assess for mild reaction which, although usually transient, should be reported.

7. If also prescribed oral anticoagulants, astemizole, seldane, digoxin, and theophyllines, monitor closely because erythromycins can inhibit cytochrome P-450 and enhance effects of these drugs or cause lethal arrhythmias.

Interventions

1. Do not administer with or immediately prior to ingestion of fruit juice or other acidic drinks because acidity may decrease activity of drug. However, adequate water (up to 8 oz) should be consumed with each dose.

2. Do not routinely administer PO medication with meals because food decreases the absorption of most erythromycins. However, provider may order medication to be given with food to reduce GI irritation.

3. Instill otic solutions at room temperature. Gently pull pinna of ear down and back for children under 3 years of age; pull pinna of ear up and back for clients over 3 years of age.

4. Observe for evidence of impaired liver or renal function; review appropriate lab data.

5. Note any evidence of hearing loss, which is usually temporary.

Evaluate

• Clinical evidence of resolution of infection (negative lab culture reports, ↓ temperature, evidence of wound healing, ↓ WBCs, improved appetite)

• Reports of symptomatic improvement

FLUOROQUINOLONES

See also the following individual entries:

Ciprofloxacin hydrochloride
Levofloxacin
Lomefloxacin hydrochloride
Ofloxacin
Sparfloxacin

Action/Kinetics: These antibiotics are synthetic, broad-spectrum antibacterial agents. The fluorine molecule confers increased activity against gram-negative organisms as well as broadens the spectrum against gram-positive organisms. These drugs act as bactericidal agents by interfering with DNA gyrase, an enzyme needed for the synthesis of bacterial DNA. Food may delay the absorption of ciprofloxacin, lomefloxacin, and norfloxacin. Both ciprofloxacin and ofloxacin may be given IV; all fluoroquinolones may be given PO.

Uses: See individual drugs; these drugs are used for a large number of gram-positive and gram-negative infections. Generally ciprofloxacin and ofloxacin are used for lower respiratory tract infections, skin and skin structure infections, and UTI. In addition ofloxacin is used for STDs and ciprofloxacin is used for bone and joint infections and infectious diarrhea. Enoxacin and norfloxacin are approved only for complicated and uncomplicated UTIs and uncomplicated urethral and cervical gonorrhea caused by *Neisseria gonorrhoeae*. Lomefloxacin has been approved for use in lower respiratory tract infections and both uncomplicated and complicated UTI.

Specific diseases for which these drugs are used include bronchitis, pneumonia (including *Legionella* and *Mycoplasma*), prostatitis, osteomyelitis, traveler's diarrhea, gonorrheal cervicitis or urethritis, prophylaxis in urological surgery, pelvic inflammatory disease, otitis media, septic arthritis, sinusitis, bacterial meningitis, bacteremia (both pseudomonal and staphylococcal), and endocarditis.

Contraindications: Hypersensitivity to the quinolone group of antibiotics, including cinoxacin and nalidixic acid. Lactation. Use in children less than 18 years of age.

Special Concerns: Lower doses are necessary in impaired renal function. Evidence suggests there may be differences in CNS toxicity between the various fluoroquinolones. Use of flouroquinolones may increase the risk of possible Achilles and other tendon inflammation and rupture.

Side Effects: See individual drugs. The following side effects are common to each of the fluoroquinolone antibiotics. *GI:* N&V, diarrhea, abdominal pain or discomfort, dry or painful mouth, heartburn, dyspepsia, flatulence, constipation, pseudomembranous colitis. *CNS:* Headache, dizziness, malaise, lethargy, fatigue, drowsiness, somnolence, depression, insomnia, ***seizures,*** paresthesia. *Dermatologic:* Rash, photosensitivity, pruritus (except for ciprofloxacin). *Hypersensitivity reactions:* Facial or ***pharyngeal edema,*** dyspnea, urticaria, itching, tingling, loss of consciousness, ***CV collapse.*** *Other:* Visual disturbances and ophthalmologic abnormalities, hearing loss, superinfection, phototoxicity, eosinophilia, crystalluria, Achilles and other tendon inflammation and rupture. Fluoroquinolones, except norfloxacin, may also cause vaginitis, syncope, chills, and edema.

OD **Overdose Management:** *Symptoms:* Extension of side effects. *Treatment:* For acute overdose, vomiting should be induced or gastric lavage performed. The client should be carefully observed and, if necessary, symptomatic and supportive treatment given. Hydration should be maintained.

Drug Interactions

Antacids / ↓ Serum levels of fluoroquinolones due to ↓ absorption from the GI tract

Anticoagulants / ↑ Effect of anticoagulant

Antineoplastic agents / ↓ Serum levels of fluoroquinolones

Cimetidine / ↓ Elimination of fluoroquinolones

Cyclosporine / ↑ Risk of nephrotoxicity

Didanosine / ↓ Serum levels of fluoroquinolones due to ↓ absorption from the GI tract

Iron salts / ↓ Serum levels of fluoroquinolones due to ↓ absorption from the GI tract

Probenecid / ↑ Serum levels of fluoroquinolones due to ↓ renal clearance

Sucralfate / ↓ Serum levels of fluoroquinolones due to ↓ absorption from the GI tract

Theophylline / ↑ Plasma levels and ↑ toxicity of theophylline due to ↓ clearance

Zinc salts / ↓ Serum levels of fluoroquinolones due to ↓ absorption from the GI tract

Laboratory Test Interferences: ↑ ALT, AST. See also individual drugs.

Dosage ─────────────────

See individual drugs.

RESPIRATORY CARE CONSIDERATIONS

See also *General Respiratory Care Considerations for All Anti-Infectives.*

Administration/Storage

1. Clients should drink liberal amounts of fluids.

2. Products containing iron or zinc and antacids containing magnesium or aluminum should not be taken simultaneously or within 4 hr before or 2 hr after dosing with fluoroquinolones.

3. Enoxacin and norfloxacin should be taken 1 hr before or 2 hr after meals; ciprofloxacin and lomefloxacin may be taken without regard to meals. Ofloxacin should not be taken with food.

Assessment

1. Document indications for therapy and type and onset of symptoms.

2. Note any previous experiences with these antibiotics and document.

3. Assess for soft tissue or extremity injury; note any instability, pain, or swelling.

4. Determine that baseline CBC, liver and renal function studies, and lab cultures have been performed.

5. List medications client currently

prescribed noting any that may interact unfavorably.

Interventions

1. Monitor VS and I&O, and encourage increased fluid intake.

2. Observe client closely for any evidence of adverse effects as hypersensitivity reactions may occur even following the first dose. The drug should be discontinued at the first sign of skin rash or other allergic manifestations.

3. If phototoxicity occurs, excessive sunlight or artificial ultraviolet light should be avoided.

4. During prolonged or chronic administration of fluoroquinolones, periodic assessment of renal, hepatic, and hematopoietic function should be performed.

5. In clients receiving anticoagulants and theophyllines, monitor closely as quinolones can cause increased drug levels with toxic drug effects, including increased bleeding or seizures.

6. Prompt cessation should occur if the client experiences onset of unusual tendon pain.

Evaluate

• Reports of symptomatic improvement

• Clinical evidence of resolution of infection (↓ WBCs, ↓ temperature, ↑ appetite)

• Laboratory evidence of negative follow-up culture reports

NARCOTIC ANALGESICS

See also the following individual entries:

Alfentanil hydrochloride
Buprenorphine hydrochloride
Butorphanol tartrate
Codeine phosphate
Codeine sulfate
Dezocine
Fentanyl citrate
Fentanyl transdermal system
Hydrocodone bitartrate and
    Acetaminophen
Hydromorphone hydrochloride
Levomethadyl acetate
    hydrochloride
Meperidine hydrochloride
Methadone hydrochloride
Morphine hydrochloride
Morphine sulfate
Nalbuphine hydrochloride
Oxycodone hydrochloride
Oxycodone terephthalate
Oxymorphone hydrochloride
Pentazocine hydrochloride with
    Naloxone hydrochloride
Pentazocine lactate
Propoxyphene hydrochloride
Propoxyphene napsylate
Remifentanil hydrochloride
Sufentanil

General Statement: The narcotic analgesics include opium, morphine, codeine, various opium derivatives, and totally synthetic substances (e.g., meperidine) with similar pharmacologic properties. The relative activity of all narcotic analgesics is measured against morphine.

Opium itself is a mixture of alkaloids obtained since ancient times from the poppy plant. Morphine and codeine are two of the pure chemical substances isolated from opium. Certain drugs (pentazocine, butorphanol, nalbuphine) have both narcotic agonist and antagonist properties. Such drugs may precipitate a withdrawal syndrome if given to clients dependent on narcotics.

Action/Kinetics

Narcotic analgesics are classified as agonists, mixed agonist-antagonists, or partial agonists depending on their activity at opiate receptors.The narcotic analgesics attach to specific receptors located in the CNS (cortex, brain stem, and spinal cord) resulting in various CNS effects. The mechanism is believed to involve decreased permeability of the cell membrane to sodium, which results in diminished transmission of pain impulses. Five categories of opioid receptors have been identified: mu, kappa, sigma, delta, and epsilon. Narcotic analgesics are believed to exert their activity at mu, kappa, and sigma receptors. Mu receptors are thought to mediate supraspinal analgesia, euphoria, and respiratory and physical depression. Pentazocine-like spinal analgesia, miosis, and sedation are mediated by kappa receptors while sigma receptors mediate dysphoria, hallucinations, as well as respiratory and vasomotor stimulation (caused by drugs with antagonist activity). In addition to an alteration of pain perception (analgesia), the drugs, especially at higher doses, induce euphoria, drowsiness, changes in mood, mental clouding, and deep sleep.

The narcotic analgesics also depress respiration. The effect is noticeable with small doses. Death by overdosage is almost always the result of respiratory arrest.

The narcotic analgesics have a nauseant and emetic effect (direct stimulation of the CTZ). They depress the cough reflex, and small doses of narcotic analgesics (codeine) are part of several antitussive preparations.

The narcotic analgesics have little effect on BP when the client is in a supine position. However, most narcotics decrease the capacity of the client to respond to stress. Morphine and other narcotic analgesics induce peripheral vasodilation, which may result in hypotension.

Many narcotic analgesics constrict the pupil. With such drugs, pupillary constriction is the most obvious sign of dependence.

The narcotic analgesics also decrease peristaltic motility. The constipating effects of these agents (Paregoric) are sometimes used therapeutically in severe diarrhea. The narcotic analgesics also increase the pressure within the biliary tract. For kinetics, see individual agents.

Uses: Severe pain, especially of coronary, pulmonary, or peripheral origin. Hepatic and renal colic. Preanesthetic medication and adjuncts to anesthesia. Postsurgical pain. Acute vascular occlusion, especially of coronary, pulmonary, and peripheral origin. Diarrhea and dysentery. Pain from MI, carcinoma, burns. Postpartum pain. Some members of this group are primarily used as antitussives. Methadone is used for heroin withdrawal and maintenance. The use of opioids to treat chronic neuropathic pain is not a first-line therapy.

Contraindications: Asthmatic conditions, emphysema, kyphoscoliosis, severe obesity, convulsive states as in epilepsy, delirium tremens, tetanus and strychnine poisoning, diabetic acidosis, myxedema, Addison's disease, hepatic cirrhosis, and children under 6 months.

Special Concerns: Use cautiously in clients with head injury or after head surgery because of morphine's capacity to elevate ICP and mask the pupillary response.

Use with caution in the elderly, in the debilitated, in young children, in individuals with increased ICP, in obstetrics, and with clients in shock or during acute alcoholic intoxication.

Morphine should be used with extreme caution in clients with pulmonary heart disease (cor pulmonale). Deaths following ordinary therapeutic doses have been reported. Use cautiously in clients with prostatic hypertrophy, because it may precipitate acute urinary retention.

Use cautiously in clients with reduced blood volume, such as in hemorrhaging clients who are more susceptible to the hypotensive effects of morphine.

Since the drugs depress the respiratory center, they should be given early in labor, at least 2 hr before delivery, to reduce the danger of respiratory depression in the newborn. When given before surgery, the narcotic analgesics should be given at least 1–2 hr preoperatively so that the danger of maximum depression of respiratory function will have passed before anesthesia is initiated.

These drugs should sometimes be withheld prior to diagnostic procedures so that the physician can use pain to locate dysfunction.

✦ = Available in Canada   ***bold italic*** = life threatening side effect

Side Effects: *Respiratory:* **Respiratory depression, apnea.** *CNS:* Dizziness, lightheadedness, sedation, lethargy, headache, euphoria, mental clouding, fainting. Idiosyncratic effects including excitement, restlessness, tremors, delirium, insomnia. *GI:* N&V, vomiting, constipation, increased pressure in biliary tract, dry mouth, anorexia. *CV:* Flushing, changes in HR and BP, circulatory collapse. *Allergic:* Skin rashes including pruritus and urticaria. Sweating, **laryngospasm,** edema. *Miscellaneous:* Urinary retention, oliguria, reduced libido, changes in body temperature. Narcotics cross the placental barrier and depress respiration of the fetus or newborn.

DEPENDENCE AND TOLERANCE: It is important to remember that all drugs of this group are addictive. Psychologic and physical dependence and tolerance develop even when clients use clinical doses. Tolerance is characterized by the fact that the client requires shorter periods of time between doses or larger doses for relief of pain. Tolerance usually develops faster when the narcotic analgesic is administered regularly and when the dose is large.

OD **Overdose Management:** *Symptoms (Acute Toxicity):* Severe toxicity is characterized by **profound respiratory depression, apnea, deep sleep, stupor or coma, circulatory collapse, seizures, cardiopulmonary arrest, and death.** Less severe toxicity results in symptoms including CNS depression, miosis, respiratory depression, deep sleep, flaccidity of skeletal muscles, hypotension, bradycardia, hypothermia, pulmonary edema, pneumonia, shock. The respiratory rate may be as low as 2–4 breaths/min. The client may be cyanotic. Urine output is decreased, the skin feels clammy, and body temperature decreases. If death occurs, it almost always results from **respiratory depression.** *Symptoms (Chronic Toxicity):* The problem of chronic dependence on narcotics occurs not only as a result of "street" use but is

also found often among those who have easy access to narcotics (physicians, nurses, pharmacists). All the principal narcotic analgesics (morphine, opium, heroin, codeine, meperidine, and others) have, at times, been used for nontherapeutic purposes.

The practitioner should be aware of the problem and be able to recognize signs of chronic dependence. These are constricted pupils, GI effects (constipation), skin infections, needle scars, abscesses, and itching, especially on the anterior surfaces of the body, where the client may inject the drug.

Withdrawal signs appear after drug is withheld for 4–12 hr. They are characterized by intense craving for the drug, insomnia, yawning, sneezing, vomiting, diarrhea, tremors, sweating, mental depression, muscular aches and pains, chills, and anxiety. Although the symptoms of narcotic withdrawal are uncomfortable, they are rarely life-threatening. This is in contrast to the withdrawal syndrome from depressants, where the life of the individual may be endangered because of the possibility of tonic-clonic seizures.

Treatment (Acute Overdose): Initial treatment is aimed at combating progressive respiratory depression by maintaining a patent airway and by assisted ventilation. Gastric lavage and induced emesis are indicated in case of oral poisoning. The narcotic antagonist naloxone (Narcan), 0.4 mg IV, is effective in the treatment of acute overdosage. Respiratory stimulants (e.g., caffeine) should not be used to treat depression from narcotic overdosage.

Drug Interactions
Alcohol, ethyl / Potentiation or addition of CNS depressant effects; concomitant use may lead to drowsiness, lethargy, stupor, respiratory collapse, coma, or death
Anesthetics, general / See *Alcohol*
Antianxiety drugs / See *Alcohol*
Antidepressants, tricyclic / ↑ Narcotic-induced respiratory depression
Antihistamines / See *Alcohol*

Barbiturates / See *Alcohol*

Cimetidine / ↑ CNS toxicity (e.g., disorientation, confusion, respiratory depression, apnea, seizures) with narcotics

CNS depressants / See *Alcohol*

MAO inhibitors / Possible potentiation of either MAO inhibitor (excitation, hypertension) or narcotic (hypotension, coma) effects; death has resulted

Methotrimeprazine / Potentiation of CNS depression

Phenothiazines / See *Alcohol*

Sedative-hypnotics, nonbarbiturate / See *Alcohol*

Skeletal muscle relaxants (surgical) / ↑ Respiratory depression and ↑ muscle relaxation

Laboratory Test Interferences: Altered liver function tests. False + or ↑ urinary glucose test (Benedict's). ↑ Plasma amylase or lipase.

Dosage

See individual drugs.

The dosage of narcotics and the reaction of a client to the dosage depend on the amount of pain. Two to four times the usual dose may be tolerated for relief of excruciating pain. However, the nurse should be aware that if, for some reason, the pain disappears, severe respiratory depression may result. This respiratory depression is not apparent while the pain is still present.

RESPIRATORY CARE CONSIDERATIONS

Administration/Storage

1. Review the list of drugs with which narcotics interact and their associated effects.

2. Request that the orders be rewritten at timed intervals as required for continued administration.

3. Record the amount of narcotic used on the narcotic inventory sheet, indicating what was administered, the date, the time, the dose, and to whom, or if the drug was wasted and include an appropriate witness as necessary, addressing all requirements for documentation.

Assessment

1. Document indications for therapy and type and onset of symptoms. Differentiate acute vs chronic syndromes.

2. Note if the client has had any prior experience with narcotic analgesics such as an adverse reaction with the drug or category of drugs prescribed.

3. Identify clinical conditions that would precipitate pain syndromes, i.e., cancer, neuropathic as in diabetic neuropathy, postherpetic neuralgia, or musculoskeletal injury.

4. Determine the cause and document the amount of pain or discomfort, its location, intensity, and duration, frequency of occurrence, and what drug has been effective in the past. The amount and type of narcotic ordered should be individualized according to the client's response.

5. Use a pain rating scale (e.g., 0–10) to assess pain quantitatively so that clients can accurately describe their level of pain and measure the level of effectiveness of drug therapy.

6. Obtain baseline VS prior to administering the drug. Generally, if the respiratory rate is less than 12 breaths/min or the SBP is less than 90 mm Hg, a narcotic should not be administered unless there is ventilatory support or specific written guidelines, with parameters for administration.

7. Note the client's weight, age, and general body size. Too large a dosage of medication for the client's weight and age can result in serious side effects.

8. Document the amount of time that has elapsed between the doses for the client to have relief from recurring pain.

9. Note precipitating factors as well as the impact of the pain on the client's ability to function.

10. Document any history of asthma or other conditions that tend to compromise respirations.

11. If the client is of childbearing age, discuss the possibility of pregnan-

cy. Narcotics cross the placental barrier and depress the respirations of the fetus. The drugs may be contraindicated under certain circumstances.

12. Baseline CBC, liver and renal functions studies, as well as electrolytes should be considered, especially when long-term therapy is anticipated.

Interventions

1. Determine when to use supportive measures, such as relaxation techniques, repositioning the client, and reassurance to assist in relieving pain. Listen to the client and/or family and attempt to answer their questions honestly.

2. Explore the problem and source of the client's pain. Use nonnarcotic analgesic medications when possible. Coadministration (such as with NSAIDs) may increase analgesic effects and permit lower doses of the narcotic analgesic.

3. Administer the medication when it is needed. *Prolonging the medication until the client experiences the maximum amount of pain reduces the effectiveness of the medication.*

4. Monitor VS and mental status and note any changes. During parenteral therapy:

• Monitor the respiratory rate for signs of respiratory depression. Obtain written parameters for administration of narcotic analgesics, as necessary.

• Narcotic analgesics depress the cough reflex. Therefore, turn clients q 2 hr, have them cough and take deep breaths to prevent atelectasis. Splinting incisions and painful areas may assist in client compliance. Ensure that narcotic is administered at least 30–60 min prior to activities or painful procedures.

• Monitor BP. Hypotension is more apt to occur in the elderly and in those who are receiving other medications with hypotension as a side effect.

• Monitor the HR. If the pulse drops below 60 beats/min in the adult or 110 beats/min in an infant, withhold the drug and report.

• Observe the client for any decrease in BP, deep sleep, or constricted pupils. Withhold the drug if any of these symptoms occur, document and report.

• Assess closely during meals to ensure that client does not choke and aspirate.

• Monitor client closely when administered as sedation for a procedure.

• Note the effects of the drug on the client's mental status. A client who has experienced pain, fear, or anxiety may become euphoric and excited. Also note any dizziness, drowsiness, pupil reactions, or hallucinations.

5. Report if the client develops N&V. If this occurs, the provider may order an antiemetic or change the medication therapy.

6. If the client is taking a narcotic medication by mouth, a snack or milk may decrease gastric irritation and lessen nausea.

7. Monitor bowel function. Narcotics, especially morphine, can have a depressant effect on the GI tract and may promote constipation. If condition permits, increase fluid intake to 2.5–3 L/day and increase intake of fruit juices, fruits, and fiber as well as level and frequency of exercise if tolerated.

8. Narcotic drugs may cause urinary retention. Monitor the client's intake and urinary output and palpate the abdomen to detect for evidence of bladder distention. Encourage the client to attempt to empty the bladder q 3–4 hr. Question clients about difficulty voiding, pain in the bladder area, sensation of not emptying the bladder, dysuria, or any unusual odors.

9. Note client complaint of difficulty with vision. Examine the client's pupillary response to light. Report if client's pupils remain constricted.

10. Monitor mental status. If the client is bedridden, put up side rails and provide other protective safety measures. Assist with ambulation, BR, and transfers.

11. When administering medication, reassure client that flushing and a feeling of warmth sometimes may occur with therapeutic doses of drug.

12. Because clients may perspire profusely when receiving a narcotic, be prepared to bathe them and change their clothes and linens frequently.

13. If a client is to be receiving a narcotic preparation over a period of time, monitor renal and liver function studies.

14. Assess hospitalized clients receiving ATC therapy for evidence of tolerance and addiction.

15. In clients with terminal disease states, dependence on drug therapy is not a consideration, whereas *adequate pain control is of the utmost concern.*

Evaluate
• Reports of effective control of severe pain without altered hemodynamics or impaired level of consciousness
• The absence of symptoms of acute toxicity, tolerance, or addiction, during short-term therapy

NARCOTIC ANTAGONISTS

See also the following individual entries:

Nalmefene hydrochloride
Naloxone hydrochloride
Naltrexone

General Statement: The narcotic antagonists are able to prevent or reverse many of the pharmacologic actions of morphine-type analgesics and meperidine. For example, respiratory depression induced by these drugs is reversed within minutes. Naloxone is considered a pure antagonist in that it does not produce morphine-like effects.

The narcotic antagonists are not effective in reversing the respiratory depression induced by barbiturates, anesthetics, or other nonnarcotic agents. Narcotic antagonists almost immediately induce withdrawal symptoms in narcotic addicts and are sometimes used to unmask dependence.

Action/Kinetics: Narcotic antagonists block the action of narcotic analgesics by displacing previously given narcotics from their receptor sites or by preventing narcotics from attaching to the opiate receptors, thereby preventing access by the analgesic. This type of antagonism is competitive.

RESPIRATORY CARE CONSIDERATIONS
Assessment
1. Determine the etiology of respiratory depression. Narcotic antagonists do not relieve the toxicity of nonnarcotic CNS depressants.
2. Assess and obtain baseline mental status and VS before administering any narcotic antagonist.
Interventions
1. Note agent being reversed. If narcotic is long acting or sustained release, anticipate that repeated doses will be required in order to continue to counteract drug effects. Monitor respirations closely after the duration of action of the narcotic antagonist. Additional doses of drug may be necessary.
2. Observe for the appearance of withdrawal symptoms after administration of the narcotic antagonist. Withdrawal symptoms are characterized by restlessness, crying out due to sudden loss of pain control, lacrimation, rhinorrhea, yawning, perspiration, vomiting, diarrhea, sweating, writhing, anxiety, pain, chills, and an intense craving for the drug.
3. Have emergency drugs and equipment readily available and observe for symptoms of airway obstruction.
4. If the client is comatose, turn frequently and position on the side to prevent aspiration.
5. Maintain a safe, protective envi-

ronment. Use side rails, supervise ambulation, and use soft supports as needed.

6. Assess VS after drug administration to determine the effectiveness of the drug.

7. If the narcotic antagonist is being used to diagnose narcotic use or dependence, observe the initial dilation of the client's pupils, followed by constriction.

8. Anticipate readministration of smaller doses of narcotic (once depressant symptoms reversed) in clients with terminal pain and conditions that warrant narcotic pain management.

Evaluate

• Effective reversal of toxic effects of narcotic analgesic as evidenced by ↑ level of consciousness and improved breathing patterns

• Confirmation of narcotic dependence as evidenced by withdrawal symptoms

NASAL DECONGESTANTS

See also the following individual entries:

Ephedrine sulfate
Epinephrine hydrochloride
Phenylephrine hydrochloride
Pseudoephedrine hydrochloride

Action/Kinetics: The most commonly used agents for relief of nasal congestion are the adrenergic drugs. They act by stimulating alpha-adrenergic receptors, thereby constricting the arterioles in the nasal mucosa; this reduces blood flow to the area, decreasing congestion. However, drugs such as ephedrine and pseudoephedrine also have beta-adrenergic effects. Both topical (sprays, drops) and oral agents may be used, although oral agents are not as effective.

Uses: PO. Nasal congestion due to hay fever, common cold, allergies, or sinusitis. To help sinus or nasal drainage. To relieve congestion of eustachian tubes. **Topical.** Nasal and nasopharyngeal mucosal congestion due to hay fever, common cold, allergies, or sinusitis. With other therapy to decrease congestion around the eustachian tubes. Relieve ear block and pressure pain during air travel.

Contraindications: Oral use in severe hypertension or CAD. Use with MAO inhibitors. Oral use of pseudoephedrine and phenylpropanolamine during lactation.

Special Concerns: Use with caution in hyperthyroidism, arteriosclerosis, increased intraocular pressure, prostatic hypertrophy, angina, diabetes, ischemic heart disease, hypertension. Also, clients receiving MAO inhibitors may manifest hypertensive crisis following the use of oral nasal decongestants. Use with caution in geriatric clients and during pregnancy and lactation. Rebound congestion may occur after topical use. OTC products containing ephedrine have been abused.

Side Effects: *Topical use:* Stinging and burning, mucosal dryness, sneezing, local irritation, rebound congestion (rhinitis medicamentosa). Systemic use may produce the following symptoms. *CV:* **CV collapse with hypotension,** arrhythmias, palpitations, precordial pain, tachycardia, transient hypertension, bradycardia. *CNS:* Anxiety, dizziness, headache, fear, restlessness, tremors, insomnia, tenseness, lightheadedness, drowsiness, psychologic disturbances, weakness, psychoses, hallucinations, **seizures,** depression. *GI:* N&V, anorexia. *Ophthalmologic:* Irritation, photophobia, tearing, blurred vision, blepharospasm. *Other:* Dysuria, sweating, pallor, breathing difficulties, orofacial dystonia.

NOTE: Ephedrine may also produce anorexia and urinary retention in men with prostatic hypertrophy.

OD **Overdose Management:** *Symptoms:* Somnolence, sedation, **coma,** profuse sweating, **hypotension, shock. Severe hypertension,** bradycardia, and rebound hypotension may occur with naphazoline and tetrahydrozoline. *Treatment:* Supportive therapy. IV phentolamine may be used in severe cases.

Drug Interactions

Furazolidone / ↑ Pressor sensitivity to drugs with both alpha- and beta-adrenergic effects (e.g., ephedrine)

Guanethidine / ↑ Effect of direct-acting agents (e.g., epinephrine) and ↓ effect of mixed-acting drugs; also, ↓ hypotensive effect of guanethidine

MAO inhibitors / Use with mixed-acting drugs (e.g., ephedrine) → severe headache, hypertension, hyperpyrexia, and possibly hypertensive crisis

Methyldopa / ↑ Risk of a pressor response

Phenothiazines / May ↓ or reverse action of nasal decongestants

Reserpine / ↑ Pressor effect of direct-acting drugs and ↓ effect of mixed-acting drugs

Theophyllines / Enhanced toxicity

Tricyclic antidepressants / ↑ Pressor effect of direct-acting agents → possibility of dysrhythmias; ↓ pressor effect of mixed-acting drugs

Urinary acidifiers / ↑ Excretion of nasal decongestants → ↓ effect

Urinary alkalinizers / ↓ Excretion of nasal decongestants → ↑ effect

Dosage

See individual drugs.

RESPIRATORY CARE CONSIDERATIONS

Administration/Storage

1. Most nasal decongestants are used topically in the form of sprays, drops, or solutions.

2. Solutions of topical nasal decongestants may become contaminated with use. This may result in the growth of bacteria and fungi. Thus, the dropper or spray tip should be rinsed in hot water after each use and covered.

3. During administration, have facial tissues and a receptacle available for used tissues.

4. Topical decongestants should not be used longer than 3–5 days and should be used sparingly, especially

in infants, children, and clients with CV disease.

Interventions

1. Use separate equipment with topical administration to prevent the spread of infection. If only one container of medication is available, use an individual dropper for each client and rinse thoroughly with hot water after each use.

2. Instruct to blow the nose gently before administering therapy. If unable to blow the nose, clear the nasal passages with a bulb-type aspirator as needed.

3. After completing the treatment, rinse the dropper or tip of spray container with hot water. Dry with a tissue and cover, using care not to introduce water into the spray container. Wipe the tip of the nasal jelly tube with a damp tissue and replace the cap.

Client/Family Teaching

1. Instruct in the appropriate technique for preparing the nasal passages.

2. Review the method of administration of the prescribed medication, whether drops, spray, or jelly.

3. Discuss and demonstrate the proper use and care of equipment.

4. Review the indications for therapy and the response that client should expect. Advise to seek medical assistance if symptoms worsen or do not improve after 3–5 days of therapy.

5. Caution that overuse or misuse of these agents may cause significant medical problems, i.e., a nasal spray used regularly for more than 3 or 4 days may precipitate rebound congestion.

6. Stress that many OTC agents contain sympathomimetics; these should be avoided in clients with hypertension, hyperthyroidism, angina, and insulin-dependent diabetes.

Evaluate

• Reports of ↓ nasal congestion
• Resolution of eustachian tube congestion and pain

• ↓ Duration and intensity of allergic manifestations

NEUROMUSCULAR BLOCKING AGENTS

See also the following individual entries:

Atracurium besylate
Cisatracurium besylate
Doxacurium chloride
Mivacurium chloride
Pancuronium bromide
Pipecuronium bromide
Rocuronium bromide
Succinylcholine chloride
Tubocurarine chloride
Vecuronium bromide

General Statement: Upon stimulation, the muscles normally contract when acetylcholine is released from storage sites embedded in the motor end plate. The drugs considered in this section interfere with nerve impulse transmission between the motor end plate and the receptors of skeletal muscle (i.e., peripheral action).

The drugs fall into two groups: competitive (nondepolarizing) agents and depolarizing agents. Competitive agents—atracurium, doxacurium, gallamine, metocurine, mivacurium, pancuronium, tubocurarine, vecuronium—compete with acetylcholine for the receptor site in the muscle cells. These agents are also called *curariform* because their mode of action is similar to that of the poison curare. The depolarizing agent—succinylcholine—initially excites skeletal muscle and then prevents the muscle from contracting by prolonging the time during which the receptors at the end plate cannot respond to acetylcholine (depolarization during refractory time).

The muscle paralysis caused by the neuromuscular blocking agents is sequential. Therapeutic doses produce muscle depression in the following order: heaviness of eyelids, difficulty in swallowing and talking, diplopia, progressive weakening of the extremities and neck, followed by relaxation of the trunk and spine. The diaphragm (respiratory paralysis) is affected last. The drugs do not affect consciousness, and their use, in the absence of adequate levels of general anesthesia, may be frightening to the client. After IV infusion, flaccid paralysis occurs within a few minutes with maximum effects within about 6 min. Maximal effects last 35–60 min and effective muscle paralysis may last for 25–90 min with complete recovery taking several hours.

There is a narrow margin of safety between a therapeutically effective dose causing muscle relaxation and a toxic dose causing respiratory paralysis. **The neuromuscular blocking agents are always administered initially by a physician.** The nurse must be prepared to maintain and monitor respiration until the effect of the drug subsides.

Uses: See individual agents. General uses include as an adjunct to general anesthesia to cause muscle relaxation; to reduce the intensity of skeletal muscle contractions in either drug-induced or electrically induced convulsions; to assist in the management of mechanical ventilation.

Contraindications: Allergy or hypersensitivity to any of these drugs.

Special Concerns: The neuromuscular blocking agents should be used with caution in clients with myasthenia gravis; renal, hepatic, endocrine, or pulmonary impairment; respiratory depression; during lactation; and in elderly, pediatric, or debilitated clients. The action of these drugs may be altered in clients by electrolyte imbalances (especially hyperkalemia), some carcinomas, body temperature, dehydration, renal disease, and in those taking digitalis.

Side Effects: *Respiratory paralysis. Severe and prolonged muscle relaxation.* CV: Cardiac arrhythmias, bradycardia, hypotension, cardiac arrest. These side effects are more frequent in neonates and premature infants. GI: Excessive salivation during light anesthesia. *Miscellaneous:* **Bronchospasms, hyperthermia,** hypersensitivity (rare). See also individual agents.

OD Overdose Management: *Symptoms:* Decreased respiratory reserve, extended skeletal muscle weakness, prolonged apnea, low tidal volume, sudden release of histamine, **CV collapse.** *Treatment:* There are no known antidotes.

• Use a peripheral nerve stimulator to monitor and assess the client's response to the neuromuscular blocking medication.

• Have anticholinesterase drugs, such as edrophonium, pyridostigmine, or neostigmine available to counteract respiratory depression due to paralysis of skeletal muscles. These drugs increase the body's production of acetylcholine. To minimize the muscarinic cholinergic side effects, atropine should also be given.

• Correct BP, electrolyte imbalance, or circulating blood volume by fluid and electrolyte therapy. Vasopressors can be used to correct hypotension due to ganglionic blockade.

Drug Interactions: The following drug interactions are for nondepolarizing skeletal muscle relaxants. See also succinylcholine.

Aminoglycoside antibiotics / Additive muscle relaxation, including prolonged respiratory depression

Amphotericin B / ↑ Muscle relaxation

Anesthetics, inhalation / Additive muscle relaxation

Carbamazepine / ↓ Duration or effect of muscle relaxants

Clindamycin / Additive muscle relaxation, including prolonged respiratory depression

Colistin / ↑ Muscle relaxation

Corticosteroids / ↓ Effect of muscle relaxants

Furosemide / ↑ or ↓ Effect of skeletal muscle relaxants (may be dose-related)

Hydantoins / ↓ Duration or effect of muscle relaxants

Ketamine / ↑ Muscle relaxation, including prolonged respiratory depression

Lincomycin / ↑ Muscle relaxation, including prolonged respiratory depression

Lithium / ↑ Recovery time of muscle relaxants → prolonged respiratory depression

Magnesium salts / ↑ Muscle relaxation, including prolonged respiratory depression

Methotrimeprazine / ↑ Muscle relaxation

Narcotic analgesics / ↑ Respiratory depression and ↑ muscle relaxation

Nitrates / ↑ Muscle relaxation, including prolonged respiratory depression

Phenothiazines / ↑ Muscle relaxation

Pipercillin / ↑ Muscle relaxation, including prolonged respiratory depression

Polymyxin B / ↑ Muscle relaxation

Procainamide / ↑ Muscle relaxation

Procaine / ↑ Muscle relaxation by ↓ plasma protein binding

Quinidine / ↑ Muscle relaxation

Ranitidine / Significant ↓ effect of muscle relaxants

Theophyllines / Reversal of effects of muscle relaxant (dose-dependent)

Thiazide diuretics / ↑ Muscle relaxation due to hypokalemia

Verapamil / ↑ Muscle relaxation, including prolonged respiratory depression

Dosage
See individual drugs.

RESPIRATORY CARE CONSIDERATIONS
Administration/Storage

1. When the drug is to be administered by a constant infusion, use a microdrip tubing administration set with an electronic infusion control device.

2. Generally, client should be sedated and intubated prior to use.

3. During drug administration, have a suction machine, oxygen, and resus-

citation equipment immediately available for emergency use.

Assessment

1. Document indications for therapy, desired outcome, and anticipated length of use.

2. Note age and condition of the client. Elderly and debilitated clients should not receive drugs in this category.

3. Determine that baseline CBC, electrolytes, CXR, ECG, and liver and renal function studies have been performed.

4. Note all other drugs the client is receiving. Often, clients requiring neuromuscular blocking agents are also receiving other drugs that may have the effect of prolonging client response to the prescribed neuromuscular blocking agent.

5. Question the client concerning changes in vision, ability to chew or to move the fingers, and document findings.

6. Note initial selective paralysis followed by paralysis in the following sequence: levator muscles of the eyelids, mastication muscles, limb muscles, abdominal muscles, glottis muscles, intercostal muscles, and the diaphragm muscles. Of note is that neuromuscular recovery occurs in the reverse order.

Interventions

1. Drugs should only be administered in a closely monitored environment and generally are used only for intubated clients.

2. Prevent overdosage during infusions by frequent evaluations (q 4 hr) with a peripheral nerve stimulator or by allowing partial return of muscle function.

3. Monitor the client's BP and pulse frequently. Respirations and pulmonary status should be monitored continuously. Ensure that cardiac monitor and ventilator alarms are set appropriately and checked at frequent intervals.

4. Observe for excessive bronchial secretions or respiratory wheezing, and suction to maintain patent airway (ET tube).

5. Perform frequent neurovascular assessments. Prolonged use of neuromuscular blocking agents may cause profound weakness and even paralysis once the drug has been discontinued. It may precipitate an acute myopathy in some individuals.

6. Observe the client closely for drug interactions. These can potentiate muscular relaxation and prove fatal. If interactions occur, report immediately and obtain orders for the appropriate medication to counteract the reaction.

7. Consciousness and pain thresholds are not affected by neuromuscular blocking agents. Most clients can still hear, feel, and see while they are receiving blocking agents. Therefore, inappropriate talking and laughing and any discussions that should not be overheard should be avoided. Adequate anesthesia and analgesics should be administered for pain or when painful procedures are necessary.

8. Clients requiring prolonged ventilatory therapy should be adequately sedated with analgesics and benzodiazepines. Anxiety levels may be very high, but client cannot communicate this.

9. Administer eye drops and eye patches to protect corneas during prolonged therapy. Explain to client and family why this is done (i.e., because the blink reflex has been suppressed).

10. Avoid the use of corticosteroids during prolonged neuromuscular blockade unless benefits outweigh the risks.

11. Perform passive range of motion to prevent loss of function and contractures with prolonged therapy.

Evaluate

• Evidence of desired level of skeletal muscle paralysis

• Successful insertion of ET tube and tolerance of mechanical ventilation

• Adequate suppression of twitch response upon peripheral nerve stimulation tests

PENICILLINS

See also the following individual entries:

Amoxicillin
Amoxicillin and Potassium
  clavulanate
Ampicillin oral
Ampicillin sodium parenteral
Ampicillin sodium/Sulbactam
  sodium
Bacampicillin hydrochloride
Carbenicillin indanyl sodium
Cloxacillin sodium
Dicloxacillin sodium
Methicillin sodium
Mezlocillin sodium
Nafcillin sodium
Oxacillin sodium
Penicillin G benzathine and
  procaine combined
Penicillin G benzathine,
  parenteral
Penicillin G potassium for
  injection
Penicillin G, sodium for injection
Penicillin G procaine suspension,
  sterile
Penicillin V potassium
Piperacillin sodium
Piperacillin sodium and
  Tazobactam sodium
Ticarcillin disodium
Ticarcillin disodium and
  Clavulanate potassium

Action/Kinetics: The bactericidal action of penicillins depends on their ability to bind penicillin-binding proteins (PBP-1 and PBP-3) in the cytoplasmic membranes of bacteria, thus inhibiting cell wall synthesis. Some penicillins act by acylation of membrane-bound transpeptidase enzymes, thereby preventing cross-linkage of peptidoglycan chains, which are necessary for bacterial cell wall strength and rigidity. Cell division and growth are inhibited and often lysis and elongation of susceptible bacteria occur. Penicillin is most effective against young, rapidly dividing organisms and has little effect on mature resting cells. Depending on the concentration of the drug at the site of infection and the susceptibility of the infectious microorganism, penicillin is either bacteriostatic or bactericidal. Penicillins are distributed throughout most of the body and pass the placental barrier. They also pass into synovial, pleural, pericardial, peritoneal, ascitic, and spinal fluids. Although normal meninges and the eyes are relatively impermeable to penicillins, they are better absorbed by inflamed meninges and eyes. **Peak serum levels, after PO:** 1 hr. **t½:** 30–110 min; protein binding: 20%–98% (see individual agents). The renal, cardiac, and hematopoietic functions, as well as the electrolyte balance, of clients receiving penicillin should be monitored at regular intervals. Excreted largely unchanged by the urine as a result of glomerular filtration and active tubular secretion.

Uses: See individual drugs. Depending on the penicillin, these drugs are effective against one or more of the following organisms. **Gram-positive organisms:** *Bacillus anthracis,* beta-hemolytic streptococci, *Corynebacterium diphtheriae, Listeria monocytogenes,* staphylococci, *Staphylococcus aureus,* streptococci, *Streptococcus faecalis, S. pneumoniae,* and *S. viridans.* **Gram-negative organisms:** *Acinetobacter* species, *Citrobacter* species, *Enterobacter* species, *Escherichia coli, Haemophilus influenzae, Klebsiella* species, *Moraxella catarrhalis, Morganella morganii, Neisseria gonorrhoeae, Neisseria meningitidis, Proteus mirabilis, Proteus vulgaris, Providencia* species, *Providencia rettgeri, Providencia stuartii, Pseudomonas aeruginosa, Salmonella* species, *Serratia* species, *Shigella* species, and *Streptobacillus moniliformis.* **Anaerobic organisms:** *Actinomyces bovis, Bacteroides* species, *Clostridium* species, *Eubacterium* species, *Fusobacterium* species, *Peptococcus* species, *Peptostreptococcus* species, *Treponema pallidum, Veillonella* species.

✿ = Available in Canada   ***bold italic*** = life threatening side effect

Contraindications: Hypersensitivity to penicillins, imipenem, and cephalosporins. PO use of penicillins during the acute stages of empyema, bacteremia, pneumonia, meningitis, pericarditis, and purulent or septic arthritis.

Special Concerns: Use of penicillins during lactation may lead to sensitization, diarrhea, candidiasis, and skin rash in the infant. Use with caution in clients with a history of asthma, hay fever, or urticaria. Clients with cystic fibrosis have a higher incidence of side effects with broad spectrum penicillins. Safety and effectiveness of carbenicillin, piperacillin, and the beta-lactamase inhibitor/penicillin combinations (e.g., amoxicillin/potassium clavulanate, ticarcillin/ potassium clavulanate) have not been determined in children less than 12 years of age. The incidence of resistant strains of staphylococci to penicillinase-resistant penicillins is increasing. Use of prolonged therapy may lead to superinfection (i.e., bacterial or fungal overgrowth of nonsusceptible organisms).

Side Effects: Penicillins are potent sensitizing agents; it is estimated that up to 10% of the US population is allergic to the antibiotic. Hypersensitivity reactions are reported to be on the increase in pediatric populations. Sensitivity reactions may be immediate (within 20 min) or delayed (as long as several days or weeks after initiation of therapy). *Allergic:* Skin rashes (including maculopapular and exanthematous), exfoliative dermatitis, erythema multiforme (rarely, ***Stevens-Johnson syndrome***), hives, pruritus, wheezing, ***anaphylaxis,*** fever, eosinophilia, ***angioedema,*** serum sickness, ***laryngeal edema, laryngospasm, prostration, angioneurotic edema, bronchospasm, hypotension, vascular collapse, death.*** *GI:* Diarrhea (may be severe), abdominal cramps or pain, N&V, bloating, flatulence, increased thirst, bitter/unpleasant taste, glossitis, gastritis, stomatitis, dry mouth, sore mouth or tongue, furry tongue, black "hairy" tongue, bloody diarrhea, rectal bleeding, enterocolitis, pseudomembranous colitis. *CNS:* Dizziness, insomnia, hyperactivity, fatigue, prolonged muscle relaxation. Neurotoxicity including lethargy, neuromuscular irritability, ***seizures,*** hallucinations following large IV doses (especially in clients with renal failure). *Hematologic:* Thrombocytopenia, leukopenia, ***agranulocytosis,*** anemia, thrombocytopenic purpura, ***hemolytic anemia,*** granulocytopenia, neutropenia, bone marrow depression. *Renal:* Oliguria, hematuria, hyaline casts, proteinuria, pyuria (all symptoms of interstitial nephritis), nephropathy. Electrolyte imbalance following IV use. *Miscellaneous:* Hepatotoxicity (cholestatic jaundice), superinfection, swelling of face and ankles, anorexia, hyperthermia, transient hepatitis, vaginitis, itchy eyes. IM injection may cause pain and induration at the injection site, ecchymosis, and hematomas. IV use may cause vein irritation, deep vein thrombosis, and thrombophlebitis.

OD **Overdose Management:** *Symptoms:* Neuromuscular hyperexcitability, convulsive seizures. Massive IV doses may cause agitation, asterixis, hallucinations, confusion, stupor, multifocal myoclonus, seizures, coma, hyperkalemia, and encephalopathy. *Treatment (Severe Allergic or Anaphylactic Reactions):* Administer epinephrine (0.3–0.5 mL of a 1:1,000 solution SC or IM, or 0.2–0.3 mL diluted in 10 mL saline, given slowly by IV). Corticosteroids should be on hand. In those instances where penicillin is the drug of choice, the physician may decide to use it even though the client is allergic, adding a medication to the regimen to control the allergic response.

Drug Interactions

Aminoglycosides / Penicillins ↓ effect of aminoglycosides

Antacids / ↓ Effect of penicillins due to ↓ absorption from GI tract

Antibiotics, Chloramphenicol, Erythromycins, Tetracyclines / ↓ Effect of penicillins

Anticoagulants / Penicillins may potentiate pharmacologic effect

Aspirin / ↑ Effect of penicillins by ↓ plasma protein binding

Chloramphenicol / Either ↑ or ↓ effects

Erythromycins / Either ↑ or ↓ effects

Heparin / ↑ Risk of bleeding following parenteral penicillins

Oral contraceptives / ↓ Effect of oral contraceptives

Phenylbutazone / ↑ Effect of penicillins by ↓ plasma protein binding

Probenecid / ↑ Effect of penicillins by ↓ excretion

Tetracyclines / ↓ Effect of penicillins

Laboratory Test Interferences: ↓ Hematocrit, hemoglobin, WBC lymphocytes, serum potassium, albumin, total proteins, uric acid. ↑ Basophils, lymphocytes, monocytes, platelets, serum alkaline phosphatase, serum sodium. ↑ AST, ALT, bilirubin, LDH following semisynthetic penicillins.

Dosage

Penicillins are available in a variety of dosage forms for PO, parenteral, inhalation, and intrathecal administration. Dosages for individual drugs are given in drug entries. Long-acting preparations are frequently used. PO doses must be higher than IM or SC doses because a large fraction of penicillin given PO may be destroyed in the stomach.

RESPIRATORY CARE CONSIDERATIONS

See also *General Respiratory Care Considerations for All Anti-Infectives*.

Administration/Storage

1. IM and IV administration of penicillin causes a great deal of local irritation. These antibiotics should thus be injected slowly.

2. IM injections are made deeply into the gluteal muscle. IV injections are usually made through the tubing of an IV infusion.

Assessment

1. Assess rigorously for allergic reactions because the incidence is higher with penicillin therapy than with other antibiotics. If a reaction occurs, the drug must be discontinued immediately. Epinephrine, oxygen, antihistamines, and corticosteroids must be immediately available.

2. Anticipate that allergic reactions are more likely to occur in clients with a history of asthma, hay fever, urticaria, or allergy to cephalosporins.

Interventions

1. Detain client in an ambulatory care site for at least 20 min after administering a penicillin injection to assess for the onset of anaphylaxis. Be prepared for prompt treatment of anaphylactic reaction.

2. Do not administer long-acting types of penicillin IV, because these types are only for IM use. They may cause emboli, CNS pathology, or cardiac pathology if administered IV.

3. Do not massage repository (long-acting) penicillin products after injection, since rate of absorption should not be increased.

4. Prevent rapid administration of IV penicillin. This method may cause local irritation and may precipitate convulsions. With some agents, high-dose therapy may precipitate aplastic anemia.

5. The elderly may be more sensitive to the effects of penicillin than are younger people. Therefore, care should be exerted when calculating the dose based on client weight and height.

6. Most penicillins are excreted in breast milk and should be prescribed cautiously to nursing mothers.

Evaluate

• Knowledge and understanding of illness and evidence of compliance with prescribed medication therapy

• Reports of symptomatic improvement

• Resolution of symptoms of infection manifested by ↓ fever, ↓ WBCs, ↑ appetite, and negative lab culture reports

SYMPATHOMIMETIC DRUGS

See also the following individual entries:

Albuterol
Bitolterol mesylate
Dobutamine hydrochloride
Dopamine hydrochloride
Ephedrine sulfate
Epinephrine
Epinephrine bitartrate
Epinephrine borate
Epinephrine hydrochloride
Isoetharine hydrochloride
Isoetharine mesylate
Isoproterenol
Isoproterenol hydrochloride
Isoproterenol sulfate
Levarterenol bitartrate
Mephentermine sulfate
Metaproterenol sulfate
Metaraminol bitartrate
Phenylephrine hydrochloride
Phenylpropanolamine
　hydrochloride
Pirbuterol acetate
Pseudoephedrine hydrochloride
Pseudoephedrine sulfate
Salmeterol xinafoate
Terbutaline sulfate

General Statement: The adrenergic drugs supplement, mimic, and reinforce the messages transmitted by the natural neurohormones— norepinephrine and epinephrine. These hormones are responsible for transmitting nerve impulses at the postganglionic neurojunctions of the sympathetic nervous system. The adrenergic drugs work in two ways: (1) by mimicking the action of norepinephrine or epinephrine (directly acting sympathomimetics) or (2) by causing or regulating the release of the natural neurohormones from their storage sites at the nerve terminals (indirectly acting sympathomimetics). Some drugs exhibit a combination of effects 1 and 2.

The myoneural junction is equipped with special receptors for the neurohormones. These receptors have been classified into two types: alpha (α) and beta (β), according to whether they respond to norepinephrine, epinephrine, or isoproterenol and to certain blocking agents. Alpha-adrenergic receptors are blocked by phenoxybenzamine and phentolamine, whereas beta-adrenergic receptors are blocked by propranolol and similar drugs.

Both alpha and beta receptors have been divided into subtypes. Thus adrenergic stimulation of receptors will manifest the following general effects:

Alpha-1-adrenergic: / Vasoconstriction, decongestion, constriction of the pupil of the eye, contraction of splenic capsule, contraction of the trigone-sphincter muscle of the urinary bladder.

Alpha-2-adrenergic: / Presynaptic to regulate amount of transmitter released; decrease tone, motility, and secretory activity of the GI tract (possibly involved in hypersecretory response also); decrease insulin secretion.

Beta-1-adrenergic: / Myocardial contraction (inotropic), regulation of heartbeat (chronotropic), improved impulse conduction, $\uparrow$ lipolysis.

Beta-2-adrenergic: / Peripheral vasodilation, bronchial dilation; $\downarrow$ tone, motility, and secretory activity of the GI tract; $\uparrow$ renin secretion.

In addition, adrenergic agents affect the exocrine glands, the salivary glands, and the CNS. The adrenergic stimulants discussed in this section act preferentially on one or more of the preceding receptor subtypes; their pharmacologic effect must be carefully monitored and balanced.

Uses: The primary determinant of usefulness of sympathomimetics is their selectivity of action. Sympathomimetic agents are mainly used for the treatment of shock induced by sudden cardiac arrest, decompensation, MI, trauma, bronchodilation, acute renal failure, drug reactions, anaphylaxis. Adrenergic drugs are also used to reverse bronchospasm caused by bronchial asthma, emphysema, exercise-induced bronchospasm, chronic bronchitis, bronchiectasis, or other obstructive pulmonary disease. Drugs with beta-receptor activity are combined with an anti-inflammatory drug for moderate asthma and with an oral corticosteroid for severe asthma. Sympathomimetic drugs having predominantly alpha-receptor activity are used for the relief of nasal and nasopharyngeal congestion due to rhinitis, sinusitis, head colds. See individual drugs.

Contraindications: Tachycardia due to arrhythmias; tachycardia or heart block caused by digitalis toxicity.

Special Concerns: Use with caution in hyperthyroidism, diabetes, prostatic hypertrophy, seizures, degenerative heart disease, especially in geriatric clients or those with asthma, emphysema, or psychoneuroses. Also, use with caution in clients with coronary insufficiency, CAD, ischemic heart disease, CHF, cardiac arrhythmias, hypertension, or history of stroke. Asthma clients who rely heavily on inhaled beta-2-agonist bronchodilators may increase their chances of death. Thus, these agents should be used to "rescue" clients but should not be prescribed for regular long-term use. Beta-2 agonists may inhibit uterine contractions.

Side Effects: See individual drugs; side effects common to most sympathomimetics are listed. *CV:* Tachycardia, arrhythmias, palpitations, BP changes, anginal pain, precordial pain, pallor, skipped beats, chest tightness, hypertension. *GI:* N&V, heartburn, anorexia, altered taste or bad taste, GI distress, dry mouth, diarrhea. *CNS:* Restlessness, anxiety, tension, insomnia, hyperkinesis, drowsiness, weakness, vertigo, irritability, dizziness, headache, tremors, general CNS stimulation, nervousness, shakiness, hyperactivity. *Respiratory:* Cough, dyspnea, dry throat, pharyngitis, *paradoxical bronchospasm,* irritation. *Other:* Flushing, sweating, *allergic reactions.*

OD **Overdose Management:** *Symptoms:* Following inhalation: Exaggeration of side effects resulting in anginal pain, hypertension, hypokalemia, *seizures.* Following systemic use: CV symptoms include bradycardia, tachycardia, palpitations, extrasystoles, *heart block,* elevated BP, chest pain, hypokalemia. CNS symptoms include anxiety, insomnia, tremor, delirium, *convulsions, collapse, and coma.* Also, fever, chills, cold perspiration, N&V, mydriasis, and blanching of the skin. *Treatment:*
• For overdosage due to inhalation: General supportive measures with sedatives given for restlessness. Cautious use of metoprolol or atenolol may be used but these drugs may induce an asthmatic attack in clients with asthma.
• For systemic overdosage: Discontinue or decrease dose. General supportive measures. For overdose due to PO agents, emesis, gastric lavage, or charcoal may be helpful. In severe cases, propranolol may be used but this may cause airway obstruction. Phentolamine may be given to block strong alpha-adrenergic effects.

Drug Interactions
Beta-adrenergic blocking agents / Inhibit adrenergic stimulation of the heart and bronchial tree; cause bronchial constriction; hypertension, asthma, not relieved by adrenergic agents
Ammonium chloride / ↓ Effect of sympathomimetics due to ↑ excretion by kidney
Anesthetics / Halogenated anesthetics sensitize heart to adrenergics—causes cardiac arrhythmias
Anticholinergics / Concomitant use aggravates glaucoma
Antidiabetics / Hyperglycemic effect of epinephrine may necessitate ↑ dosage of insulin or oral hypoglycemic agents
Corticosteroids / Chronic use with sympathomimetics may result in or aggravate glaucoma; aerosols containing sympathomimetics and corti-

---

costeroids may be lethal in asthmatic children

Digitalis glycosides / Combination may cause cardiac arrhythmias

Furazolidone / Furazolidone ↑ effects of mixed-acting sympathomimetics

Guanethidine / Direct-acting sympathomimetics ↑ effects of guanethidine, while indirect-acting sympathomimetics ↓ effects of guanethidine; also reversal of hypotensive effects of guanethidine

Lithium / ↓ Pressor effect of direct-acting sympathomimetics

MAO inhibitors / All effects of sympathomimetics are potentiated; symptoms include hypertensive crisis with possible intracranial hemorrhage, hyperthermia, convulsions, coma; death may occur

Methyldopa / ↑ Pressor response

Methylphenidate / Potentiates pressor effect of sympathomimetics; combination hazardous in glaucoma

Oxytocics / ↑ Chance of severe hypertension

Phenothiazines / ↑ Risk of cardiac arrhythmias

Reserpine / ↑ Risk of hypertension following use of direct-acting sympathomimetics and ↓ effect of indirect-acting sympathomimetics

Sodium bicarbonate / ↑ Effect of sympathomimetics due to ↓ excretion by kidney

Theophylline / Enhanced toxicity (especially cardiotoxicity); also ↓ theophylline levels

Thyroxine / Potentiation of pressor response of sympathomimetics

Tricyclic antidepressants / ↑ Effect of direct-acting sympathomimetics and ↓ effect of indirect-acting sympathomimetics

Dosage
See individual drugs.

RESPIRATORY CARE CONSIDERATIONS
Administration/Storage
1. Review the list of drugs with which adrenergic agents interact.
2. Discard colored solutions.

3. When administering IV infusions of adrenergic drugs, use an electronic infusion device, administer in a monitored environment, and assess IV site frequently to ensure patency.

Assessment
1. Determine if the client has any history of sensitivity to adrenergic drugs.
2. Document any previous experience with drugs in this class and the outcome.
3. In taking the history, note especially if the client has a history of CAD, tachycardia, endocrine disturbances, or respiratory tract problems.
4. Obtain baseline data regarding the client's general physical condition and hemodynamic status including ECG, VS, and appropriate lab data.
5. Document indications for therapy, contributing factors, and anticipated response.

Interventions
1. During the period of dosage adjustment, closely monitor and record BP and pulse.
2. Monitor I&O and continue to assess VS throughout therapy.

Client/Family Teaching
1. Discuss prescribed drug therapy and provide printed material regarding potential drug side effects.
2. Review adverse side effects and the importance of reporting.
3. Instruct not to increase the dosage of medication and not to take the medication more frequently than prescribed. Consult provider if symptoms become more severe.
4. Advise client to take the medication early in the day because these drugs may cause insomnia.
5. Explain that feelings or symptoms of fear or anxiety may be evident because these drugs mimic the body's stress response.
6. Avoid all OTC preparations without provider approval.
7. Advise client to stop smoking now in order to preserve current lung function. Offer support and formal smoking cessation classes.

SPECIAL RESPIRATORY CARE CONSIDERATIONS FOR ADRENERGIC BRONCHODILATORS

Assessment

1. Obtain a full baseline client history prior to starting the drug therapy.
2. Review the contraindications for adrenergic bronchodilators.
3. Note any previous experience with this class of drugs.
4. Assess and record VS prior to administering medications.
5. Obtain ABGs (or O_2 saturation) as a baseline against which to measure the influence of medication once therapy begins.
6. Document lung assessment and pulmonary function tests. Note characteristics of cough and sputum production.

Interventions

1. Monitor BP and pulse after therapy begins to assess client's CV response.
2. Observe the effects of the drug on the client's CNS and if pronounced, adjust the dosage and frequency of administration.
3. If the client has status asthmaticus and abnormal ABGs, continue to provide oxygen and ventilating assistance even though the symptoms appear to be relieved by the bronchodilator.
4. To prevent depression of respiratory effort, administer oxygen on the basis of the evaluation of the client's clinical symptoms and the ABGs or O_2 saturations.
5. If three to five aerosol treatments of the same agent have been administered within the last 6–12 hr, with no relief, further evaluation is warranted.
6. If the client's dyspnea worsens after repeated excessive use of the inhaler, paradoxical airway resistance may occur. Be prepared to assist with alternative therapy and respiratory support.

Client/Family Teaching

1. Explain the appropriate technique for use and care of prescribed inhalers and respiratory equipment.
2. Demonstrate how to accomplish postural drainage. Explain how to cough productively and show family how to clap and vibrate the chest to promote good respiratory hygiene.
3. Stress that regular, consistent use of the medication is essential for maximum benefit, but overuse can be life-threatening.
4. Advise that to improve lung ventilation and reduce fatigue during eating, start respiratory therapy upon arising in the morning and before meals.
5. Stress that a single aerosol treatment is usually enough to control an asthma attack. Overuse of adrenergic bronchodilators may result in reduced effectiveness, possible paradoxical reaction, and death from cardiac arrest.
6. Advise that increased fluid intake will aid in liquefying secretions, facilitating removal.
7. Consult provider if dizziness or chest pain occurs, or if there is no relief when the usual dose of medication is used.
8. Avoid OTC preparations and any other adrenergic medications unless expressly ordered.
9. Consult provider if more than three aerosol treatments in a 24-hr period are required for relief.
10. For clients using inhalable medications and bronchodilators, advise to use the bronchodilator first and to wait 5 min before administering the other medication.
11. Advise client to **stop smoking,** avoid crowds during "flu seasons," to dress warmly in cold weather, to receive the pneumonia vaccine and seasonal flu shot, and to stay in air conditioning during hot, humid days to prevent exacerbations of illness.
12. Instruct family/significant other in CPR.

Evaluate

• Knowledge and understanding of illness and evidence of compliance with prescribed medication regimen
• A positive clinical response as evidenced by ↓ symptoms for which

---

the therapy was originally prescribed

TETRACYCLINES

See also the following individual entries:

Doxycycline calcium
Doxycycline hyclate
Doxycycline monohydrate
Tetracycline
Tetracycline hydrochloride

Action/Kinetics: The tetracyclines inhibit protein synthesis by microorganisms by binding to a crucial ribosomal subunit (50S), thereby interfering with protein synthesis. The drugs block the binding of aminoacyl transfer RNA to the messenger RNA complex. Cell wall synthesis is not inhibited. The drugs are mostly bacteriostatic and are effective only against multiplying bacteria. Tetracyclines are well absorbed from the stomach and upper small intestine. They are well distributed throughout all tissues and fluids and diffuse through noninflamed meninges and the placental barrier. They become deposited in the fetal skeleton and calcifying teeth. **t½:** 7–18.6 hr (see individual agents) and is increased in the presence of renal impairment. The drugs bind to serum protein (range: 20%–93%; see individual agents). The drugs are concentrated in the liver in the bile and are excreted mostly unchanged in the urine and feces.

Uses: Used mainly for infections caused by *Rickettsia, Chlamydia,* and *Mycoplasma.* Due to development of resistance, tetracyclines are usually not used for infections by common gram-negative or gram-positive organisms.

Tetracyclines are the drugs of choice for rickettsial infections such as Rocky Mountain spotted fever, endemic typhus, and others. They are also the drugs of choice for psittacosis, lymphogranuloma venereum, and urethritis due to *Mycoplasma hominis* and *Ureaplasma urealyti-*

cum. Epididymo-orchitis due to *Chlamydia trachomatis* and/or *Neisseria gonorrhoeae.* Atypical pneumonia caused by *Mycoplasma pneumoniae.* Adjunct in the treatment of trachoma.

Tetracyclines are the drugs of choice for gram-negative bacteria causing bartonellosis, brucellosis, granuloma inguinale, cholera. They are used as alternatives for the treatment of plague, tularemia, chancroid, or *Campylobacter fetus* infections. Prophylaxis of plague after exposure. Infections caused by *Acinetobacter, Bacteroides, Enterobacter aerogenes, Escherichia coli, Shigella.* Respiratory and/or urinary tract infections caused by *Haemophilus influenzae* or *Klebsiella pneumoniae.*

As an alternative to penicillin for uncomplicated gonorrhea or disseminated gonococcal infections, especially with penicillin allergy. Acute pelvic inflammatory disease. Tetracyclines are also useful as an alternative to penicillin for early syphilis.

Although not generally used for gram-positive infections, tetracyclines may be beneficial in anthrax, *Listeria* infections, and actinomycosis. They have also been used in conjunction with quinine sulfate for chloroquine-resistant *Plasmodium falciparum* malaria and as an intracavitary injection to control pleural or pericardial effusions caused by metastatic carcinoma. As an adjunct to amebicides in acute intestinal amebiasis. Used PO to treat uncomplicated endocervical, rectal, or urethral *Chlamydia* infections.

Topical uses include skin granulomas caused by *Mycobacterium marinum;* ophthalmic bacterial infections causing blepharitis, conjunctivitis, or keratitis; and as an adjunct in the treatment of ophthalmic chlamydial infections such as trachoma or inclusion conjunctivitis. Tetracyclines are used as an alternative to silver nitrate for prophylaxis of neonatal gonococcal ophthalmia. Vaginitis. Severe acne.

Contraindications: Hypersensitivity; avoid drug during tooth development stage (last trimester of pregnancy, neonatal period, during breast-feeding, and during childhood up to 8 years) because tetracyclines interfere with enamel formation and dental pigmentation. Never administer intrathecally.

Special Concerns: Use with caution and at reduced dosage in clients with impaired kidney function.

Side Effects: *GI* (most common): N&V, thirst, diarrhea, anorexia, sore throat, flatulence, epigastric distress, bulky loose stools. Less commonly, stomatitis, dysphagia, black hairy tongue, glossitis, or inflammatory lesions of the anogenital area. Rarely, pseudomembranous colitis. PO dosage forms may cause esophageal ulcers, especially in clients with esophageal obstructive element or hiatal hernia. *Allergic* (rare): Urticaria, pericarditis, polyarthralgia, fever, rash, pulmonary infiltrates with eosinophilia, **angioneurotic edema,** worsening of SLE, **anaphylaxis,** purpura. *Skin:* Photosensitivity, maculopapular and erythematous rashes, exfoliative dermatitis (rare), onycholysis, discoloration of nails. *CNS:* Dizziness, lightheadedness, unsteadiness, paresthesias. *Hematologic:* Eosinophilia, **hemolytic anemia,** neutropenia, thrombocytopenia, thrombocytopenic purpura. *Hepatic:* Fatty liver, increases in liver enzymes; rarely, hepatotoxicity, hepatitis, hepatic cholestasis. *Miscellaneous:* Candidal superinfections including oral and vaginal candidiasis, discoloration of infants' and children's teeth, bone lesions, delayed bone growth, abnormal pigmentation of the conjunctiva, pseudotumor cerebri in adults and bulging fontanels in infants.

IV administration may cause thrombophlebitis; IM injections are painful and may cause induration at the injection site.

The administration of deteriorated tetracyclines may result in Fanconi-like syndrome characterized by N&V, acidosis, proteinuria, glycosuria, aminoaciduria, polydipsia, polyuria, hypokalemia.

Drug Interactions

Aluminum salts / ↓ Effect of tetracyclines due to ↓ absorption from GI tract

Antacids, oral / ↓ Effect of tetracyclines due to ↓ absorption from GI tract

Anticoagulants, oral / IV tetracyclines ↑ hypoprothrombinemia

Bismuth salts / ↓ Effect of tetracyclines due to ↓ absorption from GI tract

Bumetanide / ↑ Risk of kidney toxicity

Calcium salts / ↓ Effect of tetracyclines due to ↓ absorption from GI tract

Cimetidine / ↓ Effect of tetracyclines due to ↓ absorption from GI tract

Contraceptives, oral / ↓ Effect of oral contraceptives

Digoxin / Tetracyclines ↑ bioavailability of digoxin

Diuretics, thiazide / ↑ Risk of kidney toxicity

Ethacrynic acid / ↑ Risk of kidney toxicity

Furosemide / ↑ Risk of kidney toxicity

Insulin / Tetracyclines may ↓ insulin requirement

Iron preparations / ↓ Effect of tetracyclines due to ↓ absorption from GI tract

Lithium / Either ↑ or ↓ levels of lithium

Magnesium salts / ↓ Effect of tetracyclines due to ↓ absorption from GI tract

Methoxyflurane / ↑ Risk of kidney toxicity

Penicillins / Tetracyclines may mask bactericidal effect of penicillins

Sodium bicarbonate / ↓ Effect of tetracyclines due to ↓ absorption from GI tract

Zinc salts / ↓ Effect of tetracyclines due to ↓ absorption from GI tract

Laboratory Test Interferences:
False + or ↑ urinary catecholamines and urinary protein (degraded); ↑ coagulation time. False − or ↓ urinary urobilinogen, glucose tests (see *Respiratory Care Considerations*). Prolonged use or high doses may change liver function tests and WBC counts.

Dosage
See individual drugs.

RESPIRATORY CARE CONSIDERATIONS

See also *General Respiratory Care Considerations for All Anti-Infectives*.

Administration/Storage
1. Do not use outdated or deteriorated drugs because a Fanconi-like syndrome may occur (see *Side Effects*).
2. Discard unused capsules to prevent use of deteriorated medication.
3. Administer IM into large muscle mass to avoid extravasation into subcutaneous or fatty tissue.
4. Administer on an empty stomach at least 1 hr before or 2 hr after meals. Withhold antacids, iron salts, dairy foods, and other foods high in calcium for at least 2 hr after PO administration. Do not administer milk with tetracyclines.

Assessment
1. Determine any drug allergens or sensitivity. Be aware that IM form contains procaine HCl.
2. Document indications for therapy and type and onset of symptoms. List other agents prescribed and the outcome.
3. Assess for and note any evidence of impaired kidney function.
4. Determine if client has any history of colitis or other bowel problems.
5. If the client is pregnant, determine the trimester.
6. Note symptoms of infection and ensure that baseline lab studies have been performed, including CBC, BUN, creatinine, C&S, etc.
7. Document baseline VS and weights.

Interventions
1. If client experiences gastric distress following administration of medication, suggest that they be permitted to have a light meal with the medication to reduce distress. An alternative would be to reduce the individual dose of the medication but increase the frequency of administration.
2. Monitor VS and I&O. Maintain adequate I&O because renal dysfunction may result in drug accumulation, leading to toxicity. Assess client with impaired renal function for increased BUN, acidosis, anorexia, N&V, weight loss, and dehydration. Continue assessment after cessation of therapy because latent symptoms may appear.
3. To prevent or treat pruritus ani instruct and assist client to cleanse the anal area with water several times a day and/or after each bowel movement. Observe for symptoms of enterocolitis, such as diarrhea, pyrexia, abdominal distention, and scanty urine. These symptoms may necessitate discontinuing drug and substituting another antibiotic.
4. If GI disturbances occur, avoid antacids that contain calcium, magnesium, or aluminum.
5. Assess client on IV therapy for N&V, chills, fever, and hypertension resulting from too rapid administration or an excessively high dose. Slow rate of IV infusion and report if symptoms occur.
6. Observe infant for bulging fontanelle, which may be caused by a too rapid rate of IV infusion. Slow IV infusion rate and report.
7. Side effects such as sore throat, dysphagia, fever, dizziness, hoarseness, and inflammation of mucous membranes of the body may be candidal superinfections and should be reported.
8. Assess client with impaired hepatic or renal function for altered level of consciousness or other CNS disturbances, as drug may cause hepatic and renal toxicity.
9. Observe for onycholysis (loosening or detachment of the nail from the nail

bed) or discoloration and take appropriate precautions.

Evaluate

• Knowledge and understanding of illness and evidence of compliance with prescribed therapy

• Resolution of infection ($\downarrow$ temperature, $\downarrow$ WBCs, $\uparrow$ appetite)

• Reports of symptomatic improvement

• Negative C&S reports and no evidence of organism resistance to drug therapy

THEOPHYLLINE DERIVATIVES

See also the following individual entries:

    Aminophylline
    Theophylline

General Statement: Asthma is a disease characterized by difficulty in breathing, resulting from smooth muscle contraction of the bronchi and bronchioles, edema of the mucosa of the respiratory tract, or mucous secretions that adhere to the walls of the bronchi and bronchioles. The cause of asthma is not known with certainty but, in some clients, allergy is the underlying reason.

The overall objectives of drug therapy for asthma are to open blocked airways and to alter the characteristics of respiratory tract fluid. The drugs and drug classes used to treat asthma are bronchodilators, such as theophyllines and sympathomimetic amines, mucolytics, corticosteroids, and cromolyn sodium.

Action/Kinetics: The theophylline derivatives are plant alkaloids, which, like caffeine, belong to the xanthine family. They stimulate the CNS, directly relax the smooth muscles of the bronchi and pulmonary blood vessels (relieve bronchospasms), produce diuresis, inhibit uterine contractions, stimulate gastric acid secretion, and increase the rate and force of contraction of the heart. The bronchodilator activity of theophyllines is due to direct relaxation of the bronchiolar smooth muscle and pulmonary blood vessels, which relieves bronchospasm. The theophylline was thought to act by inhibiting phosphodiesterase, which resulted in an increase in cyclic adenosine monophosphate (cAMP). cAMP increased the release of endogenous epinephrine resulting in bronchodilation. However, this effect is negligible at doses used clinically. Although the exact mechanism is not known, theophyllines may act by altering the calcium levels of smooth muscle, blocking adenosine receptors, inhibiting the effect of prostaglandins on smooth muscle, and inhibiting the release of slow-reacting substance of anaphylaxis and histamine. Aminophylline, oxtriphylline, and theophylline sodium glycinate release free theophylline in vivo. Response to the drugs is highly individualized. Theophylline is well absorbed from uncoated plain tablets and PO liquids. *Theophylline salts:* **Onset:** 1–5 hr, depending on route and formulation. **Therapeutic plasma levels:** 10–20 mcg/mL. **t½:** 3–15 hr in nonsmoking adults, 4–5 hr in adult heavy smokers, 1–9 hr in children, and 20–30 hr for premature neonates. An increased **t½** may be seen in individuals with CHF, alcoholism, liver dysfunction, or respiratory infections. Because of great variations in the rate of absorption (due to dosage form, food, dose level) as well as its extremely narrow therapeutic range, theophylline therapy is best monitored by determination of the serum levels. If these determinations cannot be obtained, saliva (contains 60% of corresponding theophylline serum levels) determinations can be used. 85%–90% metabolized in the liver and various metabolites, including the active 3-methylxanthine. Theophylline is metabolized partially to caffeine in the neonate. The premature neonate excretes 50% unchanged theophylline and may accumulate the caffeine metabolite. Excretion is through the kidneys (about 10% unchanged in adults).

Uses: Prophylaxis and treatment of bronchial asthma. Reversible bronchospasms associated with chronic bronchitis, emphysema, and COPD. *Investigational:* Treatment of neonatal apnea and Cheyne-Stokes respiration.

Contraindications: Hypersensitivity to any xanthine, peptic ulcer, seizure disorders (unless on medication), hypotension, CAD, angina pectoris.

Special Concerns: Use during lactation may result in irritability, insomnia, and fretfulness in the infant. Use with caution in premature infants due to the possible accumulation of caffeine. Xanthines are not usually tolerated by small children because of excessive CNS stimulation. Geriatric clients may manifest an increased risk of toxicity. Use with caution in the presence of gastritis, alcoholism, acute cardiac diseases, hypoxemia, severe renal and hepatic disease, severe hypertension, severe myocardial damage, hyperthyroidism, glaucoma.

Side Effects: Side effects are uncommon at serum theophylline levels less than 20 mcg/mL. At levels greater than 20 mcg/mL, 75% of individuals experience side effects including N&V, diarrhea, irritability, insomnia, and headache. At levels of 35 mcg/mL or greater, individuals may manifest *cardiac arrhythmias,* hypotension, tachycardia, hyperglycemia, *seizures, brain damage, or death. GI:* N&V, diarrhea, anorexia, epigastric pain, hematemesis, dyspepsia, rectal irritation (following use of suppositories), rectal bleeding, gastroesophageal reflux during sleep or while recumbent (theophylline). *CNS:* Headache, insomnia, irritability, fever, dizziness, lightheadedness, vertigo, reflex hyperexcitability, *seizures,* depression, speech abnormalities, alternating periods of mutism and hyperactivity, *brain damage, death. CV:* Hypotension, *life-threatening ventricular arrhythmias,* palpitations, tachycardia, *peripheral vascular collapse,* extrasystoles. *Renal:* Proteinuria, excretion of erythrocytes and renal tubular cells, dehydration due to diuresis, urinary retention (men with prostatic hypertrophy). *Other:* Tachypnea, *respiratory arrest,* fever, flushing, hyperglycemia, antidiuretic hormone syndrome, leukocytosis, rash, alopecia.

NOTE: Aminophylline given by rapid IV may produce hypotension, flushing, palpitations, precordial pain, headache, dizziness, or hyperventilation. Also, the ethylenediamine in aminophylline may cause allergic reactions, including urticaria and skin rashes.

OD **Overdose Management:** *Symptoms:* Agitation, headache, nervousness, insomnia, tachycardia, extrasystoles, anorexia, N&V, fasciculations, tachypnea, *tonic-clonic seizures.* The first signs of toxicity may be seizures or ventricular arrhythmias. Toxicity is usually associated with parenteral administration but can be observed after PO administration, especially in children. *Treatment:*

• Have ipecac syrup, gastric lavage equipment, and cathartics available to treat overdose if the client is conscious and not having seizures. Otherwise a mechanical ventilator, oxygen, diazepam, and IV fluids may be necessary for the treatment of overdosage.

• For postseizure coma, an airway must be maintained and the client oxygenated. To remove the drug, perform only gastric lavage and give the cathartic and activated charcoal by a large bore gastric lavage tube. Charcoal hemoperfusion may be necessary.

• Atrial arrhythmias may be treated with verapamil and ventricular arrhythmias may be treated with lidocaine or procainamide.

• IV fluids are used to treat acid-base imbalance, hypotension, and dehydration. Hypotension may also be treated with vasopressors.

• Tepid water sponge baths or a hypothermic blanket are used to treat hyperpyrexia.

• Apnea is treated with artificial respiration.

• Serum levels of theophylline must be monitored until they fall below 20 mcg/mL as secondary rises of theophylline may occur, especially with sustained-release products.

Drug Interactions

Allopurinol / ↑ Theophylline levels

Aminogluthethimide / ↓ Theophylline levels

Barbiturates / ↓ Theophylline levels

Benzodiazepines / Sedative effect may be antagonized by theophylline

Beta-adrenergic agonists / Additive effects

Beta-adrenergic blocking agents / ↑ Theophylline levels

Calcium channel blocking drugs / ↑ Theophylline levels

Carbamazepine / Either ↑ or ↓ theophylline levels

Charcoal / ↓ Theophylline levels

Cimetidine / ↑ Theophylline levels

Ciprofloxacin / ↑ Plasma levels of theophylline with ↑ possibility of side effects

Corticosteroids / ↑ Theophylline levels

Digitalis / Theophylline ↑ toxicity of digitalis

Disulfram / ↑ Theophylline levels

Ephedrine and other sympathomimetics / ↑ Theophylline levels

Erythromycin / ↑ Effect of theophylline due to ↓ breakdown by liver

Ethacrynic acid / Either ↑ or ↓ theophylline levels

Furosemide / Either ↑ or ↓ theophylline levels

Halothane / ↑ Risk of cardiac arrhythmias

Interferon / ↑ Theophylline levels

Isoniazid / Either ↑ or ↓ theophylline levels

Ketamine / Seizures of the extensor-type

Ketoconazole / ↓ Theophylline levels

Lithium / ↓ Effect of lithium due to ↑ rate of excretion

Loop diuretics / ↓ Theophylline levels

Mexiletine / ↑ Theophylline levels

Muscle relaxants, nondepolarizing / Theophylline ↓ effect of these drugs

Oral contraceptives / ↑ Effect of theophyllines due to ↓ breakdown by liver

Phenytoin / ↓ Theophylline levels

Propofol / Theophyllines ↓ sedative effect of propofol

Quinolones / ↑ Theophylline levels

Reserpine / ↑ Risk of tachycardia

Rifampin / ↓ Theophylline levels

Sulfinpyrazone / ↓ Theophylline levels

Sympathomimetics / ↓ Theophylline levels

Tetracyclines / ↑ Risk of theophylline toxicity

Thiabendazole / ↑ Theophylline levels

Thyroid hormones / ↓ Theophylline levels in hypothyroid clients

Tobacco smoking / ↓ Effect of theophylline due to ↑ breakdown by liver

Troleandomycin / ↑ Effect of theophylline due to ↓ breakdown by liver

Verapamil / ↑ Effect of theophyllines

Laboratory Test Interferences: ↑ Plasma free fatty acids, bilirubin, urinary catecholamines, erythrocyte sedimentation rate. Interference with uric acid tests and tests for furosemide, probenecid, theobromine, and phenylbutazone.

Dosage

Individualized. Initially, dosage should be adjusted according to plasma level of drug. Usual: 10–20 mcg theophylline/mL plasma. The dose of the various salts should be equivalent based on the content of anhydrous theophylline. See individual agents.

RESPIRATORY CARE CONSIDERATIONS

Administration/Storage

1. Review the list of agents with which theophylline derivatives interact.

2. Dilute drugs and maintain proper infusion rates to minimize problems of overdosage. Use an infusion pump to regulate infusion rate of IV solutions.

3. Wait to initiate PO therapy for at least 4–6 hr after switching from IV therapy.

Assessment

1. Assess the client for any history of hypersensitivity to xanthine compounds.

2. Document indications for therapy and type and onset of symptoms. List other agents prescribed and the outcome.

3. Determine any previous experience with this class of drugs and the outcome.

4. Note if the client has any history of hypotension, CAD, angina, PUD, or seizure disorders. These drugs should be avoided or used very cautiously in these conditions.

5. Determine if the client smokes cigarettes or has a history of smoking marijuana. These habits induce hepatic metabolism of the drug. Smokers require an increase in the dosage of drug from 50%–100%.

6. Assess diet habits because these can influence the excretion of theophylline. A client eating a high-protein and/or low-carbohydrate diet will have an increased excretion of the drug. Clients eating a low-protein and/or high-carbohydrate diet will have a decrease in the excretion of theophylline. Therefore, dietary intake is an important part of the premedication assessment.

7. Obtain baseline BP and pulse prior to starting drug therapy.

8. Assess lung fields closely and describe findings. Note characteristics of the sputum, cough, and pulmonary function tests.

Interventions

1. Monitor BP and pulse closely during therapy and report any significant changes.

2. Observe closely for signs of toxicity such as nausea, anorexia, insomnia, irritability, hyperexcitability, or cardiac arrhythmias; monitor serum levels.

3. Observe small children in particular for excessive CNS stimulation; children often are unable to report side effects.

Client/Family Teaching

1. To avoid epigastric pain, take with a snack or with meals.

2. Take the medication ATC and only as prescribed, because more is *not* better.

3. Advise to report if nausea, vomiting, GI pain, or restlessness occurs. Avoid or minimize consumption of charbroiled foods (e.g., burgers).

4. **Do not smoke** because smoking may aggravate underlying medical conditions as well as interfere with drug absorption. Refer to a formal (behavior modification) smoking cessation program.

5. Explain to clients how to protect themselves from acute exacerbations of illness by avoiding crowds, dressing warmly in cold weather, obtaining the pneumonia vaccine and seasonal flu shot, covering their mouth and nose so that cold air is not directly inhaled, staying in air conditioning during excessively hot and humid weather, maintaining proper diet and nutrition and adequate fluid intake.

6. Provide written guidelines that identify the early S&S of infections, adverse side effects of drug therapy, and when to call the provider.

7. Reinforce that when secretions become thick and tacky, clients should increase their intake of fluids. This thins secretions and assists in their removal.

8. Advise client to pace activity and to avoid overexertion at all times.

9. Instruct to hold medication and report immediately any side effects or CNS depression in children and infants.

10. Review dietary restrictions and advise to limit intake of xanthine-

containing products such as coffee, colas, and chocolate.

11. Identify support groups that may assist client to understand and cope with chronic respiratory dysfunction.

Evaluate

• Knowledge and understanding of illness and level of compliance with prescribed regimen

• Evidence of a positive clinical response characterized by improved pulmonary function, ↓ wheezing, and reports of improved breathing patterns

• Laboratory confirmation that serum drug levels are within therapeutic range (10–20 mcg/mL)

(Page 96 is blank)

CHAPTER 3
A–Z Listing of Drugs

A

Acebutolol hydrochloride
(ays-**BYOU**-toe-lohl)
Pregnancy Category: B
Monitan ✽, Rhotral ✽, Sectral **(Rx)**
Classification: Beta-adrenergic blocking agent

See also *Beta-Adrenergic Blocking Agents*.
Action/Kinetics: Predominantly beta-1 blocking activity but will inhibit beta-2 receptors at higher doses. Acebutolol also has some intrinsic sympathomimetic activity. **t½:** 3–4 hr. Low lipid solubility. **Duration:** 24–30 hr. Metabolized in liver and excreted in urine and bile. Fifteen to 20% excreted unchanged.
Uses: Hypertension (either alone or with other antihypertensive agents such as thiazide diuretics). Premature ventricular contractions.
Additional Contraindications: Severe, persistent bradycardia.
Special Concerns: Dosage has not been established in children.

Dosage ―――――――――
• **Capsules**
Hypertension.
Initial: 400 mg/day (although 200 mg b.i.d. may be needed for optimum control; **then,** 400–800 mg/day (range: 200–1,200 mg/day).
Premature ventricular contractions.
Initial: 200 mg b.i.d.; **then,** increase dose gradually to reach 600–1,200 mg/day.
Dosage should be decreased in geriatric clients (should not exceed 800 mg/day) and in those with impaired kidney or liver function (decrease dose by 50% when creatinine clearance is 50 mL/min/1.73 m² and by 75% when it is less than 25 mL/min/1.73 m²).

RESPIRATORY CARE CONSIDERATIONS

See also *Respiratory Care Considerations* for *Beta-Adrenergic Blocking Agents*, and *Antihypertensive Agents*.
Administration/Storage
1. When treatment is discontinued, the drug should be withdrawn gradually over a 2-week period.
2. The bioavailability increases in elderly clients; thus, such clients may require lower maintenance doses (no more than 800 mg/day).
3. Acebutolol may be combined with another antihypertensive agent.
4. Anticipate reduced dosage in clients with impaired liver and renal function.
Evaluate
• ↓ BP
• Resolution of PVCs

Acetylcysteine
(ah-see-till-**SIS**-tay-een)
Pregnancy Category: B
Mucomyst, Mucosol, Parvolex **(Rx)**
Classification: Mucolytic

Action/Kinetics: Acetylcysteine reduces the viscosity of purulent and nonpurulent pulmonary secretions and facilitates their removal by splitting disulfide bonds. Action increases

―――――――――――――――――――――
✽ = Available in Canada   ***bold italic*** = life threatening side effect

with increasing pH (peak: pH 7–9).
Onset, inhalation: Within 1 min;
by direct instillation: immediate.
Time to peak effect: 5–10 min.

Uses: Adjunct in the treatment of
acute and chronic bronchitis, emphysema, tuberculosis, pneumonia,
bronchiectasis, atelectasis. Routine
care of clients with tracheostomy,
pulmonary complications after thoracic or CV surgery, or in posttraumatic chest conditions. Pulmonary complications of cystic fibrosis. Diagnostic bronchial asthma. Antidote in
acetaminophen poisoning to reduce
hepatotoxicity. *Investigational:* As
an ophthalmic solution for dry eye.

Contraindications: Sensitivity to
drug.

Special Concerns: Use with caution during lactation, in the elderly,
and in clients with asthma.

Side Effects: *Respiratory:* Acetylcysteine increases the incidence of
bronchospasm in clients with asthma. The drug may also increase the
amount of liquefied bronchial secretions, which must be removed by
suction if cough is inadequate. Bronchial and tracheal irritation, tightness
in chest, bronchoconstriction. *GI:*
N&V, stomatitis. *Other:* Rashes, fever, drowsiness, rhinorrhea.

Drug Interactions: Acetylcysteine
is incompatible with antibiotics and
should be administered separately.

Dosage ─────────────────
• **Nebulization, Direct Application, or Direct Intratracheal Instillation Using 10% or 20% Solution**
*Nebulization into face mask,
tracheostomy, mouth piece.*
1–10 mL of 20% solution or 2–10 mL
of 10% solution 3–4 times/day.
Closed tent or croupette.
Up to 300 mL of 10% or 20% solu-
tion/treatment.
*Direct instillation into tracheosto-
my.*
1–2 mL of 10%–20% solution q 1–4 hr.
*Percutaneous intratracheal cath-
eter.*
1–2 mL of 20% solution or 2–4 mL of

10% solution q 1–4 hr by syringe attached to catheter.
*Instillation to particular portion of
bronchopulmonary tree using small
plastic catheter into the trachea.*
2–5 mL of 20% solution instilled into
the trachea by means of a syringe
connected to a catheter.
Diagnostic procedures.
2–3 doses of 1–2 mL of 20% or 2–4 mL
of 10% solution by nebulization or
intratracheal instillation before the
procedure.
Acetaminophen overdose.
Given PO, initial: 140   mg/kg;
then, 70 mg/kg q 4 hr for a total of
17 doses.

RESPIRATORY CARE CONSIDERATIONS
Administration/Storage
1. Use nonreactive plastic, glass, or
stainless steel equipment for administration.
2. The 10% solution may be used
undiluted.
3. Use either water for injection or saline to dilute the 20% solution.
4. Administer the medication via
face mask, face tent, oxygen tent,
head tent, or by positive-pressure
breathing apparatus as indicated.
5. Administer with compressed air
for nebulization. Hand bulb nebulizers or heated nebulizers should not be
used.
6. After prolonged nebulization, dilute
the last fourth of the medication
with sterile water for injection to
prevent concentration of the medication.
7. The solution may develop a light
purple color. This does not affect
the action of the medication.
8. Closed bottles of solution remain
stable for 2 years when stored at
20°C (68°F). Open bottles should be
stored at 2°C–8°C (35°F–46°F) and
should be used within 96 hr. Once a
bottle has been opened, record the
time and date of opening so that the
drug will not be used beyond the
96-hr period.
9. Acetylcysteine is incompatible
with antibiotics and must be administered separately.

10. Have an ET tube available and a suction machine at the bedside for removal of increased bronchial secretions.

11. If nebulized into a face mask, the client's face should be washed off to remove any sticky residue.

12. Rinse nebulizer after each treatment to prevent drug concentration due to evaporation.

Assessment

1. Determine from the client and history, or through observation and assessment, when bronchial spasms occur.

2. Discuss conditions likely to cause congestion and wheezing and document.

3. Identify the previous approaches (successful and unsuccessful) used in treating client conditions.

4. Determine if the client is currently taking any antibiotic medications.

5. Document time of acetaminophen overdose. Drug should be administered within 8–10 hr following overdose to protect from hepatoxicity and death. Monitor liver function tests and acetaminophen levels.

Interventions

1. If bronchospasm occurs, have a bronchodilator, such as isoproterenol for aerosol inhalation, readily available. In clients with a history of bronchospasm, β-agonists may be administered prior to or concurrent with acetylcysteine.

2. Position the client to facilitate the removal of secretions.

3. If the client is unable to cough up secretions, provide mechanical suction for their removal.

4. Monitor VS and I&O.

5. Wash the client's face following nebulization treatment. The medication may cause the face to become sticky.

6. The administration route for acetaminophen toxicity is oral and will consist of 17 doses.

Client/Family Teaching

1. Use only as directed; do not exceed prescribed dosage.

2. Report any unusual changes in color, consistency, or characteristics of sputum.

3. Avoid any triggers that may stimulate bronchospasm (i.e., cigarette smoke, dust, chemicals, cold air).

Evaluate

• Improved airway exchange with ↓ viscosity and mobilization and expectoration of secretions

• ↓ Acetaminophen levels and associated liver toxicity when used as an antidote with overdosage

Adenosine

(ah-**DEN**-oh-seen)
Pregnancy Category: C
Adenocard, Adenoscan **(Rx)**
Classification: Antiarrhythmic

See also *Antiarrhythmic Agents.*

Action/Kinetics: Adenosine is found naturally in all cells of the body. The substance slows conduction time through the AV node, interrupts the reentry pathways through the AV node, and restores normal sinus rhythm in paroxysmal supraventricular tachycardia (including Wolff-Parkinson-White syndrome). Adenosine is competitively antagonized by caffeine, theophylline, and dipyridamole. **Onset, after IV:** 34 sec. **t½:** Less than 10 sec (taken up by erythrocytes and vascular endothelial cells). **Duration:** 1–2 min. Exogenous adenosine becomes part of the body pool and is metabolized mainly to inosine and AMP.

Uses: Conversion of sinus rhythm of paroxysmal SVT (including that associated with accessory bypass tracts). The phosphate salt is used for symptomatic relief of complications with stasis dermatitis in varicose veins. *Investigational:* With thallium-201 tomography in noninvasive assessment of clients with suspected CAD who cannot exercise adequately prior to being stress-tested. Adenosine is not effective in converting rhythms other than paroxysmal SVT. The phosphate salt has been used to treat herpes infections and to increase blood flow to brain tumors and in porphyria cutanea tarda. **Contraindications:** Second- or third-degree AV block or sick sinus syndrome (except in clients with a functioning artificial pacemaker). Also, atrial flutter, atrial fibrillation, ventricular tachycardia. History of MI or cerebral hemorrhage.

Special Concerns: At time of conversion to normal sinus rhythm, new rhythms (PVC, atrial premature contractions, sinus bradycardia, skipped beats, varying degrees of AV block, sinus tachycardia) lasting a few seconds may occur. Use with caution in clients with asthma. Safety and efficacy as a diagnostic agent have not been determined in clients less than 18 years of age.

Side Effects: *CV:* Short lasting first-, second-, or ***third-degree heart block; cardiac arrest*** , a sustained ventricular tachycardia, sinus bradycardia, ST-segment depression, sinus exit block, sinus pause, arrhythmias, T-wave changes, hypertension. prolonged asystole, Nonfatal MI, transient increase in BP, ***ventricular fibrillation***. Facial flushing (common), chest pain, sweating, palpitations, hypotension (may be significant). *CNS:* Lightheadedness, dizziness, numbness, headache, blurred vision, apprehension, paresthesia, drowsiness, emotional instability, tremors, nervousness. *GI:* Nausea, metallic taste, tightness in throat. *Respiratory:* SOB or dyspnea (common), urge to breathe deeply, chest pressure or discomfort, cough, hyperventilation, nasal congestion. *GU:* Urinary urgency, vaginal pressure. *Miscellaneous:* Pressure in head, burning sensation, neck and back pain, weakness, blurred vision, dry mouth, ear discomfort, pressure in groin, scotomas, tongue discomfort, discomfort (tingling, heaviness) in upper extremities, discomfort in throat, neck, or jaw.

Drug Interactions
Carbamazepine / ↑ Degree of heart block

Caffeine / Competitively antagonizes effect of adenosine
Digitalis / Possibility of ventricular fibrillation (rare)
Dipyridamole / ↑ Effect of adenosine
Theophylline / Competitively antagonizes effect of adenosine

Dosage ─────────────
• **Rapid IV Bolus Only**
  Antiarrhythmic.
Initial: 6 mg over 1–2 sec. If the first dose does not reverse the SVT within 1–2 min, 12 mg should be given as a rapid IV bolus. The 12-mg dose may be repeated a second time, if necessary. Doses greater than 12 mg are not recommended.
• **IV Infusion Only**
  Diagnostic aid.
Adults: 140 mcg/kg/min infused over 6 min (total dose of 0.84 mg/kg).
• **IM Only**
  Varicose veins.
Initial: 25–50 mg 1–2 times daily until symptoms subside. **Maintenance:** 25 mg 2 or 3 times weekly.

RESPIRATORY CARE CONSIDERATIONS

See also *Respiratory Care Considerations* for *Antiarrhythmic Agents.*

Administration/Storage
1. Store at room temperature. Do not refrigerate as crystallization may occur. If crystallization occurs, the product should be warmed to room temperature.
2. The solution should be clear at the time of use.
3. Discard any unused portion because the product contains no preservatives.
4. The drug should be administered directly into a vein. If it is to be given into an IV line, introduce the drug in the most proximal line and follow with a rapid saline flush.
5. When used as a diagnostic aid, the dose of thallium-201 should be given at the midpoint of the adenosine infusion (i.e., after 3 min).

Assessment
1. Document indications for thera-

py, onset of symptoms, and ECG confirmation of arrhythmia.

2. Client should be on a cardiac monitor during drug administration.

3. In stasis dermatitis carefully assess extremities and note findings.

Interventions

1. Document client complaints of chest pressure, SOB, heaviness of the arms, palpitations, or dyspnea. Note any history of MI or CVA as drug is contraindicated.

2. Report any facial flushing. Reassure client that this is a common side effect of therapy.

3. Monitor BP and pulse. If client complains of numbness, tingling in the arms, blurred vision, or appears apprehensive, report as this may be an indication to discontinue drug therapy.

4. Avoid caffeine and note if concurrently prescribed theophylline, digoxin, or dipyridamole.

5. Monitor ECG rhythm strips closely for evidence of varying degrees of AV block and increased arrhythmias during conversion to sinus rhythm. These are usually only transient.

Evaluate

• Conversion of paroxysmal SVT to NSR

• Symptomatic relief when used for stasis dermatitis

Albuterol (Salbutamol)

(al-**BYOU**-ter-ohl)

Pregnancy Category: C

Apo-Salvent Inhaler ✦, Novo-Salmol Inhaler ✦, Proventil, Proventil HFA—3M, Proventil Repetabs, Sabulin ✦, Ventolin, Ventolin Rotacaps, Volmax **(Rx)**

Classification: Direct-acting adrenergic (sympathomimetic) agent

See also *Sympathomimetic Drugs.*

Action/Kinetics: Albuterol stimulates beta-2 receptors of the bronchi, leading to bronchodilation. Causes less tachycardia and is longer-acting than isoproterenol. Has minimal beta-1 activity. Albuterol sulfate is now available as an inhaler that con-

tains no chlorofluorocarbons (Proventil HFA–3M). **Onset, PO:** 15–30 min; **inhalation,** 5–15 min. **Peak effect, PO:** 2–3 hr; **inhalation,** 60–90 min (after 2 inhalations). **Duration, PO:** 8 hr (up to 12 hr for extended-release); **inhalation,** 3–6 hr. Metabolites and unchanged drug excreted in urine and feces. Tablets not to be used in children less than 12 years of age.

Uses: Bronchial asthma; bronchospasm due to bronchitis or emphysema; bronchitis; reversible obstructive pulmonary disease in those 4 years of age and older; exercise-induced bronchospasm. Prophylaxis of bronchial asthma or bronchospasms. Parenteral for treatment of status asthmaticus. *Investigational:* Nebulized albuterol may be useful as an adjunct to treat serious acute hyperkalemia in hemodialysis clients.

Additional   Contraindications: Use during lactation.

Special Concerns: Dosage has not been established for the syrup in children less than 2 years of age, for tablets in children less than 6 years of age, and for extended-release tablets in children less than 12 years of age. Aerosol for prevention of exercise-induced bronchospasm is not recommended for children less than 12 years of age. Albuterol may delay preterm labor.

Additional Side Effects: *GI:* Diarrhea, dry mouth, increased appetite, epigastric pain. *CNS:* CNS stimulation, malaise, emotional lability, fatigue, lightheadedness, nightmares, disturbed sleep, aggressive behavior, irritability. *Respiratory:* Bronchitis, epistaxis, hoarseness (especially in children), nasal congestion, increase in sputum. *Hypersensitivity (may be immediate):* Urticaria, *angioedema,* rash, *bronchospasm. Miscellaneous:* Muscle cramps, pallor, teeth discoloration, conjunctivitis, dilated pupils, difficulty in urination, muscle spasm, voice changes, oropharyngeal edema.

A

OD **Overdose Management:** *Symptoms:* Seizures, anginal pain, hypertension, hypokalemia, tachycardia (rate may increase to 200 beats/min).

See *Sympathomimetic Drugs..*

Dosage
- **Metered Dose Inhaler**
  Bronchodilation.

Adults and children over 12 years of age: 180 mcg (2 inhalations) q 4–6 hr (Ventolin aerosol may be used in children over 4 years of age). In some clients 1 inhalation (90 mcg) q 4 hr may be sufficient.

Prophylaxis of exercise-induced bronchospasm.

Adults and children over 12 years of age: 180 mcg (2 inhalations) 15 min before exercise.

- **Solution for Inhalation**
  Bronchodilation.

Adults and children over 12 years of age: 2.5 mg t.i.d.–q.i.d. by nebulization (dilute 0.5 mL of the 0.5% solution with 2.5 mL sterile NSS and deliver over 5–15 min).

- **Capsule for Inhalation**
  Bronchodilation.

Adults and children over 4 years of age: 200 mcg q 4–6 hr using a Rotahaler inhalation device. In some clients, 400 mcg q 4–6 hr may be required.

Prophylaxis of exercise-induced bronchospasm.

Adults and children over 12 years: 200 mcg 15 min before exercise using a Rotahaler inhalation device.

- **Syrup**
  Bronchodilation.

Adults and children over 14 years of age: 2–4 mg t.i.d.–q.i.d., up to a maximum of 8 mg q.i.d. **Children, 6–14 years, initial:** 2 mg (base) t.i.d.–q.i.d.; **then,** increase as necessary to a maximum of 24 mg/day in divided doses. **Children, 2–6 years, initial:** 0.1 mg/kg t.i.d.; **then,** increase as necessary up to 0.2 mg/kg, not to exceed 4 mg t.i.d.

- **Tablets**
  Bronchodilation.

Adults and children over 12 years of age, initial: 2–4 mg (of the base) t.i.d.–q.i.d.; **then,** increase dose as needed up to a maximum of 8 mg t.i.d.–q.i.d. In geriatric clients or those sensitive to beta agonists, start with 2 mg t.i.d.–q.i.d. and then increase dose gradually, if needed, to a maximum of 8 mg t.i.d.–q.i.d. **Children, 6–12 years of age, usual, initial:** 2 mg t.i.d.–q.i.d.; **then,** if necessary, increase the dose in a stepwise fashion to a maximum of 24 mg/day in divided doses.

- **Extended-Release Tablets**
  Bronchodilation.

Adults and children over 12 years of age: 4 or 8 mg (of the base) q 12 hr up to a maximum of 32 mg/day. Clients on regular-release albuterol can be switched to the Repetabs in that a 4-mg extended-release tablet q 12 hr is equivalent to a regular 2-mg tablet q 6 hr.

RESPIRATORY CARE CONSIDERATIONS

See also *Respiratory Care Considerations* for *Sympathomimetic Drugs.*
Administration/Storage
1. Do not exceed the recommended dose without specific directions from a physician.
2. If the dose of drug used previously does not provide relief, contact the provider immediately.
3. When using albuterol inhalers, do not use other inhalation medication unless specifically prescribed.
4. The contents of the container are under pressure. Therefore, do not store near heat or open flames and do not puncture the container.
5. When given by nebulization, either a face mask or mouthpiece may be used. Compressed air or oxygen with a gas flow of 6–10 L/min should be used, with a single treatment lasting from 5 to 15 min.
6. When given by IPPB, the inspiratory pressure should be from 10 to 20 cm water, with the duration of treatment ranging from 5 to 20 min depending on the client and instrument control.

7. The MDI may also be administered on a mechanical ventilator through an adapter.

8. Extended-release tablets should be taken whole with the aid of liquids. They should not be chewed or crushed. The outer coating of Volmax Extended-Release Tablets is not absorbed and is excreted in the feces; the empty outer coating may be observed in the stool.

Assessment

1. Obtain a baseline history and assess client's CNS status before initiating therapy.

2. Assess pulmonary function and lung sounds. Note evidence of client anxiety because this may contribute to air hunger.

3. Document symptom onset, duration, frequency, and any precipitating factors.

4. Determine if the client is able to self-administer the medication.

Interventions

1. Maintain a calm, reassuring approach. If the client is acutely short of breath, do not leave unattended.

2. Instruct how to inhale through nose and exhale with pursed lip or diaphragmatic breathing in order to prolong expiration and keep the airways open longer, thus reducing the work of breathing.

3. Monitor pulmonary status (i.e., breath sounds, VS, peak flow, or ABGs) for effects of the therapy, adjusting the dose or frequency of medication, if needed.

4. Observe for evidence of allergic responses and be prepared to intervene.

Client/Family Teaching

1. Advise to take only as directed.

2. Do not put lips around inhaler; go two fingerbreadths away before attempting to activate and inhale. Use a demonstrator inhaler to show client the correct method for administration.

3. Provide a spacer with the MDI to enhance drug administration. Use and care for spacer as per enclosed directions.

4. Work with client to establish dosing regimens that fit life-style, i.e., 1–2 puffs q 6 hr or 4 puffs 4 times/day, but stress that usual dosing is q 4–6 hr with an as-needed order. Instruct client to call if requiring more puffs more frequently than prescribed.

Evaluate: Improved breathing patterns and improved airway exchange

---

Alfentanil hydrochloride
(al-**FEN**-tah-nil)
Pregnancy Category: C
Alfenta **(C-II) (Rx)**
Classification: Narcotic analgesic

See also *Narcotic Analgesics.*

Action/Kinetics: Onset: Immediate. **t½:** 1–2 hr (after IV use).

Uses: *Continuous infusion:* As an analgesic with nitrous oxide/oxygen to maintain general anesthesia. *Incremental doses:* Adjunct with barbiturate/nitrous oxide/oxygen to maintain general anesthesia. *Anesthetic induction:* As primary agent when ET intubation and mechanical ventilation are necessary.

Contraindications: Use during labor.

Special Concerns: Use in children less than 12 years of age is not recommended. Use with caution during lactation.

Additional Side Effects: Bradycardia, postoperative confusion, blurred vision, hypercapnia, shivering, and *asystole*. Neonates with respiratory distress syndrome have manifested hypotension with doses of 20 mcg/kg.

Dosage ⎯⎯⎯⎯⎯⎯⎯⎯
• **IV**

Continuous infusion, duration 45 min or more.

Initial for induction: 50–75 mcg/kg; **maintenance, with nitrous oxide/oxygen:** 0.5–3 mcg/kg/min. Following the induction dose, the infusion rate requirement should be

---

reduced by 30%–50% for the first hour of maintenance.

Induction of anesthesia, duration 45 min or more.

Initial for induction: 130–245 mcg/kg; **maintenance:** 0.5–1.5 mcg/kg/min. If a general anesthetic is used for maintenance, the concentration of inhalation agents should be reduced by 30%–50% for the first hour.

Anesthetic adjunct, 30–60 min duration, incremental injection.

Initial for induction: 20–50 mcg/kg; **maintenance:** 5–15 mcg/kg, up to a total dose of 75 mcg/kg.

Anesthetic adjunct, less than 30 min duration, incremental injection.

Initial for induction: 8–20 mcg/kg; **maintenance:** 3–5 mcg/kg (or 0.5–1 mcg/kg/min, up to a total dose of 8–40 mcg/kg). If there is a lightening of general anesthesia or the client manifests signs of surgical stress, the rate of administration of alfentanil may be increased to 4 mcg/kg/min or a bolus dose of 7 mcg/kg may be used. If the situation is not controlled following three bolus doses over 5 min, an inhalation anesthetic, a barbiturate, or a vasodilator should be used. If signs of lightening anesthesia are noted within the last 15 min of surgery, a bolus dose of 7 mcg/kg should be given rather than increasing the infusion rate. A potent inhalation anesthetic may be used as an alternative.

RESPIRATORY CARE CONSIDERATIONS

See also *Respiratory Care Considerations* for *Narcotic Analgesics*.

Administration/Storage

1. The dosage of drug must be individualized for each client and for each use.

• For elderly or debilitated clients the dosage of drug should be reduced.

• For obese clients who are more than 20% above their ideal body weight, the dosage should be based on lean body weight.

2. The injectable form may be reconstituted with either normal saline, 5% dextrose in normal saline, lactated Ringer's solution, or D5W. Direct IV administration over 1½–3 min. For continous IV administration dilute 20 cc of alfentanil in 230 mL diluent to provide a solution of 40 mcg/mL.

3. The infusion should be discontinued 10–15 min prior to the end of surgery.

4. A tuberculin syringe or equivalent should be used to administer small volumes of alfentanil.

Assessment

1. Note any history of drug hypersensitivity.

2. Obtain baseline weight and VS prior to administering the medication. (Assisted or controlled ventilation may be required.)

3. Note any evidence of muscular rigidity and report before proceeding with the next dose of medication.

4. Assess respiratory and CV status continuously during therapy.

Evaluate

• Induction and maintenance of anesthesia

• ↓ Motor activity

Alpha-1-Proteinase Inhibitor (Human) (Alpha-1-PI)

(**AL**-fah-1-**PROH**-fee-in-ayz)

Pregnancy Category: C

Prolastin **(Rx)**

Classification: Alpha-1-proteinase inhibitor

Action/Kinetics: Alpha-1-PI is the enzyme that is deficient in alpha-1-antitrypsin disease. This disease causes a progressive breakdown of elastin tissues in the alveoli, resulting in emphysema. Often fatal, alpha-1-antitrypsin disease is usually manifested in the third and fourth decades of life. Prolastin is a sterile, lyophilized product obtained from pooled human plasma that is nonreactive for the HIV antibody and the hepatitis B surface antigen. t½: 4.5 days. **Therapeutic serum levels:** Approximately 80 mg/dL, although such levels may not reflect actual functional alpha-1-PI levels.

Uses: Panacinar emphysema due to congenital alpha-1-proteinase deficiency.

Contraindications: Clients with PiMZ or PiMS phenotypes of alpha-1-antitrypsin deficiency.

Special Concerns: Safety and efficacy for use in children not determined. Use with caution in clients at risk for circulatory overload.

Side Effects: Although precautions are taken during the manufacture of this product, it is possible that hepatitis and other infectious viruses may be present. *Miscellaneous:* Delayed fever up to 12 hr following treatment, dizziness, lightheadedness, mild transient leukocytosis.

Dosage ─────────
• **IV Only**
Panacinar emphysema.
Adults: 60 mg/kg each week at a rate of 0.08 mL/kg/min (or greater).

RESPIRATORY CARE CONSIDERATIONS
Administration/Storage
1. Administer within 3 hr after reconstitution. Do not refrigerate.
2. Administer only via IV. Follow recommended procedures for reconstitution.
3. When reconstituted, Prolastin is equal to or greater than 20 mg/mL and has a pH of 6.6–7.4.
4. Prolastin should be stored at 2°C–8°C (36°F–46°F) and should not be frozen.
5. The reconstituted drug should not be mixed with other diluents except for normal saline.
6. Clients should be immunized against hepatitis B prior to using Prolastin. If time does not permit adequate immunization, a single dose of Hepatitis B Immune Globulin (Human), 0.06 mL/kg IM, should be given at the time of the initial dose of Prolastin.
7. Equipment used and any unused

reconstituted alpha-1-PI (human) should be appropriately discarded.

Assessment
1. Perform a complete history and lung assessment.
2. Obtain a hepatitis profile. If the client has not received hepatitis B immunization, document and provide appropriate therapy.

Interventions
1. Observe client for delayed fever, which may occur within 12 hr. This is usually resolved in 24 hr.
2. Note any complaints of lightheadedness or dizziness and report.

Client/Family Teaching
1. Advise that cigarette smoking may accelerate and aggravate condition by causing an increase of elastin secretion.
2. Discuss familial tendency for alpha-1-antitrypsin deficiency, and explain the need for all blood relatives to be screened and provided appropriate counseling.
3. Stress the importance of reporting weekly for medication to maintain an adequate antielastase barrier.
4. Explain that therapy must continue throughout the client's lifetime.
5. Discuss that the product is prepared from human plasma and explain the potential associated risks.

Evaluate
• ↑ Serum prolastin levels (80 mg/dL)
• Slowing of destructive process on lung tissue
• Family members identified, screened, and counseled

Alprostadil (PGE₁)
(al-**PROSS**-tah-dill)
Caverject, Prostin VR ✿, Prostin VR Pediatric **(Rx)**
Classification: Prostaglandin

Action/Kinetics: Alprostadil is the naturally occurring acidic lipid prostaglandin E₁. Alprostadil relaxes smooth muscle of the ductus arteriosus leading to increased pulmonary blood flow with increased blood oxygenation and lower body perfusion. Clients with low pO_2 values respond best. The drug may also cause vasodilation, inhibit platelet aggregation, and stimulate both intestinal and uterine smooth muscle. When injected intracavernosally, alprostadil relaxes the trabecular cavernous smooth muscles and causes dilation of penile arteries. This results in increased arterial blood flow to the corpus cavernosa and thus swelling and elongation of the penis. **Onset, systemic:** 1.5–3 hr for acyanotic congenital heart disease and 15–30 min for cyanotic congenital heart disease. **Time to peak effect:** 3 hr for coarctation of the aorta and 1.5 hr for interruption of aortic arch. **Duration:** Closure of the ductus arteriosus usually begins 1–2 hr after infusion discontinued. Alprostadil is rapidly metabolized (80% in one pass) by oxidation in the lung, and metabolites are excreted by the kidney.

Uses: For temporary maintenance of patency of the ductus arteriosus (until surgery can be performed) in neonates with congenital heart defects. Diagnosis and treatment of erectile dysfunction (male impotence) due to neurologic, vascular, psychologic, or mixed causes.

Contraindications: Respiratory distress syndrome (hyaline membrane disease). Use with caution in neonates with bleeding tendencies. History of priapism, sickle cell disease. Multiple myeloma, leukemia. In clients with anatomic deformation of the penis or in those with penile implants. Caverject should not be given to women, children, newborns, or men for whom sexual activity is not advisable or is contraindicated.

Side Effects: *Respiratory: Apnea (in 10%–12% of neonates), especially in neonates less than 2 kg at birth;* bronchial wheezing, bradypnea, hypercapnia, respiratory depression. *CNS:* Fever, *seizures,* hypothermia, jitteriness, lethargy, *cerebral bleeding,* stiffness, hyperextension of the neck, irritability. *CV:* Flushing, especially after intra-arterial dosage, bradycardia, hypotension, tachycardia, edema,

cardiac arrest, CHF, shock, arrhythmias. GI: Diarrhea, hyperbilirubinemia, gastric regurgitation. *Renal:* Hematuria, anuria. *Skeletal:* Cortical proliferation of long bones. *Hematologic: Disseminated intravascular coagulation,* thrombocytopenia, anemia, bleeding. *Miscellaneous: Sepsis, peritonitis,* hypoglycemia, hypokalemia or hyperkalemia.

Side effects when used for erectile dysfunction: Penile pain, prolonged erection, penile fibrosis, hematoma at injection site, penile disorders, including numbness, yeast infection, irritation, sensitivity, phimosis, pruritus, erythema, venous leak, penile skin tear, strange feeling in penis, discoloration of penile head, itch at tip of penis, painful erection, abnormal ejaculation.

OD **Overdose Management:** *Symptoms: Apnea,* bradycardia, flushing, hypotension, pyrexia. *Treatment:* Reduce rate of infusion if symptoms of hypotension or pyrexia occur; discontinue infusion if symptoms of apnea or bradycardia occur.

Drug Interactions: Use of alprostadil with warfarin or heparin may increase bleeding after intracavernosal injection.

Laboratory Test Interferences: ↑ Bilirubin. ↓ Glucose, serum calcium. ↑ or ↓ Potassium.

Dosage ⎯⎯⎯⎯⎯⎯⎯⎯⎯
• **Continuous IV Infusion or Umbilical Artery**
Maintain patency of ductus arteriosus.
Initial: 0.05–0.1 mcg/kg/min; **then,** after response achieved, decrease infusion rate to lowest dose that will maintain response (e.g., 0.1–0.05 to 0.025–0.01 mcg/kg/min). *NOTE:* If 0.1 mcg/kg/min is insufficient, dosage can be increased up to 0.4 mcg/kg/min.
• **Intracavernosal**
Erectile dysfunction due to vascular, psychogenic, or mixed etiology.
The dose should be individualized for each client by careful titration. **Initial:** 2.5 mcg. If there is a partial re-

sponse, increase the dose by 2.5 mcg to 5 mcg and then in increments of 5–10 mcg, depending on the erectile response, until a dose is reached that results in an erection suitable for intercourse but not exceeding 1 hr in duration. If there is no response to the initial 2.5-mcg dose, the second dose may be increased to 7.5 mcg, followed by increments of 5 to 10 mcg. **Maximum dose:** 60 mcg. The drug should not be given more than 3 times/week with at least 24 hr between each dose.

Erectile dysfunction due to pure neurogenic etiology (spinal cord injury).

Initial: 1.25 mcg. The dose may be increased by 1.25 mcg to 2.5 mcg, followed by an increment of 2.5 mcg to a dose of 5 mcg. The dose may be increased in 5-mcg increments until a dose is reached that produces an erection suitable for intercourse and not exceeding 1 hr in duration.

RESPIRATORY CARE CONSIDERATIONS

Administration/Storage

1. Administer infusions only in pediatric intensive care facilities.

2. Dilute 500 mcg with either sodium chloride injection or dextrose injection in volumes appropriate for the infant's fluid intake and suitable for the type of infusion pump available.

3. Use a Y set-up.

4. Discard any unused solutions and prepare a fresh infusion solution q 24 hr.

5. Sterile solutions should be infused for the shortest time and at the lowest dose that will produce the desired effect.

6. Have a respirator available at the cribside.

7. For use in impotence, the diluent is mixed with alprostadil powder, and the solution is swirled gently. One milliliter of the reconstituted solution contains either 10 or 20 mcg of alprostadil. The solution should be used immediately and not stored or frozen.

8. For treating impotence, alprostadil is injected into the corpus cavernosum using a small, thin needle (½ in., 27- to 30- gauge). The injection site must be cleansed with an alcohol swab. The first injection should be administered in a physician's office.

9. Store ampules at 2°C–8°C (36°F–46°F).

Assessment

1. Document indications for therapy, onset of symptoms, and any associated predisposing factors.

2. In clients with sexual dysfunction, list all medications currently prescribed and those being consumed. Note any reference to alterations in psychosocial balance.

3. Assess VS and cardiac and respiratory function and document before administering the medication.

4. Determine if the neonate has restricted pulmonary blood flow.

5. Note any evidence of bleeding tendencies or sickle cell anemia as these are contraindications to drug therapy.

Interventions

1. Monitor arterial pressure intermittently by umbilical artery catheter, auscultation, Dinemapp or with a Doppler transducer. Obtain written guidelines for arterial pressures; if the arterial pressure falls significantly, decrease the rate of flow immediately and report.

2. Observe the infant for apnea, bradycardia, pyrexia, flushing, and hypotension. These are symptoms of *overdose*. The following guidelines are appropriate.

• If the infant develops apnea or bradycardia, stop the administration of drug, change to the unmedicated solution, and start resuscitation.

• If the infant develops pyrexia or hypotension, reduce the rate of IV flow and report. The rate of IV flow will likely be reduced until the temperature and BP return to baseline values.

• Report if flushing occurs. This symptom indicates an incorrect intra-arterial placement of the catheter and it requires repositioning.

---

3. If the infant has restricted pulmonary blood flow, monitor ABGs. A positive response to alprostadil is indicated by at least a 10 mm Hg increase in blood pO_2.

4. If the infant has restricted systemic blood flow, monitor BP and serum pH. If the infant has acidosis, a positive response to alprostadil would be indicated by an increased pH, an increase in BP, and a decreased ratio of PA pressure to aortic pressure.

5. Monitor neurological status and level of consciousness; report seizures, hyperexcitability, or stiffness as drug must be stopped.

6. Treatment for impotence should be discontinued in clients who develop penile angulation, cavernosal fibrosis, or Peyronie's disease.

Evaluate

• Improved pulmonary blood flow with a resultant ↑ blood oxygenation level

• Closure of ductus arteriosus 1–2 hr following infusion

• Promotion of penile erection with intracavernosal therapy

Amantadine hydrochloride
(ah-**MAN**-tah-deen)

Pregnancy Category: C
Endantadine ✱, PMS-Amantadine ✱, Symadine, Symmetrel **(Rx)**

Classification: Antiviral and antiparkinson agent

Action/Kinetics: As an antiviral agent, amantadine is believed to prevent penetration of the virus into cells, possibly by inhibiting uncoating of the RNA virus. The reaction appears to be virus specific for influenza A but not host specific. Amantadine may also prevent the release of infectious viral nucleic acid into the host cell. The drug reduces symptoms of viral infections if given within 24–48 hr after onset of illness. For the treatment of parkinsonism, amantadine may increase the release of dopamine from dopaminergic nerve terminals in the substantia nigra of parkinson clients, resulting in an increase in dopamine levels in dopaminergic synapses. Well absorbed from GI tract. **Onset:** 48 hr. **Peak serum concentration:** 0.2 mcg/mL after 1–4 hr. **t½:** Approximately 15 hr; elimination half-life increases two- to threefold when creatinine clearance is less than 40 mL/min/1.73 m². Ninety percent excreted unchanged in urine.

Uses: Influenza A viral infections of the respiratory tract (prophylaxis and treatment of high-risk clients with immunodeficiency, CV, metabolic, neuromuscular, or pulmonary disease). Symptomatic treatment of idiopathic parkinsonism and parkinsonism syndrome resulting from encephalitis, carbon monoxide intoxication, drugs, or cerebral arteriosclerosis. The drug decreases extrapyramidal symptoms, including akinesia, rigidity, tremors, excessive salivation, gait disturbances, and total functional disability. Favorable results have been obtained in about 50% of the clients. Improvements can last for up to 30 months, although some clients report that the effect of the drug wears off in 1–3 months. A rest period or an increased dosage may reestablish effectiveness. For parkinsonism, amantadine hydrochloride is usually used concomitantly with other agents, such as levodopa and anticholinergic agents.

Amantadine is recommended for prophylaxis in the following situations:

• Short-term prophylaxis during the course of a presumed outbreak of influenza A

• Adjunct to late immunization in high-risk clients

• To reduce disruption of medical care and to decrease spread of virus in high-risk clients when influenza A virus outbreaks occur

• To supplement vaccination protection in clients with impaired immune responses

• As chemoprophylaxis during flu season for those high-risk clients for whom influenza vaccine is contraindicated due to anaphylactic response to egg protein or prior severe reactions associated with flu vaccination

Contraindications: Hypersensitivity to drug.

Special Concerns: Administer with caution to clients with liver and renal disease, history of epilepsy, CHF, peripheral edema, orthostatic hypotension, recurrent eczematoid dermatitis, or severe psychosis, in clients taking CNS stimulant drugs, to those exposed to rubella, and to nursing mothers. Safe use in lactating mothers and in children less than 1 year has not been established.

Side Effects: *GI:* N&V, constipation, anorexia, xerostomia. *CNS:* Depression, psychosis, **convulsions,** hallucinations, lightheadedness, confusion, ataxia, irritability, anxiety, headache, dizziness, fatigue, insomnia. *CV:* **CHF,** orthostatic hypotension, peripheral edema. *Miscellaneous:* Urinary retention, leukopenia, neutropenia, mottling of skin of the extremities due to poor peripheral circulation (livedo reticularis), skin rashes, visual problems, slurred speech, oculogyric episodes, dyspnea, weakness, eczematoid dermatitis.

OD   Overdose Management: *Symptoms:* Anorexia, N&V, CNS effects. *Treatment:* Gastric lavage or induction of emesis followed by supportive measures. Ensure that client is well hydrated; give IV fluids if necessary. To treat CNS toxicity, IV physostigmine, 1–2 mg given q 1–2 hr in adults or 0.5 mg at 5–10-min intervals (maximum of 2 mg/hr) in children. Sedatives and anticonvulsants may be given if needed; antiarrhythmics and vasopressors may also be required.

Drug Interactions
Anticholinergics / Additive anticholinergic effects (including hallucinations, confusion), especially with trihexyphenidyl and benztropine

CNS stimulants / May ↑ CNS and psychic effects of amantadine; use cautiously together
Hydrochlorothiazide/triamterene combination / ↓ Urinary excretion of amantadine → ↑ plasma levels
Levodopa / Potentiated by amantadine

Dosage
• **Capsules, Syrup**
  Antiviral.
Adults: 200 mg/day as a single or divided dose. **Children, 1–9 years:** 4.4–8.8 mg/kg/day up to a maximum of 150 mg/day in one or two divided doses (use syrup); **9–12 years:** 100 mg b.i.d.
  Prophylactic treatment.
Institute before or immediately after exposure and continue for 10–21 days if used concurrently with vaccine or for 90 days without vaccine.
  Symptomatic management.
Initiate as soon as possible and continue for 24–48 hr after disappearance of symptoms. Dose should be decreased in renal impairment (see package insert). Dose should be reduced to 100 mg/day for persons with active seizure disorders due to the increased risk of seizure frequency using daily doses of 200 mg.
  Parkinsonism.
When used as sole agent, usual dose is 100 mg b.i.d.; may be necessary to increase up to 400 mg/day in divided doses. When used with other antiparkinson drugs: 100 mg 1–2 times/day.
  Drug-induced extrapyramidal symptoms.
100 mg b.i.d. (up to 300 mg/day may be required in some). Dosage should be reduced in clients with impaired renal function.

RESPIRATORY CARE CONSIDERATIONS

See also *General Respiratory Care Considerations for All Anti-Infectives,* and *Antiviral Drugs.*
Administration/Storage
1. Protect capsules from moisture.

A

2. Therapy should be started for viral illness as soon as possible after symptoms begin and for 24–48 hr after symptoms disappear.

Assessment

1. Obtain a thorough history and note any evidence of seizures, CHF, and renal insufficiency.

2. With active seizure disorder drug dosage must be reduced to prevent breakthrough seizures.

3. With Parkinson's disease, following loss of effectiveness of the drug, benefits may be regained by increasing the dosage or discontinuing the drug for several weeks and then reinstituting it.

Interventions

1. Observe for an increase in seizure activity and take appropriate precautions. Ensure that dosage is reduced to 100 mg/day to prevent loss of seizure control.

2. Assess clients with a history of CHF or peripheral edema for increased edema and/or respiratory distress and report promptly.

3. Monitor I&O. Observe clients with renal impairment for crystalluria, oliguria, and increased BUN or creatinine levels.

4. Monitor CNS status and immediately report any mental status changes.

Evaluate

• ↓ Drug-induced extrapyramidal symptoms

• Improved motor control with ↓ tremor

• Improvement in symptoms of influenza A viral infections

• Influenza A prophylaxis and ↓ spread of infection to high-risk individuals during outbreaks

---

Amikacin sulfate

(am-ih-**KAY**-sin)

Pregnancy Category: D

Amikin **(Rx)**

Classification: Antibiotic, aminoglycoside

See also *Anti-Infectives,* and *Aminoglycosides.*

Action/Kinetics: Amikacin is derived from kanamycin. Its spectrum is somewhat broader than that of other aminoglycosides, including *Serratia* and *Acinetobacter* species, as well as certain staphylococci and streptococci. Amikacin is effective against both penicillinase- and non-penicillinase-producing organisms. **Peak therapeutic serum levels: IM,** 16–32 mcg/mL. **t½:** 2–3 hr. Toxic serum levels: >35 mcg/mL (peak measured after 1 hr) and >10 mcg/mL (trough measured before next dose).

Uses: Short-term treatment of gram-negative bacterial infections including *Pseudomonas, Escherichia coli, Proteus, Providencia, Klebsiella, Enterobacter, Serratia,* and *Acinetobacter.* May also be used in infections due to gentamicin or tobramycin resistant strains of *Providencia rettgeri, P. stuartii, Serratia marcescens,* and *Pseudomonas aeruginosa.*

Infections include bacterial septicemia (including neonatal sepsis); serious infections of the respiratory tract, bones, joints, skin, soft tissue, and CNS (including meningitis); intra-abdominal infections (including peritonitis); burns; postoperative infections (including postvascular surgery). Also, serious complicated and recurrent infections of the urinary tract. May be used as initial therapy in certain situations in the treatment of known or suspected staphylococcal disease. *Investigational:* Intrathecal or intraventricular use. As part of multiple drug regimen for *Mycobacterium avium* complex (commonly seen in AIDS clients).

Special Concerns: Use with caution in premature infants and neonates.

Dosage ————————

• **IM (Preferred) and IV**

Adults, children, and older infants: 15 mg/kg/day in two to three equally divided doses q 8–12 hr for 7–10 days; **maximum daily dose:** 15 mg/kg.

   Uncomplicated UTIs.

250 mg b.i.d.; **newborns:** loading dose of 10 mg/kg followed by 7.5 mg/kg q 12 hr.

Use in neonates.
Initial: Loading dose of 10 mg/kg; **then,** 7.5 mg/kg q 12 hr. Lower doses may be safer during the first 2 weeks of life.
Intrathecal or intraventricular use.
8 mg/24 hr.
As part of multiple drug regimen for M. avium complex.
15 mg/kg/day IV in divided doses q 8–12 hr.
In clients with impaired renal function.
Normal loading dose of 7.5 mg/kg; **then** administration should be monitored by serum level of amikacin (35 mcg/mL maximum) or creatinine clearance rates. Duration of treatment: **Usual:** 7–10 days.

RESPIRATORY CARE CONSIDERATIONS

See also *Respiratory Care Considerations* for *Aminoglycosides.*
Administration/Storage
1. Add 500-mg vial to 200 mL of sterile diluent, such as NSS or D5W.
2. Administer over a 300- to 600-min period for adults.
3. Administer to infants in the amount of prescribed fluid. The IV administration to infants should be over 1–2 hr.
4. Store colorless liquid at room temperature for no longer than 2 years.
5. Potency is not affected if the solution turns a light yellow.
Assessment
1. Obtain audiometric assessment with high dosage or prolonged use.
2. Note any vestibular dysfunction and monitor for eighth cranial nerve impairment R/T elevated peak drug levels.
Evaluate
• Resolution of infection
• Therapeutic serum drug levels (peak 30–35 mcg/mL; trough < 10 mcg/mL)

Amiloride hydrochloride   A

(ah-**MILL**-oh-ryd)
Pregnancy Category: B
Midamor **(Rx)**
Classification: Diuretic, potassium-sparing

Action/Kinetics: Amiloride acts on the distal tubule to inhibit $Na+$, $K+$-ATPase, thereby inhibiting sodium exchange for potassium; this results in increased secretion of sodium and water and conservation of potassium. In the proximal tubule, amiloride inhibits the $Na+/H+$ exchange mechanism. The drug also has weak diuretic and antihypertensive activity. **Onset:** 2 hr. **Peak effect:** 6–10 hr. **Peak plasma levels:** 3–4 hr. **Duration:** 24 hr. **t½:** 6–9 hr. Twenty-three percent is bound to plasma protein. Approximately 50% is excreted unchanged by kidney and 40% by the feces unchanged.
Uses: Adjunct with thiazides or loop diuretics in the treatment of hypertension or edema due to CHF, hepatic cirrhosis, and nephrotic syndrome to help restore normal serum potassium or prevent hypokalemia. Prophylaxis of hypokalemia in clients who would be at risk if hypokalemia developed (e.g., digitalized clients or clients with significant cardiac arrhythmias). *Investigational:* To reduce lithium-induced polyuria. Aerosolized amiloride may slow the progression of pulmonary function reduction in adults with cystic fibrosis.
Contraindications: Hyperkalemia (>5.5 mEq potassium/L). In clients receiving other potassium-sparing diuretics or potassium supplements. Impaired renal function. Diabetes mellitus. Use during lactation.
Special Concerns: Use with caution in metabolic or respiratory acidosis; during lactation. Geriatric clients may have a greater risk of developing hyperkalemia. Safety and efficacy have not been determined in children.

A

Side Effects: *Electrolyte:* Hyperkalemia, hyponatremia, and hypochloremia if used with other diuretics. *CNS:* Headache, dizziness, encephalopathy, tremors, paresthesias, mental confusion, insomnia, decreased libido, depression, sleepiness, vertigo, nervousness. *GI:* Nausea, anorexia, vomiting, diarrhea, changes in appetite, gas and abdominal pain, dry mouth, flatulence, abdominal fullness, GI bleeding, GI disturbance, thirst, dyspepsia, heartburn, jaundice, constipation, activation of preexisting peptic ulcer. *Respiratory:* Dyspnea, cough, SOB. *Musculoskeletal:* Weakness; muscle cramps; fatigue; joint, chest and back pain; neck or shoulder ache; pain in extremities. *GU:* Impotence, polyuria, dysuria, bladder spasms, urinary frequency. *CV:* Angina, palpitations, **arrhythmias,** orthostatic hypotension. *Hematologic:* **Aplastic anemia,** neutropenia. *Dermatologic:* Skin rash, itching, pruritus, alopecia. *Miscellaneous:* Visual disturbances, nasal congestion, tinnitus, increased intraocular pressure, abnormal liver function.

OD **Overdose Management:** *Symptoms:* Electrolyte imbalance, **dehydration.** *Treatment:* Induce emesis or gastric lavage. Treat hyperkalemia by IV sodium bicarbonate or oral or parenteral glucose with a rapid-acting insulin. Sodium polystyrene sulfonate, oral or by enema, may also be used.

Drug Interactions
ACE inhibitors / ↑ Risk of significant hyperkalemia
Digoxin / Possible ↑ renal clearance and ↓ nonrenal clearance of digoxin. Possible ↑ inotropic effect of digoxin
Lithium / ↓ Renal excretion of lithium → ↑ chance of toxicity
NSAIDs / ↓ Therapeutic effect of amiloride
Potassium products / Hyperkalemia with possibility of cardiac arrhythmias or cardiac arrest
Spironolactone, Triamterene / Hyperkalemia, hyponatremia, hypochloremia

Dosage —————
• **Tablets**
  As single agent or with other diuretics.
Adults, initial: 5 mg/day; 10 mg/day may be necessary in some clients. Doses as high as 20 mg/day may be used, if needed, with careful monitoring of electrolytes.
  Reduce lithium-induced polyuria. 10–20 mg/day.
  Slow progression of pulmonary function reduction in cystic fibrosis.
Adults: Drug is dissolved in 0.3% saline and delivered by nebulizer.

RESPIRATORY CARE CONSIDERATIONS

See also *Respiratory Care Considerations* for *Diuretics.*
Administration/Storage: Administer with food to reduce chance of GI upset.
Interventions
1. Monitor renal function studies, I&O, and weights.
2. Monitor serum electrolytes. Assess for hyperkalemia and for indications to withdraw the drug. Cardiac irregularities may be precipitated.
3. Do not encourage potassium supplementation or foods rich in potassium because drug does not promote potassium excretion.
4. Do not administer with other potassium-sparing diuretics.
Evaluate
• ↓ BP and enhanced diuresis
• Conservation of potassium
• ↓ Lithium-induced polyuria
• Maintenance of pulmonary function with cystic fibrosis

———————————————

Aminophylline
(am-in-**OFF**-ih-lin)
Pregnancy Category: C
Aminophyllin, Phyllocontin, Phyllocontin-350 ✤, Truphyllin **(Rx)**
Classification: Bronchodilator

———————————————

See also *Theophylline Derivatives.*
Action/Kinetics: Aminophylline contains 79% theophylline.
Additional Use: Neonatal apnea, respiratory stimulant in Cheyne-

Stokes respiration. Parenteral form has been used for biliary colic and as a cardiac stimulant, a diuretic, and an adjunct in treating CHF, although such uses have been replaced by more effective drugs.

Special Concerns: Use with caution when aminophylline and sodium chloride are used with corticosteroids or in clients with edema.

Additional Side Effects: The ethylenediamine in the product may cause exfoliative dermatitis or urticaria.

Dosage

• **Oral Solution, Tablets**

Bronchodilator, acute attacks, in clients not currently on theophylline therapy.

Adults and children up to 16 years of age, loading dose: Equivalent of 5–6 mg of anhydrous theophylline/kg.

Bronchodilator, acute attacks, in clients currently receiving theophylline.

Adults and children up to 16 years of age: If possible, a serum theophylline level should be obtained first. Then, base loading dose on the premise that each 0.5 mg theophylline/kg lean body weight will result in a 0.5–1.6-mcg/mL increase in serum theophylline levels. If immediate therapy is needed and a serum level cannot be obtained, a single dose of the equivalent of 2.5 mg/kg of anhydrous theophylline can be given.

Maintenance in acute attack, based on equivalent of anhydrous theophylline.

Young adult smokers: 4 mg/kg q 6 hr; **healthy, nonsmoking adults:** 3 mg/kg q 8 hr; **geriatric clients or clients with cor pulmonale:** 2 mg/kg q 8 hr; **clients with CHF or liver failure:** 2 mg/kg q 8–12 hr. **Pediatric, 12–16 years:** 3 mg/kg q 6 hr; **9–12 years:** 4 mg/kg q 6 hr; **1–9 years:** 5 mg/kg q 6 hr; **6–12 months:** Use the formula: dose (mg/kg q 8 hr) = (0.05) (age in weeks) + 1.25; **up to 6 months:** Use the formula: dose (mg/kg q 8 hr) = (0.07) (age in weeks) + 1.7.

Chronic therapy, based on equivalent of anhydrous theophylline.

Adults, initial: 6–8 mg/kg up to a maximum of 400 mg/day in three to four divided doses at 6–8-hr intervals; **then,** dose can be increased in 25% increments at 2–3 day intervals up to a maximum of 13 mg/kg or 900 mg/day, whichever is less. **Pediatric, initial:** 16 mg/kg up to a maximum of 400 mg/day in three to four divided doses at 6–8 hr intervals; **then,** dose may be increased in 25% increments at 2–3 day intervals up to the following maximum doses (without measuring serum theophylline): **16 years and older:** 13 mg/kg or 900 mg/day, whichever is less; **12–16 years:** 18 mg/kg/day; **9–12 years:** 20 mg/kg/day; **1–9 years:** 24 mg/kg/day; **up to 12 months,** Use the following formula: dose (mg/kg/day) = (0.3) (age in weeks) + 8.0.

• **Enteric-Coated Tablets**

Bronchodilator, chronic therapy, based on equivalent of anhydrous theophylline.

Adults, initial: 6–8 mg/kg up to a maximum of 400 mg/day in three to four divided doses at 6–8-hr intervals; **then,** dose may be increased, if needed and tolerated, by increments of 25% at 2–3 day intervals up to a maximum of 13 mg/kg/day or 900 mg/day, whichever is less, without measuring serum theophylline. **Pediatric, over 12 years of age, initial:** 4 mg/kg q 8–12 hr; **then,** dose may be increased by 2–3 mg/kg/day at 3-day intervals up to the following maximum doses (without measuring serum levels): **16 years and older:** 13 mg/kg/day or 900 mg/day, whichever is less; **12–16 years:** 18 mg/kg/day.

• **Enema**

For use as a bronchodilator for loading doses and for maintenance in acute attacks, see doses for oral solution and tablets.

• **IV Infusion**

A

Bronchodilator, acute attacks, for clients not currently on theophylline.
Adults and children up to 16 years, loading dose based on anhydrous theophylline: 5 mg/kg given over a period of 20 min.

Bronchodilator, acute attack, for clients currently on theophylline.
Adults and children up to 16 years, loading dose based on anhydrous theophylline: If possible, a serum theophylline level should be obtained first. Then, base loading dose on the premise that each 0.5 mg theophylline/kg lean body weight will result in a 0.5–1.6 mcg/mL increase in serum theophylline levels. If immediate therapy is needed and a serum level cannot be obtained, a single dose of the equivalent of 2.5 mg/kg of anhydrous theophylline can be given.

Maintenance for acute attacks, based on equivalent of anhydrous theophylline.
Young adult smokers: 0.7 mg/kg/hr; **nonsmoking, healthy adults:** 0.43 mg/kg/hr; **geriatric clients or clients with cor pulmonale:** 0.26 mg/kg/hr; **clients with CHF or liver failure:** 0.2 mg/kg/hr. **Pediatric, 12–16 years, nonsmokers:** 0.5 mg/kg/hr; **9–12 years,** 0.7 mg/kg/hr; **1–9 years,** 0.8 mg/kg/hr; **up to 1 year,** Based on the following formula: dose (mg/kg/hr) = (0.008) (age in weeks) + 0.21.

RESPIRATORY CARE CONSIDERATIONS

See also *Respiratory Care Considerations* for *Theophylline Derivatives.*

Administration/Storage
1. To avoid hypotension, administer IV doses of medication at a rate not to exceed 25 mg/min.
2. Only the 25 mg/mL injection (which should be further diluted) should be used for IV administration. Use an infusion pump or device to regulate infusion rates of IV solutions.
3. IM injection is not recommended due to severe, persistent pain at the site of injection.
4. A minimum of 4–6 hr should elapse when switching from IV infusion to the first dose of PO therapy.
5. Enteric-coated tablets may be incompletely and slowly absorbed.
6. Enteric-coated tablets are not recommended for children less than 12 years of age.
7. Use of aminophylline suppositories is not recommended due to the possibility of slow and unreliable absorption.

Assessment
1. Document indications for therapy, onset, duration, and characteristics of symptoms; note other therapies tried.
2. List medications currently prescribed to ensure that none interact unfavorably.
3. Perform baseline lung assessments and pulmonary function studies; note ABGs and ECG.

Interventions
1. Monitor pulse and BP closely during IV administration. Aminophylline may cause a transitory lowering of the BP. If this occurs, the dosage of drug and rate of flow should be adjusted immediately.
2. Report serum levels greater than 20 mcg/mL or symptoms of toxicity.
3. Observe and report symptoms of toxicity, i.e., N&V, restlessness, convulsions, and arrhythmias.
4. Monitor clients with a history of CAD for chest pain and ECG changes.
5. Initiate and stress the importance of smoking cessation with all clients that still smoke.
6. Instruct in pursed-lip and diaphragmatic breathing to help reduce the work of breathing by prolonging expiration and keeping the airways open longer.

Evaluate
• Improved airway exchange
• ↓ SOB; relief of PND
• Termination of acute asthma attack
• ABGs within desired range
• Therapeutic serum drug levels (10–20 mcg/mL)

Amiodarone hydrochloride

(am-ee-**OH**-dah-rohn)
Pregnancy Category: D
Cordarone **(Rx)**
Classification: Antiarrhythmic, class III

See also *Antiarrhythmic Agents*.

Action/Kinetics: The antiarrhythmic activity is due to an increase in the duration of the myocardial cell action potential and refractory period, as well as alpha- and beta-adrenergic blockade. The drug decreases sinus rate, increases PR and QT intervals, results in development of U waves, and changes T-wave contour. After IV use, amiodarone relaxes vascular smooth muscle, reduces peripheral vascular resistance (afterload), and increases cardiac index slightly. No significant changes are seen in left ventricular ejection fraction after PO use. Absorption is slow and variable. **Maximum plasma levels:** 3–7 hr after a single dose. **Onset:** Several days up to 1–3 weeks. Drug may accumulate in the liver, lung, spleen, and adipose tissue. **Therapeutic serum levels:** 0.5–2.5 mcg/mL. **t½:** Biphasic: initial t½: 2.5–10 days; final t½: 26–107 days. Effects may persist for several weeks or months after therapy is terminated. Effective plasma concentrations are difficult to predict although concentrations below 1 mg/L are usually ineffective, whereas those above 2.5 mg/L are not necessary. Neither amiodarone nor its metabolite, desethylamiodarone, is dialyzable.

Uses: Oral. This drug should be reserved for life-threatening ventricular arrhythmias unresponsive to other therapy, such as recurrent ventricular fibrillation and recurrent, hemodynamically unstable ventricular tachycardia.

IV. Initial treatment and prophylaxis of frequently recurring ventricular fibrillation and hemodynamically unstable ventricular tachycardia in clients refractory to other therapy.

Ventricular tachycardia/ventricular fibrillation clients unable to take PO medication. *Investigational:* Refractory sustained or paroxysmal atrial fibrillation, paroxysmal SVT, symptomatic atrial flutter. Also, in CHF with decreased LV ejection fraction, exercise tolerance and ventricular arrhythmias.

Contraindications: Parenteral or PO use: Marked sinus bradycardia due to severe sinus node dysfunction, second- or third-degree AV block, syncope caused by bradycardia (except when used with a pacemaker). Lactation.

Special Concerns: Safety and effectiveness in children have not been determined. The drug may be more sensitive in geriatric clients, especially on thyroid function. The IV product should be carefully monitored in geriatric clients and in those with severe left ventricular dysfunction.

Side Effects: Adverse reactions, some potentially fatal, are common with doses greater than 400 mg/day. *Pulmonary:* Pulmonary infiltrates or fibrosis, interstitial/alveolar pneumonitis, hypersensitivity pneumonitis, alveolitis, pulmonary infiltrates, pulmonary inflammation or fibrosis, *ARDS (after parenteral use),* lung edema, cough and progressive dyspnea. Oral use may cause a clinical syndrome of cough and progressive dyspnea accompanied by functional, radiographic, gallium scan, and pathologic data indicating pulmonary toxicity. *CV: **Worsening of arrhythmias, paroxysmal ventricular tachycardia,** proarrhythmias, symptomatic bradycardia, sinus arrest, SA node dysfunction, **CHF,** edema, hypotension (especially with IV use), **cardiac conduction abnormalities, coagulation abnormalities, cardiac arrest (after IV use).** IV use may result in atrial fibrillation, nodal arrhythmia, prolonged QT interval, and sinus bradycardia. *Hepatic:* Abnormal liver function tests, nonspecific hepatic disorders, cholestatic hepatitis, cirrhosis, hepatitis. *CNS:* Malaise, tremor, lack of

---

coordination, fatigue, ataxia, paresthesias, peripheral neuropathy, abnormal involuntary movements, sleep disturbances, dizziness, insomnia, headache, decreased libido, abnormal gait. *GI:* N&V, constipation, anorexia, abdominal pain, abnormal taste and smell, abnormal salivation. *Ophthalmologic:* Corneal microdeposits (asymptomatic) in clients on therapy for 6 months or more, photophobia, dry eyes, visual disturbances, blurred vision, halos, optic neuritis. *Dermatologic:* Photosensitivity, solar dermatitis, blue discoloration of skin, rash, alopecia, spontaneous ecchymosis, flushing. *Miscellaneous:* Hypothyroidism or hyperthyroidism, vasculitis, flushing, pseudotumor cerebri, epididymitis, thrombocytopenia. IV use may cause abnormal kidney function, Stevens-Johnson syndrome, respiratory syndrome, and *shock.*

OD   Overdose Management: *Symptoms:* Bradycardia, hypotension, *disorders of cardiac rhythm, cardiogenic shock,* AV block, hepatoxicity. *Treatment:* Use supportive treatment. The cardiac rhythm and BP should be monitored. A beta-adrenergic agonist or a pacemaker is used to treat bradycardia; hypotension due to insufficient tissue perfusion is treated with a vasopressor or positive inotropic agents. There is some evidence that cholestyramine hastens the reversal of side effects by increasing elimination. Drug is not dialyzable.

Drug Interactions
Anticoagulants / ↑ Anticoagulant effect → bleeding disorders
Beta-adrenergic blocking agents / ↑ Chance of bradycardia and hypotension
Calcium channel blockers / ↑ Risk of AV block with verapamil or diltiazem or hypotension with all calcium channel blockers
Cholestyramine / ↑ Elimination of amiodarone → ↓ serum levels and half-ife
Cimetidine / ↑ Serum levels of amiodarone

Cyclosporine / ↑ Levels of plasma cyclosporine → elevated creatinine levels (even with ↓ doses of cyclosporine)
Dextromethorphan / Chronic use of PO amiodarone (> 2 weeks) impairs metabolism of dextromethorphan
Digoxin / ↑ Serum digoxin levels → toxicity
Flecainide / ↑ Plasma levels of flecainide
Methotrexate / Chronic use of PO amiodarone (> 2 weeks) impairs metabolism of methotrexate
Procainamide / ↑ Serum procainamide levels → toxicity
Phenytoin / ↑ Serum phenytoin levels → toxicity; also, ↑ levels of amiodarone
Quinidine / Serum quinidine toxicity, including fatal cardiac arrhythmias
Theophylline / ↑ Serum theophylline levels → toxicity (effects may not be seen for 1 week and may last for a prolonged period after drug is discontinued)

Laboratory Test Interferences: ↑ AST, ALT, GGT. Alteration of thyroid function tests (↑ serum T_4, ↓ serum T_3).

Dosage ─────────────
Due to the drug's side effects, unusual pharmacokinetic properties, and difficult dosing schedule, amiodarone should be administered in a hospital only by physicians trained in treating life-threatening arrhythmias. Loading doses are required to ensure a reasonable onset of action.

• **IV Infusion**
Life-threatening ventricular arrhythmias.
Loading dose, rapid: 150 mg over the first 10 minutes (15 mg/min). **Then, slow loading dose:** 360 mg over the next 6 hr (1 mg/min). **Maintenance dose:** 540 mg over the remaining 18 hr (0.5 mg/min). After the first 24 hr, continue maintenance infusion rate of 0.5 mg/min (720 mg/24 hr). This may be continued with monitoring for 2 to 3 weeks.

Once arrhythmias have been suppressed, the client may be switched to PO amiodarone. The following is intended only as a guideline for PO amiodarone dosage after IV infusion. **IV infusion less than 1 week:** Initial daily dose of PO amiodarone, 800–1,600 mg. **IV infusion from 1 to 3 weeks:** Initial daily dose of PO amiodarone, 600–800 mg. **IV infusion longer than 3 weeks:** Initial daily dose of PO amiodarone, 400 mg.

• **Tablets**

Life-threatening ventricular arrhythmias.

Loading dose: 800–1,600 mg/day for 1–3 weeks (or until initial response occurs); **then,** reduce dose to 600–800 mg/day for 1 month. **Maintenance dose:** 400 mg/day (as low as 200 mg/day or as high as 600 mg/day may be needed in some clients).

RESPIRATORY CARE CONSIDERATIONS

See also *Respiratory Care Considerations* for *Antiarrhythmic Agents.*
Administration/Storage
1. Therapy should be initiated in a hospital by physicians who can treat or who have access to equipment for monitoring and treating recurrent life-threatening ventricular arrhythmias.
2. Potassium or magnesium deficiencies should be corrected before initiation of therapy since antiarrhythmics may be ineffective or arrhythmogenic in those with hypokalemia.
3. For the first rapid loading dose, 3 mL amiodarone IV (150 mg) is added to 100 mL D5W for a concentration of 1.5 mg/mL; this solution is infused at a rate of 100 mL/10 min. For the slower loading dose, 18 mL amiodarone IV (900 mg) is added to 500 mL of D5W for a concentration of 1.8 mg/mL.
4. Daily PO doses of 1,000 mg or more should be administered in divided doses with meals.

5. IV concentrations of amiodarone greater than 3 mg/mL in D5W cause a high incidence of peripheral vein phlebitis; concentrations of 2.5 mg/mL or less are not as irritating. Thus, for infusions greater than 1 hr, the IV concentration should not exceed 2 mg/mL unless a central venous catheter is used.
6. Because amiodarone adsorbs to PVC, IV infusions exceeding 2 hr must be given in glass or pollyolefin bottles containing D5W.
7. Amiodarone IV in D5W is incompatible with aminophylline, cefamandole nafate, cefazolin sodium, mezlocillin sodium, heparin sodium, and sodium bicarbonate.
8. To minimize side effects, the lowest effective dose should be determined. If side effects occur, the dose should be reduced.
9. If dosage adjustments are required, the client should be monitored for an extended period of time due to the long and variable half-life of the drug and the difficulty in predicting the time needed to achieve a new steady-state plasma drug level.
10. When initiating amiodarone therapy, other antiarrhythmic drugs should be gradually discontinued.
11. If additional antiarrhythmic therapy is required in clients on amiodarone, the initial dose of such drugs should be about one-half the usual recommended dose.
12. The injection is stored at room temperature and protected from light.
Assessment
1. Determine if client is taking any other antiarrhythmic medications.
2. Assess quality of respirations and breath sounds; note CV findings.
3. Note baseline VS and perfusion (skin temperature, color). Record pulse rate several times in similar circumstances, to establish a baseline against which to measure responses after initiating therapy.
4. Assess vision before starting therapy.
5. Determine that baseline CBC,

✦ = Available in Canada   ***bold italic*** = life threatening side effect

electrolytes, CXR, and liver and renal function studies have been performed.

6. Obtain ECG and document rhythm strips; note EPS findings when available.

Interventions

1. During administration, observe ECG for increased PR and QRS intervals, increased arrhythmias, and HR below 60 beats/min.

2. Monitor BP and assess for evidence of hypotension.

3. Note client complaints of SOB, painful breathing, or cough; assess for evidence of CHF.

4. Observe CNS symptoms such as tremor, lack of coordination, paresthesias, and dizziness.

5. Note client complaints of headaches, depression, or insomnia. Also observe for any change in behavior such as decreased interest in personal appearance or apparent hallucinations. These may indicate a need for a change in drug therapy.

6. Anticipate reduced dosages of digoxin, warfarin, quinidine, procainamide, and phenytoin if administered concomitantly with amiodarone.

7. Monitor thyroid studies because drug inhibits conversion of T_4 to T_3.

8. Schedule periodic ophthalmic examinations because small yellow-brown granular corneal deposits may develop during prolonged therapy.

Evaluate

• Termination and control of life-threatening ventricular arrhythmias

• Serum drug levels within therapeutic range (0.5–2.5 mcg/mL)

Amlodipine
(am-**LOH**-dih-peen)
Pregnancy Category: C
Norvasc **(Rx)**
Classification: Antihypertensive, antianginal (calcium channel blocking agent)

See also *Calcium Channel Blocking Agents.*

Action/Kinetics: Amlodipine increases myocardial contractility although this effect may be counteracted by reflex activity. Cardiac output is increased while there is a pronounced decrease in peripheral vascular resistance. **Peak plasma levels:** 6–12 hr. **t½, elimination:** 30–50 hr. 90% metabolized in the liver to inactive metabolites; 10% excreted unchanged in the urine.

Uses: Hypertension alone or in combination with other antihypertensives. Chronic stable angina alone or in combination with other antianginal drugs. Confirmed or suspected Prinzmetal's or variant angina alone or in combination with other antianginal drugs.

Special Concerns: Use with caution in clients with CHF and in those with impaired hepatic function or reduced hepatic blood flow. Safety and efficacy have not been determined in children.

Side Effects: *CNS:* Headache, fatigue, lethargy, somnolence, dizziness, lightheadedness, sleep disturbances, depression, amnesia, psychosis, hallucinations, paresthesia, asthenia, insomnia, abnormal dreams, malaise, anxiety, tremor, hand tremor, hypoesthesia, vertigo, depersonalization, migraine, apathy, agitation, amnesia. *GI:* Nausea, abdominal discomfort, cramps, dyspepsia, diarrhea, constipation, vomiting, dry mouth, thirst, flatulence, dysphagia, loose stools. *CV:* Peripheral edema, palpitations, hypotension, syncope, bradycardia, unspecified arrhythmias, tachycardia, ventricular extrasystoles, peripheral ischemia, *cardiac failure,* pulse irregularity, increased risk of MI. *Dermatologic:* Dermatitis, rash, pruritus, urticaria, photosensitivity, petechiae, ecchymosis, purpura, bruising, hematoma, cold/clammy skin, skin discoloration, dry skin. *Musculoskeletal:* Muscle cramps, pain, or inflammation; joint stiffness or pain, arthritis, twitching, ataxia, hypertonia. *GU:*

Polyuria, dysuria, urinary frequency, nocturia, sexual difficulties. *Respiratory:* Nasal or chest congestion, sinusitis, rhinitis, SOB, dyspnea, wheezing, cough, chest pain. *Ophthalmologic:* Diplopia, abnormal vision, conjunctivitis, eye pain, abnormal visual accommodation, xerophthalmia. *Miscellaneous:* Tinnitus, flushing, sweating, weight gain, epistaxis, anorexia, increased appetite, taste perversion, parosmia.

Dosage ————————————
• **Tablets**
   Hypertension.
Adults, usual, individualized: 5 mg/day, up to a maximum of 10 mg/day. The dose should be titrated over 7–14 days.
   Chronic stable or vasospastic angina.
Adults: 5–10 mg, using the lower dose for elderly clients and those with hepatic insufficiency. Most clients require 10 mg.

RESPIRATORY CARE CONSIDERATIONS

See also *Respiratory Care Considerations* for *Calcium Channel Blocking Agents.*
Administration/Storage
1. Food does not affect the bioavailability of amlodipine. Thus, the drug may be taken without regard to meals.
2. Elderly clients, small/fragile clients, or those with hepatic insufficiency may be started on 2.5 mg/day. This dose may also be used when adding amlodipine to other antihypertensive therapy.
Assessment
1. Note any history of CAD or CHF.
2. Review list of drugs currently prescribed to prevent any unfavorable interactions.
3. Document baseline VS, ECG, CBC, and liver and renal function studies.
Interventions
1. Monitor and record VS and I&O.

2. Anticipate reduced dose in clients with cirrhosis.
3. Monitor BP and PR interval to assess drug response.
Evaluate
• ↓ BP
• ↓ Frequency and intensity of anginal episodes

Amoxicillin (amoxycillin)
(ah-mox-ih-**SILL**-in)
Amox ✚, Amoxil, Amoxil Pediatric Drops, APO-Amoxi ✚, Biomox, Novamoxin ✚, Nu-Amoxi ✚, Polymox, Polymox Drops, Pro-Amox ✚, Trimox 125, 250, and 500, Wymox **(Rx)**

NOTE: Canadian products are all amoxicillin trihydrate.
Classification: Antibiotic, penicillin

See also *Anti-Infectives* and *Penicillins.*
Action/Kinetics: Semisynthetic broad-spectrum penicillin closely related to ampicillin. Destroyed by penicillinase, acid stable, and better absorbed than ampicillin. From 50% to 80% of a PO dose is absorbed from the GI tract. **Peak serum levels: PO:** 4–11 mcg/mL after 1–2 hr. **t½:** 60 min. Mostly excreted unchanged in urine.
Uses: Gram-positive streptococcal infections including *Streptococcus faecalis, S. pneumoniae,* and non-penicillinase-producing staphylococci. Gram-negative infections due to *Hemophilus influenzae, Proteus mirabilis, Escherichia coli,* and Neisseria gonorrhoeae.
Special Concerns: Safe use during pregnancy has not been established.

Dosage ————————————
• **Capsules, Oral Suspension, Chewable Tablets**
   Susceptible infections of ear, nose, throat, GU tract, skin and soft tissues, lower respiratory tract.
Adults: 250–500 mg q 8 hr; **pediatric under 20 kg:** 20–40 (or more) mg/kg/day in three equal doses. The pediatric dose should not exceed the maximum adult dose.

Prophylaxis of bacterial endocarditis.

3 g 60 min prior to procedure (dental, oral, or upper respiratory tract) and 1.5 g 6 hr later. Alternatively, ampicillin, 1–2 g (50 mg/kg for children) plus gentamicin, 1.5 mg/kg (2 mg/kg for children) not to exceed 80 mg, both either IM or IV 30 min before procedure followed by amoxicillin, 1.5 g (25 mg/kg for children) 6 hr after initial dose. Amoxicillin may be given as an alternate procedure for GU or GI procedures at a dose of 3 g 1 hr before procedure followed by 1.5 g 6 hr after the initial dose.

Gonococcal infections.

3 g with probenecid, 1 g, given as a single dose. In addition, tetracycline, 0.5 mg, q.i.d. for 7 days.

Gonococcal infection in pregnancy.

3 g with probenecid, 1 g, given as a single dose. In addition, erythromycin base, 0.5 g q.i.d. for 7 days.

Disseminated gonococcal infections.

3 g with probenecid, 1 g, given as a single dose; **then,** 0.5 g q.i.d. for 7 days.

Acute pelvic inflammatory disease.

3 g with probenecid, 1 g, given as a single dose. In addition, doxycycline, 100 mg b.i.d. for 10–14 days.

Sexually transmitted epididymoorchitis.

3 g with probenecid, 1 g, given as a single dose. In addition, tetracycline, 0.5 g q.i.d. for 10 days.

Bacterial vaginosis.

0.5 g q.i.d. for 7 days.

Chlamydia trachomatis during pregnancy (as an alternative to erythromycin).

0.5 g t.i.d. for 7 days.

RESPIRATORY CARE CONSIDERATIONS

See also *Respiratory Care Considerations* for *Penicillins*.

Administration/Storage

1. Dry powder is stable at room temperature for 18–30 months. Reconstituted suspension is stable for 1 week at room temperature and for 2 weeks at 2°C–8°C (36°F–46°F).

2. Chewable tablets are available for pediatric use. These may be administered with food.

Evaluate

• Resolution of infection

• Reports of symptomatic improvement

• Therapeutic peak serum drug levels (4–11 mcg/mL)

————COMBINATION DRUG————

Amoxicillin and Potassium clavulanate

(ah-mox-ih-**SILL**-in, poh-**TASS**-ee-um klav-you-**LAN**-ayt)

Pregnancy Category: B

Augmentin '125', '250', and '500', Clavulin ✦ **(Rx)**

Classification: Antibiotic, penicillin

See also *Anti-Infectives* and *Penicillins*.

Content: Each '250' Tablet contains: 250 mg amoxicillin and 125 mg potassium clavulanate. Each '500' Tablet contains 500 mg amoxicillin and 125 mg potassium clavulanate.

Each "875" tablet contains: 875 mg amoxicillin, 125 mg potassium clavulanate

Each '125' Chewable Tablet contains 125 mg amoxicillin and 31.25 mg potassium clavulanate. Each 200 Chewable Tablet contains 200 mg amoxicillin and 28.5 mg potassium clavulanate. Each '250' Chewable Tablet contains 250 mg amoxicillin and 62.5 mg potassium clavulanate.

Each 400 Chewable Tablet contains 400 mg amoxicillin and 57 mg potassium clavulanate.

Each 5 mL of the '125' Powder for Oral Suspension contains 125 mg amoxicillin and 31.25 mg potassium clavulanate. Each 5 mL of the 200 Powder for Oral Suspension contains 200 mg amoxicillin and 28.5 mg potassium clavulanate. Each 5 mL of the '250' Powder for Oral Suspension contains 250 mg amoxicillin and 62.5 mg potassium clavulanate. Each 5 mL of the 400 Powder or the 400 Powder for Oral Suspension contains 400 mg amoxicillin and 57 mg potassium clavulanate.

Action/Kinetics: *For details, see amoxicillin.* Potassium clavulanate inactivates lactamase enzymes, which are responsible for resistance to penicillins. Thus, this preparation is effective against microorganisms that have manifested resistance to amoxicillin. For potassium clavulanate: **Peak serum levels:** 1–2 hr. **t½:** 1 hr. **Uses:** For beta-lactamase-producing strains of the following organisms: *Hemophilus influenzae* and *Moraxella catarrhalis* causing lower respiratory tract infections, otitis media, and sinusitis; *Staphylococcus aureus, Escherichia coli,* and *Klebsiella,* causing skin and skin structure infections; *E. coli, Klebsiella,* and *Enterobacter,* causing UTI. *Note:* Mixed infections caused by organisms susceptible to ampicillin and organisms susceptible to amoxicillin/potassium clavulanate should not require an additional antibiotic.

Dosage ⎯⎯⎯⎯⎯⎯⎯⎯⎯
• **Oral Suspension, Chewable Tablets, Tablets**
Susceptible infections.
Adults, usual: One 500-mg tablet q 12 hr or one 250-mg tablet q 8 hr; **children less than 40 kg:** 25 mg/kg/day amoxicillin in divided doses q 12 hr.
Respiratory tract and severe infections.
Adults: One 875-mg tablet q 12 hr or one 500-mg tablet q 8 hr; **children, less than 40 kg:** 45 mg/kg/day of amoxicillin in divided doses q 12 hr (this dose is used in children for otitis media, lower respiratory tract infections, or sinusitis).
*Chancroid (*Haemophilus ducreyi infection).
Adults: One 500-mg tablet t.i.d. for 7 days (alternative to erythromycin or ceftriaxone).
Disseminated gonococcal infections.
Following therapy with an appropriate cephalosporin, (ceftriaxone, ceftizoxime, or cefotaxime) uncomplicat-ed disease therapy may be completed with one 500 mg-tablet t.i.d. for 1 week.

RESPIRATORY CARE CONSIDERATIONS

See also *Respiratory Care Considerations* for *Penicillins.*
Administration/Storage
1. Both the "250" and "500" tablets contain 125 mg clavulanic acid; therefore, two "250" tablets are not the same as one "500" tablet.
2. This combination may be taken without regard for meals; however, absorption of clavulanate potassium is enhanced if taken at the beginning of a meal.
3. The reconstituted suspension should be refrigerated and discarded after 10 days.
4. Pediatric formulations are now available in fruit flavors for the oral suspension and chewable tablets. These formulations allow twice-daily dosing, which is more convenient than three-times daily dosing and, importantly, the incidence of diarrhea is significantly reduced.
Evaluate
• Resolution of infecting organism
• Reports of symptomatic improvement
• Healing of venereal ulcers

Amphotericin B
(am-foe-**TER**-ih-sin)
Pregnancy Category: B
Fungizone, Fungizone IV **(Rx)**

Amphotericin B Lipid Complex
(am-foe-**TER**-ih-sin)
Pregnancy Category: B
Abelcet **(Rx)**
Classification: Antibiotic, antifungal

See also *Anti-Infectives.*
Action/Kinetics: This antibiotic is produced by *Streptomyces nodosus;* it is fungistatic or fungicidal depending on the concentration of the drug in body fluids and the susceptibility of

A

the fungus. Amphotericin B binds to specific chemical structures—sterols—of the fungal cellular membrane, increasing cellular permeability and promoting loss of potassium and other substances. Liposomal encapsulation or incorporation in a lipid complex can significantly affect the functional properties of the drug compared with those of the unencapsulated or non-lipid-associated drug. The liposomal amphotericin B product causes less nephrotoxicity. Amphotericin B is used either IV or topically. It is highly bound to serum protein (90%) **Peak plasma levels:** 0.5–2 mcg/mL. **t½, initial:** 24 hr; **second phase:** 15 days. Slowly excreted by kidneys.The kinetics of the drug differ in adults and children.

Uses: The drug is toxic and should be used only for clients under close medical supervision with progressive or potentially fatal fungal infections. *Amphotericin B Systemic:* Disseminated North American blastomycosis, cryptococcosis, and other systemic fungal infections, including coccidioidomycosis, histoplasmosis, mucormycosis, sporotrichosis, aspergillosis, disseminated candidiasis, and monilial overgrowth resulting from oral antibiotic therapy. Secondary therapy to treat American mucocutaneous leishmaniasis. *Liposomal Amphotericin B:* Aspergillosis in clients refractory to or intolerant of conventional amphotericin B therapy. *Investigational:* Prophylaxis of fungal infections in clients with bone marrow transplantation. *Topical:* Cutaneous and mucocutaneous infections of *Candida (Monilia)* infections.

Contraindications: Hypersensitivity to drug unless the condition is life-threatening and amenable only to amphotericin B therapy. Use to treat common forms of fungal diseases showing only positive skin or serologic tests. Use to treat noninvasive forms of fungal disease such as oral thrush, vaginal candidiasis, and esophageal candidiasis in clients with normal neutrophil counts. Lactation.

Special Concerns: The bone marrow depressant effects may result in increased incidence of microbial infection, delayed healing, and gingival bleeding. Although used in children, safety and efficacy have not been determined. Use with caution in clients receiving leukocyte transfusions.

Side Effects: After topical use. Irritation, pruritus, dry skin. Redness, itching, or burning especially in skin folds. **After IV use.** A*cute reactions occurring 1 to 3 hr after starting IV infusion:* Fever, hypotension, shaking chills, hypotension, anorexia, N&V, headache, tachypnea. Rapid infusion may cause hypotension, hypokalemia, arrhythmias, and *shock.* GI: N&V, diarrhea, dyspepsia, anorexia, abdominal cramps, epigastric pain, melena, hemorrhagic gastroenteritis, acute liver failure, hepatitis, jaundice, veno-occlusive liver disease. *CNS:* Fever, chills, headache, malaise, vertigo, leukoencephalopathy; rarely, *seizures,* encephalopathy, extrapyramidal symptoms, peripheral neuropathy, and other neurologic symptoms. *Respiratory:* Respiratory disorder, pneumonia, *respiratory failure.* Acute dyspnea, hypoxemia, interstitial infiltrates, all seen in neutropenic clients receiving amphotericin B and leukocyte transfusions. *CV:* Thrombophlebitis, phlebitis. Rarely, arrhythmias, hyper- or hypotension, tachypnea, hemoptysis, *ventricular fibrillation, cardiac arrest, cardiac failure, shock, pulmonary embolus, MI, cardiomyopathy. Renal:* Renal damage (including tubular dysfunction), azotemia, hyposthenuria, nephrocalcinosis, renal tubular acidosis, *kidney failure;* rarely, acute renal failure, decreased renal function, anuria, oliguria. *Hematologic:* Normochromic, normocytic anemia. Rarely, *coagulation defects,* thrombocytopenia, leukopenia, agranulocytosis, eosinophilia, leukocytosis. *Dermatologic:* Rarely, maculopapular rash, pruritus, exfoliative dermatitis, erythema multiforme. *Hypersensitivity:* Rarely, *bronchospasm, asthma,* *anaphylactoid reactions,* wheezing. *Miscellaneous:* Muscle and joint pain, generalized pain, weight loss, *multiple organ failure, sepsis,* infection; rarely, flushing, impotence, myasthenia. **After intrathecal use:** Blurred vision, changes in vision, difficulty in urination, numbness, tingling, pain, or weakness.

Drug Interactions

Aminoglycosides / Additive nephrotoxicity and/or ototoxicity

Antineoplastic drugs / ↑ Risk for renal toxicity, bronchospasm, and hypotension

Corticosteroids, Corticotropin / ↑ Potassium depletion caused by amphotericin B → cardiac dysfunction

Cyclosporine / ↑ Nephrotoxic effects of cyclosporine

Digitalis glycosides / ↑ Potassium depletion caused by amphotericin B → ↑ incidence of digitalis toxicity

Flucytosine / ↑ Risk of flucytosine toxicity due to ↑ cellular uptake or ↓ renal excretion

Skeletal muscle relaxants, surgical (e.g., succinylcholine, *d*-tubocurarine*)* / ↑ Muscle relaxation due to amphotericin B–induced hypokalemia

AZT / ↑ Risk of myelotoxicity and nephrotoxicity

Laboratory Test Interferences: ↑ AST, ALT, alkaline phosphatase, creatinine, BUN, NPN, BSP retention values. Hypomagnesemia, hyperkalemia, hypocalcemia, acidosis, bilirubinemia, hypoglycemia, hyperglycemia.

Dosage ——————

• **Slow IV Infusion**
   Test dose.
1 mg should be infused slowly to determine tolerance.
   Severe and rapidly progressing fungal infection.
Initial: 0.3 mg/kg/day.
Note: In impaired cardiorenal function or if a severe reaction to the test dose, therapy should be initiated with smaller daily doses (e.g., 5–10 mg). Depending on the status of the client, the dose may be increased gradually by 5–10 mg/day to a final daily dose of 0.5–0.7 mg/kg. The total daily dose should not exceed 1.5 mg/kg.
   Sporotrichosis.
20 mg/injection. Therapy may be required for up to 9 months.
   Aspergillosis.
Total dose of 3.6 g or less per day for 11 months or less.
   Rhinocerebral phycomyosis.
A cumulative dose of 3 g/day.
   Prophylaxis of fungal infections in bone marrow transplants.
0.1 mg/kg/day.

• **Liposomal Amphotericin B**
   Aspergillosis.
Adults and children: 5 mg/kg/day as a single infusion.

• **Intrathecal, Intraventricular**
   Fungal meningitis.
Initial: 0.1 mg; **then,** increase gradually up to 0.5 mg q 48 to 72 hr.

• **Bladder Irritation**
   Candidal cystitis.
5–15 mg/dL instilled periodically or continuously for 5 to 10 days.

• **Topical (Lotion, Cream, Ointment—Each 3%)**
Apply liberally to affected areas b.i.d.–q.i.d. Depending on the type of lesion, up to 4 weeks of therapy may be necessary.

RESPIRATORY CARE CONSIDERATIONS

See also *General Respiratory Care Considerations For All Anti-Infectives.*

Administration/Storage

1. *Preparation of conventional amphotericin B:* To obtain an initial concentration of 5 mg/mL, rapidly inject 10 mL sterile water for injection (without a bacteriostatic agent) directly into the lyophilized cake, using a sterile 20-gauge needle. The vial should be shaken immediately until the colloidal solution is clear. To obtain the infusion solution of 0.1 mg/mL, further dilute 1:50 with 5% dextrose injection with a pH of 4.2 or above.

——————

2. *Preparation of liposomal amphotericin B:* Shake the vial gently until there is no yellow sediment at the bottom. The appropriate dose is withdrawn from the required number of vials into one or more sterile 20-mL syringes using an 18-gauge needle. The needle is then removed from each syringe filled with liposomal amphotericin B and replaced with a 5-micron filter needle. Each filter needle is used for just one vial. Insert the filter needle on the syringe into an IV bag containing 5% dextrose injection and empty the syringe contents into the bag. The infusion concentration should be 1 mg/mL. For pediatric clients and those with CV disease, the drug may be diluted with 5% dextrose injection to a final infusion concentration of 2 mg/mL.

3. Strict aseptic technique must be used in preparation because there is no bacteriostatic agent in the medication.

4. Do not use saline solution or distilled water with bacteriostatic agent as a diluent because a precipitate may result. Use sterile water with continuous bladder irrigation.

5. Do not use the initial concentrate if any precipitate is present.

6. An in-line membrane filter with a pore diameter of 1 μm may be used. Since preparation is a colloidal suspension, anything smaller may remove the medication.

7. Protect from light during administration. However, loss of drug activity during administration is likely negligible if the solution is exposed for 8 hr or less.

8. Other drugs or electrolytes should not be mixed with lipsomal amphotericin B as compatabilities are not known. An existing IV line should be flushed with 5% dextrose injection before infusion of liposomal amphotericin B (or, a separate infusion line can be used).

9. Minimize local inflammation and danger of thrombophlebitis by administering the solution below the recommended dilution of 0.1 mg.

10. Initiate therapy in the most distal veins. When administered peripherally, changing sites with each dose may decrease phlebitis.

11. Have on hand 200–400 units of heparin sodium, since it may be ordered for the infusion to prevent thrombophlebitis.

12. Administer by slow IV infusion over 6 hr.

13. *Storage/stability of conventional amphotericin B:* Vials should be refrigerated and protected from light. After reconstitution the concentrate may be stored in the dark at room temperature for 24 hr or under refrigeration for 1 week. Any unused solution should be discarded. Diluted solutions for IV infusion should be used promptly after preparation.

14. *Storage/stability of liposomal amphotericin B:* Prior to admixture, liposomal amphotericin B should be stored at 2°C–8°C (36°F–46°F), without freezing. This product should be kept in the carton until used. The admixed liposomal amphotericin B and 5% dextrose injection may be stored for 15 hr at 2°C–8°C (36°F–46°F) and an additional 6 hr at room temperature. Any unused drug should be discarded.

15. Rub creams and lotions into lesion.

16. The cream may cause drying and slight skin discoloration; the lotion and ointment may cause staining of nail lesions, but not skin.

Assessment

1. Assess for any history of adverse effects and hypersensitivity to any anti-infectives or drugs in the antifungal category.

2. Assess mental status and note client age.

3. Review list of drugs currently prescribed to ensure none interact unfavorably.

4. Ensure that baseline CBC, liver and renal function, and laboratory cultures have been performed.

5. Assess and describe characteristics of lesions requiring therapy.

Interventions

1. Ensure correct form, liposomal or conventional, as ordered, is pre-

pared correctly for administration. Always check to ensure correct form, prior to administering.

2. Determine that a 1-mg test dose has been administered (1 mg in 20 mL D5W over 20–30 min) to assess client's tolerance to amphotericin.

3. Ascertain if client is to be pre-medicated with antipyretics, antihistamines, corticosteroids, and/or antiemetic drugs to reduce side effects. Rashes, fevers, and chills may occur frequently with this therapy.

4. Infuse IV slowly, monitor VS frequently (every 15–30 min during first dose), and interrupt if client develops any adverse effects.

5. Monitor I&O. Report a reduction in blood sediment or cloudiness in the urine.

6. Weigh client twice weekly and assess for possible malnutrition or dehydration.

7. Anticipate hypokalemia in clients concomitantly taking digoxin. Observe for toxicity and muscle weakness and monitor serum potassium and digoxin levels.

8. Intrathecal administration of amphotericin may cause inflammation of the spinal roots; assess for sensory loss or foot drop in these clients.

Evaluate
• Clinical and laboratory evidence of successful resolution of fungal infection

• Reduction in size and number of lesions

• Reports of symptomatic improvement

Ampicillin oral
(am-pih-**SILL**-in)
Pregnancy Category: B
Apo-Ampi ✿, D-Amp, Jaa Amp ✿, Novo-Ampicillin ✿, Nu-Ampi ✿, Omnipen, Penbritin ✿, Polycillin, Polycillin Pediatric Drops, Principen, Pro-Ampi ✿, Taro-Ampicillin ✿, Totacillin **(Rx)**

NOTE: The following Canadian drugs are ampicillin trihydrate: Apo-Ampi, Jaa Amp, Nu-Ampi, Pro-Ampi, Taro-Ampicillin.

---COMBINATION DRUG---

Ampicillin with Probenecid
(am-pih-**SILL**-in, proh-**BEN**-ih-sid)
Pro-Biosan ✿, Polycillin-PRB, Probampacin **(Rx)**

Ampicillin sodium, parenteral
(am-pih-**SILL**-in)
Pregnancy Category: B
Ampicin ✿, Omnipen-N, Polycillin-N, Totacillin-N **(Rx)**
Classification: Antibiotic, penicillin

See also *Anti-Infectives* and *Penicillins*.

Content: The Powder for Oral Suspension of Ampicillin with Probenecid contains 3.5 g ampicillin and 1 g probenecid per bottle.

Action/Kinetics: Synthetic, broad-spectrum antibiotic suitable for gram-negative bacteria. Acid resistant, destroyed by penicillinase. Absorbed more slowly than other penicillins. From 30% to 60% of PO dose absorbed from GI tract. **Peak serum levels: PO:** 1.8–2.9 mcg/mL after 2 hr; **IM,** 4.5–7 mcg/mL. **t½:** 80 min—range 50–110 min. Partially inactivated in liver; 25%–85% excreted unchanged in urine.

Uses: Infections of respiratory, GI, and GU tracts caused by *Shigella, Salmonella, Escherichia coli, Hemophilus influenzae, Proteus* strains, *Neisseria gonorrhoeae, N. meningitidis,* and *Enterococcus.* Also, otitis media in children, bronchitis, rat-bite fever, and whooping cough. Penicillin G-sensitive staphylococci, streptococci, pneumococci.

Additional Drug Interactions
Allopurinol / ↑ Incidence of skin rashes
Ampicillin / ↓ Effect of oral contraceptives

Dosage ————
• **Ampicillin: Capsules, Oral Suspension; Ampicillin Sodium: IV, IM**

✿ = Available in Canada   **bold italic** = life threatening side effect

Respiratory tract and soft tissue infections.

PO: 20 kg or more: 250 mg q 6 hr; **less than 20 kg:** 50 mg/kg/day in equally divided doses q 6–8 hr. **IV, IM: 40 kg or more:** 250–500 mg q 6 hr; **less than 40 kg:** 25–50 mg/kg/day in equally divided doses q 6–8 hr.

Disseminated gonococcal infections.

PO: 1 g q 6 hr.

Bacterial meningitis.

Adults: A total of 8–12 g/day given in divided doses q 3–4 hr. **Pediatric:** 100–200 mg/kg/day in divided doses q 3–4 hr.

Bacterial endocarditis prophylaxis (dental, oral, or upper respiratory tract procedures; GI or GU tract surgery or instrumentation).

Adult, IM, IV: 1–2 g (use 2 g for GI or GU tract surgery) plus gentamicin, 1.5 mg/kg (not to exceed 80 mg) IM or IV, given 30 min before procedure followed by amoxicillin, 1.5 g, 6 hr after initial dose; or, repeat parenteral dose 8 hr after initial dose. **Pediatric:** Ampicillin, 50 mg/kg with gentamicin, 2 mg/kg 30 min prior to procedure followed by amoxicillin, 25 mg/kg, after 6 hr or a parenteral dose of ampicillin is given after 8 hr.

Septicemia.

Adults/children: 150–200 mg/kg, IV for first 3 days, then IM q 3–4 hr.

• **Ampicillin with Probenecid: Oral Suspension**

Urethral, endocervical, or rectal infections due to N. gonorrhoeae.

Adults: 3.5 g ampicillin and 1 g probenecid as a single dose.

Prophylaxis of infection in rape victims.

3.5 g with 1 g probenecid.

RESPIRATORY CARE CONSIDERATIONS

See also *Respiratory Care Considerations* for *Penicillins.*

Administration/Storage

1. After reconstitution for IM or direct IV administration, the solution of sodium ampicillin **must be used within the hour.**

2. For IM use, dilute only with sterile water for injection or bacteriostatic water for injection.

3. For IVPB, ampicillin may be reconstituted with sodium chloride injection.

4. IV injections of reconstituted sodium ampicillin should be given slowly; 2 mL should be given over a period of at least 3–5 min.

5. For administration by IV drip, check compatibility and length of time that drug retains potency in a particular solution.

6. If the creatinine clearance is less than 10 mL/min, the dosing interval should be increased to 12 hr.

Assessment

1. Document indications for therapy and type, onset, and duration of symptoms.

2. Note any history of sensitivity or reactions to this drug or related compounds.

3. Obtain pretreatment CBC, liver and renal function studies, and cultures and monitor.

Interventions

1. When administering IM, tell the client that it will be painful. Rotate and document injection sites.

2. Monitor urinary output and serum potassium levels especially in the elderly.

3. Observe skin closely for rashes because they occur more often with this drug than with other penicillins. Observe for an "Ampicillin rash" which may develop which is a dull red, itchy, macular or macropapular rash and is generally benign.

4. If clients develop a latent skin rash and have symptoms of fever, fatigue, sore throat, generalized lymphadenopathy, and enlarged spleen, consider testing for mononucleosis (heterophil antibody) as this may be the cause.

Evaluate

• Resolution of S&S of infection

• Reports of symptomatic improvement

• Negative laboratory culture reports (note any evidence of resistance to drug therapy)

Amrinone lactate

(**AM**-rih-nohn)
Pregnancy Category: C
Inocor **(Rx)**
Classification: Cardiac inotropic agent

Action/Kinetics: Amrinone causes an increase in CO by increasing the force of contraction of the heart, probably by inhibiting cyclic AMP phosphodiesterase, thereby increasing cellular levels of c-AMP. It reduces afterload and preload by directly relaxing vascular smooth muscle. **Time to peak effect:** 10 min. **t½, after rapid IV:** 3.6 hr; **after IV infusion:** 5.8 hr. **Steady-state plasma levels:** 2.4 mcg/mL by maintaining an infusion of 5–10 mcg/kg/min. **Duration:** 30 min–2 hr, depending on the dose. The drug is excreted primarily in the urine both unchanged and as metabolites. Children have a larger volume of distribution and a decreased elimination half-life.

Uses: Congestive heart failure (short-term therapy in clients unresponsive to digitalis, diuretics, and/or vasodilators). Can be used in digitalized clients.

Contraindications: Hypersensitivity to amrinone or bisulfites. Severe aortic or pulmonary valvular disease in lieu of surgery. Acute MI.

Special Concerns: Safety and efficacy not established in children. Use with caution during lactation.

Side Effects: *GI:* N&V, abdominal pain, anorexia. *CV:* Hypotension, *supraventricular and ventricular arrhythmias. Allergic:* Pericarditis, pleuritis, ascites, allergic reaction to sodium bisulfite present in the product. *Other:* Thrombocytopenia, *hepatotoxicity,* fever, chest pain, burning at site of injection.

OD **Overdose Management:** *Symptoms:* Hypotension. *Treatment:* Reduce or discontinue drug administration and begin general supportive measures.

Drug Interactions: Excessive hypotension when used with disopyramide.

Dosage

- **IV**
  CHF.
Initial: 0.75 mg/kg as a bolus given slowly over 2–3 min; may be repeated after 30 min if necessary. **Maintenance, IV infusion:** 5–10 mcg/kg/min. Daily dose should not exceed 10 mg/kg although up to 18 mg/kg/day has been used in some clients for short periods.

RESPIRATORY CARE CONSIDERATIONS

Administration/Storage

1. Amrinone may be administered undiluted or diluted in 0.9% or 0.45% saline to a concentration of 1–3 mg/mL. Diluted solutions should be used within 24 hr.

2. Amrinone should not be diluted with solutions containing dextrose (glucose) prior to injection. However, the drug may be injected into running dextrose (glucose) infusions through a Y connector or directly into the tubing.

3. Administer loading dose over 2–3 min; may be repeated in 30 min.

4. Solutions should appear clear yellow.

5. Administer solution with an electronic infusion device.

6. Amrinone should not be administered in an IV line containing furosemide because a precipitate will form.

7. Protect from light and store at room temperature.

Assessment

1. Determine that baseline VS, CXR, and ECG have been performed.

2. Obtain baseline electrolytes, CBC, and platelet count.

3. Document cardiac and pulmonary assessment findings, noting any new-onset S_3, rales, or pedal edema.

4. Identify previous pharmacologic agents used for these symptoms and the results.

A

Interventions

1. Clients should be monitored closely while receiving amrinone.
2. Monitor serum potassium levels, CBC, and platelets; report any bruises or bleeding.
3. Monitor VS, I&O, weights, and urine output. Document CVP, CO, and PA pressures if Swan Ganz catheter in place.
4. Observe for any hypersensitivity reactions, including pericarditis, pleuritis, or ascites.

Evaluate

- ↓ Preload and afterload; ↑ CO
- Improvement in S&S of CHF

Amyl nitrite
(**AM**-ill)
Pregnancy Category: X
Amyl Nitrite Aspirols, Amyl Nitrite Vaporole **(Rx)**
Classification: Coronary vasodilator, antidote for cyanide poisoning

See also *Antianginal Drugs—Nitrates/Nitrites.*

Action/Kinetics: Amyl nitrite is believed to act by reducing systemic and PA pressure (afterload) and by decreasing CO due to peripheral vasodilation as opposed to causing coronary artery dilation. Vascular relaxation occurs due to stimulation of intracellular cyclic guanosine monophosphate. As an antidote to cyanide poisoning, amyl nitrite promotes formation of methemoglobin which combines with cyanide to form the nontoxic cyanmethemoglobin. **Onset (inhalation):** 30 sec. **Duration:** 3–5 min. About 33% is excreted through the kidneys.

Uses: Prophylaxis or relief of acute attacks of angina pectoris; acute cyanide poisoning. *Investigational:* Diagnostic aid to assess reserve cardiac function.

Contraindications: Lactation.

Special Concerns: Use of amyl nitrite in children has not been studied. Hypotensive effects are more likely to occur in geriatric clients.

Dosage
- **Inhalation**

Angina pectoris.
Usual: 0.3 mL (1 container crushed). Usually, 1–6 inhalations from one container produces relief. Dosage may be repeated after 3–5 min.
Antidote for cyanide poisoning.
Administer for 30–60 sec q 5 min until client is conscious; is then repeated at longer intervals for up to 24 hr.

RESPIRATORY CARE CONSIDERATIONS

See also *Respiratory Care Considerations* for *Antianginal Drugs—Nitrates/Nitrites.*

Administration/Storage

1. Administer only by inhalation.
2. Containers should be protected from light and stored at a temperature of 15°C–30°C (59°F–86°F).
3. *Amyl nitrite vapors are highly flammable. Do not use near flame or intense heat.*

Assessment

1. Take a history of common precipitating incidents that immediately precede the onset of chest pain.
2. Determine and document the degree, location, type, and duration of chest pain and where it radiates.
3. Note and identify the presence of any cardiac risk factors.
4. Determine and document source of cyanide poisoning and presenting symptoms.

Evaluate

- Improved tissue perfusion with termination of angina attack
- Antidote for cyanide poisoning

Astemizole
(ah-**STEM**-ih-zohl)
Pregnancy Category: C
Hismanil **(Rx)**
Classification: Antihistamine, miscellaneous

See also *Antihistamines.*

Action/Kinetics: Low to no sedative effect, antiemetic effect, or anticholinergic activity. The drug is metabolized in the liver to both active and inactive metabolites and is excreted through the feces. **t½:** About 1.6 days. **Onset:** 2–3 days. **Duration:**

Up to several weeks. Over 95% is bound to plasma protein. Mainly excreted through the feces.

Contraindications: Impaired hepatic function.

Special Concerns: Safety and efficacy have not been established in children less than 12 years of age. Dose should not exceed 10 mg/day.

Additional Side Effects: *Serious CV side effects, including death, cardiac arrest, QT interval prolongation, torsades de pointes and other ventricular arrhythmias* have been observed in clients exceeding the recommended dose of astemizole. Syncope may precede severe arrhythmias. Overdose may be observed with doses as low as 20–30 mg/day.

Drug Interactions: Concomitant use of astemizole with erythromycin, itraconazole, or ketoconazole may cause serious CV effects, including death, cardiac arrest, torsades de pointes, and other ventricular arrhythmias (including QT interval prolongation).

Dosage ———————————
• **Tablets**
Adults and children over 12 years: 10 mg once daily; **children, 6–12 years:** 5 mg daily..

RESPIRATORY CARE CONSIDERATIONS

See also *Respiratory Care Considerations* for *Antihistamines*.
Administration/Storage
1. The recommended dose should not be exceeded in an attempt to increase the onset of action.
2. The drug should be taken on an empty stomach at least 2 hr after a meal with no additional food taken for at least 1 hr postdosing.
Evaluate: ↓ Congestion and ↓ allergic symptoms

Atenolol
(ah-**TEN**-oh-lohl)
Pregnancy Category: C
Apo-Atenol ✦, Novo-Atenol ✦, Nu-

Atenol ✦, Taro-Atenolol ✦, Tenormin **(Rx)**
Classification: Beta-adrenergic blocking agent
———————————

See also *Beta-Adrenergic Blocking Agents*.

Action/Kinetics: Predominantly beta-1 blocking activity. Has no membrane stabilizing activity or intrinsic sympathomimetic activity. Low lipid solubility. **Peak blood levels:** 2–4 hr. **t½:** 6–9 hr. 50% eliminated unchanged in the feces.

Uses: Hypertension (either alone or with other antihypertensives such as thiazide diuretics). Angina pectoris due to hypertension, coronary atherosclerosis, and AMI. *Investigational:* Prophylaxis of migraine, alcohol withdrawal syndrome, situational anxiety, ventricular arrhythmias, prophylactically to reduce incidence of supraventricular arrhythmias in coronary artery bypass surgery.

Special Concerns: Dosage has not been established in children.

Dosage ———————————
• **Tablets**
Hypertension.
Initial: 50 mg/day, either alone or with diuretics; if response is inadequate, 100 mg/day. Doses higher than 100 mg/day will not produce further beneficial effects. Maximum effects will usually be seen within 1–2 weeks.
Angina.
Initial: 50 mg/day; if maximum response is not seen in 1 week, increase dose to 100 mg/day (some clients require 200 mg/day).
Alcohol withdrawal syndrome.
50–100 mg/day.
Prophylaxis of migraine.
50–100 mg/day.
Ventricular arrhythmias.
50–100 mg/day.
Prior to coronary artery bypass surgery.
50 mg/day started 72 hr prior to surgery.
Adjust dosage in cases of renal failure to 50 mg/day if creatinine

clearance is 15–35 mL/min/1.73 m² and to 50 mg every other day if creatinine clearance is less than 15 mL/min/1.73 m².

• **IV**
  Acute myocardial infarction.
Initial: 5 mg over 5 min followed by a second 5-mg dose 10 min later. Treatment should begin as soon as possible after client arrives at the hospital. In clients who tolerate the full 10-mg dose, a 50-mg tablet should be given 10 min after the last IV dose followed by another 50-mg dose 12 hr later. **Then,** 100 mg/day or 50 mg b.i.d. for 6–9 days (or until discharge from the hospital).

RESPIRATORY CARE CONSIDERATIONS

See also *Respiratory Care Considerations* for *Antihypertensive Agents* and *Beta-Adrenergic Blocking Agents.*

Administration/Storage
1. For IV use, the drug may be diluted in sodium chloride injection, dextrose injection, or sodium chloride and dextrose injection.
2. For hemodialysis clients, 50 mg should be given in the hospital after each dialysis.

Assessment
1. Note any client history of diabetes mellitus, pulmonary disease, or cardiac failure.
2. Document indications for therapy, type, and onset of symptoms.

Evaluate
• ↓ BP; ↓ HR
• ↓ Frequency of anginal attacks
• Prevention of reinfarction

Atovaquone
(ah-**TOV**-ah-kwohn)
Pregnancy Category: C
Mepron **(Rx)**
Classification: Antiprotozoal agent

Action/Kinetics: The mechanism of action of atovaquone against *Pneumocystis carinii* is not known. However, in *Plasmodium,* the drug appears to act by inhibiting electron transport resulting in inhibition of nucleic acid and ATP synthesis. The bioavailability of the drug is increased twofold when taken with food. The tablet formulation has been replaced by a suspension, as the latter achieves plasma levels of atovaquone that are 58% higher than those reached using tablets. Plasma levels in AIDS clients are about one-third to one-half the levels achieved in asymptomatic HIV-infected volunteers. **t½:** 2.2 days in AIDS clients; the long half-life is believed to be due to enterohepatic cycling and eventually fecal elimination. The drug is not metabolized in the liver and is not excreted appreciably through the urine; over 94% is excreted unchanged in the feces.

Uses: Acute oral treatment of mild to moderate *P. carinii* in clients who are intolerant to trimethoprim-sulfamethoxazole. The drug has not been evaluated as an agent for prophylaxis of *P. carinii.* Atovaquone is not effective for concurrent pulmonary diseases such as bacterial, viral, or fungal pneumonia or in mycobacterial diseases.

Contraindications: Hypersensitivity to atovaquone or any components of the formulation; potentially life-threatening allergic reactions are possible.

Special Concerns: Use with caution during lactation and in elderly clients. There are no efficacy studies in children. GI disorders may limit absorption of atovaquone.

Side Effects: Since many clients taking atovaquone have complications of HIV disease, it is often difficult to distinguish side effects caused by atovaquone from symptoms caused by the underlying medical condition. *Dermatologic:* Rash (including maculopapular), pruritus. *GI:* Nausea, diarrhea, vomiting, abdominal pain, constipation, dyspepsia, taste perversion. *CNS:* Headache, fever, insomnia, dizziness, anxiety, anorexia. *Respiratory:* Cough, sinusitis, rhinitis. *Hematologic:* Anemia, neutropenia. *Miscellaneous:* Asthenia, oral monilia, pain, sweating, hypoglycemia, hypotension, hyperglycemia, hyponatremia.

Drug Interactions: Since atovaquone is highly bound to plasma proteins (>99.9%), caution should be exercised when giving the drug with other highly plasma protein-bound drugs with narrow therapeutic indices as competition for binding may occur.

Laboratory Test Interferences: ↑ ALT, AST, alkaline phosphatase, amylase.

Dosage ————————

• **Suspension**

Adults: 750 mg (5 mL) given with food b.i.d. for 21 days (total daily dose: 1,500 mg).

RESPIRATORY CARE CONSIDERATIONS

Administration/Storage

1. The drug should be taken with meals as food significantly enhances the absorption of the drug. Failure to give the drug with food may result in lower plasma levels and may limit the response to therapy.

2. The drug should be dispensed in a well-closed container and stored at 15°C –25°C (59°F –77°F).

Assessment

1. Document any previous therapy for *P. carinii*, the agents used, and the outcome.

2. Assess baseline pulmonary status, CBC, and pulmonary culture results.

3. Clients with acute *P. carinii* must be carefully evaluated/screened for other related pulmonary diseases of viral, bacterial, or fungal origin and treated with additional drugs as appropriate.

Evaluate: Relief of symptoms R/T *Pneumocystis carinii*Three consectutive negative sputum cultures

Atracurium besylate
(ah-trah-**KYOUR**-ee-um)

Pregnancy Category: C

Tracrium Injection **(Rx)**

Classification: Nondepolarizing skeletal muscle relaxant

See also *Neuromuscular Blocking Agents.*

Action/Kinetics: Atracurium prevents the action of acetylcholine by competing for the cholinergic receptor at the motor end plate. It may also release histamine, leading to hypotension. **Onset:** Within 2 min. **Peak effect:** 1–2 min. **Duration:** 20–40 min with balanced anesthesia. Recovery from blockade under balanced anesthesia begins about 20–35 min after injection; recovery is usually 95% complete within 60–70 min after injection. **t½:** 20 min. Recovery occurs more rapidly than recovery from *d*-tubocurarine, metocurine, and pancuronium. Drug is metabolized in the plasma.

Uses: Skeletal muscle relaxant during surgery; adjunct to general anesthesia; assist in ET intubation. *Investigational:* Treat seizures due to drugs or electrically induced.

Contraindications: In clients with myasthenia gravis, Eaton-Lambert syndrome, electrolyte disorders, bronchial asthma.

Special Concerns: Use with caution during labor and delivery. Use with caution when significant histamine release would be dangerous (e.g., CV disease, asthma). Safety and efficacy have not been determined during lactation. Children up to 1 month of age may be more sensitive to the effects of atracurium. The drug has no known effect on pain threshold or consciousness; use only with adequate anesthesia.

Additional Side Effects: *CV:* Flushing, tachycardia. *Dermatologic:* Rash, urticaria, reaction at injection site. *Musculoskeletal:* Prolonged block, inadequate block. *Respiratory:* Dyspnea, laryngospasm. *Hypersensitivity:* Allergic reactions. Other side effects may be due to histamine release and include flushing, erythema, wheezing, urticaria, bronchial secretions, BP and HR changes.

OD **Overdose Management:** *Symptoms:* Hypotension, enhanced pharmacologic effects. *Treatment:* CV support. Ensure airway and ventilation. An anticholinesterase reversing agent (e.g., neostigmine, edrophonium, pyridostigmine) with an anticholinergic agent (e.g., atropine, glycopyrrolate) may be used.

Additional Drug Interactions

Acetylcholinesterase inhibitors / Muscle relaxation is inhibited and neuromuscular block is reversed
Aminoglycosides / ↑ Muscle relaxation
Corticosteroids / Prolonged weakness
Enflurane / ↑ Muscle relaxation
Halothane / ↑ Muscle relaxation
Isoflurane / ↑ Muscle relaxation
Lithium / ↑ Muscle relaxation
Phenytoin / ↓ Effect of atracurium
Procainamide / ↑ Muscle relaxation
Quinidine / ↑ Muscle relaxation
Succinylcholine / ↑ Onset and depth of muscle relaxation
Theophylline / ↓ Effect of atracurium
Trimethaphan / ↑ Muscle relaxation
Verapamil / ↑ Muscle relaxation

Dosage ————————————
• **IV Bolus Only**
Intubation and maintenance of neuromuscular blockade.
Adults and children over 2 years, initial: 0.4–0.5 mg/kg as IV bolus; **maintenance:** 0.08–0.1 mg/kg. The first maintenance dose is usually required 20–45 min after the initial dose. Maintenance doses should be given every 15–25 min under balanced anesthesia, slightly longer under isoflurane or enflurane anesthesia.
Following use of succinylcholine for intubation under balanced anesthesia.
Initial: 0.3–0.4 mg/kg; if using potent inhalation anesthetics, further reductions may be required.
Use in neuromuscular disease, severe electrolyte disorders, or carcinomatosis.
Dosage reductions should be considered where potentiation of neuromuscular blockade or difficulty with reversal have been noted.
Use after steady-state enflurane or isoflurane anesthesia established.
0.25–0.35 mg/kg (about ⅓ less than the usual initial dose).

Use in infants 1 month to 2 years of age under halothane anesthesia.
0.3–0.4 mg/kg. More frequent maintenance doses may be required.
• **IV Infusion**
Balanced anesthesia.
IV infusion: 9–10 mcg/kg until the level of neuromuscular blockade is reestablished; **then,** rate of infusion is adjusted according to client needs (usually 5–9 mcg/kg/min although some clients may require as little as 2 mcg/kg/min and others as much as 15 mcg/kg/min).
For cardiopulmonary bypass surgery in which hypothermia is induced.
Reduce rate of infusion by 50%.

_____

RESPIRATORY CARE CONSIDERATIONS

See also *Respiratory Care Considerations* for *Neuromuscular Blocking Agents.*

Administration/Storage

1. Atracurium should be used only by those skilled in airway management and ventilatory support. Equipment and personnel must be available immediately for endotracheal intubation and support of ventilation. Anticholinesterase reversal agents should be immediately available.
2. Initial dosage should be reduced to 0.25–0.35 mg/kg if drug is being used with steady-state enflurane or isoflurane (smaller reductions if halothane is being used).
3. Dosage should be reduced in clients with myasthenia gravis or other neuromuscular diseases, electrolyte disorders, or carcinomatosis.
4. Infusion solutions are prepared by admixing atracurium with either 5% dextrose injection, 0.9% sodium chloride injection, or 5% dextrose and 0.9% sodium chloride injection. Atracurium should *not* be mixed with alkaline solutions, including lactated Ringer's injection.
5. Maintenance doses can be given by continuous infusion of a diluted solution to clients 2 years of age to adulthood.
6. Solutions containing 0.2 or 0.5

mg/mL can be stored either under refrigeration or at room temperature for 24 hr without significant loss of potency.

7. To preserve potency, the drug should be refrigerated at 2°C–8°C (36°F–46°F).

8. IM administration may cause tissue irritation.

9. Drug does not affect consciousness or pain threshold. Concomitant antianxiety agents and analgesics should be employed.

10. IV atropine may be used to treat bradycardia due to atracurium.

Assessment

1. Document indications for therapy and onset, duration, and characteristics of symptoms.

2. Utilize a peripheral nerve stimulator to assess neuromuscular response and recovery.

3. Obtain baseline ECG, VS, and lab studies.

Interventions

1. Monitor VS and ECG. Drug can cause vagal stimulation resulting in bradycardia, hypotension, and cardiac arrhythmias.

2. Document length of time client is receiving the drug. It should be used only on a short-term basis and in a continuously monitored environment.

3. Remember that client may be fully conscious and aware of surroundings and conversations.

4. Drug does not affect pain or anxiety so administer analgesics and antianxiety agents as indicated.

Evaluate

• Desired level of skeletal muscle relaxation

• Facilitation of ET intubation and tolerance of mechanical ventilation

• Control of electrically or pharmacologically induced seizures

---

Atropine sulfate

(**AH**-troh-peen)

Pregnancy Category: C

Atropair, Atropine-1 Ophthalmic, Atropine A.K. ✦, Atropine Minims ✦, Atropine Sulfate Ophthalmic, Atropine-Care Ophthalmic, Atropisol Ophthalmic, Dioptic's Atropine ✦, Isopto Atropine Ophthalmic, Minims Atropine ✦, R.O.-Atropine ✦ **(Rx)**

Classification: Cholinergic blocking agent

See also *Cholinergic Blocking Agents.*

Action/Kinetics: Atropine blocks the action of acetylcholine on postganglionic cholinergic receptors in smooth muscle, cardiac muscle, exocrine glands, urinary bladder, and the AV and SA nodes in the heart. Ophthalmologically, atropine blocks the effect of acetylcholine on the sphincter muscle of the iris and the accommodative muscle of the ciliary body. This results in dilation of the pupil (mydriasis) and paralysis of the muscles required to accommodate for close vision (cycloplegia). This enables the physician to examine the inner structure of the eye, including the retina. It also permits examination of refractive errors of the lens without the client automatically accommodating. **Peak effect:** Mydriasis, 30–40 min; *cycloplegia,* 1–3 hr. **Recovery:** Up to 12 days. **Duration, PO:** 4–6 hr. t½: 2.5 hr. Metabolized by the liver although 30%–50% is excreted through the kidneys unchanged.

Uses: PO: Adjunct in peptic ulcer treatment. Irritable bowel syndrome. Adjunct in treatment of spastic disorders of the biliary tract. Urologic disorders, urinary incontinence. During anesthesia to control salivation and bronchial secretions. Has been used for parkinsonism but more effective drugs are available.

Parenteral: Antiarrhythmic, adjunct in GI radiography. Prophylaxis of arrhythmias induced by succinylcholine or surgical procedures. Reduce sinus bradycardia (severe) and syncope in hyperactive carotid sinus reflex. Prophylaxis and treatment of toxicity due to cholinesterase inhibitors, including organophosphate pesticides. Treatment of curariform

---

A

block. As a preanesthetic or in dentistry to decrease secretions.

Ophthalmologic: Cycloplegic refraction or pupillary dilation in acute inflammatory conditions of the iris and uveal tract. *Investigational:* Treatment and prophylaxis of posterior synechiae; pre- and postoperative mydriasis; treatment of malignant glaucoma.

Additional Contraindications: Ophthalmic use: Infants less than 3 months of age, primary glaucoma or a tendency toward glaucoma, adhesions between the iris and the lens, geriatric clients and others where undiagnosed glaucoma or excessive pressure in the eye may be present, in children who have had a previous severe systemic reaction to atropine.

Special Concerns: Use with caution in infants, small children, geriatric clients, diabetes, hypo- or hyperthyroidism, narrow anterior chamber angle, individuals with Down syndrome.

Additional Side Effects: *Ophthalmologic:* Blurred vision, stinging, increased intraocular pressure, contact dermatitis. Long-term use may cause irritation, photophobia, eczematoid dermatitis, conjunctivitis, hyperemia, or edema.

OD **Overdose Management:** *Treatment of Ocular Overdose:* Eyes should be flushed with water or normal saline. A topical miotic may be necessary.

Dosage _____
• **Tablets**
Anticholinergic or antispasmodic.
Adults: 0.3–1.2 mg q 4–6 hr. **Pediatric, over 41 kg:** same as adult; **29.5–41 kg:** 0.4 mg q 4–6 hr; **18.2–29.5 kg:** 0.3 mg q 4–6 hr; **10.9–18.2 kg:** 0.2 mg q 4–6 hr; **7.3–10.9 kg:** 0.15 mg q 4–6 hr; **3.2–7.3 kg:** 0.1 mg q 4–6 hr.
Prophylaxis of respiratory tract secretions and excess salivation during anesthesia.
Adults: 2 mg.
Parkinsonism.
Adults: 0.1–0.25 mg q.i.d.
• **IM, IV, SC**

Anticholinergic.
Adults, IM, IV, SC: 0.4–0.6 mg q 4–6 hr. **Pediatric, SC:** 0.01 mg/kg, not to exceed 0.4 mg (or 0.3 mg/m²).
To reverse curariform blockade.
Adults, IV: 0.6–1.2 mg given at the same time or a few minutes before 0.5–2 mg neostigmine methylsulfate (use separate syringes).
Treatment of toxicity from cholinesterase inhibitors.
Adults, IV, initial: 2–4 mg; **then,** 2 mg repeated q 5–10 min until muscarinic symptoms disappear and signs of atropine toxicity begin to appear. **Pediatric, IM, IV, initial:** 1 mg; **then,** 0.5–1 mg q 5–10 min until muscarinic symptoms disappear and signs of atropine toxicity appear.
Treatment of mushroom poisoning due to muscarine.
Adults, IM, IV: 1–2 mg q hr until respiratory effects decrease.
Treatment of organophosphate poisoning.
Adults, IM, IV, initial: 1–2 mg; **then,** repeat in 20–30 min (as soon as cyanosis has disappeared). Dosage may be continued for up to 2 days until symptoms improve.
Arrhythmias.
Pediatric, IV: 0.01–0.03 mg/kg.
Prophylaxis of respiratory tract secretions, excessive salivation, succinylcholine- or surgical procedure-induced arrhythmias.
Pediatric, up to 3 kg, SC: 0.1 mg; **7–9 kg:** 0.2 mg; **12–16 kg:** 0.3 mg; **20–27 kg:** 0.4 mg; **32 kg:** 0.5 mg; **41 kg:** 0.6 mg.
• **Ophthalmic Solution**
Uveitis.
Adults: 1–2 gtt instilled into the eye(s) up to q.i.d. **Children:** 1–2 gtt of the 0.5% solution into the eye(s) up to t.i.d.
Refraction.
Adults: 1–2 gtt of the 1% solution into the eye(s) 1 hr before refracting. **Children:** 1–2 gtt of the 0.5% solution into the eye(s) b.i.d. for 1–3 days before refraction.
• **Ophthalmic Ointment**
Instill a small amount into the conjunctival sac up to t.i.d.

RESPIRATORY CARE CONSIDERATIONS

See also *Respiratory Care Considerations* for *Cholinergic Blocking Agents*.

Administration/Storage

1. For ophthalmic use, atropine sulfate is available in 0.5%, 1%, or 2% solutions or 1% ointment.
2. After instillation of the ophthalmic ointment, compress the lacrimal sac by digital pressure for 1–3 min. This tends to decrease systemic effects.
3. Have physostigmine available in the event of overdose.

Assessment

1. Document presenting symptoms and indications for therapy.
2. Check for a history of angle-closure glaucoma before administering the drug in the eye because atropine may precipitate an acute crisis.
3. Obtain VS and ECG; monitor cardiopulmonary status during IV therapy.

Evaluate

- ↑ HR
- Desired pupillary dilatation
- ↓ GI activity
- Reversal of muscarinic effects of anticholinesterase agents
- ↓ Salivation

Azithromycin

(az-**zith**-roh-**MY**-sin)
Pregnancy Category: B
Zithromax **(Rx)**
Classification: Antibiotic, macrolide

Action/Kinetics: Azithromycin is an azalide antibiotic (subclass of macrolides) derived from erythromycin. The drug acts by binding to the 50S ribosomal subunit of susceptible organisms, thus interfering with microbial protein synthesis. It is rapidly absorbed and distributed widely throughout the body. Food decreases the absorption of azithromycin. **t½, terminal:** 68 hr. A loading dose will achieve steady-state levels more quickly. The major route of elimina-

tion is biliary excretion of unchanged drug with a small amount being excreted through the kidneys.

Uses: Mild to moderate infections in clients 16 years of age or older as described in what follows. Acute bacterial exacerbations of COPD due to *Hemophilus influenzae, Moraxella catarrhalis,* or *Streptococcus pneumoniae.* Community-acquired pneumonia due to *Strep. pneumoniae* or *H. influenzae* in clients who can take outpatient PO therapy. As an alternative to first-line therapy to treat streptococcal pharyngitis or tonsillitis due to *Streptococcus pyogenes.* Uncomplicated skin and skin structure infections due to *Staphylococcus aureus, Staphyloccus pyogenes,* or *Streptococcus agalactiae.* Abscesses usually require surgical drainage. Nongonococcal urethritis and cervicitis due to *Chlamydia trachomatis.* Used alone or with rifabutin for prophylaxis of *Mycobacterium avium* complex (MAC) disease in clients with advanced HIV infections. Pediatric infections, including acute otitis media caused by *H. influenza, Strep. pneumoniae,* and M. catarrhalis.

Contraindications: Hypersensitivity to azithromycin, any macrolide antibiotic, or erythromycin. In clients who are not eligible for outpatient PO therapy (e.g., known or suspected bacteremia, immunodeficiency, functional asplenia, nosocomially acquired infections, geriatric or debilitated clients).

Special Concerns: Use with caution in clients with impaired hepatic or renal function and during lactation. Safety and efficacy for acute otitis media have not been determined in children less than 6 months of age; also, safety and efficacy for pharyngitis/tonsillits have not been determined in children less than 2 years of age. Recommended doses should not be relied upon to treat gonorrhea or syphilis.

Side Effects: *GI:* N&V, diarrhea, loose stools, abdominal pain, dyspepsia, flatulence, melena, cholestatic jaundice, pseudomembranous colitis. In children, gastritis, constipation, and anorexia have also been noted. *CNS:* Dizziness, headache, somnolence, fatigue, vertigo. In children, hyperkinesia, agitation, nervousness, insomnia, fever, and malaise have been noted. *CV:* Chest pain, palpitations, **ventricular arrhythmias (including ventricular tachycardia and torsades de pointes in clients with prolonged QT intervals observed with other macrolides).** *GU:* Monilia, nephritis, vaginitis. *Allergic:* Angioedema, photosensitivity, rash, **anaphylaxis.** *Hematologic:* Leukopenia, neutropenia, decreased platelet count. *Miscellaneous:* Superinfection, conjunctivitis (in children).

Drug Interactions: See also *Drug Interactions for Erythromycins.*
Aluminum- and magnesium-containing antacids / ↑ *Peak serum levels of azithromycin but not the total amount absorbed*
Tacrolimus / Azithromycin may ↑ plasma levels of tacrolimus → ↑ risk of toxicity
Laboratory Test Interferences: ↑ Serum CPK, potassium, ALT, GGT, AST, serum alkaline phosphatase, bilirubin, BUN, creatinine, blood glucose, LDH, and phosphate.

Dosage ———————————
• **Capsules, Suspension, Tablets**
Adults: Upper and lower respiratory tract infections due to COPD, pneumonia, pharyngitis/tonsillitis; uncomplicated skin and skin structure infections.
Adults and children over 16 years of age: 500 mg as a single dose on day 1 followed by 250 mg once daily on days 2–5 for a total dose of 1.5 g.
Nongonococcal urethritis and cervicitis due to C. trachomatis, chancroid, chlamydia.
1 g given as a single dose.
• **Tablets**
Prophylaxis of M. avium *complex in advanced HIV infections.*

1,200 mg once a week (two 600-mg tablets).
• **Oral Suspension**
Pediatric: otitis media.
10 mg/kg (not to exceed 500 mg) on day 1, followed by 5 mg/kg (not to exceed 250 mg/day) on days 2–5.
Pediatric: pharyngitis/tonsillitis.
12 mg/kg/day for 5 days, not to exceed 500 mg/day.

RESPIRATORY CARE CONSIDERATIONS

See also *Respiratory Care Considerations* for *Erythromycins.*
Administration/Storage: The capsules should be given at least 1 hr prior to a meal or at least 2 hr after a meal. Tablets may be taken with or without food, although increased tolerability has been observed if taken with food.
Assessment
1. Determine any history of sensitivity to erythromycins and note any previous experience with macrolide antibiotics and the results.
2. Determine if client is currently prescribed warfarin or theophylline. Azithromycin may cause an increase in serum concentrations of these drugs so levels should be monitored throughout therapy.
3. Obtain documentation that clients with sexually transmitted cervicitis or urethritis are tested for gonorrhea and syphilis at the time of diagnosis. Ensure that appropriate drug therapy is instituted if necessary.
4. Obtain baseline liver and renal function studies and appropriate cultures when warranted.
Evaluate
• Resolution of S&S of infection
• Laboratory confirmation of negative culture reports

———————————————

Aztreonam for injection
(as-**TREE**-oh-nam)
Pregnancy Category: B
Azactam for Injection **(Rx)**
Classification: Monobactam antibiotic

———————————————

See also *Anti-Infectives.*

Action/Kinetics: Aztreonam belongs to a class of antibiotics called *monobactams*. It is a synthetic drug that is bactericidal against gram-negative aerobic pathogens. The drug acts by inhibiting cell wall synthesis due to a high affinity of the drug for penicillin binding protein 3; this results in cell lysis and death. Widely distributed to all body fluids. **Time to peak serum levels:** 0.6–1.3 hr. **t½:** 1.5–2 hr. The t½ is prolonged in clients with impaired renal function. Approximately 60%–75% excreted unchanged in the urine within 8 hr.

Uses: Complicated and uncomplicated urinary tract infections (including pyelonephritis and cystitis) due to *Escherichia coli, Klebsiella pneumoniae, Proteus mirabilis, Pseudomonas aeruginosa, Enterobacter cloacae, Klebsiella oxytoca, Citrobacter* species, and *Serratia marcescens.* Lower respiratory tract infections (including bronchitis and pneumonia) due to *E. coli, K. pneumoniae, P. aeruginosa, Hemophilus influenzae, P. mirabilis, Enterobacter* species, and *S. marcescens.* Septicemia due to *E. coli, K. pneumoniae, P. aeruginosa, P. mirabilis, S. marcescens* and *Enterobacter* species. Skin and skin structure infections (including postoperative wounds, ulcers, and burns) caused by *E. coli, P. mirabilis, S. marcescens, Enterobacter* species, *P. aeruginosa, K. pneumoniae*, and *Citrobacter* species. Intra-abdominal infections (including peritonitis) due to *E. coli, K. pneumoniae, Enterobacter* species, *P. aeruginosa, Citrobacter* species, and *Serratia* species. Gynecologic infections (including endometritis and pelvic cellulitis) due to *E. coli, K. pneumoniae, P. mirabilis,* and *Enterobacter* species. As an adjunct to surgery to manage infections caused by susceptible organisms. As an alternative to spectinomycin in clients with acute uncomplicated gonorrhea who are resistant to penicillin. Concomitant initial therapy with other anti-infective drugs and aztreonam in seriously ill clients is recommended before the causative organism is known and who are at risk for an infection due to gram-positive aerobic pathogens.

Contraindications: Allergy to aztreonam. Lactation.

Special Concerns: Safety and effectiveness have not been determined in children and infants. Use with caution in clients allergic to penicillins or cephalosporins and in those with impaired hepatic or renal function.

Side Effects: *GI:* N&V, diarrhea, abdominal cramps, mouth ulcers, numb tongue, halitosis, *Clostridium difficile*-associated diarrhea or GI bleeding. *CNS:* Confusion, **seizures,** vertigo, paresthesia, insomnia, dizziness. *Hematologic:* Anemia, neutropenia, thrombocytopenia, leukocytosis, thrombocytosis, pancytopenia. *Dermatologic:* Rash, purpura, erythema multiforme, urticaria, petechiae, pruritus, diaphoresis, exfoliative dermatitis. *CV:* Hypotension, transient ECG changes, flushing. *Following parenteral use:* Phlebitis and thrombophlebitis after IV use; discomfort and swelling at the injection site after IM use. *Miscellaneous:* **Anaphylaxis,** hypersensitivity reactions, headache, weakness, fever, malaise, hepatitis, jaundice, muscle aches, tinnitus, diplopia, nasal congestion, altered taste, sneezing, vaginal candidiasis, vaginitis, breast tenderness, chest pain, eosinophilia.

OD **Overdose Management:** *Treatment:* Hemodialysis or peritoneal dialysis to reduce serum levels.

Drug Interactions: Antibiotics that increase levels of beta-lactamase (e.g., cefoxitin, imipenem) may inhibit the activity of aztreonam.

Laboratory Test Interferences: ↑ AST, ALT, alkaline phosphatase, serum creatinine, PT, PTT. Positive Coombs' test.

Dosage

- **IM, IV**

    Urinary tract infections.

B

Adults: 0.5–1 g q 8–12 hr, not to exceed 8 g/day. **Children:** 30 mg/kg q 6–8 hr.

Moderate to severe systemic infections.
1–2 g q 8–12 hr, not to exceed 8 g/day.

Severe systemic or life-threatening infections.
2 g q 6–8 hr, not to exceed 8 g/day.

P. aeruginosa infections in children.
50 mg/kg q 4–6 hr.

NOTE: Dose must be reduced in clients with impaired renal function.

RESPIRATORY CARE CONSIDERATIONS

See also *General Respiratory Care Considerations For All Anti-Infectives.*

Administration/Storage
1. The IV route should be used for doses greater than 1 g or in clients with septicemia.
2. Therapy should be continued for at least 48 hr after the client becomes asymptomatic or until laboratory tests indicate that the infection has been eradicated.
3. For use as a bolus, the 15-mL vial should be diluted with 6–10 mL sterile water for injection. For IM use, the 15-mL vial should be diluted with at least 3 mL of either sterile water for injection, sodium chloride injection, bacteriostatic water for injection, or bacteriostatic sodium chloride injection. Final dilution should not exceed 20 mg/mL.
4. An IV bolus injected slowly over 3–5 min may be used to initiate therapy. IV infusion should be given over 20–60 min.
5. For IM use, the drug should be given in a large muscle mass.
6. Aztreonam is incompatible with cephradine, nafcillin sodium, and metronidazole. Data for other drugs are not available and therefore use of other admixtures is not recommended.

Assessment
1. Note any allergy to penicillins or cephalosporins.
2. Obtain baseline CBC and liver and renal function studies and monitor throughout therapy.
3. Anticipate reduced dosage in clients with impaired renal function (see package insert).
4. Monitor renal function if used with an aminoglycoside (especially if high doses are used or if therapy is prolonged).

Evaluate
• Resolution of infecting organism
• Reports of symptomatic improvement

B

Bacampicillin hydrochloride
(bah-kam-pih-**SILL**-in)
Pregnancy Category: B
Penglobe ✦, Spectrobid **(Rx)**
Classification: Antibiotic, penicillin

See also *Anti-Infectives* and *Penicillins.*

Action/Kinetics: Bacampicillin is a semisynthetic, acid-resistant penicillin that is hydrolyzed to the active ampicillin in the GI tract. Food does not affect absorption of the drug. The drug is 98% absorbed from the GI tract and is approximately 20% plasma protein bound. **Peak serum levels:** Obtained in 0.9 hr are approximately 3 times those seen with equivalent doses of ampicillin. Seventy-five percent is excreted in the urine as active ampicillin within 8 hr.

Uses: Upper and lower respiratory tract infections caused by beta-hemolytic streptococcus, *Staphylococcus pyogenes,* pneumococci, non-penicillinase-producing staphylococci, and *Haemophilus influenzae.*

UTIs caused by *Escherichia coli, Proteus mirabilis,* and enterococci. Skin infections caused by streptococci and susceptible staphylococci. Acute uncomplicated urogenital infections caused by Neisseria gonorrhoeae.

Contraindications: History of penicillin allergy. Concomitant use with disulfiram (Antabuse).

Drug Interactions: Bacampicillin should not be used concomitantly with disulfiram.

Laboratory Test Interferences: False + reaction to Clinitest, Benedict's solution, and Fehling's solution. ↑ AST.

Dosage
• **Tablets**

Upper respiratory tract infections, otitis media, UTIs, skin and skin structure infections.

Adults (25 kg or more): 400 mg q 12 hr; **pediatric:** 25 mg/kg/day in equally divided doses q 12 hr. Dose may be doubled in cases of lower respiratory tract infections, severe infections, or in treating less susceptible organisms.

Gonorrhea.

Males and females: 1.6 g with 1 g probenecid as a single dose. No pediatric dosage has been established.

RESPIRATORY CARE CONSIDERATIONS

See also *General Respiratory Care Considerations for All Anti-Infectives.*

Evaluate
• Negative C&S results
• Resolution of infection and reports of improvement

Bacitracin intramuscular
(bass-ih-**TRAY**-sin)
Bacitracin Sterile **(Rx)**

Bacitracin ointment
(bass-ih-**TRAY**-sin)
Baciguent, Bacitin ✿ **(OTC)**

Bacitracin ophthalmic ointment
(bass-ih-**TRAY**-sin)
AK-Tracin, Bacitracin Ophthalmic Ointment **(Rx)**
Classification: Antibiotic, miscellaneous

See also *Anti-Infectives.*

Action/Kinetics: This antibiotic is produced by *Bacillus subtilis.* The drug interferes with synthesis of cell wall, preventing incorporation of amino acids and nucleotides. Bacitracin is bactericidal, bacteriostatic, and active against protoplasts. It is not absorbed from the GI tract. When given parenterally, drug is well distributed in pleural and ascitic fluids.

Bacitracin has high nephrotoxicity. Its systemic use is restricted to infants (see *Uses*). Renal function must be carefully evaluated prior to, and daily, during use. **Peak plasma levels: IM,** 0.2–2 mcg/mL after 2 hr. From 10% to 40% is excreted in the urine after IM administration.

Uses: Parenteral: Limited to the treatment of staphylococcal pneumonia and staphylococcus-induced empyema in infants. **Topical:** Prophylaxis or treatment of infections in minor cuts, wounds, burns, and skin abrasions. As an aid to healing and for treating superficial infections of the skin due to susceptible organisms. **Ophthalmic:** Effective against species of *Staphylococcus, S. aureus, Streptococcus, S. pneumoniae, S. pyogenes, Corynebacterium, Neisseria, N. gonorrhoeae,* and beta-hemolytic streptococci.

Contraindications: Hypersensitivity or toxic reaction to bacitracin. Pregnancy. Epithelial herpes simplex keratitis, vaccinia, varicella, mycobacterial eye infections, fungal diseases of the eye. Topical antibiotics should not be used in deep-seated ocular infections or in those that are likely to become systemic.

Special Concerns: Ophthalmic ointments may retard corneal epithelial healing. Prolonged or repeat-

---

ed use may result in bacterial or fungal overgrowth of nonsusceptible organisms leading to a secondary infection.

Side Effects: Parenteral use: *Nephrotoxicity due to tubular and glomerular necrosis, renal failure;* toxic reactions; N&V. **Topical use:** Allergic contact dermatitis, superinfection. **Ophthalmic use:** Transient burning, stinging, itching, irritation, inflammation, angioneurotic edema, urticaria, vesicular and maculopapular dermatitis.

Drug Interactions

Aminoglycosides / Additive nephrotoxicity and neuromuscular blocking activity

Anesthetics / ↑ Neuromuscular blockade → possible muscle paralysis

Neuromuscular blocking agents / Additive neuromuscular blockade → possible muscle paralysis

Dosage ————————————

• **IM Only**

Infants, 2.5 kg and below: 900 units/kg/day in two to three divided doses; **infants over 2.5 kg:** 1,000 units/kg/day in two to three divided doses.

• **Ophthalmic Ointment (500 units/g)**

Acute infections.

½ in. in lower conjunctival sac q 3–4 hr until improvement occurs. Treatment should be reduced before the drug is discontinued.

Mild to moderate infections.

½ in. b.i.d.–t.i.d.

• **Topical Ointment (500 units/g)**

Apply a small amount equal to the surface area of a fingertip 1–3 times/day after cleaning the affected area. Should not be used for more than 1 week.

RESPIRATORY CARE CONSIDERATIONS

See also *General Respiratory Care Considerations for All Anti-Infectives.*

Administration/Storage: Do not mix bacitracin with glycerin or other polyalcohols that cause drug to deteriorate. When used topically, the affected area may be covered with a sterile bandage.

Assessment

1. Document indications for therapy, type, onset, and duration of symptoms.

2. List any previous experiences with this type of infection (especially of ocular origin), agents used, and the outcome.

3. Recurrent ophthalmic infections should be cultured and carefully assessed by an ophthalmologist.

Interventions

1. Monitor and maintain adequate I&O with parenteral use of drug.

2. Withhold drug and report when output is inadequate. Monitor renal function studies.

3. Test pH of urine daily; pH should be kept at 6 or greater to decrease renal irritation.

4. Have sodium bicarbonate or other alkali available to administer if urine pH drops below 6.

5. Do not administer concurrently or sequentially with a topical or systemic nephrotoxic drug.

6. Cleanse area thoroughly before applying bacitracin as a wet dressing or ointment.

Evaluate

• Resolution of S&S of infection
• Restoration of skin integrity
• Negative lab C&S reports

Beclomethasone dipropionate

(be-kloh-**METH**-ah-zohn)

Pregnancy Category: C

Aerosol Inhaler: Beclodisk ✤, Becloforte Inhaler ✤, Beclovent, Vanceril, Vanceril DS **(Rx)**, **Intranasal:** Beconase AQ Nasal, Beconase Inhalation, Vancenase AQ 84 mcg Double Strength, Vancenase AQ Forte, Vancenase AQ Nasal, Vancenase Nasal Inhaler **(Rx)**, **Topical:** Propaderm ✤

Classification: Glucocorticoid

See also *Corticosteroids.*

Action/Kinetics: Rapidly inactivated, thereby resulting in few systemic effects.

NOTE: If a client is on systemic steroids, transfer to beclomethasone may be difficult because recovery from impaired renal function may be slow.

Uses: Intranasal use for relief of symptoms of seasonal or perennial rhinitis in clients not responsive to more conventional therapy, to prevent recurrence of nasal polyps following surgical removal, and to treat allergic or nonallergic (vasomotor) rhinitis (spray formulations). Inhalation therapy for chronic use in bronchial asthma. In glucocorticoid-dependent clients, beclomethasone often permits a decrease in the dosage of the systemic agent. Withdrawal of systemic corticosteroids must be carried out gradually.

Contraindications: Status asthmaticus, acute episodes of asthma, hypersensitivity to drug or aerosol ingredients.

Special Concerns: Safe use during lactation and in children under 6 years of age not established.

Side Effects: *Intranasal:* Headache, pharyngitis, coughing, epistaxis, nasal burning, pain, conjunctivitis, myalgia, tinnitus. Rarely, ulceration of the nasal mucosa and nasal septum perforation.

Dosage ————————————
• **Metered Dose Inhaler**
Asthma.
Adults: 2 inhalations (total of 84 mcg beclomethasone) t.i.d.–q.i.d. In some clients, 2–4 inhalations (84–168 mcg) b.i.d. have been effective. **Pediatric, 6–12 years:** 1–2 inhalations (42–84 mcg) t.i.d.–q.i.d., not to exceed 10 inhalations (420 mcg) daily. Dosage has not been determined in children less than 6 years of age.
Severe asthma.
Adults, initial: 12–16 inhalations (504–672 mcg beclomethasone) daily; **then,** decrease dose according to response. **Maximum daily dose:** 20

inhalations (840 mcg beclomethasone).

NOTE: Vanceril DS can be used once daily for treatment of asthma.

In clients also receiving systemic glucocorticosteroids, beclomethasone should be started when client's condition is relatively stable.
• **Nasal Aerosol or Spray**
Allergic or nonallergic rhinitis, Prophylaxis of nasal polyps.
Adults and children over 12 years: 1 inhalation (42 mcg) in each nostril b.i.d.–q.i.d. (i.e., total daily dose: 168–336 mcg). If no response after 3 weeks, discontinue therapy. **Maintenance, usual:** 1 inhalation in each nostril t.i.d. (252 mcg/day). For nasal polyps, treatment may be required for several weeks or more before a therapeutic effect can be assessed fully. Two sprays of the double-strength product (Vancenase AQ 84 mcg Double Strength) are administered once daily.

Vancenase AQ Forte may be used once daily for treatment of rhinitis.

RESPIRATORY CARE CONSIDERATIONS

See also *Respiratory Care Considerations* for *Corticosteroids.*
Administration/Storage
1. To administer beclomethasone with an inhaler, use the following procedure and instruct clients to:
• Shake metal cannister thoroughly immediately prior to use.
• -Exhale as completely as possible, usually to functional residual capacity, or to residual volume.
• -Place mouthpiece of inhaler approximately one inch in front of open mouth, or place in mouth with teeth apart and tongue flat.
• -Inhale deeply and slowly while actuating inhaler by pressing down on cannister.
• -Inhale to total lung capacity and hold breath for 10 seconds if possible. Remove mouthpiece.
• -Exhale normally, then shake cannister, administer subsequent

breaths after 30 to 60 seconds, if indicated.

• -If using a bronchodilator, take bronchodilator first, then use corticosteroid after 2 to 5 minute wait.

• -It is always preferable to use a reservoir or spacer device when administering corticosteroids via MDI.

• -Always rinse mouth and throat with water after last puff.

2. To prevent explosion of contents under pressure, do not store or use near heat or open flame, or throw into a fire or incinerator. Keep secure from children.

3. If the cannister is cold, the therapeutic effect may be decreased.

Assessment

1. Note any history of sensitivity to corticosteroids or fluorocarbon propellants.

2. Document indications for therapy and pretreatment pulmonary assessments and pulmonary function tests.

Interventions

1. For clients who are receiving systemic steroid therapy, initiate beclomethasone therapy *very* slowly, withdrawing the systemic steroids as ordered. The benefit of inhaled steroids is that it requires a much lower dose since it goes to the target organ and does not require weaning.

2. Assess for and report any signs of adrenal insufficiency (such as muscular pain, lassitude, and depression) even if the client's respiratory function has improved.

3. Symptoms of adrenal insufficiency, such as hypotension and weight loss, are indications that the dosage of systemic steroid should be boosted temporarily, and then withdrawn more gradually.

Client/Family Teaching

1. Instruct in the use, care, and storage of the inhaler. Caution the client to rinse out their mouth and to wash the mouth piece, spacer, and sprayer and to dry it after each use.

2. Observe client technique to ensure proper administration. A spacer may facilitate administration. With nasal administration advise to aim toward the eye and not the septum to decrease nasal irritation. Use a demonstrator, if available, to enhance client understanding.

3. Explain that the inhaler is not effective for acute asthma attacks but should be used regularly as prescribed to prevent the occurrence of these attacks.

4. Stress the importance of complying with the prescribed drug therapy even though it may take 1–4 weeks for any improvement in respiratory function to be realized.

5. More than 1 mg in adults or more than 500 mcg in children may precipitate hypothalamic-pituitary axis depression, resulting in adrenal insufficiency. Therefore, advise clients not to overuse the inhaler or exceed prescribed dosage.

6. Report any symptoms of localized fungal infections in the mouth. Gargling and rinsing after treatments and rinsing of the spacer and/or administration port may help prevent these infections. These must be reported immediately and will require antifungal medication and possibly discontinuation of the drug.

7. Advise clients also receiving bronchodilators by inhalation that they should use the bronchodilator first to open the airways and then use beclomethasone 15 minutes later. This increases the penetration of steroid and reduces the potential toxicity from inhaled fluorocarbon propellants of both inhalers.

8. Once clients have had a systemic steroid withdrawn, they should be provided with a supply of PO glucocorticoids. These are to be taken immediately if subjected to unusual stress or severe asthma attack. All usage should be noted and reported.

9. Carry a card indicating the diagnosis, treatment, and possible need for systemic glucocorticoids, in the event of exposure to unusual stress or severe asthma attack.

10. Instruct in several relaxation techniques to perform during stressful situations.

Evaluate

• Control of the symptoms of asthma
• Successful ↓ in or withdrawal of systemic steroids

- Relief of rhinitis
- Prophylaxis of nasal polyps

Benazepril hydrochloride
(beh-**NAYZ**-eh-prill)
Pregnancy Category: D
Lotensin **(Rx)**
Classification: Antihypertensive, ACE inhibitor

See also *Angiotensin-Converting Enzyme Inhibitors*

Action/Kinetics: Both supine and standing BPs are reduced in clients with mild-to-moderate hypertension with no compensatory tachycardia. Benazepril also has an antihypertensive effect in clients with low-renin hypertension. Food does not affect the extent of absorption. Benazepril is almost completely converted to the active benazeprilat, which has greater ACE inhibitor activity. **Onset:** 1 hr. **Duration:** 24 hr. **Peak plasma levels, benazepril:** 30–60 min. **Peak plasma levels, benazeprilat:** 1–2 hr if fasting and 2–4 hr if not fasting. **t½, benazeprilat:** 10–11 hr. **Peak reduction in BP:** 2–4 hr after dosing. **Peak effect with chronic therapy:** 1–2 weeks. The drug is highly bound to plasma protein and is excreted through the urine with about 20% of a dose excreted as benazeprilat.

Uses: Used alone or in combination with thiazide diuretics to treat hypertension.

Contraindications: Hypersensitivity to benazepril or any other ACE inhibitor.

Special Concerns: Use with caution during lactation. Safety and effectiveness have not been determined in children.

Side Effects: *CNS:* Headache, dizziness, fatigue, anxiety, insomnia, nervousness. *GI:* N&V, constipation, abdominal pain, melena. *CV:* Symptomatic hypotension, postural hypotension, syncope, angina pectoris, palpitations, peripheral edema, ECG changes. *Dermatologic:* Dermatitis, pruritus, rash, flushing, dia-

phoresis. *GU:* Decreased libido, impotence, UTI. *Respiratory:* Cough, asthma, bronchitis, dyspnea, sinusitis, bronchospasm. *Neuromuscular:* Paresthesias, arthralgia, arthritis, asthenia, myalgia. *Hematologic:* Occasionally, eosinophilia, leukopenia, neutropenia, decreased hemoglobin. *Miscellaneous:* Angioedema, which may be associated with involvement of the tongue, glottis, or larynx; hypertonia; proteinuria; hyponatremia; infection.

Drug Interactions
Diuretics / Excessive ↓ in BP
Lithium / ↑ Serum lithium levels with ↑ risk of lithium toxicity
Potassium-sparing diuretics, potassium supplements / ↑ Risk of hyperkalemia

Laboratory Test Interferences: ↑ Serum creatinine, BUN, serum potassium. ↓ Hemoglobin. ECG changes.

Dosage ———————
- **Tablets**
  Clients not receiving a diuretic.
  Initial: 10 mg once daily; **maintenance:** 20–40 mg/day given as a single dose or in two equally divided doses. Total daily doses greater than 80 mg have not been evaluated.
  Clients receiving a diuretic.
  Initial: 5 mg/day.
  Creatinine clearance < 30 mL/min/1.73 m². The recommended starting dose is 5 mg/day; **maintenance:** titrate dose upward until BP is controlled or to a maximum total daily dose of 40 mg.

RESPIRATORY CARE CONSIDERATIONS

See also *Respiratory Care Considerations* for *Angiotensin-Converting Enzyme Inhibitors,* and *Antihypertensive Agents.*

Administration/Storage
1. Dosage adjustment should be based on measuring peak (2–6 hr after dosing) and trough responses. If once daily dosing does not provide an adequate trough response, increas-

ing the dose or giving divided doses should be considered.

2. If BP cannot be controlled by benazepril alone, a diuretic can be added.

3. If a client is receiving a diuretic, the diuretic, if possible, should be discontinued 2–3 days before beginning benazepril therapy.

4. The drug may be taken without regard to food.

Assessment

1. Note any previous experience with this class of drugs.

2. Obtain baseline electrolytes, liver, and renal function studies and monitor throughout therapy.

Evaluate: Control of hypertension with a minimum of side effects

---

Bepridil hydrochloride

(**BEH**-prih-dill)
Pregnancy Category: C
Vascor **(Rx)**
Classification: Antianginal, calcium channel blocking drug

See also *Calcium Channel Blocking Agents.*

Action/Kinetics: Bepridil inhibits the transmembrane influx of calcium ions into cardiac and vascular smooth muscle. The drug increases the effective refractory period of the atria, AV node, His-Purkinje fibers, and ventricles. The drug dilates peripheral arterioles and reduces total peripheral resistance; it reduces HR and arterial pressure at rest and at a given level of exercise. The drug is rapidly and completely absorbed following PO use. **Onset:** 60 min. **Time to peak plasma levels:** 2–3 hr. Greater than 99% bound to plasma protein. Food does not affect either the peak plasma levels or the extent of absorption. **Therapeutic serum levels:** 1–2 ng/mL. **t½, distribution:** 2 hr; **terminal elimination:** 24 hr.

Steady-state blood levels do not occur for 8 days. The drug is metabolized in the liver, and metabolites are excreted through both the kidney (70%) and the feces (22%).

Uses: Chronic stable angina (classic effort-associated angina) in clients who have failed to respond to other antianginal medications or who are intolerant to such medications. It may be used alone or with beta blockers or nitrates. An additive effect occurs if used with propranolol.

Contraindications: Clients with a history of serious ventricular arrhythmias, sick sinus syndrome, second- or third-degree heart block (except in the presence of a functioning ventricular pacemaker), hypotension (less than 90 mm Hg systolic), uncompensated cardiac insufficiency, congenital QT interval prolongation, and in those taking other drugs that prolong the QT interval (e.g., quinidine, procainamide, tricyclic antidepressants). Use in clients with MI during the previous 3 months. During lactation.

Special Concerns: Safety and effectiveness have not been determined in children. Use with caution in clients with CHF, left bundle block, sinus bradycardia (less than 50 beats/min), serious hepatic or renal disorders. New arrhythmias can be induced. Geriatric clients may require more frequent monitoring.

Side Effects: *CV: Induction of new serious arrhythmias such as torsades de pointes type ventricular tachycardia, prolongation of QTc and QT interval, increased PVC rates, new sustained VT and VT/VF,* sinus tachycardia, sinus bradycardia, hypertension vasodilation, palpitations. *GI:* Nausea (common), dyspepsia, GI distress, diarrhea, dry mouth, anorexia, abdominal pain, constipation, flatulence, gastritis, increased appetite. *CNS:* Nervousness, dizziness, drowsiness, insomnia, depression, vertigo, akathisia, anxiousness, tremor, hand tremor, syncope, paresthesia. *Respiratory:* Cough, pharyngitis, rhinitis, dyspnea, respiratory infection. *Body as a whole:* Asthenia, headache, flu syndrome, fever, pain, superinfection. *Dermatologic:* Rash, skin irritation, sweating. *Miscellaneous:* Tinnitus, arthritis, blurred vision, taste change, loss of libido, impotence, agranulocytosis.

Drug Interactions

Cardiac glycosides / Exaggeration of the depression of AV nodal conduction

Digoxin / Possible ↑ serum digoxin levels

Potassium-wasting diuretics / Hypokalemia, which causes an ↑ risk of serious ventricular arrhythmias

Procainamide / ↑ Risk of serious side effects due to exaggerated prolongation of the QT interval

Quinidine / ↑ Risk of serious side effects due to exaggerated prolongation of the QT interval

Tricyclic antidepressants / ↑ Risk of serious side effects due to exaggerated prolongation of the QT interval

Laboratory Test Interferences: ↑ ALT, transaminase. Abnormal liver function tests.

Dosage —————
- **Tablets**

  Chronic stable angina.

Adults, initial: 200 mg once daily; after 10 days the dosage may be adjusted upward depending on the response of the client (e.g., ability to perform ADL, QT interval, HR, frequency and severity of angina). **Maintenance:** 300 mg/day, not to exceed 400 mg/day. The minimum effective dose is 200 mg.

RESPIRATORY CARE CONSIDERATIONS

See also *Respiratory Care Considerations* for *Calcium Channel Blocking Agents.*

Administration/Storage

1. Can be taken with meals or at bedtime if nausea occurs.

2. Bepridil should be taken at about the same time each day. If a dose is missed, the next dose should *not* be doubled.

3. Geriatric clients may require more frequent monitoring.

Assessment

1. Determine which antianginal

agents have been used in the past and their effects.

2. Perform baseline CBC, serum electrolytes (especially K) and ECG prior to initiating drug therapy.

3. List drugs currently prescribed to determine any potential drug interactions. Notify provider if client prescribed any medications that prolong the QT interval (e.g., procainamide, quinidine, tricyclic antidepressants).

4. QT intervals should be checked prior to initiating therapy with bepridil, 1–3 weeks after beginning therapy, and periodically thereafter, and especially after any dosage adjustment. Prolongation of QT intervals may predispose client to serious ventricular arrhythmias.

5. Document any evidence of AV block, arrhythmias, MI, and implanted ventricular pacemaker.

Interventions

1. Clients requiring diuretics should take a potassium-sparing agent.

2. Monitor VS. Observe closely for evidence of new arrhythmias, especially torsades de pointes tachycardia.

3. Clients should continue taking nitroglycerin if prescribed.

Evaluate

- Prophylaxis and control of angina
- Therapeutic serum drug levels (1–2 ng/mL)

Beractant

(beh-**RACK**-tant)

Survanta **(Rx)**

Classification: Lung surfactant

Action/Kinetics: Beractant, derived from natural bovine lung extract, contains phospholipids, fatty acids, neutral lipids, and surfactant-associated proteins (to which colfosceril palmitate, tripalmitin, and palmitic acid are added). The proteins in the product—SP-B and SP-C—are hydrophobic, low molecular weight, and surfactant associated. Beractant replenishes pulmonary surfactant and restores surface activity to the

B

lungs of premature infants to reduce respiratory distress syndrome. The drug is intended for intratracheal use only. Significant improvement is observed in the arterial-alveolar oxygen ratio and mean airway pressure. Beractant significantly decreases the incidence of respiratory distress syndrome, mortality due to respiratory distress syndrome, and air leak complications.

Uses: Prevention and treatment ("rescue") of respiratory distress syndrome (hyaline membrane disease) in premature infants.

Special Concerns: Beractant can quickly affect oxygenation and lung compliance; thus, it should only be used in a highly supervised setting with immediate availability of physicians experienced with intubation, ventilator management, and general care of premature infants.

Side Effects: Commonly, side effects are associated with the dosing procedure and include transient bradycardia, oxygen desaturation, ET tube reflux, vasoconstriction, pallor, hypotension, hypertension, ET tube blockage, hypocarbia, hypercarbia, and *apnea*. Other symptoms include *intracranial hemorrhage,* rales, moist breath sounds, and nosocomial sepsis.

OD   Overdose   Management: *Symptoms: Acute airway obstruction.*

Dosage ⎯⎯⎯⎯⎯⎯⎯⎯⎯⎯⎯
• **Intratracheal Only**
4 mL/kg (100 mg phospholipids/kg birth weight).

RESPIRATORY CARE CONSIDERATIONS
Administration/Storage
1. For prevention of respiratory distress syndrome in premature infants weighing less than 1,250 g at birth or with evidence of surfactant deficiency, beractant should be given as soon as possible, preferably within 15 min of birth.
2. To treat infants with confirmed respiratory distress syndrome and who require mechanical ventilation, beractant should be given as soon as

possible, preferably within 8 hr of birth.
3. Four doses can be given within the first 48 hr of life; doses should be given no sooner than q 6 hr.
4. Beractant should be refrigerated at 2°C–8°C (36°F–46°F) and warmed at room temperature for at least 20 min or in the hand for at least 8 min before administration. The drug does not have to be reconstituted or sonicated before use. If a prevention dose is required, preparation should begin before the infant is born. The drug should not be warmed and then returned to the refrigerator for future use more than once.
5. Before administration the vial should be visually inspected for discoloration (beractant is off-white to light brown). If settling occurs during storage, the vial should be swirled gently (not shaken) to redisperse although some foaming may occur at the surface during handling.
6. Each vial is for single use only; any residual drug should thus be discarded.
7. Instill beractant through a 5 French end-hole catheter that has been inserted into the ET tube of the infant with the tip of the catheter protruding just beyond the end of the ET tube above the infant's carina. The length of the catheter should be shortened before inserting it through the ET tube. The drug should not be given into a mainstem bronchus.
8. To ensure homogeneous distribution, each dose should be divided into four quarter-doses with each quarter-dose given with the infant in a different position—head and body inclined slightly down, head turned to the right; head and body inclined slightly down, head turned to the left; head and body inclined slightly up, head turned to the right; and head and body inclined slightly up, head turned to the left.
9. For the first dose, determine the total dose based on the infant's birth weight and withdraw the entire contents of the vial into the plastic syringe using at least a 20-gauge needle. The premeasured 5 French end-hole

catheter is attached to the syringe and the catheter filled with beractant. Any excess should be discarded through the catheter so that only the total dose to be given remains in the syringe. Before giving the drug, proper placement and patency of the ET tube must be ensured (the tube may be suctioned before giving the drug). The infant should be allowed to stabilize before proceeding with dosing.

10. If the first dose is to be used for prevention strategy, the dose should be administered to the stabilized infant as soon as possible after birth (preferably within 15 min). The infant is positioned appropriately and the first quarter-dose is gently injected through the catheter over 2–3 sec. After the first quarter-dose is given, the catheter is removed from the ET tube. To prevent cyanosis, manually ventilate with sufficient oxygen using a hand-bag (ambu type) at a rate of 60 breaths/min with sufficient positive pressure to provide adequate air exchange and chest wall excursion.

11. If rescue strategy is to be undertaken, the first dose should be given as soon as possible after the infant is placed on a ventilator for management of hyaline membrane disease. Studies have been undertaken in which the infant's ventilator settings were changed to a rate of 60/min (inspiratory time 0.5 sec and FiO_2 1) immediately before instilling the first quarter-dose. The infant is positioned appropriately and the first quarter-dose is gently injected through the catheter over 2–3 sec. The catheter is removed from the ET tube and the infant is returned to the mechanical ventilator.

12. When using both prevention and rescue strategies, the infant is ventilated for 20 sec or until stable. The infant is repositioned for instillation of the next quarter-dose. The remaining quarter-doses are given using the same procedures. After instillation of each quarter-dose, the

catheter is removed and the infant is ventilated for 30 sec or until stabilized. After the final quarter-dose is instilled, the catheter is removed without flushing. The infant should not be suctioned for 1 hr after dosing unless signs of significant obstruction of the airway occur. After the dosing procedure is completed, usual ventilator management and clinical care should be resumed.

13. If repeat doses are necessary, the dose is also 100 mg phospholipids/kg with the dose based on the infant's birth weight (the infant should not be reweighed). Additional doses are determined by evidence of continuing respiratory distress. Repeat doses should not be given sooner than 6 hr after the preceding dose if the infant remains intubated and requires a FiO_2 of at least 30 to maintain a pO_2 of less than or equal to 80 torr. Radiographic confirmation of respiratory distress syndrome should be made before giving additional doses to infants who received a prevention dose.

14. Repeat doses are given by the same procedure as described for prevention strategy. However, studies have used different ventilator settings. For repeat doses, the FiO_2 was increased by 0.2 or an amount sufficient to prevent cyanosis. The ventilator delivered a rate of 30/min with an inspiratory time of less than 1 sec. If the infant's pretreatment rate was greater than or equal to 30, it was left unchanged during instillation. Manual hand-bag ventilation should *not* be used to give repeat doses.

15. Unopened vials should be stored in the refrigerator at 2°C–8°C (36°F–46°F) and protected from light. Vials should be stored in the carton until ready for use.

16. Ross Laboratories offers audiovisual instructional materials concerning administration procedures and dosing requirements.

17. Studies continue regarding different methods of administering beractant and other exogenous surfac-

B

tants. So, other protocols, other then described here, may be appropriate.

Assessment

1. Note indications for medication therapy (prevention, rescue, or both).

2. The infant HR, color, chest expansion, facial expression, oximeter readings, and ET tube patency and position should be documented and monitored carefully before and during beractant therapy.

3. Ascertain that the ET tube tip is in the trachea and not in the esophagus or right or left mainstem bronchus, before inserting the 5 French end-hole catheter, to ensure appropriate drug dispersion to all lung areas.

4. Document baseline birth weight, ABGs, CXR, and physical assessment findings.

Interventions

1. Follow administration guidelines carefully. Beractant is for intratracheal administration only. It should only be administered by trained personnel in a highly supervised environment permitting continuous client observation.

2. Auscultate lung fields frequently and avoid suctioning for 1 hr after dosing unless symptoms of significant airway obstruction are evident.

3. Monitor ECG, arterial BP, and oxygen saturation continuously. After beractant treatment, frequent ABGs should be measured to prevent postdosing hyperoxia and hypocarbia.

4. Monitor (during dosing) for any evidence of transient bradycardia and decreased oxygen saturation. If evident, the dosing procedure should be stopped and the client treated symptomatically until stabilized; then the dosing procedure may be resumed.

5. Observe closely for air leaks and mucous plugs. If mucous plug is unrelieved by suctioning, the ET tube must be replaced immediately.

Evaluate

• Improved airway exchange with ↓ pulmonary air leaks

• Oxygen saturation readings between 90% and 95%; improved pulmonary parameters more consistent with survival

• Prevention or successful treatment of respiratory distress syndrome in premature infants

Betamethasone
(bay-tah-**METH**-ah-zohn)
Celestone **(Rx)**

Betamethasone dipropionate
(bay-tah-**METH**-ah-zohn)
Topical: Alphatrex, Diprolene, Diprolene Glycol ✦, Diprosone, Maxivate, Occlucort ✦, Rhoprolene ✦, Rhoprosone ✦, Taro-Sone ✦, Topilene ✦, Topisone ✦ **(Rx)**

Betamethasone sodium phosphate
(bay-tah-**METH**-ah-zohn)
Celestone Phosphate, Cel-U-Jec **(Rx)**

Betamethasone sodium phosphate and Betamethasone acetate
(bay-tah-**METH**-ah-zohn)
Celestone Soluspan **(Rx)**

Betamethasone valerate
(bay-tah-**METH**-ah-zohn)
Topical: Betacort ✦, Betaderm ✦, Betagel ✦, Betatrex, Betnovate ✦, Betnovate-1/2 ✦, Celestoderm-V ✦, Celestoderm-V/2 ✦, Dermabet, Ectosone Mild ✦, Ectosone Regular, Ectosone Scalp Lotion ✦, Prevex B ✦, Rivasone ✦, Valisone, Valisone Reduced Strength, Valnac **(Rx)**
Classification: Glucocorticoid

See also *Corticosteroids*.

Action/Kinetics: Causes low degree of sodium and water retention, as well as potassium depletion. The injectable form contains both rapid-acting and repository forms of betamethasone (mixture of betamethasone sodium phosphate and betamethasone acetate). Not recommended for replacement therapy in any acute or chronic adrenal cortical insufficiency because it does not have strong sodium-retaining effects. Long-acting. **t½:** over 300 min.

Additional Use: Prevention of respiratory distress syndrome in premature infants.

Special Concerns: Safe use during pregnancy and lactation has not been established.

Dosage ─────────────

BETAMETHASONE

• **Syrup, Tablets**
0.6–7.2 mg/day.

BETAMETHASONE SODIUM PHOSPHATE

• **IV, Intra-articular, Intralesional, Soft Tissue Injection**
Initial: up to 9 mg/day; **then,** adjust dosage at minimal level to reduce symptoms.

BETAMETHASONE SODIUM PHOSPHATE AND BETAMETHASONE ACETATE(contains 3 mg/mL each of the acetate and sodium phosphate)

• **IM**
Initial: 0.5–9 mg/day (dose ranges are ⅓–½ the PO dose given q 12 hr.)

• **Intra-articular,   Intrabursal, Intradermal, Intralesional**
Bursitis, peritendinitis, tenosynovitis.
1 mL.
Rheumatoid arthritis and osteoarthritis.
0.25–2 mL, depending on size of the joint.
Foot disorders, bursitis.
0.25–0.5 mL under heloma durum or heloma molle; 0.5 mL under calcaneal spur or over hallux rigidus or digiti quinti varus. Tenosynovitis or periostitis of cuboid: 0.5 mL.
Acute gouty arthritis.
0.5–1 mL.

• **Intradermal**
0.2 mL/cm² not to exceed 1 mL/week.

BETAMETHASONE DIPROPIONATE, BETAMETHASONE VALERATE

• **Topical Aerosol, Cream, Lotion, Ointment**
Apply sparingly to affected areas and rub in lightly.

RESPIRATORY CARE CONSIDERATIONS

See *Respiratory Care Considerations for Corticosteroids.*

Administration/Storage: Avoid injection into deltoid muscle because SC atrophy of tissue may occur.

Assessment: Document indications for therapy, type, onset, and duration of symptoms, and any agents prescribed with the outcome.

Client/Family Teaching

1. Report any S&S of infection, i.e., increased fever and any redness, odor, or purulent drainage of wound.

2. Cover topical area to avoid sun burn.

3. Advise not to overuse joint after injection as this may further injure joint.

4. Carefully monitor weight; report any sudden weight gain or presence of edema.

Evaluate

• ↓ Pain and inflammation with improved mobility of extremity

• Prevention of respiratory distress syndrome in premies

• Evidence of improved skin integrity and healing of lesions

Betaxolol hydrochloride
(beh-**TAX**-oh-lohl)
Pregnancy Category: C
Betoptic, Betoptic S, Kerlone **(Rx)**
Classification: Beta-adrenergic blocking agent

See also *Beta-Adrenergic Blocking Agents.*

Action/Kinetics: Inhibits beta-1-adrenergic receptors although beta-2 receptors will be inhibited at high doses. Has some membrane stabilizing activity but no intrinsic sympathomimetic activity. Low lipid solubility. When used in the eye, betaxolol reduces the production of aqueous humor, thus, reducing intraocular pressure. It has no effect on pupil size or accommodation. **t½:** 14–22 hr. Metabolized in the liver with most excreted through the urine; about 15% is excreted unchanged.

Uses: PO: Hypertension, alone or with other antihypertensive agents (especially diuretics). **Ophthalmic:** Ocular hypertension and chronic open-angle glaucoma (used alone or in combination with other antiglaucoma drugs).

Special Concerns: Use with caution during lactation. Safety and effectiveness have not been determined in children. Geriatric clients are at greater risk of developing bradycardia.

Dosage ─────────
• **Tablets**
  Hypertension.
Initial: 10 mg once daily either alone or with a diuretic. If the desired effect is not reached, the dose can be increased to 20 mg although doses higher than 20 mg will not increase the therapeutic effect. In geriatric clients the initial dose should be 5 mg/day.
• **Ophthalmic Solution, Suspension**
Adults: 1–2 gtt b.i.d. If used to replace another drug, continue the drug being used and add 1 gtt of betaxolol b.i.d. The previous drug should be discontinued the following day. If transferring from several antiglaucoma drugs being used together, adjust one drug at a time at intervals of not less than 1 week. The agents being used can be continued and add 1 gtt betaxolol b.i.d. The next day, another agent should be discontinued. The remaining antiglaucoma drug dosage can be decreased or discontinued depending on the response of the client.

RESPIRATORY CARE CONSIDERATIONS

See also *Respiratory Care Considerations* for *Beta-Adrenergic Blocking Agents* and *Antihypertensive Agents*.
Administration/Storage
1. The full antihypertensive effect is usually observed within 7–14 days.
2. As the PO dose is increased, the HR decreases.
3. PO drug therapy with betaxolol

should be discontinued gradually over a 2-week period.
4. Ophthalmic products should be stored at room temperature not to exceed 30°C (86°F).
5. The ophthalmic suspension should be shaken well before use.
Evaluate
• ↓ BP (PO)
• ↓ Intraocular pressure (Ophth)

Bisoprolol fumarate
(**BUY**-soh-**proh**-lol)
Pregnancy Category: C
Zebeta **(Rx)**
Classification: Beta-adrenergic blocking agent

See also *Beta-Adrenergic Blocking Agents.*
Action/Kinetics: At clinical doses, bisoprolol inhibits beta-1-adrenergic receptors; at higher doses beta-2 receptors are also inhibited. The drug has no intrinsic sympathomimetic activity and has no membrane stabilizing activity. **t½:** 9–12 hr. Over 90% of PO dose is absorbed. Approximately 50% is excreted unchanged through the urine and the remainder as inactive metabolites; a small amount (less than 2%) is excreted through the feces.
Uses: For hypertension alone or in combination with other antihypertensive agents. *Investigational:* Angina pectoris, SVTs, PVCs.
Special Concerns: Use with caution during lactation. Safety and efficacy have not been determined in children. Since bisoprolol is rather selective for beta-1 receptors, it may be used with caution in clients with bronchospastic disease who do not respond to, or who cannot tolerate, other antihypertensive therapy.
Laboratory Test Interferences: ↑ AST, ALT, uric acid, creatinine, BUN, serum potassium, glucose, and phosphorus. ↓ WBCs and platelets.

Dosage ─────────
• **Tablets**
  Antihypertensive.
Dose must be individualized. **Adults, initial:** 5 mg once daily (in

some clients, 2.5 mg/day may be appropriate). **Maintenance:** If the 5-mg dose is inadequate, the dose may be increased to 10 mg/day and then, if needed, to 20 mg once daily. In clients with impaired renal or hepatic function, the initial daily dose should be 2.5 mg with caution used in titrating the dose upward.

RESPIRATORY CARE CONSIDERATIONS

See also *Respiratory Care Considerations* for *Beta-Adrenergic Blocking Agents.*

Administration/Storage

1. Food does not affect the bioavailability of bisoprolol; thus, the drug may be given without regard to meals.

2. The half-life of bisoprolol is increased in clients with a creatinine clearance below 40 mL/min and in those with cirrhosis; thus, the dose must be adjusted.

3. Since bisoprolol is not dialyzable, dose adjustments are not necessary in clients undergoing hemodialysis.

Assessment

1. Document indications for therapy, previous agents used, and the outcome.

2. Obtain baseline CBC, electrolytes, and liver and renal function studies.

3. Once baseline parameters have been determined, continue to monitor BP in both arms with client lying, sitting, and standing.

4. Document cardiac rhythm and any evidence of arrhythmia by ECG.

Evaluate

- ↓ BP
- Relief of angina
- Restoration of stable cardiac rhythm

Bitolterol mesylate
(bye-**TOHL**-ter-ohl)
Pregnancy Category: C
Tornalate Aerosol **(Rx)**
Classification: Bronchodilator

See also *Sympathomimetic Drugs.*

Action/Kinetics: Bitolterol is considered a prodrug in that it is converted by esterases in the body to the active colterol. Colterol is said to combine with beta-2-adrenergic receptors, producing dilation of bronchioles. Minimal beta-1-adrenergic activity. **Onset following inhalation:** 3–4 min. **Time to peak effect:** 30–60 min. **Duration:** 5–8 hr.

Uses: Prophylaxis and treatment of bronchial asthma and bronchospasms. Treatment of bronchitis, emphysema, bronchiectasis, and COPD. May be used with theophylline and/or steroids.

Special Concerns: Safety has not been established for use during lactation and in children less than 12 years of age. Use with caution in ischemic heart disease, hypertension, hyperthyroidism, diabetes mellitus, cardiac arrhythmias, seizure disorders, or in those who respond unusually to beta-adrenergic agonists. There may be decreased effectiveness in steroid-dependent asthmatic clients. Hypersensitivity reactions may occur.

Additional Side Effects: *CNS:* Hyperactivity, hyperkinesia, lightheadedness. *CV:* Premature ventricular contractions. *Other:* Throat irritation.

Drug Interactions: Additive effects with other beta-adrenergic bronchodilators.

Laboratory Test Interferences: ↑ AST. ↓ Platelets, WBCs. Proteinuria.

Dosage

- **Metered Dose Inhaler**
  Bronchodilation.
  Adults and children over 12 years: 2 inhalations at an interval of 1–3 min q 8 hr (if necessary, a third inhalation may be taken). The dose should not exceed 3 inhalations q 6 hr or 2 inhalations q 4 hr.
  Prophylaxis of bronchospasm.
  Adults and children over 12 years: 2 inhalations q 8 hr.

B

RESPIRATORY CARE CONSIDERATIONS

See also *Respiratory Care Considerations* for *Sympathomimetic Drugs*.

Administration/Storage

1. Bitolterol is available in a MDI. With the inhaler in an upright position, the client should breathe out completely in a normal fashion. As the client is breathing in slowly and deeply, the canister and mouthpiece should be squeezed between the thumb and forefinger, activating the medication. The breath should be held for 10 sec and then slowly exhaled. A spacer may facilitate administration.

2. The medication should not be stored above 120°F (49°C).

3. The inhaler delivers 0.37 mg bitolterol per actuation.

Client/Family Teaching

1. Use a demonstrator to assist client in proper administration. Add a spacer to enhance drug dispersion.

2. Advise not to exceed prescribed dosage and to seek medical assistance if symptoms worsen.

Evaluate

• Improved airway exchange with ↓ airway resistance

• Asthma and bronchospasm prophylaxis

Bretylium tosylate

(breh-**TILL**-ee-um **TOZ**-ill-ayt)

Pregnancy Category: C

Bretylate Parenteral ✿, Bretylol **(Rx)**

Classification: Antiarrhythmic, class III

Action/Kinetics: Bretylium inhibits catecholamine release at nerve endings by decreasing excitability of the nerve terminal. Initially there is a release of norepinephrine, which may cause tachycardia and a rise in BP; this is followed by a blockade of release of catecholamines. The drug also increases the duration of the action potential and the effective refractory period, which may assist in reversing arrhythmias. **Peak plasma concentration and effect:** 1 hr after IM injection. Antifibrillatory effect within a few minutes after IV use. Suppression of ventricular tachycardia and ventricular arrhythmias takes 20–120 min, whereas suppression of PVCs does not occur for 6–9 hr. **Therapeutic serum levels:** 0.5–1.5 mcg/mL. **t½:** Approximately 5–10 hr. **Duration:** 6–8 hr. From 0% to 8% is protein bound. Up to 90% of drug is excreted unchanged in the urine after 24 hr.

Uses: Life-threatening ventricular arrhythmias that have failed to respond to other antiarrhythmics. Prophylaxis and treatment of ventricular fibrillation. For short-term use only. *Investigational:* Second-line drug (after lidocaine) for advanced cardiac life support during CPR.

Contraindications: Severe aortic stenosis, severe pulmonary hypertension.

Special Concerns: Safety and efficacy in children have not been established. Dosage adjustment is required in clients with impaired renal function.

Side Effects: *CV:* Hypotension (including postural hypotension), transient hypertension, increased frequency of PVCs, bradycardia, precipitation of anginal attacks, initial increase in arrhythmias, sensation of substernal pressure. *GI:* N&V (especially after rapid IV administration), diarrhea, abdominal pain, hiccoughs. *CNS:* Vertigo, dizziness, lightheadedness, syncope, anxiety, paranoid psychosis, confusion, mood swings. *Miscellaneous:* Renal dysfunction, flushing, hyperthermia, SOB, nasal stuffiness, diaphoresis, conjunctivitis, erythematous macular rash, lethargy, generalized tenderness.

OD **Overdose Management:** *Symptoms:* Marked hypertension followed by hypotension. *Treatment:* Hypertension can be treated by nitroprusside or another short-acting IV antihypertensive. Hypotension can be treated with appropriate fluid therapy and pressor agents such as norepinephrine or dopamine.

Drug Interactions:

Digitoxin, Digoxin / Bretylium may aggravate digitalis toxicity due to initial release of norepinephrine

Procainamide, Quinidine / Concomitant use with bretylium ↓ inotropic effect of bretylium and ↑ hypotension

Dosage ——————————
• **IV**
Ventricular fibrillation, hemodynamically unstable ventricular tachycardia.
Adults: 5 mg/kg of undiluted solution given rapidly. Can increase to 10 mg/kg if ventricular fibrillation persists; repeat as needed. **Maintenance, IV infusion:** 1–2 mg/min; or, 5–10 mg/kg q 6 hr of diluted drug infused over more than 8 min.
Children: 5 mg/kg/dose IV followed by 10 mg/kg at 15–30-min intervals for a maximum total dose of 30 mg/kg; **maintenance:** 5–10 mg/kg q 6 hr.
Other ventricular arrhythmias.
• **IV Infusion**
5–10 mg/kg of diluted solution over more than 8 min. **Maintenance:** 5–10 mg/kg q 6 hr over a period of 8 min or more or 1–2 mg/min by continuous IV infusion. **Children:** 5–10 mg/kg/dose q 6 hr.
• **IM**
Other ventricular arrhythmias.
Adults: 5–10 mg/kg of undiluted solution followed, if necessary, by the same dose at 1–2-hr intervals; **then,** give same dosage q 6–8 hr.

RESPIRATORY CARE CONSIDERATIONS

See also *Respiratory Care Considerations* for *Antiarrhythmic Agents*.
Administration/Storage
1. For IV infusion, bretylium is compatible with 5% dextrose injection, 0.9% sodium chloride, 5% dextrose and 0.45% sodium chloride, 5% dextrose in 0.9% sodium chloride, 5% dextrose in lactated Ringer's, 5% sodium bicarbonate, 20% mannitol, 1/6 molar sodium lactate, lactated Ringer's, calcium chloride (54.5 mEq/L) in 5% dextrose, and potassium chloride (40 mEq/L) in 5% dextrose.
2. For direct IV, administer undiluted over 15–30 sec; may repeat in 15–30 min if symptoms persist. May further dilute 500 mg in 50 cc and infuse over 10–30 min.
3. For IM injection, use the drug undiluted.
4. Rotate the injection sites so that no more than 5 mL of drug is given at any site. This avoids localized atrophy, necrosis, fibrosis, vascular degeneration, or inflammation.
5. The client should be kept supine during therapy or closely observed for postural hypotension.
6. The client should be placed on an oral antiarrhythmic medication as soon as possible.
Assessment
1. Document indications for therapy and pretreatment ECG and vital signs.
2. Note if client is taking digitalis. Bretylium tosylate may aggravate digitalis toxicity.
Interventions
1. Monitor VS and rhythm strips as the dose of bretylium to be administered is titrated based on the client's response to therapy.
2. To reduce N&V, administer the IV drug slowly over 10 min with the client supine.
3. Bretylium often causes a fall in supine BP within 1 hr of IV administration. If the SBP falls below 75 mm Hg, anticipate the need to use pressor agents.
4. Once the IV is finished, the client should continue to remain supine until the BP has stabilized.
5. Supervise clients once ambulation is permitted because they may develop lightheadedness and vertigo.
6. If clients develop side effects, stay with them, reassuring and reorienting as needed.
Evaluate
• Termination of life-threatening ventricular arrhythmia
• Restoration of stable cardiac rhythm
• Therapeutic serum drug levels (0.5–1.5 mcg/mL)

✦ = Available in Canada   ***bold italic*** = life threatening side effect

Brompheniramine maleate
(brohm-fen-**EAR**-ah-meen)
Pregnancy Category: B
Brombay, Chlorphed, Conjec-B, Cophene-B, Diamine T.D., Dimetane Extentabs, Dimetane-Ten, Histaject Modified, Nasahist B, ND Stat Revised, Oraminic II, Sinusol-B, Veltane (Rx; Dimetane and Dimetane Extentabs are OTC)
Classification: Antihistamine, alkylamine type

See also *Antihistamines.*
Action/Kinetics: Fewer sedative effects. t½: 25 hr. **Time to peak effect:** 3–9 hr. **Duration:** 4–25 hr.
Uses: Perennial and seasonal allergic rhinitis, allergic conjunctivitis, allergic and nonallergic pruritic symptoms.
Special Concerns: Use is not recommended for neonates. Geriatric clients may be more sensitive to the usual adult dose.

Dosage
• **Capsules, Elixir, Tablets**
Adults and children over 12 years: 4 mg q 4–6 hr, not to exceed 24 mg/day. **Pediatric, 6–12 years:** 2 mg q 4–6 hr, not to exceed 12 mg/day; **2–6 years:** 1 mg q 4–6 hr, not to exceed 6 mg/day.
• **Extended-Release Tablets**
Adults and children over 12 years: 8 mg q 8–12 hr or 12 mg q 12 hr; **pediatric, 6–12 years:** 8–12 mg q 12 hr.
• **IM, IV, SC**
Adults: usual, 10 mg (range: 5–20 mg) q 8–12 hr (maximum daily dose: 40 mg); **pediatric, under 12 years:** 0.125 mg/kg (3.75 mg/m²) 3–4 times/day.

RESPIRATORY CARE CONSIDERATIONS

See also *Respiratory Care Considerations* for *Antihistamines.*
Administration/Storage
1. Do not use solutions containing preservatives for IV injection.
2. For children aged 6–12 years, sustained-release preparations require the supervision of a physician.
3. For IV administration, the 10-mg/mL preparations may be used undiluted or diluted 1:10 with sterile saline for injection. Administer over 1 min.
4. The 10-mg/mL preparations may also be added to 5% glucose, NSS, or whole blood for IV use.
5. The 100-mg/mL preparation is not recommended for IV use.
6. For IM or SC use, the drug may be used undiluted or diluted 1:10 with NSS.

Evaluate
• Relief of allergic manifestations
• ↓ Nasal congestion

Budesonide
(byou-**DES**-oh-nyd)
Pregnancy Category: C
Entocort ✿, Pulmicort ✿, Pulmicort Turbuhaler, Rhinocort **(Rx)**
Classification: Corticosteroid

See also *Corticosteroids.*
Action/Kinetics: Budesonide is used intranasally and exerts a direct local anti-inflammatory effect with minimal systemic effects. However, exceeding the recommended dose may result in suppression of hypothalamic-pituitary-adrenal function. Metabolism of absorbed drug is rapid.
Uses: Treat symptoms of seasonal or perennial allergic rhinitis in both adults and children. Also, nonallergic perennial rhinitis in adults.
Contraindications: Hypersensitivity to the drug. Untreated localized nasal mucosa infections. Lactation. Use in children less than 6 years of age.
Special Concerns: Use with caution in clients already on alternate day corticosteroids (e.g., prednisone). Use with caution in clients with active or quiescent tuberculosis infections of the respiratory tract or in untreated fungal, bacterial, or systemic viral infections or ocular herpes simplex. Use with caution in clients with recent nasal septal ulcers, recurrent epistaxis, nasal surgery, or trauma. Exposure to chicken pox or measles should be avoided.

Side Effects: *Respiratory:* Nasopharyngeal irritation, nasal irritation, pharyngitis, increased cough, hoarseness, nasal pain,burning, stinging, dryness, epistaxis, bloody mucus, rebound congestion, ***bronchial asthma,*** , occasional sneezing attacks (especially in children), rhinorrhea, reduced sense of smell, throat discomfort, ulceration of the nasal mucosa, sore throat, dyspnea, localized infections of nose and pharynx with *Candida albicans,* wheezing (rare). *CNS:* Lightheadedness, headache, nervousness. *GI:* Nausea, loss of sense of taste, bad taste in mouth, dry mouth, dyspepsia. *Miscellaneous:* Watery eyes, ***immediate and delayed hypersensitivity reactions,*** moniliasis, facial edema, rash, pruritus, herpes simplex, alopecia, arthralgia, myalgia, contact dermatitis (rare).

OD **Overdose Management:** *Symptoms:* Symptoms of hypercorticism, including menstrual irregularities, acneiform lesions, and cushingoid features (all are rarely seen, however). *Treatment:* Discontinue the drug slowly using procedures that are acceptable for discontinuing oral corticosteroids.

Dosage
• **Inhalation Aerosol**
Seasonal or perennial rhinitis.
Adults and children 6 years of age and older, initial: 256 mcg/day given as either 2 sprays in each nostril in the morning and evening or 4 sprays in each nostril in the morning. Doses greater than 256 mcg/day are not recommended. **Maintenance:** Reduce initial dose to the smallest amount necessary to control symptoms; decrease dose q 2–4 weeks as long as desired effect is maintained. If symptoms return, the dose may be increased briefly to the initial dose.

RESPIRATORY CARE CONSIDERATIONS

See also *Respiratory Care Considerations* for *Corticosteroids.*

Administration/Storage
1. Prior to using the drug, the nasal passages should be cleared of secretions. If nasal passages are blocked, a decongestant should be administered before using budesonide.
2. Maximum benefit is usually not seen for 3–7 days, although a decrease in symptoms can usually be seen within 24 hr. If no improvement is noted within 3 weeks, therapy should be discontinued.
3. The canister should be shaken well before using.
4. The aerosol should be stored with the valve downward. Once the aluminum pouch is opened, the canister should be used within 6 months. The drug should not be stored in areas of high humidity.

Assessment
1. Note indications for therapy, onset of symptoms, and frequency of occurrence.
2. List drugs currently prescribed to ensure that none interact unfavorably.

Client/Family Teaching
1. Review the appropriate method and frequency for administration and observe client self-administer. The use of a spacer may enhance administraton.
2. Caution to avoid persons with chicken pox or communicable diseases.
3. Advise to rinse mouth and spacer thoroughly after each use to prevent oral fungal infections.
4. Review side effects stressing those which require immediate medical intervention.
5. Explain that symptoms of hoarseness may be evident but should subside upon completion of therapy.
6. Caution that drug is a steroid and that chronic use in excessive amounts may lead to adverse systemic reactions.
7. Assist to identify triggers and remind client to avoid irritant to prevent development of symptoms.

Evaluate: Relief of nasal congestion and allergic manifestations

---

Bumetanide
(byou-**MET**-ah-nyd)
Pregnancy Category: C
Bumex, Burinex ✦ **(Rx)**
Classification: Loop diuretic

See also *Diuretics, Loop.*

Action/Kinetics: Bumetanide inhibits reabsorption of both sodium and chloride in the proximal tubule as well as the ascending loop of Henle. It may also have some activity in the proximal tubule to promote phosphate excretion. **Onset, PO:** 30–60 min. **Peak effect, PO:** 1–2 hr. **Duration, PO:** 4–6 hr (dose-dependent). **Onset, IV:** Several minutes. **Peak effect, IV:** 15–30 min. **Duration, IV:** 3.5–4 hr. **t½:** 1–1.5 hr. Metabolized in the liver although 45% excreted unchanged in the urine.

Uses: Edema associated with CHF, nephrotic syndrome, hepatic disease. Adjunct to treat acute pulmonary edema. Especially useful in clients refractory to other diuretics. *Investigational:* Treatment of adult nocturia. The drug is not effective in males with prostatic hypertrophy.

Contraindications: Anuria. Hepatic coma or severe electrolyte depletion until the condition is improved or corrected. Hypersensitivity to the drug. Lactation.

Special Concerns: Safety and efficacy in children under 18 have not been established. Geriatric clients may be more sensitive to the hypotensive and electrolyte effects and are at greater risk in developing thromboembolic problems and circulatory collapse. SLE may be activated or made worse. Clients allergic to sulfonamides may show cross sensitivity to bumetanide. Sudden changes in electrolyte balance may cause hepatic encephalopathy and coma in clients with hepatic cirrhosis and ascites.

Side Effects: *Electrolyte and fluid changes:* Excess water loss, ***dehydration,*** electrolyte depletion including hypokalemia, hypochloremia, hyponatremia; hypovolemia, thromboembolism, ***circulatory collapse.*** *Otic:* Tinnitus, reversible and irreversible hearing impairment, deafness, vertigo (with a sense of fullness in the ears). *CV:* ***Reduction in blood volume may cause circulatory collapse and vascular thrombosis and embolism, especially in geriatric clients.*** Hypotension, ECG changes, chest pain. *CNS:* Asterixis, encephalopathy with preexisting liver disease, vertigo, headache, dizziness. *GI:* Upset stomach, dry mouth, N&V, diarrhea, GI pain. *GU:* Premature ejaculation, difficulty maintaining erection, renal failure. *Musculoskeletal:* Arthritic pain, weakness, muscle cramps, fatigue. *Hematologic:* Agranulocytosis, thrombocytopenia. *Allergic:* Pruritus, urticaria, rashes. *Miscellaneous:* Sweating, hyperventilation, rash, nipple tenderness, photosensitivity, pain following parenteral use.

OD **Overdose Management:** *Symptoms: **Profound loss of water, electrolyte depletion, dehydration, decreased blood volume, circulatory collapse (possibility of vascular thrombosis and embolism).*** Symptoms of electrolyte depletion include: anorexia, cramps, weakness, dizziness, vomiting, and mental confusion. *Treatment:* Replace electrolyte and fluid losses and monitor urinary electrolyte levels as well as serum electrolytes. Emesis or gastric lavage. Oxygen or assisted ventilation may be necessary. General supportive measures.

Laboratory Test Interferences: Alterations in LDH, AST, ALT, alkaline phosphatase, creatinine clearance, total serum bilirubin, serum proteins, cholesterol. Changes in hemoglobin, PT, hematocrit, WBCs, platelet and differential counts, phosphorus, carbon dioxide content, bicarbonate, and calcium. ↑ Urinary glucose and protein, serum creatinine. Also, hyperuricemia, hypochloremia, hypokalemia, azotemia, hyponatremia, hyperglycemia.

Dosage

• **Tablets**

Adults: 0.5–2 mg once daily; if response is inadequate, a second or third dose may be given at 4–5-hr intervals up to a maximum of 10 mg/day.

• **IV, IM**

Adults: 0.5–1 mg; if response is inadequate, a second or third dose may be given at 2–3-hr intervals up to a maximum of 10 mg/day. PO dosing should be started as soon as possible.

RESPIRATORY CARE CONSIDERATIONS

See also *Respiratory Care Considerations* for *Diuretics, Loop.*

Administration/Storage

1. Solutions for IM or IV use should be freshly prepared and used within 24 hr.

2. Ampules may be reconstituted with 5% dextrose in water, 0.9% sodium chloride, or lactated Ringer's solution.

3. IV solutions should be administered slowly over 1–2 min.

4. IV or IM administration should be reserved for clients in whom PO use is not practical or in whom absorption from the GI tract is impaired.

5. The recommended PO medication schedule is on alternate days or for 3–4 days with a 1–2-day rest period in between.

6. Bumetanide, at a 1:40 ratio of bumetanide:furosemide, may be ordered for clients allergic to furosemide.

7. In severe chronic renal insufficiency, a continuous infusion of bumetanide, 12 mg over 12 hr, may be more effective and cause fewer side effects than intermittent bolus therapy.

Assessment

1. Document indications for therapy and pretreatment findings.

2. Note any sulfonamide allergy as there may be cross sensitivity.

3. Obtain hepatic and renal function studies as well as serum electrolyte levels and monitor throughout therapy; assess for hypokalemia.

4. Review history and note any evidence of lupus, hearing impairment, or thromboembolic events.

5. *NOTE:* 1 mg of bumetanide is essentially equivalent to 40 mg of furosemide.

Interventions

1. Monitor BP and pulse regularly. Rapid diuresis may cause dehydration and circulatory collapse (especially in the elderly). Hypotension may also occur when drug is administered with antihypertensive drugs.

2. Observe for ototoxicity, especially if the client is receiving other ototoxic drugs and assess hearing periodically.

Evaluate

• ↓ Peripheral and sacral edema
• Enhanced diuresis

Buprenorphine hydrochloride
(byou-pren-**OR**-feen)
Pregnancy Category: C
Buprenex **(C-V) (Rx)**
Classification: Narcotic agonist/antagonist

See also *Narcotic Analgesics.*

Action/Kinetics: Semisynthetic opiate possessing both narcotic agonist and antagonist activity. It has limited activity at the mu receptor. **IM, onset:** 15 min; **Peak effect:** 1 hr; **Duration:** 6 hr. **t½:** 2–3 hr. May also be given IV with shorter onset and peak effect. Buprenorphine is about equipotent with naloxone as a narcotic antagonist.

Uses: Moderate to severe pain.

Special Concerns: Use during lactation only if benefits outweigh risks. Use in children less than 2 years of age has not been established. Use with caution in clients with compromised respiratory function, in head injuries, in impairment of liver or renal function, Addison's disease, prostatic hypertrophy, biliary tract dysfunction, urethral stricture, myxedema, and hypothyroidism. Administration to individuals physically dependent on narcotics may result in precipitation of a withdrawal syndrome.

B

Side Effects: *CNS:* Sedation, dizziness, confusion, headache, euphoria, slurred speech, depression, paresthesia, psychosis, malaise, hallucinations, coma, dysphoria, agitation, seizures. *GI:* N&V, constipation, dyspepsia, loss of appetite, dry mouth. *Ophthalmologic:* Miosis, blurred vision, double vision, conjunctivitis. *CV:* Hypotension, bradycardia, tachycardia, Wenckebach block. *Respiratory:* Decreased respiratory rate, cyanosis, dyspepsia. *Dermatologic:* Sweating, rash, pruritus, flushing. *Other:* Urinary retention, chills, tinnitus.

Drug Interactions: Additive CNS depression with alcohol, general anesthetics, antianxiety agents, sedative-hypnotics, phenothiazines, and other narcotic analgesics.

Dosage ———————————
- **IM, Slow IV**
  Analgesia.
Over 13 years of age: 0.3 mg q 6 hr. Up to 0.6 mg may be given; doses greater than 0.6 mg not recommended. **Children, 2–12 years of age:** 2–6 mcg/kg q 4–6 hr. Single doses greater than 6 mcg/kg should not be given.

RESPIRATORY CARE CONSIDERATIONS

See also *Respiratory Care Considerations* for *Narcotic Analgesics.*
Administration/Storage
1. Buprenorphine may be mixed with isotonic saline, lactated Ringer's solution, and 5% dextrose and 0.9% saline.
2. May be administered undiluted IV, slowly.
3. Buprenorphine may be mixed with solutions containing haloperidol, glycopyrrolate, scopolamine hydrobromide, hydroxyzine chloride, or droperidol.
4. Buprenorphine should not be mixed with solutions containing diazepam or lorazepam.
5. Storage in excessive heat and light should be avoided.
6. Not all children may clear buprenorphine faster than adults. Thus,

fixed interval or "round the clock" dosing should not be undertaken until the proper interdose interval has been established.
7. Some pediatric clients may not need to be remedicated for 6–8 hr.
8. Have naloxone available to reverse drug-induced respiratory depression.

Assessment
1. Document indications for therapy, onset, location, and intensity of symptoms.
2. Determine if the client has evidence of respiratory depression and report because drug is contraindicated.
3. Report any evidence of head injuries immediately.
4. If the client has been receiving narcotics, observe for withdrawal symptoms and document.
5. Note any evidence of liver or renal dysfunction, diseases of the biliary tract, or prostatic hypertrophy.
Evaluate: Relief of pain

Butorphanol tartrate
(byou-**TOR**-fah-nohl)
Pregnancy Category: C
Stadol, Stadol NS **(Rx)**
Classification: Narcotic agonist/antagonist

See also *Narcotic Analgesics.*
Action/Kinetics: Butorphanol has both narcotic agonist and antagonist properties. Its analgesic potency is said to be up to 7 times that of morphine and 30–40 times that of meperidine. Overdosage responds to naloxone. After IV use, CV effects include increased PA pressure, pulmonary wedge pressure, LV end-diastolic pressure, system arterial pressure, pulmonary vascular resistance, and increased cardiac work load. **Onset, IM:** 10–15 min; **IV:** rapid; **nasal:** within 15 min. **Duration, IM, IV:** 3–4 hr; **nasal:** 4–5 hr. **Peak analgesia, IM, IV:** 30–60 min; **nasal:** 1–2 hr; **IM:** 2.1–8.8 hr; **nasal:** 2.9–9.2 hr. The t½ is increased up to 25% in clients over 65 years of age. Butorphanol is metabolized in the

liver and excreted by the kidney. The drug has about 1/40 the narcotic antagonist activity as naloxone. A metered-dose nasal spray is now available for this drug.

Uses: Parenteral and nasal: Moderate to severe pain, especially after surgery. **Parenteral:** Preoperative medication (as part of balanced anesthesia). Pain during labor. **Nasal:** Treatment of migraine headaches.

Contraindications: The nasal form should not be used during labor or delivery.

Special Concerns: Safe use during pregnancy, during labor for premature infants, or in children under 18 years not established. Use with extreme caution in clients with AMI, ventricular dysfunction, and coronary insufficiency (morphine or meperidine are preferred). Use in clients physically dependent on narcotics will result in precipitation of a withdrawal syndrome. Geriatric clients may be more sensitive to side effects, especially dizziness.

Additional Side Effects: The most common side effects are somnolence, dizziness, N&V. The nasal product commonly causes nasal congestion and insomnia.

Additional Drug Interactions: Barbiturate anesthetics may increase respiratory and CNS depression of butorphanol.

Dosage ———————————
• **IM**
Analgesia.
Adults, usual: 2 mg q 3–4 hr, as necessary; **range:** 1–4 mg q 3–4 hr. Single doses should not exceed 4 mg.
Preoperative/preanesthetic.
Adults: 2 mg 60–90 min before surgery. Individualize dosage.
Labor.
Adults: 1–2 mg if at full term and during early labor. May be repeated after 4 hr.
• **IV**
Analgesia.
Adults, usual: 1 mg q 3–4 hr;

range: 0.5–2 mg q 3–4 hr. **Not recommended for use in children.**
Balanced anesthesia.
Adults: 2 mg just before induction or 0.5–1 mg in increments during anesthesia. The increment may be up to 0.06 mg/kg, depending on drugs previously given. Total dose range: less than 4 mg to less than 12.5 mg.
Labor.
Adults: 1–2 mg if at full term and during early labor. May be repeated after 4 hr.
• **Nasal Spray**
Analgesia.
Adults: 1 spray (1 mg) in one nostril. If pain relief is not reached within 60–90 min, an additional 1 mg may be given. The two-dose sequence may be repeated in 3–4 hr if necessary. In severe pain, 2 mg (1 spray in each nostril) may be given initially followed in 3–4 hr by additional 2-mg doses if needed. **Geriatric clients, initial:** 1 mg; wait 90–120 min before determining if a second 1-mg dose is required.

RESPIRATORY CARE CONSIDERATIONS

See also *Respiratory Care Considerations* for *Narcotic Analgesics*.
Administration/Storage
1. Geriatric clients should receive one-half the usual dose at twice the usual interval.
2. For clients with renal/hepatic impairment, increase the initial dosage interval to 6–8 hr with subsequent intervals determined by client response.
3. If the drug is to be administered by direct IV infusion, it may be given undiluted. Administer it at a rate of 2 mg or less over a 3–5-min period of time.
4. Have naloxone available for treatment of overdose.
5. The nasal product should be stored below 86°F (30°C).
Assessment
1. Determine if the client is likely to be dependent on narcotics. Antagonist

property of drug may precipitate withdrawal symptoms.

2. Monitor VS and CNS status during therapy.

3. Document any history of CV problems as morphine may be a preferred drug to use.

Evaluate
• Relief of pain
• Treatment of migraine headache

C

Calcium chloride
(**KAL**-see-um **KLOH**-ryd)
Pregnancy Category: C
Calciject ✹ **(Rx)**
Classification: Calcium salt

See also *Calcium Salts.*
Uses: Mild hypocalcemia due to neonatal tetany, tetany due to parathyroid deficiency or vitamin D deficiency, and alkalosis. Prophylaxis of hypocalcemia during exchange transfusions. Intestinal malabsorption. Treat effects of serious hyperkalemia as measured by ECG. Cardiac resuscitation after open heart surgery when epinephrine fails to improve weak or ineffective myocardial contractions. Adjunct to treat insect bites or stings to relieve muscle cramping. Depression due to magnesium overdosage. Acute symptoms of lead colic. Rickets, osteomalacia. Reverse symptoms of verapamil overdosage.
Contraindications: Use to treat hypocalcemia of renal insufficiency.
Special Concerns: Use usually restricted in children due to significant irritation and possible tissue necrosis and sloughing caused by IV calcium chloride.
Additional Side Effects: Peripheral vasodilation with moderate decreases in BP. Extravasation can cause severe necrosis, sloughing, or abscess formation following IM or SC use.

Dosage

• **IV Only**
  Hypocalcemia, replenish electrolytes.
Adults: 0.5–1 g q 1–3 days (given at a rate not to exceed 13.6–27.3 mg/min). **Pediatric:** 25 mg/kg (0.2 mL/kg up to 1–10 mL/kg) given slowly.
  Magnesium intoxication.
0.5 g promptly; observe for recovery before other doses given.
  Cardiac resuscitation.
0.5– **Pediatric:** 0.2 mL/kg.
  Hyperkalemia.
Sufficient amount to return ECG to normal.
  NOTE: The preparation contains 27.2% calcium and 272 mg calcium/g (13.6 mEq/g).

RESPIRATORY CARE CONSIDERATIONS

See also *Respiratory Care Considerations* for *Calcium Salts.*
Administration/Storage
1. *Never administer IM.*
2. May administer undiluted IV push.
Evaluate
• Serum calcium level within desired range
• ↓ Serum magnesium and potassium levels
• Control of twitching and spasm with tetany

Calcium gluconate
(**KAL**-see-um **GLUE**-koh-nayt)
Kalcinate (Rx, injection; OTC, tablets)
Classification: Calcium salt

See also *Calcium Salts.*
Uses: Mild hypocalcemia due to neonatal tetany, tetany due to parathyroid deficiency or vitamin D deficiency, and alkalosis. Prophylaxis of hypocalcemia during exchange transfusions. Intestinal malabsorption. Adjunct to treat insect

bites or stings to relieve muscle cramping. Depression due to magnesium overdosage. Acute symptoms of lead colic. Rickets, osteomalacia. Reverse symptoms of verapamil overdosage. Decrease capillary permeability in allergic conditions, nonthrombocytopenic purpura, and exudative dermatoses (e.g., dermatitis herpetiformis). Pruritus due to certain drugs. Hyperkalemia to antagonize cardiac toxicity (as long as client is not receiving digitalis).

Contraindications: Intramuscular, intramyocardial, or SC use due to severe tissue necrosis, sloughing, and abscess formation.

Dosage ─────────

• **Chewable Tablets, Tablets**
Treatment of hypocalcemia.
Adults: 8.8–16.5 g/day in divided doses; **pediatric:** 0.5–0.72 g/kg/day in divided doses.
Nutritional supplement.
Adults: 8.8–16.5 g/day in divided doses.

• **IV Only**
Treatment of hypocalcemia.
Adults: 2.3–9.3 mEq (5–20 mL of the 10% solution) as needed (range: 4.65–70 mEq/day). **Children:** 2.3 mEq/kg/day (or 56 mEq/m²/day) given well diluted and slowly in divided doses. **Infants:** No more than 0.93 mEq (2 mL of the 10% solution).
Emergency elevation of serum calcium.
Adults: 7–14 mEq (15–30.1 mL). **Children:** 1–7 mEq (2.2–15 mL). **Infants:** Less than 1 mEq (2.2 mL). Depending on client response, the dose may be repeated q 1–3 days.
Hypocalcemic tetany.
Children: 0.5–0.7 mEq/kg (1.1–1.5 mL/kg) t.i.d.–q.i.d. until tetany is controlled. **Infants:** 2.4 mEq/kg/day (5.2 mL/kg/day) in divided doses.
Hyperkalemia with cardiac toxicity.
2.25–14 mEq (4.8–30.1 mL) while

monitoring the ECG. If needed, the dose can be repeated after 1–2 min.
Magnesium intoxication.
Initial: 4.5–9 mEq (9.7–19.4 mL). Subsequent dosage based on client response.
Exchange transfusion.
Adults: 1.35 mEq (2.9 mL) concurrent with each 100 mL citrated blood. **Neonates:** 0.45 mEq (1 mL)/100 mL citrated blood.

• **IM**
Hypocalcemic tetany.
Adults: 4.5–16 mEq (9.7–34.4 mL) until a therapeutic response is noted.
Magnesium intoxication.
If IV administration is not possible: 2–5 mEq (4.3–10.8 mL) in divided doses as needed.
NOTE: The preparation contains 9% calcium and 90 mg calcium/g (4.5 mEq/g).

RESPIRATORY CARE CONSIDERATIONS

See also *Respiratory Care Considerations* for *Calcium Salts.*
Administration/Storage
1. IV rate should not exceed 0.5–2 mL/min.
2. Can also be given by intermittent IV infusion at a rate not exceeding 200 mg (19.5 mg calcium ion)/min. Can also be used by continuous IV infusion.
3. If a precipitate is noted in the syringe, do not use.
4. If a precipitate is noted in the vials or ampules, heat to 80°C (146°F) in a dry heat oven for 1 hr to dissolve. Shake vigorously and allow to cool to room temperature. Do not use if precipitate remains.
Evaluate
• Restoration of serum calcium levels
• ↓ Serum magnesium and potassium levels

─────────────

Captopril
(**KAP**-toe-prill)
Pregnancy Category: C (first trimester); D (second and third trimesters)

─────────────

Apo-Capto ✤, Capoten, Novo-
Capto ✤, Nu-Capto ✤, Syn-Captopril
✤ (Rx)

Classification: Antihypertensive,
inhibitor of angiotensin synthesis

See also *Angiotensin-Converting Enzyme Inhibitors.*

Action/Kinetics: Onset: 15 min.
Peak serum levels: 30–90 min;
presence of food decreases absorption
by 30%–40%. **Plasma protein binding:** 25%–30%. **Time to peak effect:** 60–90 min. **Duration:** 6–12 hr.
t½, normal renal function: 2 hr;
t½, impaired renal function:
3.5–32 hr. More than 95% of absorbed dose excreted in urine
(40%–50% unchanged). Food decreases bioavailability of captopril
by 30%–40%.

Uses: Antihypertensive, step I therapy in clients with normal renal function. Concomitant use with diuretic
therapy may, however, cause precipitous hypotension. In combination with diuretics and digitalis in
treatment of CHF not responding to
conventional therapy. To improve
survival following MI in clinically
stable clients with LV dysfunction
manifested as an ejection fraction of
40% or less. Treatment of diabetic
nephropathy (proteinuria > 500
mg/day) in those with type I insulin-
dependent diabetes and retinopathy.
Investigational: Rheumatoid arthritis, hypertensive crisis, neonatal and
childhood hypertension, hypertension related to scleroderma renal crisis, diagnosis of anatomic renal
artery stenosis, diagnosis of primary
aldosteronism, Raynaud's syndrome,
hypertension of Takayasu's disease,
idiopathic edema, and Bartter's syndrome.

Contraindications: In clients with
a history of angioedema related to
previous use of ACE inhibitors.

Special Concerns: Use with caution in cases of impaired renal function. Use in children only if other
antihypertensive therapy has proven
ineffective in controlling BP. Use
with caution during lactation. May
cause a profound drop in BP following the first dose.

Side Effects: *Dermatologic:* Rash
(usually maculopapular) with pruritus
and occasionally fever, eosinophilia,
and arthralgia. Alopecia, erythema
multiforme, photosensitivity, exfoliative dermatitis, *Stevens-Johnson syndrome,* reversible pemphigoid-like
lesions, bullous pemphigus, onycholysis, flushing, pallor, scalded
mouth sensation. *GI:* N&V, anorexia,
constipation or diarrhea, gastric irritation, abdominal pain, dysgeusia,
peptic ulcers, aphthous ulcers, dyspepsia, dry mouth, glossitis, pancreatitis. *Hepatic:* Jaundice, cholestasis,
hepatitis. *CNS:* Headache, dizziness,
insomnia, malaise, fatigue, paresthesias, confusion, depression, nervousness, ataxia, somnolence. *CV:*
Hypotension, angina, *MI,* Raynaud's
phenomenon, chest pain, palpitations, tachycardia, *CVA, CHF, cardiac arrest,* orthostatic hypotension,
rhythm disturbances. *Renal:* Renal
insufficiency or failure, proteinuria,
urinary frequency, oliguria, polyuria,
nephrotic syndrome, interstitial
nephritis. *Respiratory:* **Bronchospasm,**
cough, dyspnea, asthma, *pulmonary
embolism, pulmonary infarction.* He-
matologic: Agranulocytosis, neutropenia, thrombocytopenia, pancytopenia, *aplastic or hemolytic anemia.*
Other: Decrease or loss of taste perception with weight loss (reversible), angioedema, asthenia,
syncope, fever, myalgia, arthralgia,
vasculitis, blurred vision, impotence,
hyperkalemia, hyponatremia, myasthenia, gynecomastia, rhinitis,
eosinophilic pneumonitis.

OD **Overdose Management:**
Symptoms: Hypotension is the most
common with a systolic BP of <80 mm
Hg a possibility. *Treatment:* Volume
expansion with NSS (IV) is the treatment of choice to restore BP.

Additional Drug Interactions:
Probenecid increases blood levels of
captopril due to decreased renal excretion.

Laboratory Test Interferences:
False + test for urine acetone.

Dosage
• Tablets
Hypertension.
Adults, initial: 25 mg b.i.d.–t.i.d. If unsatisfactory response after 1–2 weeks, increase to 50 mg b.i.d.–t.i.d.; if still unsatisfactory after another 1–2 weeks, thiazide diuretic should be added (e.g., hydrochlorothiazide, 25 mg/day). Dosage may be increased to 100–150 mg b.i.d.–t.i.d., not to exceed 450 mg/day.

Accelerated or malignant hypertension.
Stop current medication (except for the diuretic) and initiate captopril at a dose of 25 mg b.i.d.–t.i.d. The dose may be increased q 24 hr until a satisfactory response is obtained or the maximum dose reached. Furosemide may be indicated.

Heart failure.
Initial: 25 mg t.i.d.; **then,** if necessary, increase dose to 50 mg t.i.d. and evaluate response; **maintenance:** 50–100 mg t.i.d., not to exceed 450 mg/day.

NOTE: For adults, an initial dose of 6.25–12.5 mg (0.15 mg/kg t.i.d. in children) should be given b.i.d.–t.i.d. to clients who are sodium- and water-depleted due to diuretics, who will continue to be on diuretic therapy, and who have renal impairment.

Left ventricular dysfunction after MI.
Therapy may be started as early as 3 days after the MI. **Initial dose:** 6.25 mg; **then,** begin 12.5 mg t.i.d. and increase to 25 mg t.i.d. over the next several days. The target dose is 50 mg t.i.d. over the next several weeks. Other treatments for MI may be used concomitantly (e.g., aspirin, beta blockers, thrombolytic drugs).

Diabetic nephropathy.
25 mg t.i.d. for chronic use. Other antihypertensive drugs (e.g., beta blockers, centrally-acting drugs, diuretics, vasodilators) may be used with captopril if additional drug therapy is needed to reduce BP.

Hypertensive crisis.
Initial: 25 mg; **then,** 100 mg 90–120 min later, 200–300 mg/day for 2–5 days (then adjust dose). Sublingual captopril, 25 mg, has also been used successfully.

Rheumatoid arthritis.
75–150 mg/day in divided doses.

NOTE: For all uses, doses should be reduced in clients with renal impairment.

RESPIRATORY CARE CONSIDERATIONS

See also *Respiratory Care Considerations* for *Angiotensin-Converting Enzyme Inhibitors* and *Antihypertensive Agents.*

Administration/Storage
1. Captopril should not be discontinued without the provider's consent.
2. The dose should be given 1 hr before meals.
3. If possible, previous antihypertensive medication should be discontinued 1 week before starting captopril.
4. If a solution of captopril is desired, tablets can be used for its preparation.

Assessment
1. Obtain baseline hematologic studies and renal and liver function tests prior to beginning therapy.
2. Determine if the client is taking diuretics, nitroglycerin, or other antianginal nitrates. These may act in synergism with captopril and may cause a more pronounced response.
3. Document any intolerance to other ACE inhibitors.
4. Determine the potential for the client to understand and comply with the prescribed therapy.
5. Document ejection fraction (at or below 40%) in stable, post-MI clients.
6. Note any evidence of heart failure, diabetes, or arthritis as drug usually is very effective with these clients.

Interventions
1. Observe client closely for a pre-

cipitous drop in BP within 3 hr after initial dose of captopril if client has been on diuretic therapy and a sodium-restricted diet.

2. If BP falls rapidly, place the client in a supine position and be prepared to assist with an IV infusion of saline.

3. Check for proteinuria monthly after the onset of treatment and for at least 9 months during therapy.

4. Withhold potassium-sparing diuretics and report as hyperkalemia may result.

5. Be alert to hyperkalemia occurring several months after administration of spironolactone and captopril.

Evaluate
- ↓ BP
- Improvement in symptoms of CHF (↓ preload, ↓ afterload)
- Improved mortality post-MI

Carbenicillin indanyl sodium

(kar-ben-ih-**SILL**-in)
Pregnancy Category: B
Geocillin, Geopen Oral ✿ **(Rx)**
Classification: Antibiotic, penicillin

See also *Anti-Infectives* and *Penicillins*.

Action/Kinetics: The drug is acid stable. **Peak serum levels: PO:** 6.5 mcg/mL after 1 hr. **t½:** 60 min. Rapidly excreted unchanged in urine.

Uses: Upper and lower UTIs or bacteriuria due to *Escherichia coli, Proteus vulgaris and P. mirabilis, Morganella morganii, Providencia rettgeri, Enterobacter, Pseudomonas,* and enterococci. Prostatitis due to *E. coli, Streptococcus faecalis* (enterococci), *P. mirabilis,* and *Enterobacter* species.

Additional Contraindications: Pregnancy.

Special Concerns: Safe use in children not established. Use with caution in clients with impaired renal function.

Additional Side Effects: Neurotoxicity in clients with impaired renal function.

Additional Drug Interactions: When used in combination with gentamicin or tobramycin for *Pseudomonas* infections, effect of carbenicillin may be enhanced.

Dosage
- **Tablets**

UTIs due to E. coli, Proteus, Enterobacter.
382–764 mg q.i.d.
UTIs due to Pseudomonas *and enterococci.*
764 mg q.i.d.
Prostatitis due to E. coli, P. mirabilis, Enterobacter, *and enterococci.*
764 mg q.i.d.

RESPIRATORY CARE CONSIDERATIONS

See also *General Respiratory Care Considerations* for *All Anti-Infectives,* and *Penicillins.*

Administration/Storage
1. Protect from moisture.
2. Store at temperature of 30°C (86F) or less.

Interventions
1. Provide frequent mouth care to minimize nausea and unpleasant aftertaste.
2. Monitor renal function studies and assess client with impaired renal function for evidence of neurotoxicity, manifested by hallucinations, impaired sensorium, muscular irritability, and seizures.
3. Monitor CBC and assess for any hemorrhagic manifestations, such as ecchymosis, petechiae, and frank bleeding of gums and/or rectum.

Evaluate
- Negative lab C&S results
- Resolution of infection and reports of symptomatic improvement

Carteolol hydrochloride

(kar-**TEE**-oh-lohl)
Pregnancy Category: C
Cartrol, Ocupress **(Rx)**
Classification: Beta-adrenergic blocking agent

See also *Beta-Adrenergic Blocking Agents.*

Action/Kinetics: Carteolol has both beta-1 and beta-2 receptor blocking activity. The drug has no membrane-stabilizing activity but does have moderate intrinsic sympathomimetic effects. Low lipid solubility. **t½:** 6 hr. **Duration, ophthalmic use:** 12 hr. Approximately 50%–70% excreted unchanged in the urine.

Uses: PO. Hypertension. *Investigational:* Reduce frequency of anginal attacks. **Ophthalmic.** Chronic open-angle glaucoma and intraocular hypertension alone or in combination with other drugs.

Contraindications: Severe, persistent bradycardia. Bronchial asthma or bronchospasm, including severe COPD.

Special Concerns: Dosage has not been established in children.

Additional Side Effects: Ophthalmic use. Transient irritation, burning, tearing, conjunctival hyperemia, edema, blurred or cloudy vision, photophobia, decreased night vision, ptosis, blepharoconjunctivitis, abnormal corneal staining, corneal sensitivity.

Dosage
• **Tablets**
Hypertension.
Initial: 2.5 mg once daily either alone or with a diuretic. In the event of an inadequate response, the dose may be increased gradually to 5 mg and then 10 mg/day as a single dose. **Maintenance:** 2.5–5 mg once daily. Doses greater than 10 mg/day are not likely to increase the beneficial effect and may decrease the response. The dosage interval should be increased in clients with renal impairment.
Reduce frequency of anginal attacks.
10 mg/day.
• **Ophthalmic Solution**
Usual: 1 gtt in affected eye b.i.d. If the response is unsatisfactory, concomitant therapy may be initiated.

RESPIRATORY CARE CONSIDERATIONS

See also *Respiratory Care Considerations* for *Beta-Adrenergic Blocking Agents* and *Antihypertensive Agents*.
Assessment
1. Document indications for therapy and note baseline findings.
2. Assess renal function; anticipate reduced dose with impairment.
Evaluate
• ↓ BP
• ↓ Frequency of anginal attacks
• ↓ Intraocular pressure

Carvedilol
(kar-**VAY**-dih-lol)
Pregnancy Category: C
Coreg **(Rx)**
Classification: Alpha/beta-adrenergic blocking agent

See also *Adrenergic Blocking Agents*.
Action/Kinetics: Carvedilol has both alpha- and beta-adrenergic blocking activity. As a result, the drug decreases cardiac output, reduces exercise- or isoproterenol-induced tachycardia, reduces reflex orthostatic hypotension, causes vasodilation, and reduces peripheral vascular resistance. Significant beta-blocking activity occurs within 60 min while alpha-blocking action is observed within 30 min. BP is lowered more in the standing than in the supine position. The drug also significantly lowers plasma renin activity when given for at least 4 weeks. Carvedilol is rapidly absorbed after PO administration, but there is a significant first-pass effect. **Terminal t½:** 7–10 hr. Food delays the rate of absorption. Over 98% of the drug is bound to plasma protein. Plasma levels average 50% higher in geriatric compared with younger clients. The drug is extensively metabolized in the liver, with metabolites excreted primarily via the bile into the feces.
Uses: Essential hypertension used either alone or in combination with other antihypertensive drugs, especially thiazide diuretics. *Investigational:* Congestive heart failure,

angina pectoris, idiopathic cardiomyopathy.

Contraindications: Clients with New York Heart Association Class IV decompensated cardiac failure, bronchial asthma, or related bronchospastic conditions, second- or third-degree AV block, cardiogenic shock, severe bradycardia, drug hypersensitivity. Use in those with hepatic impairment. Lactation.

Special Concerns: Use with caution in hypertensive clients with CHF controlled with digitalis, diuretics, or an ACE inhibitor. Use with caution in peripheral vascular disease, in surgical procedures using anesthetic agents that depress myocardial function, in diabetics receiving insulin or oral hypoglycemic drugs, in those subject to spontaneous hypoglycemia, or in thyrotoxicosis. Clients with a history of severe anaphylactic reaction to a variety of allergens may be more reactive to repeated challenge while taking beta blockers. Safety and efficacy have not been established in children less than 18 years of age.

Side Effects: *CV:* Bradycardia, postural hypotension, dependent or peripheral edema, AV block, extrasystoles, hypertension, hypotension, palpitations, peripheral ischemia, syncope, angina, arrhythmias, atrial fibrillation, bundle branch block, *cardiac failure,* myocardial ischemia, CV disorder. *CNS:* Dizziness, somnolence, insomnia, ataxia, hypesthesia, paresthesia, vertigo, depression, nervousness, migraine, neuralgia, paresis, amnesia, confusion. *GI:* Diarrhea, abdominal pain, bilirubinemia, constipation, flatulence, dry mouth. *Respiratory:* Rhinitis, pharyngitis, dyspnea, *asthma, bronchospasm,* cough, allergy, respiratory alkalosis, eosinophilia. *GU:* Urinary tract infection, decreased libido and impotence in males, albuminuria, hematuria, frequency of micturition. *Dermatologic:* Pruritus; erythematous, maculopapular, and psoriaform rashes. *Metabolic:* Hypertriglyceridemia, hypercholesterolemia, hyperglycemia, hyperuricemia, glyco-

suria, increased weight. *Hematologic:* Thrombocytopenia, anemia, leukopenia, atypical lymphocytes. *Miscellaneous:* Fatigue, injury, back pain, viral infection, asthenia, hot flushes, leg cramps, malaise, increased sweating, myalgia, abnormal vision, tinnitus, decreased hearing.

OD **Overdose Management:** *Symptoms:* Severe hypotension, bradycardia, cardiac insufficiency, *cardiogenic shock, cardiac arrest, generalized seizures,* respiratory problems, bronchospasms, vomiting, lapse of consciousness. *Treatment:* Place the client in a supine position and monitor carefully and treat under intensive care conditions. Treatment should continue for a long enough period of time consistent with the 7- to 10-hr half-life of the drug.

• Gastric lavage or induced emesis shortly after ingestion
• For excessive bradycardia, atropine, 2 mg IV. If the bradycardia is resistant to therapy, perform pacemaker therapy.
• To support cardiovascular function, give glucagon, 5–10 mg IV rapidly over 30 sec, followed by a continuous infusion of 5 mg/hr. Sympathomimetics (dobutamine, isoproterenol, epinephrine) may be given.
• For peripheral vasodilation, give epinephrine or norepinephrine with continuous monitoring of circulatory conditions.
• For bronchospasm, give beta sympathomimetics as aerosol or IV or give aminophylline IV.
• In the event of seizures, give a slow IV injection of diazepam or clonazepam.

Drug Interactions
Antidiabetic agents / The beta-blocking effect may ↑ the hypoglycemic effect of insulin and oral hypoglycemics
Calcium channel blocking agents / ↑ Risk of conduction disturbances
Clonidine / Potentiation of BP and heart rate lowering effects
Digoxin / ↑ Digoxin levels
Rifampin / ↓ Plasma levels of carvedilol

Laboratory Test Interferences: ↑ Hepatic enzymes, BUN, NPN, alkaline phosphatase. ↓ HDL. Hyperkalemia, hypokalemia.

Dosage
• **Tablets**
Essential hypertension.
Initial: 6.25 mg b.i.d. If this is tolerated, using standing systolic pressure measured about 1 hr after dosing, maintain the dose for 7–14 days. **Then,** increase to 12.5 mg b.i.d., if necessary, based on trough BP, using standing systolic pressure 2 hr after dosing. This dose should be maintained for 7–14 days and can then be adjusted upward to 25 mg b.i.d. if necessary and tolerated. The total daily dose should not exceed 50 mg.
Congestive heart failure.
12.5–50 mg b.i.d.
Angina pectoris.
25–50 mg b.i.d.
Idiopathic cardiomyopathy.
6.25–25 mg b.i.d.

RESPIRATORY CARE CONSIDERATIONS

See also *Respiratory Care Considerations* for *Antihypertensive Agents* and *Adrenergic Blocking Agents.*
Administration/Storage:
1. The full antihypertensive effect is seen within 7–14 days.
2. The drug should be taken with food to slow absorption and decrease the incidence of orthostatic effects.
3. Addition of a diuretic can produce additive effects and exaggerate the orthostatic effect.
Assessment
1. Document indications for therapy, type and onset of symptoms, and other agents trialed with the outcome.
2. Note any history or evidence of bronchospastic conditions, asthma, advanced AV block, or severe bradycardia as drug is contraindicated.
3. Obtain baseline CBC and liver and renal function studies.
Evaluate: Desired reduction of BP

Cefaclor
(**SEF**-ah-klor)
Pregnancy Category: B
Ceclor, Ceclor CD **(Rx)**
Classification: Cephalosporin, second-generation

See also *Anti-Infectives* and *Cephalosporins.*
Action/Kinetics: Peak serum levels: 5–15 mcg/mL after 1 hr. **t½: PO,** 36–54 min. Well absorbed from GI tract. From 60% to 85% excreted in urine within 8 hr.
Uses: Otitis media due to *Streptococcus pneumoniae, Hemophilus influenzae, Streptococcus pyogenes,* and staphylococci. Upper respiratory tract infections (including pharyngitis and tonsillitis) caused by *S. pyogenes.* Lower respiratory tract infections (including pneumonia) due to *S. pneumoniae, H. influenzae,* and *S. pyogenes.* Skin and skin structure infections due to *Staphylococcus aureus* and *S. pyogenes.* UTIs (including pyelonephritis and cystitis) caused by *Escherichia coli, Proteus mirabilis, Klebsiella,* and coagulase-negative staphylococci. The extended-release dosage form has been approved for treating acute exacerbations of chronic bronchitis, secondary bacterial infections of acute bronchitis, pharyngitis, tonsillitis, and uncomplicated skin and skin structure infections. *Investigational:* Acute uncomplicated UTIs in select populations using a single dose of 2 g.
Special Concerns: Safety for use in infants less than 1 month of age has not been established.
Additional Side Effects: Cholestatic jaundice, lymphocytosis.

Dosage
• **Capsules, Oral Suspension**
Adults: 250 mg q 8 hr. Dose may be doubled in more severe infections or those caused by less susceptible organisms. Total daily dose should not exceed 4 g. The extended-release product allows twice-daily dosing.

Children: 20 mg/kg/day in divided doses q 8 hr. Dose may be doubled in more serious infections, otitis media, or for infections caused by less susceptible organisms. For otitis media and pharyngitis, the total daily dose may be divided and given q 12 hr. Total daily dose should not exceed 1 g.

RESPIRATORY CARE CONSIDERATIONS

See also *General Respiratory Care Considerations for All Anti-Infectives,* and *Cephalosporins.*

Administration/Storage
1. The suspension should be refrigerated after reconstitution and discarded after 2 weeks.
2. The total daily dose for otitis media and pharyngitis can be divided and given q 12 hr.

Assessment
1. Document indications for therapy, type, onset, and duration of symptoms, and any other agents prescribed.
2. Note any allergic reactions to PCNs as a cross-sensitivity reaction may occur.

Evaluate: Resolution of infection and reports of symptomatic improvement

---

Cefadroxil monohydrate
(sef-ah-**DROX**-ill)
Pregnancy Category: B
Duricef **(Rx)**
Classification: Cephalosporin, first-generation

See also *Anti-Infectives* and *Cephalosporins.*

Action/Kinetics: Peak serum levels: PO, 15–33 mcg/mL after 90 min. **t½: PO,** 70–80 min. Ninety percent of drug is excreted unchanged in urine within 24 hr.

Uses: UTIs caused by *Escherichia coli, Proteus mirabilis,* and *Klebsiella.* Skin and skin structure infections due to staphylococci or streptococci. Pharyngitis and tonsillitis due to group A beta-hemolytic streptococci.

Special Concerns: Safe use in children not established. Creatinine clearance determinations must be carried out in clients with renal impairment.

Dosage
• **Capsules, Oral Suspension, Tablets**
Pharyngitis, tonsillitis.
Adults: 1 g/day in single or two divided doses for 10 days. **Children:** 30 mg/kg/day in single or two divided doses (for beta-hemolytic streptococcal infection, dose should be given for 10 days).
Skin and skin structure infections.
Adults: 1 g/day in single or two divided doses. **Children:** 30 mg/kg/day in divided doses q 12 hr.
UTIs.
Adults: 1–2 g/day in single or two divided doses for uncomplicated lower UTI (e.g., cystitis). For all other UTIs, the usual dose is 2 g/day in two divided doses. **Children:** 30 mg/kg/day in divided doses q 12 hr.
For clients with creatinine clearance rates below 50 mL/min.
Initial: 1 g; **maintenance,** 500 mg at following dosage intervals: q 36 hr for creatinine clearance rates of 0–10 mL/min; q 24 hr for creatinine clearance rates of 10–25 mL/min; q 12 hr for creatinine clearance rates of 25–50 mL/min.

RESPIRATORY CARE CONSIDERATIONS

See also *General Respiratory Care Considerations for All Anti-Infectives* , and *Cephalosporins.*

Administration/Storage
1. Cefadroxil can be given without regard to meals.
2. The suspension should be shaken well before using.
3. For beta-hemolytic streptococcal infections, treatment should be continued for 10 days.

Assessment
1. Document indications for therapy, type and onset of symptoms, and pretreatment culture results.
2. Note any history of PCN allergy.

Evaluate
- Reports of symptomatic improvement
- Negative follow-up lab culture reports

Cefamandole nafate
(sef-ah-**MAN**-dole)
Pregnancy Category: B
Mandol **(Rx)**
Classification: Cephalosporin, second-generation

See also *Anti-Infectives,* and *Cephalosporins.*

Action/Kinetics: Cefamandole nafate has a particularly broad spectrum of activity. **Peak serum levels: IM,** 12–36 mcg/mL after 30–120 min. **t½: IM,** 60 min; **IV,** 30 min. From 65% to 85% excreted unchanged in urine.

Uses: Infections of the urinary tract, lower respiratory tract, bones, joints, skin, and skin structures. Mixed infections of the respiratory tract, skin, and in pelvic inflammatory disease. Peritonitis, septicemia, prophylaxis in surgery. Also, with aminoglycosides in gram-positive or gram-negative sepsis.

Special Concerns: Safety and effectiveness have not been determined in infants less than 1 month of age.

Additional Side Effects: Hypoprothrombinemia leading to bleeding and/or bruising; cholestatic jaundice, decreased creatinine clearance in clients with prior renal impairment.

Additional Drug Interactions: Concomitant use with ethanol produces a disulfiram-type reaction and hypotension.

Dosage
• **IV or Deep IM Injection Only**
In gluteus or lateral thigh to minimize pain.
Infections.
Adults, usual: 0.5–1 g q 4–8 hr. **Infants and children:** 50–100 mg/kg/day in equally divided doses q 4–8 hr.
Severe infections.

Adults: Up to 2 g q 4 hr. **Infants and children:** Up to 150 mg/kg/day (not to exceed adult dose) divided for infections as in the above.
Preoperative.
Adults, initial: 1–2 g 30–60 min prior to surgery; **then,** 1–2 g q 6 hr for 1–2 days (3 days for prosthetic arthroplasty). For cesarean section, the first dose should be given just prior to surgery or just after the cord has been clamped. **Pediatric (3 months and older):** 50–100 mg/kg/day in divided doses, using same schedule as for adults.
Impaired renal function.
Initial: 1–2 g; then a maintenance dosage is given, depending on creatinine clearance, according to schedule provided by manufacturer.

RESPIRATORY CARE CONSIDERATIONS

See also *General Respiratory Care Considerations for All Anti-Infectives,* and *Cephalosporins.*

Administration/Storage
1. Review package insert for details on how to reconstitute drug.
2. Reconstituted solutions of cefamandole nafate are stable for 24 hr at room temperature and for 96 hr when stored in the refrigerator. Cefamandole solutions reconstituted with dextrose or sodium chloride are stable for 6 months when frozen immediately after reconstitution.
3. For direct IV administration, dilute 1 g in 10 mL of solution and administer over 3–5 min. May be further diluted and administered over 15–30 min.
4. Peripheral IV site *must* be changed every 2–3 days to prevent phlebitis.
5. Carbon dioxide gas forms when reconstituted solutions are kept at room temperature. This gas does not affect the activity of the antibiotic and may be dissipated or used to aid in the withdrawal of the contents of the vial.
6. Use separate IV fluid containers and separate injection sites for each

drug when cefamandole is administered concomitantly with another antibiotic such as an aminoglycoside.

7. Follow manufacturer guidelines for dosage with impaired renal function.

Evaluate: Resolution of infection

Cefazolin sodium
(sef-**AYZ**-oh-lin)
Pregnancy Category: B
Ancef, Kefzol, Zolicef **(Rx)**
Classification: Cephalosporin, first-generation

See also *Anti-Infectives* and *Cephalosporins.*

Action/Kinetics: Peak serum concentration: IM 17–76 mcg/mL after 1 hr. **t½:** IM, IV: 90–130 min. From 80% to 100% excreted unchanged in urine.

Uses: Infections of the urinary tract, biliary tract, respiratory tract, bones, joints, soft tissue, and skin. Endocarditis, septicemia, prophylaxis in surgery.

Special Concerns: Safety in infants under 1 month of age has not been determined.

Additional Side Effects: When high doses are used in renal failure clients: extreme confusion, *tonic-clonic seizures,* mild hemiparesis.

Dosage ————————————
• **IM, IV Only**
Mild infections due to gram-positive cocci.
Adults: 250–500 mg q 8 hr.
Mild to moderate infections.
Children over 1 month: 25–50 mg/kg/day in three to four doses.
Moderate to severe infections.
Adults: 0.5–1 g q 6–8 hr.
Acute, uncomplicated UTIs.
Adults: 1 g q 12 hr. *For severe infections,* up to 100 mg/kg/day may be used.
Endocarditis, septicemia.
Adults: 1–1.5 g q 6 hr (rarely, up to 12 g/day).
Pneumococcal pneumonia.
Adults: 0.5 g q 12 hr.
Preoperative.

Adults: 1 g 30–60 min prior to surgery.
During surgery.
Adults: 0.5–1 g.
Postoperative.
Adults: 0.5–1 g q 6–8 hr for 24 hr (may be given up to 5 days, especially in open heart surgery or prosthetic arthroplasty).
Impaired renal function.
Initial: 0.5 g; **then,** maintenance doses are given, depending on creatinine clearance, according to schedule provided by manufacturer.

RESPIRATORY CARE CONSIDERATIONS

See also *General Respiratory Care Considerations for All Anti-Infectives,* and *Cephalosporins.*

Administration/Storage
1. Dissolve the solute by shaking vial.
2. For direct IV administration, dilute dose in 10 mL of sterile water and infuse over 3–5 min. For intermittent use, further dilute 500 mg–1 g in 50–100 mL NSS or D5%/W and administer over 30–60 min. Assess carefully for phlebitis.
3. Discard reconstituted solution after 24 hr at room temperature and after 96 hr when refrigerated.
4. Note any evidence of renal dysfunction and follow manufacturer guidelines for dosage.

Assessment: Document indications for therapy, type and onset of symptoms, and pretreatment culture results.

Evaluate
• Resolution of infection
• Negative posttreatment C&S reports

Cefepime hydrochloride
(**SEF**-eh-pim)
Pregnancy Category: B
Maxipime **(Rx)**
Classification: Cephalosporin

See also *Cephalosporins.*
Action/Kinetics: Cefepime has a spectrum of activity against both gram-negative and gram-positive

pathogens, including those resistant to other β-lactam antibiotics. It has a high affinity for the multiple penicillin-binding proteins that are essential for cell wall synthesis. **Peak serum levels, after IV:** 78 mcg/mL. **t½, terminal:** 2 hr. About 85% of the drug is excreted unchanged in the urine.

Uses: Uncomplicated and complicated UTIs (including pyelonephritis) caused by *Escherichia coli* and *Klebsiella pneumoniae;* when the infection is severe or caused by *E. coli, K. pneumoniae,* or *Proteus mirabilis;* when the infection is mild to moderate, including infections associated with concurrent bacteremia with these microorganisms. Uncomplicated skin and skin structure infections caused by *Staphylococcus aureus* (methicillin-susceptible strains only) or *Streptococcus pyogenes.* Moderate to severe pneumonia due to *Streptococcus pneumoniae,* including cases associated with concurrent bacteremia, *Pseudomonas aeruginosa, K. pneumoniae,* or *Enterobacter* species.

Contraindications: Use in those who have had an immediate hypersensitivity reaction to cefepime, cephalosporins, penicillins, or any other β-lactam antibiotics.

Special Concerns: Use with caution during lactation. Safety and efficacy have not been determined in children less than 12 years of age.

Side Effects: *See Cephalosporins.* The most common side effects include rash, phlebitis, pain, and/or inflammation.

Laboratory Test Alteration: ↑ ALT, AST, alkaline phosphatase, BUN, creatinine, potassium, total bilirubin. ↓ Hematocrit, neutrophils, platelets, WBCs. ↑ or ↓ Calcium, phosphorus. Positive Coomb's test. Abnormal PTT, PT.

Drug Interactions
Aminoglycosides / ↑ Risk of nephrotoxicity and ototoxicity
Furosemide / ↑ Risk of nephrotoxicity

Dosage ───────────
• **IM, IV**
   Mild to moderate uncomplicated or complicated UTIs, including pyelonephritis, due to E. coli, K. pneumoniae, *or* P. mirabilis.
Adults and children over 12 years: 0.5–1 g IV or IM (for *E. coli* infections) q 12 hr for 7–10 days.
   Severe uncomplicated or complicated UTIs, including pyelonephritis, due to E. coli *or* K. pneumoniae.
Adults and children over 12 years: 2 g IV q 12 hr for 10 days.
   Moderate to severe pneumonia due to S. pneumoniae, P. aeruginosa, K. pneumoniae, *or* Enterobacter *species.*
Adults and children over 12 years: 1–2 g IV q 12 hr for 10 days.
   Moderate to severe uncomplicated skin and skin structure infections due to S. aureus *or* S. pyogenes.
Adults and children over 12 years: 2 g IV q 12 hr for 10 days.

RESPIRATORY CARE CONSIDERATIONS

See also *Respiratory Care Considerations* for *Cephalosporins.*

Administration/Storage
1. The dose should be adjusted (see package insert) for clients with impaired renal function (C_{CR} less than 60 mL/min).
2. To reconstitute for IV use, dilute with 50–100 mL of 0.9% sodium chloride injection, 5% and 10% dextrose injection, M/6 sodium lactate injection, 5% dextrose and 0.9% sodium chloride injection, lactated Ringer's and 5% dextrose injection, or Normosol-R or Normosol-M in 5% dextrose injection and administer over 30 min. Cefepime is compatible at concentrations of 1–40 mg/mL with the above solutions.
3. Solutions of cefepime should not be added to ampicillin at a concentration of 40 mg/mL and should not be added to aminophylline, gentamicin, metronidazole, netilmicin sulfate, tobramycin, or vancomycin.

However, if necessary, each of these antibiotics can be given separately.

4. To reconstitute for IM use, dilute with 0.9% sodium chloride injection, 5% dextrose injection, 0.5% or 1% lidocaine HCl or bacteriostatic water for injection with parabens or benzyl alcohol.

5. The reconstituted drug is to be protected from light and stored at a room temperature of 20°C–25°C (68°F–77°F) for 24 hr or refrigerated at 2°C–8°C (36°F–46°F) for 7 days.

Assessment

1. Document indications for therapy and onset, location, duration, and characteristics of symptoms. List other agents prescribed and the outcome.

2. Note any previous sensitivity to PCN, cephalosporins, or other β-lactam antibiotics.

3. Obtain baseline CBC, liver and renal function studies, and appropriate cultures.

4. Anticipate reduced dosing with renal dysfunction.

5. List other agents prescribed; aminoglycosides and furosemide may increase the risk of nephrotoxicity or ototoxicity.

Evaluate: Reports of symptomatic improvement with resolution of infective organism

Cefixime oral

(seh-**FIX**-eem)
Pregnancy Category: B
Suprax **(Rx)**
Classification: Cephalosporin, third-generation

See also *Anti-Infectives* and *Cephalosporins.*

Action/Kinetics: Stable in the presence of beta-lactamase enzymes. **Peak serum levels:** 2–6 hr. **t½:** averages 3–4 hr. About 50% excreted unchanged in the urine and approximately 10% in the bile. In addition to the microorganisms listed under *Uses* for cephalosporins, cefixime is effective against *Moraxella catarrhalis, Streptococcus agalactiae, Haemophilus parainfluenzae, Pas-*

teurella multocida, Salmonella species, and *Shigella* species. The following microorganisms are resistant to cefixime: most strains of *Bacteroides fragilis* and clostridia, *Pseudomonas* species, strains of group D. *streptococci* including enterococci, *Listeria monocytogenes,* and most strains of staphylococci and Enterobacter.

Uses: Uncomplicated UTIs caused by *E. coli* and *P. mirabilis.* Otitis media due to *H. influenzae* (beta-lactamase positive and negative strains), *Moraxella catarrhalis,* and *S. pyogenes.* Pharyngitis and tonsillitis caused by *S. pyogenes.* Acute bronchitis and acute exacerbations of chronic bronchitis caused by *S. pneumoniae* and *H. influenzae* (beta-lactamase positive and negative strains). Uncomplicated cervical or urethral gonorrhea due to *N. gonorrhoeae* (both penicillinase- and non-penicillinase-producing strains).

Special Concerns: Safe use in infants less than 6 months old has not been established.

Additional Side Effects: *GI:* Flatulence. *Hepatic:* Elevated alkaline phosphatase levels. *Renal:* Transient increases in BUN or creatinine.

Additional Laboratory Test Interference: False + test for ketones using nitroprusside test.

Dosage ————
• **Oral Suspension, Tablets**
Adults: Either 400 mg once daily or 200 mg q 12 hr. **Children:** Either 8 mg/kg once daily or 4 mg/kg q 12 hr. Clients on renal dialysis or in whom creatinine clearance is 21–60 mL/min, the dose should be 75% of the standard dose (i.e., 300 mg/day). If the creatinine clearance is less than 20 mL/min, the dose should be 50% of the standard dose (i.e., 200 mg/day).

Uncomplicated gonorrhea.
One 400-mg tablet.

RESPIRATORY CARE CONSIDERATIONS

See also *Respiratory Care Considerations* for *Cephalosporins.*

Administration/Storage

1. Therapy should be at least 10 days when treating *S. pyogenes*.
2. Children older than 12 years or weighing more than 50 kg should be given the adult dose.
3. Otitis media should be treated using the suspension as higher blood levels are achieved compared with the tablet given at the same dose.
4. Once reconstituted, the suspension should be kept at room temperature where it maintains potency for 14 days.

Assessment

1. Take a drug history, noting any prior sensitivity to cephalosporins or penicillins.
2. Assess client financial status and health care coverage because prescription cost may be prohibitive.

Interventions

1. Anticipate reduced dose with impaired renal function.
2. Use the suspension in children and when treating otitis media.
3. Cefixime may alter results of urine glucose and ketone testing; finger sticks may provide more accurate blood sugar recordings during drug therapy.

Evaluate: Resolution of infection and reports of symptomatic improvement

Cefmetazole sodium

(sef-**MET**-ah-zole)
Pregnancy Category: B
Zefazone **(Rx)**
Classification: Cephalosporin, second-generation

See also *Anti-Infectives* and *Cephalosporins*.

Uses: Urinary tract, lower respiratory tract, skin and skin structure, and intra-abdominal infections. Preoperatively to decrease incidence of postoperative infections following cesarean section, cholecystectomy (high risk), colorectal surgery, abdominal or vaginal hysterectomy.

Dosage

- **IV**

    Infections.
    2 g q 6–12 hr for 5–14 days.
    Prophylaxis, abdominal hysterectomy or high-risk cholecystectomy.
    1 g 30–90 min prior to surgery and again 8 and 16 hr following surgery.
    Prophylaxis, vaginal hysterectomy.
    2 g 30–90 min prior to surgery or 1 g 30–90 min prior to surgery and again 8 and 16 hr following surgery.
    Prophylaxis, cesarean section.
    2 g in a single dose after clamping cord or 1 g after clamping cord and again 8 and 16 hr later.
    Prophylaxis, colorectal surgery.
    2 g 30–90 min prior to surgery or 2 g 30–60 min prior to surgery and again 8 and 16 hr following surgery.

RESPIRATORY CARE CONSIDERATIONS

See also *Respiratory Care Considerations* for *Cephalosporins*.

Administration/Storage

1. The drug should be reconstituted with sterile water for injection, bacteriostatic water for injection, or 0.9% sodium chloride injection.
2. After reconstitution, the drug is stable for 24 hr at room temperature, for 7 days if refrigerated, and for 6 weeks if frozen.
3. If necessary, the reconstituted solution may be further diluted to concentrations of 1–20 mg/mL with 0.9% sodium chloride injection, 5% dextrose injection, or lactated Ringer's injection. Infuse over 15–30 min. Such solutions are stable as described in 2.
4. Thawed solutions should not be refrozen.
5. Any unused solutions or frozen material should be discarded.

Assessment

1. Document indications for therapy and the recommended administration frequency and dosage.
2. Obtain baseline renal function studies and anticipate reduced dose and frequency of administration of

cefmetazole with impaired renal function.

3. Note any history of PCN sensitivity reactions.

Evaluate
• Resolution of existing infection
• Infection prophylaxis during surgery

Cefonicid sodium
(seh-**FON**-ih-sid)
Pregnancy Category: B
Monocid **(Rx)**
Classification: Cephalosporin, second-generation

See also *Anti-Infectives* and *Cephalosporins*.

Uses: Infections of the lower respiratory tract, urinary tract, bones, joints, skin, and skin structures. Septicemia. Prophylaxis in surgery, especially colorectal surgery, vaginal hysterectomy, cholecystectomy, prosthetic arthroplasty, open heart surgery, cesarean section after the cord has been clamped.

Dosage ———
• **IV, Deep IM**
Uncomplicated UTIs.
Adults: 0.5 g once daily.
Mild to moderate infections.
Adults: 1 g once daily.
Severe or life-threatening infections.
Adults: 2 g once daily.
Prophylaxis in surgery.
Adults: 1 g 1 hr prior to surgery; dosage may be repeated for 2 more days if required.
In renal impairment.
Initial: 7.5 mg/kg given **IV or IM; then,** follow schedule provided by manufacturer.

RESPIRATORY CARE CONSIDERATIONS

See also *Respiratory Care Considerations* for *Cephalosporins*.

Administration/Storage
1. If 2 g is required IM, give half the dose in different large muscle masses.
2. For IV bolus, give cefonicid slowly over 3–5 min either through IV tubing or directly, assess for phlebitis, and change peripheral site every 48–72 hr.

3. For IV infusion, reconstitute in 50–100 mL of appropriate diluent and infuse over 30 min (see package insert). Solutions are stable for 24 hr at room temperature and 72 hr if refrigerated.

Assessment
1. Document indications for therapy, type and onset of symptoms, and pretreatment lab studies.
2. Anticipate reduced dose with renal dysfunction.
3. Note any previous history of PCN sensitivity.

Evaluate
• Resolution of existing infection
• Infection prophylaxis during surgery

Cefoperazone sodium
(sef-oh-**PER**-ah-zohn)
Pregnancy Category: B
Cefobid **(Rx)**
Classification: Cephalosporin, third-generation

See also *Anti-Infectives* and *Cephalosporins*.

Action/Kinetics: Peak serum levels: 73–153 mcg/mL. **t½:** 102–156 min. Approximately 30% excreted unchanged in the urine.

Uses: Infections of skin, skin structures, urinary tract, and respiratory tract. Intra-abdominal infections including peritonitis. Bacterial septicemia, pelvic inflammatory disease, endometritis, other infections of the female genital tract.

Special Concerns: Use with caution in hepatic disease or biliary obstruction. Safety and effectiveness have not been determined in children.

Additional Side Effects: Hypoprothrombinemia resulting in bleeding and/or bruising.

Additional Drug Interactions: Concomitant use with ethanol may cause an Antabuse-like reaction.

Dosage
• **IM, IV**

Adults, usual: 2–4 g/day in divided doses q 12 hr (up to 12–16 g/day has been used in severe infections or for less sensitive organisms).

NOTE: This drug is significantly excreted in the bile; thus, the daily dose should not exceed 4 g in hepatic disease or biliary obstruction.

RESPIRATORY CARE CONSIDERATIONS

See also *Respiratory Care Considerations* for *Cephalosporins.*

Administration/Storage

1. Dilute each gram in 20–40 mL of solution and infuse over 15–30 min.
2. Following reconstitution, the solution should be allowed to stand for dissipation of any foaming and to determine if complete solubilization has occurred. Vigorous shaking may be necessary to dissolve higher concentrations.
3. Reconstituted drug may be frozen; however, after thawing, any unused portion should be discarded.
4. The unreconstituted powder should be protected from light and stored in the refrigerator.
5. If used for neonates, cefoperazone should not be reconstituted with diluents containing benzyl alcohol.

Assessment

1. Complete a history and note any PCN sensitivity. Assess for bruising, hematuria, black stools, or other evidence of bleeding.
2. Obtain baseline coagulation studies and monitor during therapy as drug may cause hypoprothrombinemia.
3. Assess need for prophylactic vitamin K administration (usually 10 mg/week).
4. If client is receiving treatment for skin lesions, inspect lesions closely, noting size, location, and extent of involvement.
5. Assess for any evidence/history of excessive use of alcohol.
6. Determine if client has liver or biliary disease as dose should be reduced.

Evaluate
• ↓ Size and number of skin lesions with evidence of wound healing
• Resolution of infection

Cefotaxime sodium
(sef-oh-**TAX**-eem)
Pregnancy Category: B
Claforan **(Rx)**
Classification: Cephalosporin, third-generation

See also *Anti-Infectives* and *Cephalosporins.*

Action/Kinetics: Treatment should be continued for a minimum of 10 days for group A beta-hemolytic streptococcal infections to minimize the risk of glomerulonephritis or rheumatic fever. The IV route is preferable for clients with severe or life-threatening infections; for clients after surgery; or for those manifesting malnutrition, trauma, malignancy, heart failure, or diabetes, especially if shock is present or possible. **t½:** 1 hr. From 20% to 36% is excreted unchanged in the urine.

Uses: Infections of the GU tract, lower respiratory tract (including pneumonia), skin, skin structures, bones, joints, and CNS (including ventriculitis and meningitis). Intra-abdominal infections (including peritonitis), gynecologic infections (including endometritis, pelvic cellulitis, pelvic inflammatory disease), septicemia, bacteremia, and prophylaxis in surgery. Used with aminoglycosides for gram-positive or gram-negative sepsis where the causative agent has not been identified.

Dosage
• **IV, IM**
  Uncomplicated infections.
Adults: 1 g q 12 hr.
  Moderate to severe infections.
Adults: 1–2 g q 8 hr.
  Septicemia.
Adults, IV: 2 g q 6–8 hr.

✦ = Available in Canada   ***bold italic*** = life threatening side effect

Life-threatening infections.
Adults, IV: 2 g q 4 hr up to 12 g/day.
Gonorrhea.
Adults, IM: Single dose of 1 g.
Preoperative prophylaxis.
Adults: 1 g 30–90 min prior to surgery.
Cesarean section.
IV: 1 g when the umbilical cord is clamped; **then,** give 1 g 6 and 12 hr after the first dose.
Pediatric, 1 month to 12 years, IM, IV: 50–180 mg/kg/day in four to six divided doses; **1–4 weeks, IV:** 50 mg/kg q 8 hr; **0–1 week, IV:** 50 mg/kg q 12 hr. *NOTE:* Use adult dose in children 50 kg or over.

RESPIRATORY CARE CONSIDERATIONS

See also *Respiratory Care Considerations* for *Cephalosporins.*
Administration/Storage
1. Cefotaxime should not be mixed with aminoglycosides for continuous IV infusion. If they are to be given to the same client, each should be given separately.
2. Cefotaxime is maximally stable at a pH of 5–7; solutions should not be prepared with diluents having a pH greater than 7.5 (e.g., sodium bicarbonate injection).
3. Dry cefotaxime should be stored below 30°C (86°F) and should be protected from excess heat and light to prevent darkening.
4. Add recommended amount of diluent, shake to dissolve, and observe for particles or discoloration of solution. Do not administer if particles are present or if solution is discolored. The normal color of solution ranges from light yellow to amber.
5. For IM use, reconstitute with sterile water for injection or bacteriostatic water for injection. Inject deeply into large muscle. Divide doses of 2 g and administer into different sites.
6. For direct IV administration, 1 or 2 g cefotaxime should be mixed with 10 mL sterile water for injection and administered over 3–5 min. For intermittent administration, further dilute in

50–100 mL of solution and infuse over 30 min.
7. Discontinue IV administration of other solutions during administration of cefotaxime.
8. After reconstitution, the drug remains stable for 24 hr at room temperature, 5 days refrigerated, and 13 weeks frozen. Thaw frozen samples at room temperature before use. Do not refreeze unused portions.
9. Anticipate reduced dosage in clients with impaired renal function.
Assessment
1. For clients receiving therapy for joint infections, carefully assess the extent of their ROM and freedom of movement.
2. In clients with gynecologic infections, determine how long symptoms have been evident and how extensive the infection is prior to treatment.
3. Obtain appropriate lab studies prior to initiating therapy. Review culture results to determine any organism resistance to this drug.
Interventions
1. Maintain careful documentation of the type and extent of infection and subjective complaints.
2. Monitor and record I&O.
3. Inspect site of injections for pain and redness. IM administration of these medications may cause thrombophlebitis.
Evaluate
• Resolution of infection and reports of symptomatic improvement
• Negative lab culture reports

Cefotetan disodium
(sef-oh-**TEE**-tan)
Pregnancy Category: B
Cefotan **(Rx)**
Classification: Cephalosporin, second-generation

See also *Anti-Infectives* and *Cephalosporins.*
Action/Kinetics: Administered parenterally only. **t½:** 3–4.6 hr. From 50% to 80% is excreted unchanged in the urine.
Uses: Infections of the urinary tract,

lower respiratory tract, skin and skin structures, bones, and joints. Also gynecologic and intra-abdominal infections. Prophylaxis of postoperative infections (e.g., due to abdominal or vaginal hysterectomy, transurethral surgery, GI or biliary tract surgery, cesarean section).

Special Concerns: Safety and effectiveness have not been determined in children.

Additional Side Effects: Concomitant use with ethanol produces a disulfiram-type reaction and hypotension.

Additional Laboratory Test Interference: The drug may affect measurement of creatinine levels by the Jaffe reaction.

Dosage

• **IV or IM**
  Usual infections.
Adults: 1–2 g q 12 hr for 5–10 days.
  UTIs.
Adults: Either 0.5 g q 12 hr, or 1–2 g q 12–24 hr.
  Severe infections.
Adults, IV: 2 g q 12 hr.
  Life-threatening infections.
Adults, IV: 3 g q 12 hr.
  Prophylaxis of postoperative infection.
Adults, IV: 1–2 g 30–60 min prior to surgery.

RESPIRATORY CARE CONSIDERATIONS

See also *Respiratory Care Considerations* for *Cephalosporins*.

Administration/Storage

1. Cefotetan disodium must be administered parenterally, because it is not absorbed from the GI tract.
2. IM injections should be made well within a large muscle (e.g., the gluteus maximus).
3. The IV route is preferred for clients with bacterial septicemia, bacteremia, or other severe or life-threatening infections. The IV route is also preferred for poor-risk clients as the result of malnutrition, surgery, diabetes, trauma, heart failure, ma-

lignancy, or if shock is present or impending.
4. Direct IV administration may be completed over 3–5 min following reconstitution (1 g in 10 mL of sterile water for injection). May further dilute in 50–100 mL D5%/W or NSS and infuse over 30–60 min.
5. For IM use, reconstitute with sterile water for injection, NSS, bacteriostatic water for injection, or 0.5%–1% lidocaine HCl.
6. Reconstituted solutions maintain potency for 24 hr at room temperature, for 96 hr if refrigerated, and for 1 week if frozen.
7. Cefotetan should not be mixed with solutions containing aminoglycosides.
8. Dosage should be reduced in impaired renal function and depends on creatinine clearance.

Assessment

1. Obtain a complete history and assess for bruising, hematuria, black stools, or other evidence of bleeding.
2. Note any evidence or history of PCN reaction or excessive use of alcohol.
3. Obtain baseline coagulation studies and monitor during therapy as drug may cause hypoprothrombinemia.
4. Assess need for prophylactic vitamin K administration (usually 10 mg/week).

Evaluate

• Resolution of infection with reports of symptomatic improvement
• Infection prophylaxis during surgery

Cefoxitin sodium
(seh-**FOX**-ih-tin)
Pregnancy Category: B
Mefoxin **(Rx)**
Classification: Cephalosporin, second-generation

See also *Anti-Infectives* and *Cephalosporins*.

Action/Kinetics: Broad-spectrum cephalosporin that is penicillinase-

and cephalosporinase-resistant and is stable in the presence of beta-lactamases. **Peak serum concentration:** IM, 20–30 min. t½: IM, IV, 41–65 min; 85% of drug excreted unchanged in urine after 6 hr.

Uses: Infections of the urinary tract (including gonorrhea), bones, joints, lower respiratory tract (including lung abscesses and pneumonia), skin, and skin structures. Intra-abdominal infections (including intra-abdominal abscesses and peritonitis), gynecologic infections (including pelvic inflammatory disease, pelvic cellulitis, and endometritis), septicemia, and prophylaxis in surgery. Oral bacterial *Eikenella corrodens* infections. *NOTE:* Many gram-negative infections resistant to certain cephalosporins and penicillins respond to cefoxitin.

Additional Side Effects: Higher doses have caused increased incidence of eosinophilia and increased AST levels in children over 3 months of age.

Additional Laboratory Test Interference: High concentrations may interfere with the measurement of creatinine by the Jaffe method.

Dosage ————————————
• **IM, IV**
Uncomplicated infections (cutaneous, pneumonia, urinary tract).
Adults, IV, IM: 1 g q 6–8 hr.
Severe infections.
Adults, IV: 1 g q 4 hr or 2 g q 6–8 hr.
Gas gangrene.
Adults, IV: 2 g q 4 hr or 3 g q 6 hr.
Gonorrhea.
Adults: 2 g IM with 1 g probenecid PO.
Prophylaxis in surgery.
Adults, IV, IM: 2 g 30–60 min before surgery followed by 2 g q 6 hr after first dose for 24 hr only (72 hr for prosthetic arthroplasty).
Cesarean section, prophylaxis.
2 g **IV** when cord is clamped; **then,** give two additional doses IV or IM 4 and 8 hr later. Subsequent doses may be given q 6 hr for no more than 1 day.
Transurethral prostatectomy, prophylaxis.

1 g before surgery; **then,** 1 g q 8 hr for up to 5 days.
Impaired renal function.
Initial: 1–2 g; **then,** follow maintenance schedule provided by manufacturer.
Infections.
Children over 3 months: 80–160 mg/kg/day in four to six divided doses. Total daily dosage should not exceed 12 g.
Prophylaxis.
Children: 30–40 mg/kg q 6 hr.

RESPIRATORY CARE CONSIDERATIONS

See also *Respiratory Care Considerations* for *Cephalosporins.*

Administration/Storage
1. Do not mix with other antibiotics during administration.
2. Reconstituted solutions are stable for 24 hr at room temperature, 1 week in the refrigerator, and 26 weeks when frozen.
3. Store drug vials below 30°C (86°F).
4. Reconstituted solutions are white to light amber. Color does not affect potency. Consult pharmacist if unsure of drug potency.
5. For IM injections, lidocaine hydrochloride 0.05% (without epinephrine) may be used as diluent, by provider's order, to reduce pain at injection site.
6. For direct IV administration dilute 1 g in 10 mL sterile water and infuse over 3–5 min. For intermittent administration, further dilute in 50–100 mL of solution and infuse over 15–30 min.
7. Do not administer cefoxitin rapidly, because it is irritating to veins.

Interventions
1. Monitor I&O, withhold medication, and report any significant reduction in urinary output.
2. Assess infusion site for pain and redness as medication can cause thrombophlebitis.

Evaluate
• Resolution of infection and reports of symptomatic relief
• Infection prophylaxis during surgery

Cefpodoxime proxetil
(sef-poh-**DOX**-eem)

Pregnancy Category: B

Vantin **(Rx)**

Classification: Cephalosporin, second-generation

See also *Anti-Infectives* and *Cephalosporins.*

Action/Kinetics: From 29% to 33% is recovered unchanged from the urine.

Uses: Acute, community-acquired pneumonia due to *Streptococcus pneumoniae* or *Hemophilus influenzae* (only non-beta-lactamase-producing strains). Acute otitis media caused by *S. pneumoniae, H. influenzae* (including beta-lactamase-producing strains), and *Moraxella catarrhalis.* Pharyngitis or tonsillitis due to *Streptococcus pyogenes.* Acute, uncomplicated urethral and cervical gonorrhea caused by *Neisseria gonorrhoeae* (including penicillinase-producing strains). Acute, uncomplicated anorectal infections in women due to *N. gonorrhoeae* (including penicillinase-producing strains). Uncomplicated skin and skin structure infections due to *Staphylococcus aureus* (including penicillinase-producing strains) or *S. pyogenes.* Uncomplicated UTIs (cystitis) due to *Escherichia coli, Klebsiella pneumoniae, Proteus mirabilis,* or *Staphyloccus saprophyticus.* Acute bacterial exacerbation of chronic bronchitis caused by *S. pneumoniae,* non-beta-lactamase-producing *H. influenzae,* or M. catarrhalis.

Dosage ─────────────

• **Tablets, Suspension**

Acute community-acquired pneumonia.

Adults and children over 13 years: 200 mg q 12 hr for 14 days.

Acute bacterial exacerbations of chronic bronchitis.

Adults and children over 13 years: 200 mg q 12 hr for 10 days.

Uncomplicated gonorrhea (men and women) and rectal gonococcal infections (women).

Adults and children over 13 years: Single dose of 200 mg.

Skin and skin structure infections.

Adults and children over 13 years: 400 mg q 12 hr for 7–14 days.

Pharyngitis, tonsillitis.

Adults and children over 13 years: 100 mg q 12 hr for 5–10 days.

Children, 6 months–12 years: 5 mg/kg (maximum of 100 mg/dose) q 12 hr (maximum daily dose: 200 mg) for 5–10 days.

Uncomplicated UTIs.

Adults and children over 13 years: 100 mg q 12 hr for 7 days.

Acute otitis media.

Children, 6 months–12 years: 5 mg/kg (maximum of 200 mg/dose) q 12 hr or 10 mg/kg q 24 hr for 10 days. The maximum daily dose should not exceed 400 mg.

─────────────

RESPIRATORY CARE CONSIDERATIONS

See also *General Respiratory Care Considerations for All Anti-Infectives,* and *Cephalosporins.*

Administration/Storage

1. Dosage adjustment is not required in clients with cirrhosis.

2. In severe renal impairment (creatinine clearance less than 30 mL/min), the dosing interval should be increased to q 24 hr. If the client is maintained on hemodialysis, a dosage frequency of 3 times/week after hemodialysis should be used.

3. If only the serum creatinine level is available, the following formula can be used to estimate creatinine clearance (mL/min): males: weight (kg) × (140 - age)/72 × serum creatinine (mg/100 mL); females: 0.85 × male value.

4. The suspension is prepared by adding a total of 58 mL of distilled water to the 50 mg/mL product or 57 mL of distilled water to the 100 mg/5 mL product. After tapping the bottle gently to loosen the powder, add 25 mL of water and shake vigorously

for 15 sec to wet the powder. The remainder of the water is then added and the bottle is shaken vigorously for 3 min or until all particles are suspended.

5. After reconstitution, the suspension is stored in the refrigerator and any unused portion should be discarded after 14 days.

6. The reconstituted suspension should be shaken well before using.

Assessment

1. Determine any previous sensitivity reactions to cephalosporins or penicillins as cross-sensitivity can occur.

2. Document source of infection and ensure that baseline cultures have been performed.

3. Note any history or evidence of renal dysfunction.

4. Obtain a serologic test for syphilis in clients being treated for gonorrhea.

Interventions

1. Closely monitor VS and I&O.

2. Discontinue drug therapy and report if seizures occur.

3. Clients with persistent diarrhea should be evaluated for other causes, such as *C. difficile*.

Evaluate

• Resolution of infection

• Negative culture reports

• Reports of symptomatic improvement

Cefprozil

(**SEF**-proh-zill)

Pregnancy Category: B

Cefzil **(Rx)**

Classification: Cephalosporin, second-generation

See also *Anti-Infectives* and *Cephalosporins*.

Action/Kinetics: Sixty percent is recovered in the urine unchanged.

Uses: Pharyngitis and tonsillitis due to *Streptococcus pyogenes*. Acute bacterial sinusitis due to *Streptococcus pneumoniae, Staphylococcus aureus, Haemophilus influenzae,* and *Morazella catarrhalis*. Otitis media caused by *S. pneumoniae, H. in-*

fluenzae, and *M. catarrhalis*. Uncomplicated skin and skin structure infections due to *S. aureus* (including penicillinase-producing strains) and *S. pyogenes*. Secondary bacterial infection of acute bronchitis and acute bacterial exacerbation of chronic bronchitis due to *S. pneumoniae, H. influenzae* (beta-lactamase positive and negative strains), and M. catarrhalis.

Dosage ─────────────

• **Suspension, Tablets**

Pharyngitis, tonsillitis, acute sinusitis.

Adults and children over 13 years of age: 500 mg q 24 hr for at least 10 days (especially for *S. pyogenes* infections). **Children, 2–12 years of age:** 7.5 mg/kg q 12 hr for at least 10 days (especially for *S. pyogenes* infections).

Secondary bacterial infections of acute bronchitis and acute bacterial exacerbation of chronic bronchitis.

Adults and children over 13 years of age: 500 mg q 12 hr for 10 days.

Uncomplicated skin and skin structure infections.

Adults and children over 13 years of age: Either 250 mg q 12 hr, 500 mg q 24 hr, or 500 mg q 12 hr (all for a duration of 10 days).

Otitis media.

Infants and children 6 months–12 years: 15 mg/kg q 12 hr for 10 days.

RESPIRATORY CARE CONSIDERATIONS

See also *General Respiratory Care Considerations for All Anti-Infectives,* and *Cephalosporins*.

Administration/Storage

1. In clients with impaired renal function (creatinine clearance of 0–30 mL/min), the dose should be 50% of the standard use given at standard intervals.

2. After reconstitution, store the suspension in a refrigerator and discard any unused portion after 14 days.

Interventions

1. Monitor VS and I&O.

2. Anticipate reduced dose with impaired renal function.

Evaluate
• Reports of symptomatic improvement
• Resolution of infection

Ceftazidime
(sef-**TAY**-zih-deem)
Pregnancy Category: B
Ceptaz ✦, Fortaz, Tazicef, Tazidime
(Rx)
Classification: Cephalosporin, third-generation

See also *Anti-Infectives* and *Cephalosporins*.
Action/Kinetics: Only for IM or IV use. t½: 2–3 hr. From 80% to 90% is excreted unchanged in the urine.
Uses: Bacterial septicemia. Infections of the lower respiratory tract, skin and skin structures, bones and joints, CNS (including meningitis), and urinary tract. Also, intra-abdominal (including peritonitis) and gynecologic infections (including endometritis, pelvic cellulitis). Use with aminoglycosides, clindamycin, or vancomycin in severe or life-threatening infections or in the immunocompromised client.
Special Concerns: A sodium carbonate formulation should be used if the drug is indicated for children less than 12 years of age.

Dosage
• **IM, IV**
Usual infections.
Adults: 1 g q 8–12 hr.
UTIs, uncomplicated.
Adults, IM, IV: 0.25 g q 12 hr.
UTIs, complicated.
Adults, IM, IV: 0.5 g q 8–12 hr.
Uncomplicated pneumonia, skin and skin structure infections.
Adults, IM, IV: 0.5–1 g q 8 hr.
Bone and joint infections.
Adults, IV: 2 g q 12 hr.
Serious gynecologic or intra-abdominal infections, meningitis, severe or life-threatening infections (especially in immunocompromised clients).

Adults, IV: 2 g q 8 hr.
Pseudomonal lung infections in cystic fibrosis clients.
IV: 30–50 mg/kg q 8 hr, not to exceed 6 g/day. **Neonates, 0–4 weeks, IV:** 30 mg/kg q 12 hr. **Infants and children, 1 month–12 years, IV:** 30–50 mg/kg q 8 hr not to exceed 6 g/day.

RESPIRATORY CARE CONSIDERATIONS

See also *General Respiratory Care Considerations for All Anti-Infectives* and *Cephalosporins*.
Administration/Storage
1. Ceftazidime must be administered parenterally, because it is not absorbed from the GI tract.
2. If administering IM, use large muscle mass and inject deeply.
3. The IV route is preferred for clients with bacterial septicemia, peritonitis, bacterial meningitis, or other severe or life-threatening infections. Also, IV should be used for clients considered to be poor risks due to malnutrition, surgery, diabetes, trauma, heart failure, malignancy, or if shock is present or imminent.
4. For direct IV administration, reconstitute 1 g in 10 mL sterile water for injection and administer over 3–5 min.
5. For intermittent administration, further dilute in 50–100 mL of solution and administer over 30–60 min. It is compatible with 0.9% sodium chloride injection, Ringer's injection, lactated Ringer's injection, 5% or 10% dextrose injection, M/6 sodium lactate injection, 5% dextrose and 0.225%, 0.45%, or 0.9% sodium chloride injection, 10% invert sugar in water for injection. Sodium bicarbonate injection should not be used for reconstitution; however, a sodium carbonate formulation should be used for children less than 12.
6. For use as an IV infusion, the 1- or 2-g infusion pack is reconstituted with 100 mL sterile water for injection (or a compatible IV solution).
7. For IM administration, reconstitute in sterile water for injection,

bacteriostatic water for injection, or 0.5%–1% lidocaine HCl injection.

8. Ceftazidime should not be added to solutions containing aminoglycosides.

9. Dosage must be reduced in clients with impaired renal function (see package insert).

Assessment

1. Note any PCN allergy.

2. Obtain renal function studies; anticipate reduced dosage with impaired function.

Evaluate

• Resolution of infection

• Negative lab culture reports

Ceftibuten

(sef-**TYE**-byou-ten)

Cedax **(Rx)**

Classification: Cephalosporin

See also *Cephalosporins,*

Action/Kinetics: Ceftibuten is resistant to beta-lactamase. It has the broadest gram-negative spectrum of any of the current PO cephalosporins. The drug is well absorbed from the GI tract. Food delays the time to peak serum concentration, lowers the peak cencentration, and decreases the total amount of drug absorbed. **Peak serum levels:** 2 to 3 hours. **t½:** 2 hr. It is excreted in the urine.

Uses: Acute bacterial exacerbations of chronic bronchitis due to *Haemophilus influenzae* (including beta-lactamase-producing strains), *Moraxella catarrhalis* (including beta-lactamase-producing strains), and penicillin-susceptible strains of *Streptococcus pneumoniae.* Acute bacterial otitis media due to *H. influenzae, M. catarrhalis,* and *Staphylococcus pyogenes.* Pharyngitis and tonsillitis due to *S. pyogenes.*

Special Concerns: Although ceftibuten has been approved for pharyngitis or tonsillitis, only penicillin has been shown to be effective in preventing rheumatic fever. The drug has not been approved to treat urinary infections.

Side Effects: See *Cephalosporins.* Ceftibuten is usually well tolerated.

The most common side effect is diarrhea.

Dosage ───────────

• **Capsules, Oral Suspension**

All uses.

Adults and children over 12 years of age: 400 mg once daily for 10 days. The maximum daily dose is 400 mg. The dose should be adjusted in clients with a creatine clearance less than 50 mL/min as follows. If the creatinine clearance is between 30 and 49 mL/min, the recommended dose is 4.5 mg/kg or 200 mg once daily. If the creatinine clearance is between 5 and 29 mL/min, the recommended dose is 2.25 mg/kg or 100 mg once daily. In clients undergoing hemodialysis 2 or 3 times/week, a single 400-mg dose of ceftibuten capsules or a single dose of 9 mg/kg (maximum of 400 mg) of PO suspension can be given at the end of each hemodialysis session.

Children: pharyngitis, tonsillitis, acute bacterial otitis media.

9 mg/kg, up to a maximum of 400 mg daily, for a total of 10 days. Children over 45 kg should receive the maximum daily dose of 400 mg.

RESPIRATORY CARE CONSIDERATIONS

See also *Respiratory Care Considerations* for *Cephalosporins.*

Administration/Storage

1. The pediatric suspension is available as either 90 mg/5 mL or 180 mg/5 mL.

2. The suspension must be given at least 2 hr before or 1 hr after a meal.

3. The directions for mixing ceftibuten suspension must be carefully followed, depending on the final concentration and the bottle size. First, the bottle should be tapped to loosen powder. Then, the appropriate amount of water is added in two portions, shaking well after each portion.

4. After mixing, the suspension may be kept for 14 days under refrigeration. The container must be kept tightly closed and must be shaken well before each use. Any unused

drug should be discarded after 14 days.

Assessment

1. Document indications for therapy and type, onset, duration, and characteristics of symptoms.

2. Obtain baseline cultures and renal function studies; anticipate reduced dosage with impaired renal function.

3. Review conditions requiring treatment as drug is only approved for chronic bronchitis, bacterial otitis media, and pharyngitis or tonsillitis, with limitations based on the infective organisms.

Evaluate

• Resolution of underlying infection
• Reports of symptomatic improvement

Ceftizoxime sodium

(sef-tih-**ZOX**-eem)
Pregnancy Category: B
Cefizox **(Rx)**
Classification: Cephalosporin, third-generation

See also *Anti-Infectives* and *Cephalosporins*.

Action/Kinetics: t½: Approximately 1–2 hr. Approximately 80% excreted unchanged in the urine.

Uses: Infections of the urinary tract, lower respiratory tract, skin, skin structures, bones, and joints. Intra-abdominal infections, septicemia, meningitis (caused by *Haemophilus influenzae* or *Streptococcus pneumoniae),* gonorrhea (including uncomplicated cervical and urethral gonorrhea caused by *Neisseria*). Pelvic inflammatory disease caused by *Neisseria gonorrhoeae, Escherichia coli,* or Streptococcus agalactiae.

Additional Side Effects: Transient increased levels of eosinophils, AST, ALT, and CPK have been seen in children over 6 months of age.

Dosage ─────────────
• **IM, IV**

Uncomplicated urinary tract and other infections.
Adults: 0.5 g q 12 hr.
Severe or resistant infections.
Adults: 1 g q 8 hr or 2 g q 8–12 hr.
Life-threatening infections.
Adults: Up to 3–4 g q 8 hr.
Pelvic inflammatory disease.
2 g q 8 hr IV (doses up to 2 g q 4 hr have been used).
• **IV**
Uncomplicated gonorrhea.
Adults: 1 g as a single dose **IM. Pediatric, over 6 months:** 50 mg/kg q 6–8 hr up to 200 mg/kg/day (not to exceed the maximum adult dose).
Impaired renal function.
Initial, IM, IV: 0.5–1 g; **then,** use maintenance schedule in package insert.

RESPIRATORY CARE CONSIDERATIONS

See also *General Respiratory Care Considerations for All Anti-Infectives* and *Cephalosporins*.

Administration/Storage

1. For IM doses of 2 g, divide the dose equally and give in different large muscle masses.

2. For direct IV administration, reconstitute 1 g in 10 mL sterile water and give slowly over 3–5 min.

3. For intermittent administration, further dilute in 50–100 mL of D5W or NSS and infuse over 30 min.

4. Reconstituted solutions are stable at room temperature for 8 hr and, if refrigerated, for 48 hr.

Evaluate

• Negative C&S reports
• Resolution of S&S of infection

Ceftriaxone sodium

(sef-try-**AX**-ohn)
Pregnancy Category: B
Rocephin **(Rx)**
Classification: Cephalosporin, third-generation

See also *Anti-Infectives* and *Cephalosporins*.

Action/Kinetics: t½: Approximately 6–8 hr. Significantly protein bound. One-third to two-thirds excreted unchanged in the urine.

Uses: Infections of the lower respiratory tract, urinary tract, skin, skin structures, bones, joints, abdomen. Also, uncomplicated gonorrhea (cervical, urethral, rectal) including both penicillinase- and non-penicillinase-producing strains of *Neisseria gonorrhoeae* and pharyngeal gonorrhea caused by non-penicillinase-producing strains of *N. gonorrhoeae*. Pelvic inflammatory disease, pediatric meningitis, prophylaxis of infections in surgery, bacterial septicemia. *Investigational:* Neurologic complications, arthritis, and carditis associated with Lyme disease (infection caused by *Borrelia burgdorferi)* in clients refractory to penicillin G.

Additional Side Effects: Increase in serum creatinine, presence of casts in the urine, alteration of PTs (rare).

Dosage ——————————

• **IV, IM**

General infections.
Adults, usual: 1–2 g/day in single or divided doses q 12 hr, not to exceed 4 g/day. Therapy is maintained for 4–14 days, depending on the infection. **Pediatric:** *Other than meningitis:* 50–75 mg/kg/day not to exceed total daily dose of 2 g given in divided doses q 12 hr.

Meningitis.
Pediatric: 100 mg/kg/day, not to exceed total daily dose of 4 g given once daily or in equally divided doses q 12 hr for 7–14 days.

Prophylaxis of infection in surgery.
1 g 30–120 min prior to surgery.

Uncomplicated gonorrhea.
Adults, IM: 125 mg as a single dose plus doxycycline.

Pharyngeal gonorrhea due to non-penicillinase-producing strains of N. gonorrhoeae.
250 mg as a single IM dose.

Gonococcal infections in children.
Less than 45 kg: 125 mg given once. **Infants:** 25–50 mg/kg/day not

to exceed 125 mg IV or IM in a single daily dose for 7 days.

Gonococcal infection during pregnancy.
Adults: 250 mg as a single IM dose plus erythromycin.

Disseminated gonococcal infection.
Adults: 1 g IM or IV q 24 hr.

Gonococcal meningitis or endocarditis.
Adults: 1–2 g IV q 12 hr for 10–14 days (meningitis) or 4 weeks (endocarditis).

Gonococcal ophthalmia.
Adults and children over 20 kg: 1 g given as a single IM dose.

Acute pelvic inflammatory disease.
250 mg IM plus doxycycline or tetracycline.

Lyme disease.
IV: 2–4 g/day for 14 days. Dosage adjustment is not required for renal or hepatic impairment; however, monitor blood levels in dialysis clients.

RESPIRATORY CARE CONSIDERATIONS

See also *General Respiratory Care Considerations for All Anti-Infectives* and *Cephalosporins.*

Administration/Storage
1. IM injections should be deep into the body of a large muscle.
2. IV infusions should contain concentrations of 10–40 mg/mL. Reconstitute 500 mg in 4.8 mL of sterile water, NSS, or D5W. Then further dilute in 50–100 mL D5W or NSS and infuse over 30–60 min.
3. The drug should not be mixed with other antibiotics.
4. Stability of solutions for IM or IV use varies depending on the diluent used; the package insert should be checked carefully.
5. Dosage should be maintained for at least 2 days after symptoms of infection have disappeared (usual course of therapy is 4–14 days, although complicated infections may require longer therapy).
6. Dosage should be continued for at

least 10 days when treating *Strepto-coccus pyogenes* infections.

Assessment

1. Note if client has any history of GI disease, especially colitis, because drug should be used cautiously in this setting.

2. Note any previous reaction to PCNs.

3. Obtain baseline coagulation studies and monitor as drug may alter PTs. May administer vitamin K (10 mg/week) prophylactically if bleeding occurs.

4. Document indications for therapy and include pretreatment findings.

Evaluate

• Resolution of S&S of infection

• Negative lab culture reports

Cefuroxime axetil

(sef-your-**OX**-eem)
Pregnancy Category: B
Ceftin **(Rx)**

Cefuroxime sodium

(sef-your-**OX**-eem)
Pregnancy Category: B
Kefurox, Zinacef **(Rx)**
Classification: Cephalosporin, second-generation

See also *Anti-Infectives* and *Cephalosporins*.

Action/Kinetics: Cefuroxime axetil is used PO, whereas cefuroxime sodium is used either IM or IV. **IM, IV:** t½, 1–2 hr; 66%–100% is excreted unchanged in the urine. The half-life will be prolonged in clients with renal failure.

Uses: PO (axetil). Pharyngitis, tonsillitis, otitis media, sinusitis, acute bacterial exacerbations of chronic bronchitis and secondary bacterial infections of acute bronchitis, uncomplicated UTIs, uncomplicated skin and skin structure infections, uncomplicated gonorrhea (urethral and endocervical) caused by non-penicillinase-producing strains of *Neisseria gonorrhoeae*. The suspension is indicated for children from 3 months to 12 years to treat pharyngi-

tis, tonsillitis, acute bacterial otitis media, and impetigo.

IM, IV (sodium). Infections of the urinary tract, lower respiratory tract (including pneumonia), skin and skin structures, bones, and joints. Septicemia, meningitis, uncomplicated and disseminated gonococcal infections due to penicillinase- or non-penicillinase-producing strains of *N. gonorrhoeae* in men and women. Mixed infections in which several organisms have been identified. Prophylaxis of postoperative infections in surgical procedures such as vaginal hysterectomy.

Additional Side Effects: Decrease in H&H.

Additional Laboratory Test Interference: False – reaction in the ferricyanide test for blood glucose.

Dosage ————————

• **Tablets (Cefuroxime Axetil)**

Pharyngitis, tonsillitis.

Adults and children over 13 years: 250 mg q 12 hr for 10 days. **Children:** 125 mg q 12 hr for 10 days.

Acute bacterial exacerbations of chronic bronchitis and secondary bacterial infections of acute bronchitis, uncomplicated skin and skin structure infections.

Adults and children over 13 years: 250 or 500 mg q 12 hr for 10 days.

Uncomplicated UTIs.

Adults and children over 13 years: 125 or 250 mg q 12 hr for 7–10 days. **Infants and children less than 12 years:** 125 mg b.i.d.

Acute otitis media.

Children: 250 mg b.i.d. for 10 days.

Uncomplicated gonorrhea.

Adults and children over 13 years: 1,000 mg as a single dose.

• **Suspension (Cefuroxime Axetil)**

Pharyngitis, tonsillitis.

Children, 3 months to 12 years: 20 mg/kg/day in 2 divided doses, not to exceed 500 mg total dose/day, for 10 days.

Acute otitis media, impetigo.
Children, 3 months to 12 years: 30 mg/kg/day in 2 divided doses, not to exceed 1,000 mg total dose/day, for 10 days.

- **IM, IV (Cefuroxime Sodium)**

Uncomplicated infections, including urinary tract, pneumonia, disseminated gonococcal, skin and skin structure.
Adults: 750 mg q 8 hr. **Pediatric, over 3 months:** 50–100 mg/kg/day in divided doses q 6–8 hr (not to exceed adult dose for severe infections).

Severe or complicated infections; bone and joint infections.
Adults: 1.5 g q 8 hr. **Pediatric, over 3 months:** b*one and joint infections,* **IV:** 150 mg/kg/day in divided doses q 8 hr (not to exceed adult dose).

Life-threatening infections or those due to less susceptible organisms.
Adults: 1.5 g q 6 hr.

Bacterial meningitis.
Adults: Up to 3 g q 8 hr. **Pediatric, over 3 months, initial, IV:** 200–240 mg/kg/day in divided doses q 6–8 hr; **then,** after clinical improvement, 100 mg/kg/day.

Gonorrhea (uncomplicated).
1.5 g as a single IM dose given at two different sites together with 1 g PO probenecid.

Prophylaxis in surgery.
Adults, IV: 1.5 g 30–60 min before surgery; if procedure is of long duration, **IM, IV,** 0.75 g q 8 hr.

Open heart surgery, prophylaxis.
IV: 1.5 g when anesthesia is initiated; **then,** 1.5 g q 12 hr for a total of 6 g.

RESPIRATORY CARE CONSIDERATIONS

See also *General Respiratory Care Considerations for All Anti-Infectives* and *Cephalosporins.*

Administration/Storage

1. Use IV route for severe or life-threatening infections such as septicemia or in poor-risk clients, especially in presence of shock.
2. For direct IV, reconstitute 750 mg with 8 mL sterile water and give over 3–5 min. For intermittent IV administration, further dilute in 100 mL of dextrose or saline solution and infuse over 30 min.
3. For direct intermittent IV administration, slowly inject the drug over 3 to 5 min, or give it through the tubing through which the client receives other IV solutions. For intermittent IV infusion with a Y-type administration set, the dose can be given through the tubing through which the client is receiving other medications; however, during drug infusion, administration of other solutions should be discontinued. For continuous IV infusion, the drug may be added to 0.9% sodium chloride injection, 5% or 10% dextrose injection, 5% dextrose and 0.45% or 0.9% sodium chloride injection, and M/6 sodium lactate injection.
4. Cefuroxime sodium should not be added to solutions of aminoglycosides; if both drugs are required, each should be given separately to the client.
5. For IM use, inject deep into a large muscle mass.
6. Prior to reconstitution, protect the drug from light. The powder and reconstituted drug may darken without affecting potency.
7. Cefuroxime axetil for PO use is available in tablet and suspension forms. Tablets should be swallowed whole and not crushed, as the crushed tablet has a strong, bitter, persistent taste.
8. To reconstitute the suspension, loosen the powder by shaking the bottle. Add the appropriate amount of water (depending on bottle size). Invert the bottle and shake vigorously.
9. The suspension must be given with food.
10. The tablet and suspension are not bioequivalent and are not substitutable on a milligram-per-milligram basis.
11. Therapy should be continued for at least 10 days in infections due to *Streptococcus pyogenes.*
12. Dosage in adults and children should be reduced in impaired renal function.

Assessment:

1. Document indications for therapy and note baseline assessments.

2. Assess for any clinical and lab evidence of anemia and renal dysfunction. Anticipate reduced dosage with impaired renal function.

Evaluate

- Resolution of S&S of infection
- Normal H&H
- Infection prophylaxis during surgery

Cephalexin hydrochloride monohydrate

(sef-ah-**LEX**-in)
Pregnancy Category: B
Keftab **(Rx)**

Cephalexin monohydrate

(sef-ah-**LEX**-in)
Pregnancy Category: B
Apo-Cephalex ✦, Biocef, Keflex, Novo–Lexin ✦, Nu-Cephalex ✦ **(Rx)**
Classification: Cephalosporin, first-generation

See also *Anti-Infectives* and *Cephalosporins.*

Action/Kinetics: Peak serum levels: PO, 9–39 mcg/mL after 1 hr. **t½, PO:** 30–72 min. Absorption delayed in children. The HCl monohydrate does not require conversion in the stomach before absorption. Ninety percent of drug excreted unchanged in urine within 8 hr.

Uses: Respiratory tract infections caused by *Streptococcus pneumoniae* and group A β-hemolytic streptococci. Otitis media due to *S. pneumoniae, Hemophilus influenzae, Moraxella catarrhalis* (use monohydrate only), staphylococci, and streptococci. Genitourinary tract infections (including acute prostatitis) due to *Escherichia coli, Proteus mirabilis,* and *Klebsiella.* Bone infections caused by *P. mirabilis* and staphylococci. Skin and skin structure infections due to staphylococci and streptococci.

Special Concerns: Safety and effectiveness of the HCl monohydrate have not been determined in children.

Additional Side Effects: Nephrotoxicity, cholestatic jaundice.

Dosage ——————

- **Capsules, Oral Suspension, Tablets**

General infections.

Adults, usual: 250 mg q 6 hr up to 4 g/day. **Pediatric:** *Monohydrate,* 25–50 mg/kg/day in four equally divided doses.

Infections of skin and skin structures, streptococcal pharyngitis, uncomplicated cystitis, over 15 years.

Adults: 500 mg q 12 hr. Large doses may be needed for severe infections or for less susceptible organisms. For streptococcal pharyngitis in children over 1 year and for skin and skin structure infections, the total daily dose should be divided and given q 12 hr. In severe infections, the dose should be doubled.

Otitis media.

Pediatric: 75–100 mg/kg/day in four divided doses.

RESPIRATORY CARE CONSIDERATIONS

See also *General Respiratory Care Considerations for All Anti-Infectives* and *Cephalosporins.*

Administration/Storage

1. After reconstitution, the drug should be refrigerated and the unused portion discarded after 14 days.

2. If the total daily dose is more than 4 g, parenteral drug therapy should be undertaken.

3. Treatment should be continued for at least 10 days for beta-hemolytic streptococcal infections.

4. Dosage may have to be reduced in clients with impaired renal function or increased for severe infections. Action of drug can be prolonged by the concurrent administration of PO probenecid.

Evaluate

- Resolution of infection

• Reports of symptomatic improvement

Cephalothin sodium
(sef-**AL**-oh-thin)
Pregnancy Category: B
Keflin ✤, Keflin Neutral **(Rx)**
Classification: Cephalosporin, first-generation

See also *Anti-Infectives* and *Cephalosporins*.
Action/Kinetics: Poorly absorbed from GI tract; must be given parenterally. **Peak serum levels: IM,** 6–21 mcg/mL after 30 min. **t½, IM, IV:** 30–60 min. Fifty-five percent to 90% excreted unchanged in urine. Its low nephrotoxicity, ototoxicity, and neurotoxicity make the drug suitable for clients with impaired renal function.
Uses: Infections of the GU tract, GI tract, respiratory tract, skin, soft tissues, bones, and joints. Meningitis, septicemia (including endocarditis), and prophylaxis in surgery.
Additional Side Effects: Nephrotoxicity, severe phlebitis, hemolytic anemia, increased PT.
Laboratory Test Interferences: Large doses may produce false + results in urinary protein tests that use sulfosalicylic acid.

Dosage
• **Deep IM, IV**
  General infections.
Adults, usual: 0.5–1 g q 4–6 hr. **Pediatric:** 80–160 mg/kg/day in divided doses.
  UTIs, uncomplicated pneumonia, furunculosis with cellulitis.
Adults: 0.5 g q 6 hr (for severe infections increase the dose to 1 g or give 0.5 g q 4 hr).
  Life-threatening infections.
Adults: 2 g q 4 hr (up to 12 g/day for bacteremia, septicemia).
  Preoperative and during surgery.
Adults: 1–2 g 30–60 min prior to surgery and during surgery. **Pediatric:** *Prophylaxis in surgery:* 20–30 mg/kg using adult schedule.
  Postoperative.
Adults: 1–2 g q 6 hr for 24 hr.
  Impaired renal function.

Initial: 1–2 g; **then,** use manufacturer's guidelines for maintenance doses.

RESPIRATORY CARE CONSIDERATIONS

See also *General Respiratory Care Considerations for All Anti-Infectives* and *Cephalosporins*.
Administration/Storage
1. Dilute according to directions on package insert. For direct IV administration, dilute 1 g in 10 mL of solution and infuse over 3–5 min. For intermittent IV administration further dilute 1 g in 50 mL of dextrose or saline solution and infuse over 15–30 min.
2. Discard reconstituted solution after 12 hr at room temperature and after 96 hr when refrigerated.
3. Dissolve precipitate by warming vial in hand and shaking. Do not overheat.
4. For prolonged IV infusion, the medication should be replaced with a freshly prepared solution every 24 hr to ensure stability.
5. For direct IV administration, add a small needle into larger veins.
6. Alter dose and follow manufacturer's guidelines for clients with impaired renal function.
Assessment
1. Monitor PT and assess for bleeding. May administer vitamin K (10 mg/week) if bleeding occurs.
2. Monitor I&O and renal function studies; assess for any allergic reactions.
Evaluate
• Resolution of infection
• Infection prophylaxis during surgery

Cephapirin sodium
(sef-ah-**PIE**-rin)
Pregnancy Category: B
Cefadyl **(Rx)**
Classification: Cephalosporin, first-generation

See also *Anti-Infectives* and *Cephalosporins*.

Action/Kinetics: Peak serum levels: IM, 9.4 mcg/mL after 30 min. **t½, IM, IV:** 21–47 min. Virtually entirely excreted in the urine within 6 hr, with 41%–60% excreted unchanged.

Uses: Infections of the respiratory tract, urinary tract, skin, and skin structures. Septicemia, endocarditis, osteomyelitis, prophylaxis in surgery.

Special Concerns: Before use in children less than 3 months, assess benefits versus risks.

Additional Side Effects: Increase in serum bilirubin.

Dosage ⸻

- **IM, IV only**
  General infections.
  Adults: 0.5–1 g q 4–6 hr up to 12 g/day for serious or life-threatening infections.
  Preoperatively.
  Adults: 1–2 g 30–60 min before surgery.
  During surgery.
  Adults: 1–2 g.
  Postoperatively.
  Adults: 1–2 g q 6 hr for 24 hr. **Pediatric, over 3 months:** 40–80 mg/kg/day in four equally divided doses.

  In clients with impaired renal function, a dose of 7.5–15 mg/kg q 12 hr may be adequate.

RESPIRATORY CARE CONSIDERATIONS

See also *General Respiratory Care Considerations for All Anti-Infectives* and *Cephalosporins*.

Administration/Storage
1. For direct IV administration reconstitute 1 g in 10 mL of solution and infuse over 3–5 min. For intermittent infusions, further dilute in 50–100 mL of solution and infuse over 15–20 min.
2. Discard after 12 hr when kept at room temperature and after 10 days when refrigerated at 4°C (39°F).
3. Concurrent administration with probenecid may inhibit excretion of cephapirin.

Assessment
1. Note any previous reactions to antibiotics.
2. Anticipate reduced dose with impaired renal function.

Evaluate
- Resolution of infection
- Infection prophylaxis during surgery

Cephradine
(**SEF**-rah-deen)
Pregnancy Category: B
Anspor, Velosef **(Rx)**
Classification: Cephalosporin, first-generation

See also *Anti-Infectives* and *Cephalosporins*.

Action/Kinetics: Similar to that of cephalexin. Rapidly absorbed from GI tract or IM injection site (30 min–2 hr); 60%–90% excreted after 6 hr. **Peak serum levels: PO,** 8–24 mcg/mL after 30–60 min; **IM,** 5.6–13.6 mcg/mL after 1–2 hr. **t½:** 42–120 min; 80%–95% excreted in urine unchanged.

Uses: Infections of the respiratory tract (including lobar pneumonia, tonsillitis, pharyngitis), urinary tract (including prostatitis and enterococcal infections), skin, skin structures, and bone. Otitis media, septicemia, prophylaxis in surgery, following cesarean section to prevent infection. In severe infections, therapy is usually initiated parenterally.

Special Concerns: Safe use during pregnancy has not been established. Safe use of the parenteral form in infants under 1 month of age and the PO form in children less than 9 months of age have not been established.

Additional Laboratory Test Interference: False + reactions using sulfosalicylic acid for urinary protein tests. High concentrations may interfere with measurement of creatinine by the Jaffe method.

Dosage ⸻
- **Capsules, Oral Suspension**

Skin and skin structures, respiratory tract infections.
Adults, usual: 250 mg q 6 hr or 500 mg q 12 hr.

Lobar pneumonia.
Adults: 500 mg q 6 hr or 1 g q 12 hr.

Uncomplicated UTIs.
Adults, usual: 500 mg q 12 hr.

More serious infections and prostatitis.
500 mg q 6 hr or 1 g q 12 hr (severe, chronic infections may require up to 1 g q 6 hr).

Pediatric, over 9 months: 25–50 mg/kg/day in equally divided doses q 6–12 hr (75–100 mg/kg/day for otitis media).

• **Deep IM, IV**
General infections.
Adults: 2–4 g/day in equally divided doses q.i.d.

Surgical prophylaxis.
Adults: 1 g 30–90 min before surgery; **then,** 1 g q 4–6 hr for one to two doses (or up to 24 hr postoperatively).

Cesarean section, prophylaxis.
IV: 1 g when the umbilical cord is clamped; **then,** give two additional 1-g doses **IV or IM** 6 and 12 hr after the initial dose. **Pediatric, over 1 year:** 50–100 mg/kg/day in equally divided doses q.i.d.

RESPIRATORY CARE CONSIDERATIONS

See also *General Respiratory Care Considerations for All Anti-Infectives* and *Cephalosporins.*

Administration/Storage
1. Dilute according to directions on package insert.
2. For direct IV administration dilute 1 g in 10 mL of D5%/W or NSS and infuse over 3–5 min. For intermittent infusions further reconstitute in 50–100 mL of dextrose or saline solution and infuse over 30–60 min. Discontinue other IV solutions during IV administration of cephalosporins.
3. Do not mix with lactated Ringer's solution.
4. Discard reconstituted solution after 10 hr at room temperature and after 48 hr when refrigerated at 5°C.

5. A slightly yellow solution may be retained for use; if unsure of solution potency, consult with pharmacist.
6. Be especially careful to inject into muscle, because sterile abscesses from accidental SC injection have occurred.
7. Before and after reconstitution, protect from excessive heat and light.
8. To ensure stability, replace medication infusion solution during prolonged IV administration q 10 hr.
9. Administer PO medication without regard to meals.
10. Rotate and document injection sites carefully.

Assessment
1. Note any previous reaction to PCN.
2. Anticipate reduced dose in clients with impaired renal function.

Evaluate
• Resolution of S&S of infection
• Infection prophylaxis in surgery
• Negative lab culture reports

Cetirizine hydrochloride
(seh-**TIH**-rah-zeen)
Pregnancy Category: B
Zyrtec **(Rx)**
Classification: Antihistamine

See also *Antihistamines,*

Action/Kinetics: Cetirizine is a potent H$_1$-receptor antagonist. The drug has a mild bronchodilator effect and protects against histmine-induced bronchospasm. Cetirizine has negligible anticholinergic and antiserotonergic activity. It is rapidly absorbed after PO administration; however, food delays the time to peak serum levels but does not decrease the total amount of drug absorbed. It penetrates poorly to the CNS, but high levels are distributed to the skin. **t½:** 8 hr (longer in elderly clients and in those with impaired liver or renal function). Cetirizine is excreted mostly unchanged (70%) in the urine; 10% is excreted in the feces.

Uses: Adults and children over 12 years of age for relief of symptoms associated with seasonal allergic rhinitis due to ragweed, grass, and tree pollens; perennial allergic rhinitis due to allergens such as dust mites, animal dander, and molds; and chronic idiopathic urticaria.

Contraindications: Lactation.

Special Concerns: Due to the possibility of sedation, use with caution in situations requiring mental alertness. Safety and efficacy have not been determined in children less than 12 years of age.

Side Effects: See *Antihistamines*. The most common side effects are somnolence, dry mouth, fatigue, pharyngitis, and dizziness.

OD **Overdose Management:** *Symptoms*: Somnolence. *Treatment*: Treatment is symptomatic and supportive. Dialysis is not effective in removing the drug from the body.

Dosage
• **Tablets**
Seasonal or perennial allergic rhinitis, chronic urticaria.
Adults and children over 12 years of age, initial: Depending on the severity of the symptoms, 5 or 10 mg (most common initial dose) once daily. In clients with decreased renal function (creatinine clearance 11–31 mL/min), in hemodialysis clients (creatinine clearance less than 7 mL/min), and in those with impaired hepatic function, the dose is 5 mg once daily.

RESPIRATORY CARE CONSIDERATIONS

See also *Respiratory Care Considerations* for *Antihistamines*.

Administration/Storage
1. The drug may be given with or without food.
2. The time of administration may be varied depending on the needs of the client.

Assessment
1. Document indications for therapy, type, onset, and characteristics of symptoms, and triggers (if known).

2. Note any hypersensitivity to hydroxyzine.

Client/Family Teaching
1. Advise to use caution when performing activities that require mental alertness until drug effects realized, as drug may cause drowsiness.
2. Drug may cause dry mouth and fatigue; report any adverse effects that inhibit compliance with therapy.
3. Avoid alcohol or any other CNS depressants.
4. Review allergens that trigger symptoms, e.g., ragweed, dust mites, molds, animal dander, etc., and instruct in how to control and avoid contact.

Evaluate
• Relief of symptoms associated with seasonal and perennial allergic rhinitis
• ↓ Occurrence, duration, and severity of hives with significant reduction in pruritus

Chloral hydrate
(**KLOH**-ral **HY**-drayt)
Pregnancy Category: C
Aquachloral Supprettes, PMS-Chloral Hydrate ✦ **(C-IV) (Rx)**
Classification: Nonbenzodiazepine, nonbarbiturate sedative-hypnotic

Action/Kinetics: Chloral hydrate is metabolized to trichloroethanol, which is the active metabolite causing CNS depression. Chloral hydrate produces only slight hangover effects and is said not to affect REM sleep. High doses lead to severe CNS depression, as well as depression of respiratory and vasomotor centers (hypotension). Both psychologic and physical dependence develop. **Onset:** Within 30 min. **Duration:** 4–8 hr. **t½, trichloroethanol:** 7–10 hr. The drug is readily absorbed from the GI tract and is distributed to all tissues; it passes the placental barrier and appears in breast milk as well. Metabolites excreted by kidney.

Uses: Short-term hypnotic. Daytime sedative and sedation prior to EEG procedures. Preoperative sedative and postoperative as adjunct to analgesics. Prevent or reduce symptoms of alcohol withdrawal.

Contraindications: Marked hepatic or renal impairment, severe cardiac disease, lactation. Drugs should not be given PO to clients with esophagitis, gastritis, or gastric or duodenal ulcer.

Special Concerns: Use by nursing mothers may cause sedation in the infant. A decrease in dose may be necessary in geriatric clients due to age-related decrease in both hepatic and renal function.

Side Effects: *CNS:* Paradoxical paranoid reactions. Sudden withdrawal in dependent clients may result in "chloral delirium." ***Sudden intolerance to the drug following prolonged use may result in respiratory depression, hypotension, cardiac effects, and possibly death.*** *GI:* N&V, diarrhea, bad taste in mouth, gastritis, increased peristalsis. *GU:* Renal damage, decreased urine flow and uric acid excretion. *Miscellaneous:* Skin reactions, hepatic damage, allergic reactions, leukopenia, eosinophilia.

Chronic toxicity is treated by gradual withdrawal and rehabilitative measures such as those used in treatment of the chronic alcoholic. Poisoning by chloral hydrate resembles acute barbiturate intoxication; the same supportive treatment is indicated (see *Barbiturates*).

Drug Interactions
Anticoagulants, oral / ↑ Effect of anticoagulants by ↓ plasma protein binding
CNS depressants / Additive CNS depression; concomitant use may lead to drowsiness, lethargy, stupor, respiratory collapse, coma, or death
Furosemide (IV) / Concomitant use results in diaphoresis, tachycardia, hypertension, flushing

Laboratory Test Interferences: ↑ 17-Hydroxycorticosteroids. Interference with fluorescence tests for catecholamines and copper sulfate test for glucose.

Dosage —————————
• **Capsules, Syrup**
Daytime sedative.
Adults: 250 mg t.i.d. after meals.
Preoperative sedative.
Adults: 0.5–1.0 g 30 min before surgery.
Hypnotic.
Adults: 0.5–1 g 15–30 min before bedtime. **Pediatric:** 50 mg/kg (1.5 g/m²) at bedtime (up to 1 g may be given as a single dose).
Daytime sedative.
Pediatric: 8.3 mg/kg (250 mg/m²) up to a maximum of 500 mg t.i.d. after meals.
Premedication prior to EEG procedures.
Pediatric: 20–25 mg/kg.
• **Suppositories, Rectal**
Daytime sedative.
Adults: 325 mg t.i.d. **Pediatric:** 8.3 mg/kg (250 mg/m²) t.i.d.
Hypnotic.
Adults: 0.5–1 g at bedtime. **Pediatric:** 50 mg/kg (1.5 g/m²) at bedtime (up to 1 g as a single dose).

RESPIRATORY CARE CONSIDERATIONS
Administration/Storage
1. PO: give capsules after meals with a full glass of water. Give the syrup with half a glass of juice, water, or ginger ale.
2. PO syrups have an unpleasant taste, which can be reduced by chilling the syrup before administration.
3. Have emergency drugs and equipment available should the client require supportive, physiologic treatment of acute poisoning.
Assessment
1. Document indications for therapy and evaluate sleep habits and patterns.
2. Assess mental status and response to stimuli.
3. Note any history of cardiac disease, liver or renal dysfunction. Drug is metabolized to an alcohol component.
Interventions
1. Monitor level and pattern of alertness and compare with the premedication history.

2. Observe respiratory and cardiac responses. Document any evidence of vasomotor depression and dilatation of cutaneous blood vessels.

3. Periodically perform liver and renal function studies to determine any evidence of impairment.

4. Observe for psychologic and physical dependence and report if evident. Symptoms of dependence resemble those of acute alcoholism, but with more severe gastritis.

5. Offer measures to promote comfort and relaxation.

6. Protect from injury. Assist with ambulation, side rails up, call bell within reach, and night light.

7. Administer analgesics as needed for pain relief.

Evaluate
• Desired level of sedation
• Control of symptoms of alcohol withdrawal
• Improved sleep patterns

Chloramphenicol
(klor-am-**FEN**-ih-kohl)
Chloromycetin (Cream and Otic), Mychel, Pentamycetin ✿, PMS-Chloramphenicol **(Rx)**

Chloramphenicol ophthalmic
(klor-am-**FEN**-ih-kohl)
AK Chlor, Chloromycetin Ophthalmic, Chloroptic Ophthalmic, Chloroptic S.O.P. Ophthalmic, Diochloram ✿, Ophtho-Chloram ✿, Sopamycetin ✿ **(Rx)**

Chloramphenicol sodium succinate
(klor-am-**FEN**-ih-kohl)
Chloromycetin Sodium Succinate, Mychel-S **(Rx)**
Classification: Anti-infective

See also *Anti-Infectives.*
General Statement: This antibiotic was originally isolated from *Streptomyces venezuellae* and is now produced synthetically. The antibiotic can be extremely toxic (due to protein synthesis inhibition in rapidly proliferating cells, as in bone marrow) and should not be used for trivial infections.

Action/Kinetics: Chloramphenicol interferes with or inhibits protein synthesis in bacteria by binding to 50S ribosomal subunits. Therapeutic serum concentrations: *peak,* 10–20 mcg/mL; *trough:* 5–10 mcg/mL (less for neonates). **Peak serum concentration: IM,** 2 hr. **t½:** 4 hr. Drug is metabolized in the liver; 75%–90% of drug excreted in urine within 24 hr, as parent drug (8%–12%) and inactive metabolites. The drug is mostly bacteriostatic. Chloramphenicol is well absorbed from the GI tract and is distributed to all parts of the body, including CSF, pleural, and ascitic fluids; saliva; milk; and aqueous and vitreous humors.

Uses: *Not to be used for trivial infections, prophylaxis of bacterial infections, or to treat colds, flu, or throat infections.* **Systemic Use.** Treatment of choice for typhoid fever but not for typhoid carrier state. Serious infections caused by *Salmonella, Rickettsia, Chlamydia,* and lymphogranuloma-psittacosis group. Meningitis due to *Haemophilus influenzae.* Brain abscesses due to *Bacteroides fragilis.* Cystic fibrosis anti-infective. Meningococcal or pneumococcal meningitis. **Topical Use.** Otitis externa. Prophylaxis of infection in minor cuts, wounds, skin abrasions, burns; promote healing in superficial infections of the skin. **Ophthalmic Use.** Superficial ocular infections due to *Staphylococcus aureus; Streptococcus* species, including *S. pneumoniae; Escherichia coli, H. influenzae, H. aegyptius, H. ducreyi, Klebsiella* species, *Neisseria* species, *Enterobacter* species, *Moraxella* species, and *Vibrio* species. Chloramphenicol should be used only for serious ocular infections for which less dangerous drugs are either contraindicated or ineffective.

Contraindications: Hypersensitivity to chloramphenicol; pregnancy, especially near term and during labor; lactation. Avoid simultaneous administration of other drugs that may depress bone marrow. Ophthalmically in the presence of dendritic keratitis, vaccinia, varicella, mycobacterial or fungal eye infections, or following removal of a corneal foreign body. Topical products should not be used near or in the eye.

Special Concerns: Use with caution in clients with intermittent porphyria or G6PD deficiency. To avoid gray syndrome, use with caution and in reduced doses in premature and full-term infants. Ophthalmic ointments may retard corneal epithelial healing.

Side Effects: *Hematologic* (most serious): ***Aplastic anemia, hypoplastic anemia,*** thrombocytopenia, granulocytopenia, ***hemolytic anemia,*** pancytopenia, hemoglobinuria (paroxysmal nocturnal). *Hematologic studies should be undertaken before and every 2 days during therapy. GI:* N&V, diarrhea, glossitis, stomatitis, unpleasant taste, enterocolitis, pruritus ani. *Allergic:* Fever, angioedema, macular and vesicular rashes, urticaria, hemorrhages of the skin, intestine, bladder, mouth. ***Anaphylaxis.*** *CNS:* Headache, delirium, confusion, mental depression. *Neurologic:* Optic neuritis, peripheral neuritis. *Following topical use:* Burning, itching, irritation, redness of skin. Hypersensitive clients may exhibit ***angioneurotic edema,*** urticaria, vesicular and maculopapular dermatoses. *Miscellaneous:* Superinfection. Jaundice (rare). Herxheimer-like reactions when used for typhoid fever (may be due to release of bacterial endotoxins). ***Gray syndrome in infants:*** Rapid respiration, ashen gray color, failure to feed, abdominal distention with or without vomiting, progressive pallid cyanosis, vasomotor collapse, death. Can be reversed when drug is discontinued. *NOTE: Neonates should be observed closely, since the drug accumulates in the bloodstream and the infant is thus subject to greater hazards of toxicity.*

After ophthalmic use: Temporary blurring of vision, stinging, itching, burning, redness, irritation, swelling, decreased vision, persistent or worse pain.

Drug Interactions

Acetaminophen / ↑ Effect of chloramphenicol due to ↑ serum levels

Anticoagulants, oral / ↑ Effect of anticoagulants due to ↓ breakdown by liver

Antidiabetics, oral / ↑ Effect of antidiabetics due to ↓ breakdown by liver

Barbiturates / ↑ Effect of barbiturates due to ↓ breakdown by liver; also, ↓ serum levels of chloramphenicol

Chymotrypsin / Chloramphenicol will inhibit chymotrypsin

Cyclophosphamide / Delayed or ↓ activation of cyclophosphamide

Iron preparations / ↑ Serum iron levels

Penicillins / Either ↑ or ↓ effect when combined to treat certain microorganisms

Phenytoin / ↑ Effect of phenytoin due to ↓ breakdown by liver; also, chloramphenicol levels may be ↑ or ↓

Rifampin / ↓ Effect of chloramphenicol due to ↑ breakdown by liver

Vitamin B₁₂ / ↓ Response to vitamin B_{12} when treating pernicious anemia

Dosage ─────────────
• **IV: Chloramphenicol**

Adults: 50 mg/kg/day in four equally divided doses q 6 hr. Can be increased to 100 mg/kg/day in severe infections, but dosage should be reduced as soon as possible. **Neonates and children with immature metabolic function:** 25 mg/kg once daily in divided doses q 12 hr. **Neonates, less than 2 kg:** 25 mg/kg once daily. **Neonates, over 2 kg, over 7 days of age:** 50 mg/kg/day q 12 hr in divided doses. **Neonates, over 2 kg, from birth to 7 days of age:** 50 mg/kg once daily. **Children:** 50–75 mg/kg/day in divided doses q 6 hr (50–100 mg/kg/day in divided doses q 6 hr for meningitis). *NOTE:* Carefully follow dosage for premature and newborn infants less than 2 weeks of age because blood levels differ significantly from those of other age groups.

• **Chloramphenicol Sodium Succinate—IV Only**

Same dosage as chloramphenicol (see the preceding). Switch to **PO** as soon as possible.

• **Chloramphenicol Ophthalmic Ointment 1%**

0.5-in. ribbon placed in lower conjunctival sac q 3–4 hr for acute infections and b.i.d.–t.i.d. for mild to moderate infections.

• **Chloramphenicol Ophthalmic Solution 0.5%**

1–2 gtt in lower conjunctival sac 2–6 times/day (or more for acute infections).

• **Chloramphenicol Otic Solution 0.5%**

2–3 gtt in ear t.i.d.

• **Chloramphenicol   Topical Cream 1%**

Apply 1–4 times/day.

RESPIRATORY CARE CONSIDERATIONS

See also *General Respiratory Care Considerations for All Anti-Infectives.*

Administration/Storage

1. Administer IV as a 10% solution over at least a 60-sec interval. Reconstitute 1 g in 10 mL of water for injection or 5% dextrose injection. May further dilute in 50–100 mL of dextrose or saline solution and infuse over 30–60 min.

2. When used topically for skin infections, a sterile bandage may be used if necessary.

3. To instill in the eye, place the head back and place the medication in the conjunctival sac and close the eyes. Light finger pressure should be applied on the lacrimal sac for 1 min.

4. To avoid contamination, the tip of the ophthalmic products should not touch any surface.

5. Contact lenses should not be worn if treating bacterial conjunctivitis. If contact lenses are required, however, the lenses should not be inserted for at least 15 min after using any solutions that contain benzalkonium chloride (may be absorbed by the lens).

Assessment

1. Note any history of hypersensitivity to chloramphenicol or previous reaction to other agents.

2. Document indications for therapy, type, onset, and duration of symptoms, and any other agents prescribed.

3. If client is a nursing mother, transmission of the drug to breast milk can result in the infant receiving the drug as well. Infants have underdeveloped capacity to metabolize chloramphenicol.

4. Take a complete history. Clients who are diabetic and taking oral hypoglycemic agents may have to use insulin during treatment with chloramphenicol.

5. Chloramphenicol may produce a false positive reaction with Fehling's or Benedict's solutions, both of which contain copper sulfate. In diabetic clients, use Lab-Stix to test the urine or, if available, do finger sticks for enhanced accuracy of glucose determinations.

6. If client is concomitantly receiving drugs that cause bone marrow depression, use of chloramphenicol is contraindicated.

7. Be certain that baseline hematologic studies are completed before drug treatment begins.

8. Arrange for frequent hematologic studies to detect early signs of bone marrow depression. This may also develop weeks to months following drug therapy.

9. Anticipate reduced dosage in clients with impaired renal function and in newborn infants.

Interventions

1. Become familiar with drugs that enhance the effects of chloramphenicol and monitor closely for ev-

---

idence of severe toxicity in clients on concurrent therapy.

2. Client should receive the drug only as necessary; avoid repeated courses of therapy with chloramphenicol because the drug is highly toxic.

3. Monitor client for the development of any of the following:

• *Bone marrow depression* characterized by weakness, fatigue, sore throat, and bleeding; discontinuation of the drug may be indicated.

• *Optic neuritis* characterized by bilaterally reduced visual acuity, an indication to discontinue the drug immediately.

• *Peripheral neuritis* characterized by pain and disturbance of sensation, both of which are indications to discontinue the drug immediately.

• Development of *gray syndrome* in premature and newborn infants, characterized by rapid respiration, failure to feed, abdominal distention with or without vomiting, loose green stools, progressive cyanosis, and vasomotor collapse. Withhold drug and report if evident.

4. Assess for toxic and irritative effects, such as N&V, unpleasant taste, diarrhea, and perineal irritation following PO administration. Differentiation of drug-induced diarrhea from that caused by a superinfection is critical and may be accomplished by assessment and analysis of all presenting symptoms.

Evaluate
• Resolution of infection
• Therapeutic serum drug levels (peak 10–20 mcg/mL; trough 5–10 mcg/mL)

Chlorothiazide
(klor-oh-**THIGH**-ah-zyd)
Pregnancy Category: C
Diurigen, Diuril **(Rx)**

Chlorothiazide sodium
(klor-oh-**THIGH**-ah-zyd)
Pregnancy Category: C
Sodium Diuril **(Rx)**
Classification: Diuretic, thiazide type

See also *Diuretics, Thiazides.*

Action/Kinetics: Onset: 2 hr for PO, 15 min for IV; **Peak effect:** 4 hr for PO, 30 min for IV; **Duration:** 6–12 hr. **t½:** 45–120 min. Incompletely absorbed from the GI tract. Produces a greater diuretic effect if given in divided doses. Also found in Diupres.

Special Concerns: Geriatric clients may be more sensitive to the usual adult dose.

Additional Side Effects: Hypotension, renal failure, renal dysfunction, interstitial nephritis. Following IV use: Alopecia, hematuria, exfoliative dermatitis, toxic epidermal necrolysis, erythema multiforme, *Stevens-Johnson syndrome.*

Dosage ——————
• **Oral Suspension, Tablets, IV**
  Diuretic.
Adults: 0.5–2 g 1–2 times/day either PO or IV (reserved for clients unable to take PO medication or in emergencies). Some clients may respond to the drug given 3–5 days each week.
  Antihypertensive.
Adults, IV, PO: 0.5–1 g/day in one or more divided doses. **Pediatric, 6 months and older, PO:** 22 mg/kg/day (10 mg/lb/day) in two divided doses; **6 months and younger, PO:** 33 mg/kg/day (15 mg/lb/day) in two divided doses. Thus, children up to 2 years of age may be given 125–375 mg/day in two doses while children 2–12 years of age may be given 375 mg–1 g/day in two doses. IV use in children is not recommended.

RESPIRATORY CARE CONSIDERATIONS

See also *Respiratory Care Considerations* for *Diuretics, Thiazides,* and *Antihypertensive Agents.*

Administration/Storage

1. To obtain an isotonic solution for injection, add 18 mL sterile water for injection to 500 mg powder and administer over 5 min.

2. IV use is not recommended for children and should be reserved for

those adults unable to take medication PO or in emergency situations.

3. Unused reconstituted solutions should be discarded after 24 hr.

4. Simultaneous administration of whole blood or derivatives with chlorothiazide should be avoided.

5. The IV solution is compatible with sodium chloride or dextrose solutions.

6. Should not be given SC or IM.

Assessment

1. List drugs currently prescribed.

2. Note any sulfa allergy.

Evaluate

• ↓ BP

• Enhanced diuresis with ↓ edema

Chlorpheniramine maleate
(klor-fen-**EAR**-ah-meen)
Pregnancy Category: B
Syrup, Tablets, Chewable Tablets: Aller-Chlor, Chlo-Amine, Chlorate, Chlor-Niramine, Chlortab 4, Chlor-Trimeton, Chlor-Tripolon ✤, Genallerate, Pfeiffer's Allergy, Phenetron, Trymegen. **Extended-release Capsules, Extended-release Tablets:** Chlorspan-12, Chlortab 8, Chlor-Trimeton Repetabs, Chlor-Tripolon ✤, Phenetron Telachlor, Teldrin. **Injectables:** Chlor-100, Chlor-Pro, Chlor-Pro 10, Chlor-Trimeton (OTC and Rx)
Classification: Antihistamine, alkylamine type

See also *Antihistamines.*

Action/Kinetics: Sedation less pronounced. **t½:** 21–27 hr. **Time to peak effect:** 6 hr. **Duration:** 4–8 hr. **Additional Contraindications:** Not recommended for children under 6 years of age.

Special Concerns: Geriatric clients may be more sensitive to the adult dose. The parenteral route is not recommended for neonates.

Dosage

• **Syrup, Tablets, Chewable Tablets**

Adults: 4 mg q 6 hr as needed. **Pediatric, 6–11 years:** 2 mg q 4–6 hr, not to exceed 12 mg/day; **2–5 years:** 1 mg q 4–6 hr.

• **Extended-Release Capsules, Extended-Release Tablets**

Adults: 8–12 mg q 8–12 hr as needed; **pediatric, 12 years and older:** 8 mg q 12 hr as needed.

• **IM, IV, SC**

Adults: 5–40 mg as a single dose as needed, up to 40 mg/day; **pediatric, SC:** 0.0875 mg/kg (2.5 mg/m²) q 6 hr as needed.

RESPIRATORY CARE CONSIDERATIONS

See also *Respiratory Care Considerations* for *Antihistamines.*

Administration/Storage

1. If administered with food, the absorption of drug is delayed.

2. The injection containing 10 mg/mL may be administered IV, IM, or SC. To administer IV, use 10 mg/mL and give over 1 min.

3. The injection containing 100 mg/mL should only be administered IM or SC.

4. Expect the onset of action to occur within 15–30 min and to last 3–6 hr.

Evaluate: ↓ Nasal congestion and associated allergic manifestations

---

Chlorthalidone
(klor-**THAL**-ih-dohn)
Pregnancy Category: B
Apo-Chlorthalidone ✤, Novo-Thalidone ✤, Hygroton, Thalitone, Uridon ✤ **(Rx)**
Classification: Diuretic, thiazide

See also *Diuretics, Thiazides.*

Action/Kinetics: Onset: 2–3 hr. **Peak effect:** 2–6 hr. **Duration:** 24–72 hr. **t½:** 40 hr. Bioavailability may be dose-dependent.

Additional Use: Particularly good for potentiating and reducing dosage of other antihypertensive agents.

Special Concerns: Geriatric clients may be more sensitive to the usual adult dose.

Additional Side Effects: Exfoliative dermatitis, toxic epidermal necrosis.

Dosage
- **Tablets**

Edema.

Adults, initial: 50–100 mg/day (30–60 mg Thalitone) or 100–200 mg (60 mg Thalitone) on alternate days. Some clients require 150 or 200 mg (90–120 mg Thalitone). **Maximum daily dose:** 200 mg (120 mg Thalitone). **Pediatric:** All uses, 2 mg/kg (60 mg/m²) 3 times/week.

Hypertension.

Adults, initial: Single dose of 25 mg (15 mg Thalitone); if response is not sufficient, dose may be increased to 50 mg (30 mg Thalitone). For additional control, increase the dose to 100 mg/day (except Thalitone) or a second antihypertensive drug may be added to the regimen. **Maintenance:** Determined by client response.*NOTE:* Doses greater than 25 mg/day are likely to increase potassium excretion but not cause further benefit in sodium excretion or BP reduction.

RESPIRATORY CARE CONSIDERATIONS

See Respiratory Care Considerations for Diuretics, Thiazides, , and Antihypertensive Agents..

Administration/Storage

1. Administer in the morning with food.

2. Dosage should be initiated with the lowest possible dose. Maintenance doses may be lower than initial doses.

3. Doses higher than 25 mg/day will increase potassium excretion but will not cause further benefit in sodium excretion or reduction of BP.

Assessment

1. Note indications for therapy, other agents trialed, and the outcome.

2. Obtain baseline CBC, electrolytes, glucose, BUN, and creatinine and monitor.

Evaluate

- Enhanced diuresis
- ↓ Edema
- ↓ BP

Ciprofloxacin hydrochloride

(sip-row-**FLOX**-ah-sin)
Pregnancy Category: C
Ciloxan Ophthalmic, Cipro, Cipro Cystitis Pack, Cipro I.V. **(Rx)**
Classification: Fluoroquinolone anti-infective

See also *Fluoroquinolones.*

Action/Kinetics: Ciprofloxacin is effective against both gram-positive and gram-negative organisms. Rapidly and well absorbed following PO administration. Food delays absorption of the drug. **Maximum serum levels:** 2–4 mcg/mL 1–2 hr after dosing. **t½:** 4 hr for PO use and 5–6 hr for IV use. Peak serum levels above 5 mcg/mL should be avoided. About 40%–50% of a PO dose and 50%–70% of an IV dose is excreted unchanged in the urine.

Uses: Systemic. UTIs caused by *Escherichia coli, Enterobacter cloacae, Citrobacter diversus, Citrobacter freundii, Klebsiella pneumoniae, Proteus mirabilis, Providencia rettgeri, Pseudomonas aeruginosa, Morganella morganii, Serratia marcescens, Serratia epidermidis,* and *Streptococcus faecalis.* Uncomplicated cervical and urethral gonorrhea due to *Neisseria gonorrhoeae.* Chancroid due to *Haemophilus ducreyi*; uncomplicated or disseminated gonococcal infections.

Lower respiratory tract infections caused by *E. coli, E. cloacae, K. pneumoniae, P. mirabilis, P. aeruginosa, Haemophilus influenzae, H. parainfluenzae,* and *Streptococcus pneumoniae.*

Bone and joint infections due to *E. cloacae, P. aeruginosa,* and *S. marcescens.*

Skin and skin structure infections caused by *E. coli, E. cloacae, Citrobacter freundii, M. morganii, K. pneumoniae, P. aeruginosa, P. mirabilis, Proteus vulgaris, Providencia stuartii, Staphylococcus pyogenes, Staphylococcus epidermidis,* and penicillinase- and non-penicillinase-producing strains of *Staphylococcus aureus.*

Infectious diarrhea caused by enterotoxigenic strains of *E. coli.* Also, *Campylobacter jejuni, Shigella flexneri,* and *Shigella sonnei.*

Typhoid fever (enteric fever) due to *Salmonella typhi.* Efficacy in eradicating the chronic typhoid carrier state has not been shown.

Investigational: Clients, over 14 years of age, with cystic fibrosis who have pulmonary exacerbations due to susceptible microorganisms. Malignant external otitis. In combination with rifampin and other tuberculostatics for tuberculosis.

Ophthalmic. Superficial ocular infections due to *Staphylococcus* species (including *S. aureus*), *Streptococcus* species (including *S. pneumoniae, S. pyogenes*), *E. coli, H. ducreyi, H. influenzae, H. parainfluenzae, K. pneumoniae, N. gonorrhoeae, Proteus* species, *Klebsiella* species, *Acinetobacter calcoaceticus, Enterobacter aerogenes, P. aeruginosa, S. marcescens, Chlamydia trachomatis, Vibrio* species, and *Providencia* species.

Contraindications: Hypersensitivity to quinolones. Use in children. During lactation, consideration should be given either to discontinuing nursing or the drug. Ophthalmic use in the presence of dendritic keratitis, varicella, vaccinia, and mycobacterial and fungal eye infections and after removal of foreign bodies from the cornea.

Special Concerns: Safety and effectiveness of ophthalmic, PO, or IV use has not been determined in children. Use with caution during lactation.

Additional Side Effects

See also *Side Effects* for *Fluoroquinolones.*

GI: N&V, abdominal pain/discomfort, diarrhea, dry/painful mouth, dyspepsia, heartburn, constipation, flatulence, pseudomembranous colitis, oral candidiasis, ***intestinal perforation,*** anorexia, GI bleeding, bad

taste in mouth. *CNS:* Headache, dizziness, fatigue, lethargy, malaise, drowsiness, restlessness, insomnia, nightmares, hallucinations, tremor, lightheadedness, irritability, confusion, ataxia, mania, weakness, psychotic reactions, depression, depersonalization, seizures. *GU:* Nephritis, hematuria, cylindruria, renal failure, urinary retention, polyuria, vaginitis, urethral bleeding, acidosis, renal calculi, interstitial nephritis, vaginal candidiasis. *Skin:* Urticaria, photosensitivity, hypersensitivity, flushing, erythema nodosum, cutaneous candidiasis, hyperpigmentation, rash, paresthesia, edema (of lips, neck, face, conjunctivae, hands), angioedema, toxic epidermal necrolysis, exfoliative dermatitis, ***Stevens-Johnson syndrome.*** *Ophthalmic:* Blurred or disturbed vision, double vision, eye pain, nystagmus. *CV:* Hypertension, syncope, angina pectoris, palpitations, atrial flutter, ***MI, cerebral thrombosis,*** ventricular ectopy, ***cardiopulmonary arrest,*** postural hypotension. *Respiratory:* Dyspnea, ***bronchospasm, pulmonary embolism, edema of larynx or lungs,*** hemoptysis, hiccoughs, epistaxis. *Hematologic:* Eosinophilia, pancytopenia, leukopenia, anemia, leukocytosis, ***agranulocytosis,*** bleeding diathesis. *Miscellaneous:* Superinfections; fever; chills; tinnitus; joint pain or stiffness; back, neck, or chest pain; flare-up of gout; flushing; worsening of myasthenia gravis; ***hepatic necrosis;*** cholestatic jaundice; hearing loss, dysphasia.

After ophthalmic use: Irritation, burning, itching, angioneurotic edema, urticaria, maculopapular and vesicular dermatitis, crusting of lid margins, conjunctival hyperemia, bad taste in mouth, corneal staining, keratitis, keratopathy, allergic reactions, photophobia, decreased vision, tearing, lid edema. Also, a white, crystalline precipitate in the superficial part of corneal defect (onset within 1–7 days after initiating therapy; lasts about 2 weeks and does not affect continued use of the medication).

Additional Drug Interactions
Azlocillin / ↓ Excretion of ciprofloxacin → possible ↑ effect
Caffeine / ↓ Excretion of caffeine → ↑ pharmacologic effects
Cyclosporine / ↑ Nephrotoxic effect of cyclosporine
Hydantoins / ↓ Phenytoin serum levels
Theophylline / Should not be taken with ciprofloxacin

Laboratory Test Interferences: ↑ ALT, AST, alkaline phosphatase, serum bilirubin, LDH, serum creatinine, BUN, serum gamma-glutamyltransferase, serum amylase, uric acid, blood monocytes, potassium, PT, triglycerides, cholesterol. ↓ H&H. Either ↑ or ↓ blood glucose, platelets.

Dosage ————
• **Tablets**
   UTIs.
250 mg (mild to moderate) to 500 mg (severe/complicated) q 12 hr for 7–14 days.
   Urethral or cervical gonococcal infections, uncomplicated.
250 mg in a single dose.
   Infectious diarrhea.
500 mg q 12 hr for 5–7 days.
   Skin, skin structures, lower respiratory tract, bone and joint infections.
500 mg (mild to moderate) to 750 mg (severe or complicated) q 12 hr for 7–14 days. Treatment may be required for 4–6 weeks in bone and joint infections.
   Typhoid fever.
500 mg (mild to moderate) q 12 hr for 10 days.
   Chancroid (H. ducreyi infection).
500 mg b.i.d. for 3 days.
   Disseminated gonococcal infections.
500 mg b.i.d. to complete a full week of therapy after initial treatment with ceftriaxone, 1 g IM or IV q 24 hr for 24–48 hr after improvement begins.
   Uncomplicated gonococcal infections.

500 mg in a single dose plus doxycycline.
   NOTE: Dose must be reduced in clients with a creatinine clearance less than 50 mL/min. The PO dose should be 250–500 mg q 12 hr if the C_{Cr} is 30–50 mL/min and 250–500 mg q 18 hr (IV: 200–400 mg q 18–24 hr) if the C_{Cr} is 5–29 mL/min. If the client is on hemodialysis or peritoneal dialysis, the PO dose should be 250–500 mg q 24 hr after dialysis.
• **Cipro Cystitis Pack**
   Uncomplicated UTI infections.
100 mg b.i.d. for 3 days. The pack contains six 100-mg tablets of ciprofloxacin and is intended to increase compliance.
• **IV Infusion**
   UTIs.
200 mg (mild to moderate) to 400 mg (severe or complicated) q 12 hr for 7–14 days.
   Skin, skin structures, respiratory tract, bone and joint infections.
400 mg (for mild to moderate infections) q 12 hr for 7–14 days.
• **Ophthalmic Solution**
   Acute infections.
Initial, 1–2 gtt q 15–30 min; **then,** reduce dosage as infection improves.
   Moderate infections.
1–2 gtt 4–6 (or more) times/day.

RESPIRATORY CARE CONSIDERATIONS

See also *Respiratory Care Considerations for All Anti-infectives* and *Fluoroquinolones.*

Administration/Storage
1. Although food delays the absorption of the drug, it may be taken with or without meals. The recommended time for dosing is 2 hr after a meal.
2. Clients on theophylline or probenecid require close observation and potential medication adjustments.
3. Do not administer to children.
4. Following instillation of the ophthalmic solution, light finger pressure should be applied to the lacrimal sac for 1 min.
5. The IV solution dose should be

reconstituted to 0.5–2 mg/mL and then given over a period of 60 min. To minimize discomfort and irritation, slowly infuse a dilute solution into a large vein.

6. The IV product can be diluted with 0.9% sodium chloride injection or 5% dextrose injection. Such dilutions are stable up to 14 days at refrigerated or room temperatures and should not be frozen.

7. Ciprofloxin in admixture is incompatible with aminophylline, amoxicillin sodium, amoxicillin sodium/potassium clavulanate, clindamycin, and mezlocillin.

Assessment

1. Note indications for therapy. Ensure that C&S obtained prior to use.

2. Determine age. Not for use in children under 18 as irreversible collagen destruction has been noted.

3. Note medications currently prescribed. Fatal reactions have been reported in clients receiving concurrent administration of IV ciprofloxacin and theophylline.

Evaluate

• Improvement in symptoms of infection as evidenced by ↓ fever, ↓ WBCs, ↑ appetite

• Negative lab culture reports

Cisatracurium besylate
(sis-ah-trah-**KYOU**-ree-um)
Pregnancy Category: B
Nimbex **(Rx)**
Classification: Neuromuscular blocking agent

See also *Neuromuscular Blocking Agents.*

Action/Kinetics: Cisatracurium is a nondepolarizing neuromuscular blocking agent. The drug binds competitively to cholinergic receptors on the motor end-plate, resulting in antagonism of the action of acetylcholine and therefore neuromuscular blockade. The neuromuscular blocking potency of cisatracurium is about three times greater than that for atracurium. Compared with other neuromuscular blocking agents, cisatracurium is considered to be both intermediate onset and duration. **Time to maximum blockade**: 2 min. **Time to recovery**: Approximately 55 min. Continuous infusion for up to 3 hr may be undertaken without tachyphylaxis or cumulative neuromuscular blockade. The time required for recovery following successive maintenance doses does not change with the number of doses given, provided that partial recovery is allowed to occur between doses. Onset, duration, and recovery are faster in children. About 95% of a dose is excreted as metabolites and unchanged drug (10%) in the urine and 4% is eliminated through the feces. Laudanosine, a major biologically active metabolite with no neuromuscular activity, may cause transient hypotension and cerebral excitatory effects (in high doses).

Uses: Neuromuscular blocking agent for in-patients and out-patients as an adjunct to general anesthesia, to facilitate tracheal intubation, and to cause skeletal muscle relaxation during surgery or mechanical ventilation in the intensive care unit.

Contraindications: Hypersensitivity to cisatracurium or other bis-benzylisoquinolinium agents or hypersensitivity to benzyl alcohol. Use for rapid-sequence ET intubation due to its intermediate onset of action.

Special Concerns: Since the drug has no effect on consciousness, pain threshold, or cerebration, administration should not be undertaken before unconsciousness. The drug may cause a profound effect in those with myasthenia gravis or the myasthenic syndrome. Burn clients may require higher doses. Onset time is faster (about 1 min) and recovery is slower (by about 1 min) in clients with impaired hepatic function. The time to maximum blockage is about 1 min slower in geriatric clients and in those with impaired renal function. Use with caution during lactation.

Safety and efficacy have not been determined in children less than 2 years of age.

Side Effects: Bradycardia, hypotension, flushing, bronchospasm, rash.

OD Overdose Management: *Symptoms:* Neuromuscular blockade beyond the time needed for surgery and anesthesia. *Treatment:* Maintain a patent airway and control ventilation until recovery of normal function is assured. Once recovery begins, the process may be facilitated by using neostigmine or edrophonium with an anticholinergic drug. These antidotes should not be given when complete blockade is evident.

Drug Interactions

Aminoglycosides / ↑ Effect of cisatracurium

Bacitracin / ↑ Effect of cisatracurium

Carbamazepine / Resistance to neuromuscular blockage → *slightly shorter duration.*

Clindamycin / ↑ Effect of cisatracurium

Colistin, sodium colistimethate / ↑ Effect of cisatracurium

Enflurane/nitrous oxide/oxygen / ↑ Duration of cisatracurium

Isoflurane/nitrous oxide/oxygen / ↑ Duration of cisatracurium

Lincomycin / ↑ Effect of cisatracurium

Lithium / ↑ Effect of cisatracurium

Local anesthetics / ↑ Effect of cisatracurium

Magnesium salts / ↑ Effect of cisatracurium

Phenobarbital / Resistance to neuromuscular blockade → slightly shorter duration

Polymyxins / ↑ Effect of cisatracurium

Procainamide / ↑ Effect of cisatracurium

Quinidine / ↑ Effect of cisatracurium

Succinylcholine / Time to onset of maximum block of cisatracurium is about 2 min faster

Tetracyclines / ↑ Effect of cisatracurium

Dosage ⎯⎯⎯⎯⎯⎯⎯⎯

• **IV Bolus**
  Neuromuscular blockade.

Adults, initial: Depending on the desired time to intubation and the anticipated length of surgery, either 0.15 or 0.2 mg/kg is used. These doses are components of a propofol/nitrous oxide/oxygen induction-intubation technique. **Maintenance during prolonged surgery:** 0.03 mg/kg given 40–50 min following an initial dose of 0.15 mg/kg and 50–60 min following an initial dose of 0.2 mg/kg.

Children, 2–12 years of age: 0.1 mg/kg over 5–10 sec during either halothane or opioid anesthesia. When given during stable opioid/nitrous oxide/oxygen anesthesia, 0.1 mg/kg produces maximum effects in about 2.8 min and a clinically effective blockade for 28 min.

• **IV Infusion**
  Neuromuscular blockade during extended surgery or use in the intensive care unit.

In the operating room or intensive care unit, following an initial bolus dose, a diluted solution can be given by continuous infusion to both adults and children over 2 years of age. The rate of administration is dependent on the response of the client determined by peripheral nerve stimulation. An infusion rate of 3 mcg/kg/min can be used to counteract rapid spontaneous recovery of neuromuscular blockade. Thereafter, an infusion rate of 1–2 mcg/kg/min is usually adequate to maintain blockade. The infusion rate should be reduced by 30%–40% when given during stable isoflurane or enflurane anesthesia.

RESPIRATORY CARE CONSIDERATIONS

See also *Respiratory Care Considerations* for *Neuromuscular Blocking Agents,*

Administration/Storage

1. Due to slower times of onset in geriatric clients and those with impaired renal function, the interval

between administration of the drug and intubation should be extended.

2. Spontaneous recovery following infusion will proceed at a rate comparable to that following administration of a bolus dose.

3. Cisatracurium is acidic; thus, it may not be compatible with alkaline solutions with a pH greater than 8.5 (e.g., barbiturate solutions).

4. Cisatracurium is compatible with 5% dextrose injection, 0.9% sodium chloride injection, 5% dextrose and 0.9% sodium chloride injection, sufentanil, alfentanil hydrochloride, fentanyl, midazolam hydrochloride, and droperidol. The drug is not compatible with propofol or ketorolac for Y-site administration.

5. Vials should be refrigerated at 2°C–8°C (36°F–46°F) and protected from light. Once removed from the refrigerator, vials should be used within 21 days, even if rerefrigerated.

6. Cisatracurium diluted in 5% dextrose injection, 0.9% sodium chloride injection, or 5% dextrose and 0.9% sodium chloride injection may be refrigerated or stored at room temperature for 24 hr without significant loss of potency. Dilutions to 0.1 or 0.2 mg/mL in 5% dextrose and lactated Ringer's injection may be refrigerated for 24 hr. Due to chemical instability, cisatracurium should not be diluted in lactated Ringer's injection.

Assessment

1. Document indications for therapy, other agents trialed, and anticipated duration of therapy.

2. Note any hypersensitivity to benzyl alcohol.

3. Obtain baseline neurologic assessment and note findings.

Interventions

1. Drug should only be administered by those trained in administration of neuromuscular blocking agents.

2. Client requires constant monitoring and respiratory support.

3. Medicate with analgesics for pain and agents for anxiety based on assessed need.

4. Utilize a peripheral nerve stimulator to evaluate response to therapy and to ensure partial recovery between doses.

Evaluate
- Facilitation of ET intubation
- Desired level of skeletal muscle relaxation

Clarithromycin
(klah-**rith**-roh-**MY**-sin)
Pregnancy Category: C
Biaxin **(Rx)**
Classification: Antibiotic, macrolide

See also *Anti-Infectives*.

Action/Kinetics: Clarithromycin is a macrolide antibiotic that acts by binding to the 50S ribosomal subunit of susceptible organisms, thus interfering with or inhibiting microbial protein synthesis. The drug is rapidly absorbed from the GI tract although food slightly delays the onset of absorption as well as the formation of the active metabolite but does not affect the extent of the bioavailability. **Peak serum levels:** When fasting, 2 hr for the tablet and 3 hr for the suspension. **Steady-state peak serum levels:** 1 mcg/mL within 2–3 days after 250 mg q 12 hr and 2–3 mcg/mL after 500 mg q 12 hr. Clarithromycin and 14-OH clarithromycin (active metabolite) are readily distributed to body tissues and fluids. **t½, elimination:** 3–7 hr (depending on the dose) for clarithromycin and 5–6 hr for 14-OH clarithromycin. Up to 30% of a dose is excreted unchanged in the urine.

Uses: Mild to moderate infections caused by susceptible strains of the following. **Adults.** Pharyngitis/tonsillitis due to *Streptococcus pyogenes.* Acute maxillary sinusitis or acute bacterial exacerbaton of chronic bronchitis due to *Sreptococcus pneumoniae, Haemophilus influenzae,* and *Moraxella catarrhalis.* Pneumonia due to *Mycoplasma pneumoniae* or *S. pneumoniae.* Uncomplicated skin and skin structure infections due to *Staphylococcus aureus* or *S.*

pyogenes. The active metabolite, 14-OH clarithromycin, has significant activity (twice the parent compound) against *H. influenzae.* Treatment of disseminated mycobacterial infections due to *Mycobacterium avium* (commonly seen in AIDS clients) and *M. intracellulare.* Prevention of disseminated *M. avium* complex in individuals with advanced HIV.

Used with omeprazole for the eradication of *Helicobacter pylori* infection in clients with active duodenal ulcers associated with *H. pylori* infection. Clarithromycin with ranitidine bismuth citrate (Tritec) is also used for this purpose.

Children. Pharyngitis or tonsillitis due to *S. pyogenes.* Acute maxillary sinusitis due to *S. pneumoniae, H. influenzae,* and *M. catarrhalis.* Acute otitis media due to *H. influenzae, M. catarrhalis, S. pneumoniae.* Uncomplicated skin and skin structure infections due to *S. aureus* or *S. pyogenes.* Disseminated mycobacterial infections due to *M. avium* or *M. intracellulare.* Prevention of disseminated *M. avium* complex disease in clients with advanced HIV infection. Community-acquired pneumonia caused by *M. pneumoniae, Chlamydia pneumoniae,* and *S. pneumoniae.*

Contraindications: Hypersensitivity to clarithromycin, other macrolide antibiotics, or erythromycin. Clients taking astemizole or terfenadine who have preexisting cardiac abnormalities (e.g., arrhythmias, bradycardia, QT interval prolongation, ischemic heart disease, CHF) or electrolyte disturbances.

Special Concerns: Use with caution in severe renal impairment with or without concomitant hepatic impairment and during lactation. Safety and effectiveness in children less than 6 months of age have not been determined.

Side Effects: *GI:* Diarrhea, nausea, abnormal taste, dyspepsia, abdominal discomfort or pain, pseudomembranous colitis, glossitis, stomatitis, oral moniliasis, vomiting. *CNS:* Headache, dizziness, behavioral changes, confusion, depersonaliza-

tion, disorientation, hallucinations, insomnia, nightmares, vertigo. *Allergic:* Urticaria, mild skin eruptions and, rarely, **anaphylaxis and Stevens-Johnson syndrome.** *Hepatic:* Hepatocellular cholestatic hepatitis with or without jaundice, increased liver enzymes, **hepatic failure.** *Miscellaneous:* Hearing loss (usually reversible), alteration of sense of smell (usually with taste perversion).

In children, the most common side effects are diarrhea, vomiting, abdominal pain, rash, and headache.

Drug Interactions

See also Drug Interactions for Erythromycins.

Anticoagulants / ↑ Anticoagulant effects

Astemizole / Combination not to be used in clients who have preexisting cardiac abnormalities or electrolyte disturbances

Carbamazepine / ↑ Blood levels of carbamazepine

Cisapride / Possibility of serious cardiac arrhythmias, including ventricular tachycardia, ventricular fibrillation, torsade de pointes, and QT prolongation

Cyclosporine ↑ Levels of cyclosporine → ↑ risk of nephrotoxicity and neurotoxicity

Digoxin / ↑ Plasma levels of digoxin due to ↓ metabolism of digoxin by the gut flora

Ergot alkaloids / Acute ergot toxicity, including severe peripheral vasospasm and dysesthesia

Tacrolimus / ↑ Plasma tacrolimus levels → ↑ risk of toxicity

Terfenadine / ↑ Plasma levels of the active acid metabolite of terfenadine; ↑ risk of cardiac arrhythmias, including QT interval prolongation

Theophylline / ↑ Serum levels of theophylline

Triazolam / ↑ Risk of somnolence and confusion

AZT / ↓ Steady-state AZT levels in HIV-infected clients; however, peak serum AZT levels may be ↑ or ↓

Laboratory Test Interferences: ↑ ALT, AST, GGT, alkaline phosphatase, LDH, total bilirubin, BUN, serum creatinine, PT. ↓ WBC count.

Dosage
- **Tablets, Oral Suspension**
  Pharyngitis, tonsillitis.
250 mg q 12 hr for 10 days.
  Lower respiratory tract infections.
250–500 mg q 12 hr for 7–14 days.
  Acute exacerbation of chronic bronchitis due to S. pneumoniae or M. catarrhalis; pneumonia due to S. pneumoniae or M. pneumoniae; skin and skin structure infections.
250 mg q 12 hr for 7–14 days.
  Acute maxillary sinusitis, acute exacerbation of chronic bronchitis due to H. influenzae.
500 mg q 12 hr for 7–14 days.
  Disseminated M. avium complex or prophylaxis of M. avium complex.
Adults: 0.5 g b.i.d.; **children:** 7.5 mg/kg b.i.d. up to 500 mg b.i.d.
NOTE: The usual daily dose for children is 15 mg/kg q 12 hr for 10 days.
  Community-acquired pneumonia in children.
15 mg/kg/day of the suspension, divided and given q 12 hr for 10 days.
  Active duodenal ulcers associated with H. pylori *infection.*
Clarithromycin, 500 mg t.i.d., with omeprazole, 40 mg, each morning for 2 weeks. **Then,** omeprazole is given alone at a dose of 20 mg/day for 2 more weeks. Or, clarithromycin, 500 mg t.i.d., with ranitidine bismuth citrate, 400 mg b.i.d., for 2 weeks. **Then,** ranitidine bismuth citrate is given alone at a dose of 400 mg b.i.d. for 2 more weeks.

RESPIRATORY CARE CONSIDERATIONS

See also *Respiratory Care Considerations* for *Erythromycins.*
Administration/Storage
1. The drug may be given with or without meals and can be given with milk. However, food delays both the onset of absorption and the formation of 14-OH clarithromycin (the active metabolite).

2. Decreased doses or prolonging the dosing interval should be considered in clients with severe renal impairment with or without coexisting impaired hepatic function.
3. Drug may cause a bitter taste.
4. The reconstituted suspension should be shaken well before each use; it should be used within 14 days and should not be refrigerated. The suspension can be taken with milk.
Assessment
1. Note any sensitivity to erythromycin or any of the macrolide antibiotics.
2. Obtain baseline CBC *and* liver and renal function studies.
3. Determine that appropriate lab cultures are done prior to initiation of drug therapy.
4. List drugs client currently prescribed noting any potential interactions.
5. Document indications for therapy and note type, severity, onset, and duration of symptoms.
Interventions: Monitor I&O and observe client for any evidence of persistent diarrhea. Report if evident as an antibiotic-associated colitis may be precipitated by *C. difficile* and require alternative management.
Evaluate
- Clinical evidence and reports of symptomatic improvement
- Negative follow-up culture reports

Clindamycin hydrochloride hydrate
(klin-dah-**MY**-sin)
Cleocin Hydrochloride, Dalacin C ✽ **(Rx)**

Clindamycin palmitate hydrochloride
(klin-dah-**MY**-sin)
Cleocin Pediatric, Dalacin C Palmitate ✽ **(Rx)**

Clindamycin phosphate
(klin-dah-**MY**-sin)

Pregnancy Category: B (vaginal cream, topical gel, lotion, solution) Cleocin Vaginal Cream, Cleocin Phosphate, Cleocin T, Clinda-Derm, C/T/S, Dalacin C Phosphate ✦, Dalacin T Topical ✦, Dalacin Vaginal Cream ✦ **(Rx)**

Classification: Antibiotic, clindamycin and lincomycin

See also *Anti-Infectives.*

General Statement: Clindamycin is a semisynthetic antibiotic. Its spectrum resembles that of the erythromycins and includes a variety of gram-positive organisms, particularly staphylococci, streptococci, and pneumococci, and some gram-negative organisms. Should not be used for trivial infections.

Action/Kinetics: Suppresses protein synthesis by microorganism by binding to ribosomes (50S subunit) and preventing peptide bond formation. Is both bacteriostatic and bactericidal. **Peak serum concentration: PO,** 4 mcg/mL after 300 mg; **IM,** 4.9 mcg/mL after 300 mg; **IV,** 14.7 mcg/mL after 300 mg. **t½:** 2.4–3 hr. In serious infections the rate of IV administration is adjusted to maintain appropriate serum drug concentrations: 4–6 mcg/mL.

Uses: Systemic. Serious respiratory tract infections (e.g., empyema, lung abscess, pneumonia) caused by staphylococci, streptococci, and pneumococci. Serious skin and soft tissue infections, septicemia, intra-abdominal infections, pelvic inflammatory disease, female genital tract infections. May be the drug of choice for *Bacteroides fragilis.* In combination with aminoglycosides for mixed aerobic and anaerobic bacterial infections. Staphylococci-induced acute hematogenous osteomyelitis. Adjunct to surgery for chronic bone/joint infections. *Investigational:* Alternative to sulfonamides in combination with pyrimethamine in the acute treatment of CNS toxoplasmosis in AIDS clients. In combination with primaquine to treat *Pneumocystis carinii* pneumonia. Chlamydial infections in women. Bacterial vaginosis due to *Gardnerella vaginalis.* **Topical Use.** Used topically for inflammatory acne vulgaris. Vaginally to treat bacterial vaginosis. *Investigational:* Treatment of rosacea (lotion used).

Contraindications: Hypersensitivity to either clindamycin or lincomycin. Not for use in treating viral and minor bacterial infections. Use in clients with a history of regional enteritis, ulcerative colitis, or antibiotic-associated colitis. Lactation.

Special Concerns: Use with caution in infants up to 1 month of age. Use with caution in clients with GI disease, liver or renal disease, history of allergy or asthma. Safety and efficacy of topical products have not been established in children less than 12 years of age.

Side Effects: *GI:* N&V, diarrhea, bloody diarrhea, abdominal pain, GI disturbances, tenesmus, flatulence, bloating, anorexia, weight loss, esophagitis. Nonspecific colitis, pseudomembranous colitis (may be severe). *Allergic:* Morbilliform rash (most common). Also, maculopapular rash, urticaria, pruritus, fever, hypotension. Rarely, polyarteritis, anaphylaxis, erythema multiforme. *Hematologic:* Leukopenia, neutropenia, eosinophilia, thrombocytopenia, **agranulocytosis.** *Miscellaneous:* Superinfection. Also sore throat, fatigue, urinary frequency, headache.

Following IV use: Thrombophlebitis, erythema, pain, swelling. *Following IM use:* Pain, induration, sterile abscesses.

Following topical use: Erythema, irritation, dryness, peeling, itching, burning, oiliness of skin.

Following vaginal use: Cervicitis, vaginitis, vulvar irritation, urticaria, rash.

NOTE: The injection contains benzyl alcohol, which has been associated with *a fatal "gasping syndrome"* in infants.

Drug Interactions
Antiperistaltic antidiarrheals (opi-

ates, Lomotil) / ↑ Diarrhea due to ↓ removal of toxins from colon
Ciprofloxacin HCl / Additive antibacterial activity
Erythromycin / Cross-interference → ↓ effect of both drugs
Kaolin (e.g., Kaopectate) / ↓ Effect due to ↓ absorption from GI tract
Neuromuscular blocking agents / ↑ Effect of blocking agents
Laboratory Test Interferences: ↓ Levels of AST, ALT, NPN, alkaline phosphatase, bilirubin, BSP retention, and ↓ platelet count.

Dosage

• **PO only: Capsules, Oral Solution**
Adults: Clindamycin HCl, Clindamycin palmitate HCl: 150–450 mg q 6 hr, depending on severity of infection. **Pediatric: Clindamycin HCl hydrate:** 8–20 mg/kg/day divided into three to four equal doses; clindamycin palmitate HCl: 8–25 mg/kg/day divided into three to four equal doses. **Children less than 10 kg:** Minimum recommended dose is 37.5 mg t.i.d.

• **IV**
Clindamycin phosphate. Adults: 0.6–2.7 g/day in two to four equal doses depending on severity of infection.
Life-threatening infections.
4.8 g. **Pediatric over 1 month:** 15–40 mg/kg/day in three to four equal doses depending on severity of infections.
Severe infections.
No less than 300 mg/day, regardless of body weight.
Acute pelvic inflammatory disease.
IV: 600 mg q.i.d. plus gentamicin, 2 mg/kg IV; **then,** gentamicin, 1.5 mg/kg t.i.d. IV. IV therapy should be continued for 2 days after client improves. The 10–14-day treatment cycle should be completed using clindamycin, **PO:** 450 mg q.i.d.

• **Topical Gel, Lotion, or Solution**

Apply thin film b.i.d. to affected areas. One or more pledgets may also be used.

• **Vaginal Cream (2%)**
One applicatorful (containing about 100 mg clindamycin phosphate), preferably at bedtime, for 7 consecutive days.

RESPIRATORY CARE CONSIDERATIONS

See also *General Respiratory Care Considerations for All Anti-Infectives.*

Administration/Storage

1. Give parenteral clindamycin only to hospitalized clients.
2. Dilute IV injections to maximum concentration of 12 mg/mL, with no more than 1,200 mg administered in 1 hr.
3. Single IM injections greater than 600 mg are not advisable. Inject deeply into muscle to prevent induration, pain, and sterile abscesses.
4. Do not refrigerate; otherwise, solution may become thickened.
5. Administer IV over a period of 20–60 min, depending on dose and therapeutic serum concentration to be attained.
6. Dosage should be reduced in severe renal impairment.
7. The lotion should be shaken well just before using.

Assessment

1. Take a complete history. Document indications for therapy and type and onset of symptoms.
2. Auscultate lungs and note extensiveness of respiratory tract infections.
3. Document presence and extent of serious skin and soft tissue infections, septicemia, and female genital tract infections.
4. List any client complaints indicative of pelvic inflammatory disease or intra-abdominal infections.
5. Note any history of liver or renal disease, allergies, or history of GI problems.
6. Obtain baseline liver and renal function studies.

Interventions

1. Be prepared to manage pseudomembranous colitis, which can occur 2–9 days or several weeks after initiation of therapy. Provide fluids, electrolytes, protein supplements, systemic corticosteroids, and oral antibiotics as prescribed.

2. Do not administer, and caution client against using, antiperistaltic agents if diarrhea occurs because these can prolong or aggravate the condition.

3. Do not administer kaolin concomitantly because this will reduce absorption of antibiotic. If kaolin is required, administer 3 hr before antibiotic.

4. Do not use any acne or topical mercury preparations containing a peeling agent in an area affected by medication because severe irritation may occur.

5. Administer on an empty stomach to ensure optimum absorption. Drug should be administered only as long as necessary.

6. During IV administration observe for hypotension and keep client in bed for 30 min following therapy. Advise that a bitter taste may also be evident.

7. Observe for drug interactions caused by concurrent administration of neuromuscular blocking agents. Be alert to hypotension, bronchospasms, cardiac disturbances, hyperthermia, and respiratory depression.

8. Observe closely for:
- Skin rash because this is the most frequently reported side effect
- Clients with renal and/or hepatic impairment and newborns for organ dysfunction
- GI disturbances, such as abdominal pain, diarrhea, anorexia, N&V, bloody or tarry stools, and excessive flatulence. Discontinuation of drug may be indicated.

Evaluate

- Resolution of infection
- Reports of symptomatic improvement
- Negative lab culture reports

- Therapeutic serum drug concentrations with IV therapy (4–6 mcg/mL)

Clonidine hydrochloride
(**KLOH**-nih-deen)

Pregnancy Category: C
Apo-Clonidine ✹; Catapres; Catapres-TTS-1, -2, and -3; Dixarit ✹; Novo-Clonidine ✹, Nu-Clonidine ✹ **(Rx)**

Classification: Antihypertensive, centrally acting antiadrenergic

See also *Antihypertensive Agents.*

Action/Kinetics: Stimulates alpha-adrenergic receptors of the CNS, which results in inhibition of the sympathetic vasomotor centers and decreased nerve impulses. Thus, bradycardia and a fall in both SBP and DBP occur. Plasma renin levels are decreased, while peripheral venous pressure remains unchanged. The drug has few orthostatic effects. Although sodium chloride excretion is markedly decreased, potassium excretion remains unchanged. Tolerance to the drug may develop. **Onset, PO:** 30–60 min; **transdermal:** 2–3 days. **Peak plasma levels, PO:** 3–5 hr; **transdermal:** 2–3 days. **Maximum effect, PO:** 2–4 hr. **Duration, PO:** 12–24 hr; **transdermal:** 7 days (with system in place). **t½:** 12–16 hr. Approximately 50% excreted unchanged in the urine; 20% excreted through the feces.

The transdermal dosage form contains the following levels of drug: Catapres-TTS-1 contains 2.5 mg clonidine (surface area 3.5 cm²), with 0.1 mg released daily; Catapres-TTS-2 contains 5 mg clonidine (surface area 7 cm²), with 0.2 mg released daily; and Catapres-TTS-3 contains 7.5 mg clonidine (surface area 10.5 cm²), with 0.3 mg released daily.

Uses: Mild to moderate hypertension. A diuretic or other antihypertensive drugs, or both, are often used concomitantly. *Investigational:* Diabetic diarrhea, alcohol withdrawal, treatment of Gilles de la Tourette syndrome, detoxification of opiate dependence, constitutional growth delay in children, hypertensive urgency (DBP greater than 120 mm Hg), menopausal flushing, diagnosis of pheochromocytoma, facilitate cessation of smoking, ulcerative colitis, postherpetic neuralgia, reduce allergen-induced inflammation in clients with extrinsic asthma.

Special Concerns: Use with caution in presence of severe coronary insufficiency, recent MI, cerebrovascular disease, or chronic renal failure. Use with caution during lactation. Safe use in children not established. Geriatric clients may be more sensitive to the hypotensive effects; a decreased dosage may also be necessary in these clients due to age-related decreases in renal function.

Side Effects: *CNS:* Drowsiness (common), sedation, dizziness, headache, fatigue, malaise, nightmares, nervousness, restlessness, anxiety, mental depression, increased dreaming, insomnia, hallucinations, delirium, agitation. *GI:* Dry mouth (common), constipation, anorexia, N&V, parotid pain, weight gain. *CV:* CHF, Raynaud's phenomenon, abnormalities in ECG, palpitations, tachycardia and bradycardia, orthostatic symptoms, conduction disturbances, sinus bradycardia. *Dermatologic:* Urticaria, skin rashes, *angioneurotic edema,* pruritus, thinning of hair, alopecia. *GU:* Impotence, urinary retention, decreased sexual activity, loss of libido, nocturia, difficulty in urination. *Musculoskeletal:* Muscle or joint pain, leg cramps, weakness. *Other:* Gynecomastia, increase in blood glucose (transient), increased sensitivity to alcohol, dryness of mucous membranes of nose; itching, burning, dryness of eyes; skin pallor, fever.

Transdermal products: Localized skin reactions, pruritus, erythema, allergic contact sensitization and contact dermatitis, localized vesiculation, hyperpigmentation, edema, excoriation, burning, papules, throb-

bing, blanching, generalized macular rash.

NOTE: Rebound hypertension may be manifested if clonidine is withdrawn abruptly.

OD **Overdose Management:** *Symptoms:* Hypotension, bradycardia, respiratory and CNS depression, hypoventilation, hypothermia, apnea, miosis, agitation, irritability, lethargy, *seizures, cardiac conduction defects, arrhythmias,* transient hypertension, diarrhea, vomiting. *Treatment:* Maintain oxygenation and ventilation; perform gastric lavage followed by activated charcoal. Magnesium sulfate may be used to hasten the rate of transport through the GI tract. IV atropine sulfate (0.6 mg for adults; 0.01 mg/kg for children), epinephrine, tolazoline, or dopamine to treat persistent bradycardia. IV fluids and elevation of the legs are used to reverse hypotension; if unresponsive to these measures, dopamine (2–20 mcg/kg/min) or tolazoline (1 mg/kg IV, up to a maximum of 10 mg/dose) may be used. To treat hypertension, diazoxide, IV furosemide, or an alpha-adrenergic blocking drug may be used.

Drug Interactions
Alcohol / ↑ Depressant effects
Beta-adrenergic blocking agents / Paradoxical hypertension; also, ↑ severity of rebound hypertension following clonidine withdrawal
CNS depressants / ↑ Depressant effect
Levodopa / ↓ Effect of levodopa
Tolazoline / Blocks antihypertensive effect
Tricyclic antidepressants / Blocks antihypertensive effect

Laboratory Test Interferences: Transient ↑ blood glucose and serum CPK. Weakly + Coombs' test. Alteration of electrolyte balance.

Dosage ——————————
• **Tablets**
  Hypertension.
Initial: 0.1 mg b.i.d.; **then,** increase by 0.1–0.2 mg/day until desired re-

sponse is attained; **maintenance:** 0.2–0.6 mg/day in divided doses (maximum: 2.4 mg/day). Tolerance necessitates increased dosage or concomitant administration of a diuretic. Gradual increase of dosage after initiation minimizes side effects.

NOTE: In hypertensive clients unable to take PO medication, clonidine may be administered sublingually at doses of 0.2–0.4 mg/day. **Pediatric:** 0.005–0.025 mg/kg/day (5–25 mcg/kg/day) in divided doses q 6 hr; increase dose at 5–7-day intervals.

Gilles de la Tourette syndrome.
0.15–0.2 mg/day.

Withdrawal from opiate dependence.
0.015–0.016 mg/kg/day (15–16 mcg/kg/day).

Alcohol withdrawal.
0.3–0.6 mg q 6 hr.

Diabetic diarrhea.
0.15–1.2 mg/day.

Constitutional growth delay in children.
0.0375–0.15 mg/m²/day.

Hypertensive urgency.
Initial: 0.1–0.2 mg; **then,** 0.05–0.1 mg q hr to a maximum of 0.8 mg.

Menopausal flushing.
0.1–0.4 mg.

Diagnosis of pheochromocytoma.
0.3 mg.

Postherpetic neuralgia.
0.2 mg/day.

Reduce allergen-induced inflammation in extrinsic asthma.
0.15 mg for 3 days.

Facilitate cessation of smoking.
0.15–0.4 mg/day or 0.2 mg/24 hr patch.

Ulcerative colitis.
0.3 mg t.i.d.

• **Transdermal**
Hypertension.
Initial: Use 0.1-mg system; **then,** if after 1–2 weeks adequate control has not been achieved, can use another 0.1-mg system or a larger system. The antihypertensive effect may not be seen for 2–3 days. The system should be changed q 7 days.

Diabetic diarrhea.

0.3 mg/24 hr patch.
Menopausal flushing.
0.1 mg/24 hr patch.
Facilitate cessation of smoking.
0.2 mg/24 hr patch.

RESPIRATORY CARE CONSIDERATIONS

See also *Respiratory Care Considerations* for *Antihypertensive Agents*.

Administration/Storage

1. If the transdermal system is used, apply the medication to a hairless area of skin, such as upper arm or torso changing the system q 7 days.

2. Use a different site with each application.

3. It may take 2–3 days to achieve effective blood levels using the transdermal system. Therefore, any prior drug dosage should be reduced gradually.

4. If the drug is to be taken PO, administer the last dose of the day at bedtime to ensure overnight control of BP.

5. Clients with severe hypertension may require other antihypertensive drug therapy in addition to transdermal clonidine.

6. If the drug is to be discontinued, it should be done gradually over a period of 2–4 days.

Assessment

1. Document indications for therapy, onset and type of symptoms, and previous treatments.

2. Obtain baseline CBC and liver and renal function studies.

3. Note client's occupation as this drug may interfere with the ability to work and should be noted.

4. List drugs currently prescribed to prevent any unfavorable interactions.

5. Note evidence of alcohol, drug, or nicotine addiction. These agents usually work well for BP control in this group of clients (especially the once-a-week patch).

Interventions

1. Monitor BP closely during the initial therapy. A decrease in BP occurs within 30–60 min after administration of clonidine and may persist for 8 hr.

2. Weigh the client daily, in the morning, in clothing of the same weight, to determine if there is edema caused by sodium retention. Any fluid retention should disappear after 3–4 days.

3. Note any fluctuations in BP to determine whether it is preferable to use clonidine alone or concomitantly with a diuretic. A stable BP reduces orthostatic effects of postural changes.

4. Observe for a paradoxical hypertensive response if client is also receiving propranolol.

5. Note any evidence of depression that may be precipitated by the drug, especially in those clients with a history of mental depression.

6. If the client is concomitantly receiving tolazoline or a tricyclic antidepressant, be aware that these drugs may block the antihypertensive action of clonidine. An increased dosage of clonidine may be indicated.

Evaluate
• Control of BP
• Control of withdrawal symptoms from opiates
• Reduction in menopausal symptoms

Cloxacillin sodium
(klox-ah-**SILL**-in)
Apo-Cloxi ✿, Cloxapen, Novo-Cloxin ✿, Nu-CLoxi ✿, Orbenin ✿, Taro-Cloxacillin ✿, Tegopen **(Rx)**
Classification: Antibiotic, penicillin

See also *Anti-Infectives* and *Penicillins*.

Action/Kinetics: Resistant to penicillinase and is acid stable. **Peak plasma levels:** 7–15 mcg/mL after 30–60 min. **t½:** 30 min. Protein binding: 88%–96%. Well absorbed from GI tract. Mostly excreted in urine, but some excreted in bile.

Uses: Infections caused by penicillinase-producing staphylococci, including pneumococci, group A beta-hemolytic streptococci, and penicillin G-sensitive staphylococci.

Dosage
• **Capsules, Oral Solution**
Skin and soft tissue infections, mild to moderate URTIs.
Adults and children over 20 kg: 250 mg q 6 hr; **pediatric, less than 20 kg:** 50 mg/kg/day in divided doses q 6 hr.
Lower respiratory tract infections or disseminated infections.
Adults and children over 20 kg: 0.5 g q 6 hr; **pediatric, less than 20 kg:** 100 (or more) mg/kg/day in divided doses q 6 hr. Alternatively, a dose of 50–100 mg/kg/day (up to a maximum of 4 g/day) divided q 6 hr may be used for infants and children.

RESPIRATORY CARE CONSIDERATIONS

See also *Respiratory Care Considerations* for *Penicillins*.

Administration/Storage
1. Add amount of water stated on label in two portions; shake well after each addition.
2. Shake well before pouring each dose.
3. Refrigerate reconstituted solution and discard unused portion after 14 days.
4. Administer 1 hr before or 2 hr after meals because food interferes with absorption of drug.

Assessment
1. Note any previous sensitivity to PCN.
2. Obtain baseline CBC, liver function studies, and cultures.

Evaluate
• Eradication of infection and reports of symptomatic improvement
• ↓ Fever, ↓ WBCs, ↑ appetite, and negative lab culture reports

Codeine phosphate
(**KOH**-deen)
Pregnancy Category: C
Paveral ✿ **(C-II) (Rx)**

Codeine sulfate
(**KOH**-deen)

Pregnancy Category: C
(C-II) (Rx)
Classification: Narcotic analgesic, morphine type

See also *Narcotic Analgesics*.

Action/Kinetics: Codeine resembles morphine pharmacologically but produces less respiratory depression and N&V. It is moderately habit-forming and constipating. Dosages over 60 mg often cause restlessness and excitement and irritate the cough center. However, in lower doses, it is a potent antitussive and is an ingredient in many cough syrups. **Onset:** 10–30 min. **Peak effect:** 30–60 min. **Duration:** 4–6 hr. t½: 3–4 hr. Codeine is two-thirds as effective PO as parenterally.

It is often used to supplement the effect of nonnarcotic analgesics such as aspirin and acetaminophen. Codeine is also found in many combination cough/cold products.

Uses: Relief of mild to moderate pain. Antitussive to relieve chemical or mechanical respiratory tract irritation.

Contraindications: Premature infants or during labor when delivery of a premature infant is expected.

Special Concerns: May increase the duration of labor. Use with caution and reduce the initial dose in clients with seizure disorders, acute abdominal conditions, renal or hepatic disease, fever, Addison's disease, hypothyroidism, prostatic hypertrophy, ulcerative colitis, urethral stricture, following recent GI or GU tract surgery, and in the young, geriatric, or debilitated clients.

Additional Drug Interactions: Combination with chlordiazepoxide may induce coma.

Dosage ———————
• **Solution, Tablets, IM, IV, SC**
Analgesia.
Adults: 15–60 mg q 4–6 hr, not to exceed 360 mg/day. **Pediatric, over 1 year:** 0.5 mg/kg q 4–6 hr. IV should not be used in children.
Antitussive.
Adults: 10–20 mg q 4–6 hr, up to maximum of 120 mg/day. **Pediatric,**

2–6 years: 2.5–5 mg PO q 4–6 hr, not to exceed 30 mg/day; **6–12 years:** 5–10 mg q 4–6 hr, not to exceed 60 mg/day.

RESPIRATORY CARE CONSIDERATIONS

See also *Respiratory Care Considerations* for *Narcotic Analgesics*.
Evaluate
• Relief of pain
• Control of coughing with improved sleeping patterns

Colfosceril palmitate (Dipalmitoylphosphatidyl choline, DPPC)

(kohl-**FOSS**-sir-ill)
Exosurf Neonatal **(Rx)**
Classification: Lung surfactant

Action/Kinetics: Colfosceril contains dipalmitoylphosphatidyl-choline (DPPC), which reduces surface tension in the lungs, as well as cetyl alcohol, which acts as a spreading agent for DPPC on the air–fluid surface. The product also contains tyloxapol, which is a nonionic surfactant that assists in dispersion of DPPC and cetyl alcohol, and sodium chloride to adjust osmolality. The drug can rapidly affect oxygenation and lung compliance. DPPC is reabsorbed from the alveoli into lung tissue where it is broken down and reutilized for further phospholipid synthesis and secretion.

Uses: Prophylaxis of respiratory distress syndrome in infants with birth weights of less than 1,350 g and in infants with birth weights greater than 1,350 g who manifest pulmonary immaturity. Treatment of infants who have developed respiratory distress syndrome. Such infants should be on mechanical ventilation and should have been diagnosed as having respiratory distress syndrome.

Special Concerns: Use of colfosceril should be undertaken only by medical personnel trained and experienced in airway and clinical management of unstable premature infants. Although colfosceril is effective in reducing mortality due to premature birth, infants may still develop severe complications resulting in either death or survival but with permanent handicaps. Benefits versus risks should be carefully assessed before using colfosceril in infants weighing 500–700 g.

Side Effects: *Respiratory:* ***Pulmonary hemorrhage, pulmonary air leak (pneumothorax, pneumomediastinum, pneumopericardium, pulmonary interstitial emphysema), mucous plugs in the ET tube, apnea,*** congenital pneumonia, nosocomial pneumonia. *CV:* ***Intraventricular hemorrhage,*** patent ductus arteriosus, hypotension, bradycardia, tachycardia, exchange transfusion, persistent fetal circulation. *Changes in blood gases:* Fall or rise in oxygen saturation, fall or rise in transcutaneous pO_2, fall or rise in transcutaneous pCO_2. *Miscellaneous:* ***Necrotizing enterocolitis,*** major anomalies, hyperbilirubinemia, gagging, thrombocytopenia, ***seizures.***

Dosage

- **Intratracheal**
    Prophylaxis.
    5 mL/kg (as two 2.5-mL/kg half-doses) as soon as possible after birth. A second and third dose should be given 12 and 24 hr later to infants who are still on mechanical ventilation.
    Rescue treatment.
    5 mL/kg (as two 2.5-mL/kg half-doses) as soon as possible after the diagnosis of respiratory distress syndrome is confirmed. A second 5-mL/kg dose is given after 12 hr to infants who are still on mechanical ventilation. The safety and effectiveness of additional doses are not known.

RESPIRATORY CARE CONSIDERATIONS

Administration/Storage

1. The drug should be reconstituted, according to the directions provided by the manufacturer, immediately prior to use with the diluent provided (preservative-free sterile water for injection). The reconstituted product is a milky white suspension.
2. The reconstituted suspension should be uniformly dispersed before administration. If the vial contains large flakes or particulate matter, it should not be used.
3. Five different-sized ET tube adapters are provided with each vial of colfosceril. The adapters are clean but not sterile. The adapters should be used according to the instructions provided by the manufacturer.
4. Colfosceril is administered directly into the trachea through the side-port on the special ET tube adapter without interruption of mechanical ventilation.
5. Each half-dose is given slowly over 1–2 min in small bursts timed with inspiration.
6. The first 2.5-mL/kg dose is given with the infant in the midline position; after the first half-dose is given, the infant's head and torso are first turned 45° to the right for 30 sec and then 45° to the left for 30 sec while continuing mechanical ventilation. This allows for gravity to help with lung distribution of the drug.
7. Refluxing of colfosceril into the ET tube may occur if the drug is given rapidly. If reflux is noted, administration of the drug should be stopped and the peak inspiratory pressure should be increased on the ventilator by 4–5 cm water until the ET tube clears.
8. Colfosceril administration should be undertaken only by experienced neonatologists and other individuals experienced at neonatal intubation and ventilatory management.
9. Studies continue regarding different methods of administering colfosceril and other exogenous surfactants. So, other protocols, other than described here, may be appropriate.

Assessment

1. Review indications for drug therapy to ensure that infant meets criteria

and document as rescue or prophylactic treatment.

2. The infant's color, chest expansion, facial expression, oximeter readings, HR, and ET tube patency and position should be documented and monitored carefully before and during colfosceril dosing.

3. Ascertain that the ET tube tip is in the trachea and not in the esophagus or right or left mainstem bronchus to ensure drug dispersion to all lung areas.

4. Document baseline weight, ABGs, VS, CXR, and physical assessment findings.

Interventions

1. Confirm brisk and symmetrical chest movement and equal breath sounds in the two axillae with each mechanical inspiration prior to and at the conclusion of each dosing.

2. The infant should be suctioned before administration of the drug but not for 2 hr after colfosceril administration (unless clinically necessary).

3. It is essential that continuous monitoring of ECG, arterial BP, and transcutaneous oxygen saturation be undertaken during dosing. After either prophylactic or rescue treatment, frequent ABGs should be measured to prevent postdosing hyperoxia and hypocarbia.

4. The volume of the 5-mL/kg dose may cause a transient impairment of gas exchange due to physical blockage of the airway. Thus, infants may show a decrease in oxygen saturation during dosing, especially if they are on low ventilator settings prior to dosing. If this occurs, the peak inspiratory pressure on the ventilator should be increased by 4–5 cm water for 1–2 min. Also, the FiO$_2$ should be increased for 1–2 min.

5. If chest expansion improves significantly after dosing, the peak ventilator inspiratory pressure should be reduced immediately. Failure to do this may cause lung overdistention and fatal pulmonary air leak.

6. If the infant becomes pink and oxygen saturation is more than 95%, the FiO$_2$ should be reduced in small but repeated steps until saturation is 90%–95%. Failure to do this may cause hyperoxia.

7. If arterial or transcutaneous CO$_2$ levels are less than 30 mm Hg, the ventilator rate must be reduced immediately. Failure to do this can result in significant hypocarbia, which reduces cerebral blood flow.

8. After the dose has been administered, the position of the ET tube should be confirmed by listening for equal breath sounds in the two axillae. Particular attention should be paid to chest expansion, skin color, transcutaneous O$_2$ saturation, and ABGs (samples should be taken frequently). The infant should be closely monitored for at least 30 min after dosing.

9. Observe closely for air leaks and mucous plugs. If mucous plug is unrelieved by suctioning, the ET tube must be replaced immediately.

Evaluate

• Oxygen saturation between 90% and 95% and improved pulmonary parameters more consistent with survival

• ↓ Pulmonary air leaks and prevention of alveolar collapse

Cortisone acetate (Compound E)

(**KOR**-tih-zohn)

Cortone ✽, Cortone Acetate, Cortone Acetate Sterile Suspension **(Rx)**

Classification: Corticosteroid, glucocorticoid-type

See also *Corticosteroids*.

Action/Kinetics: Possesses both glucocorticoid and mineralocorticoid activity. Short-acting. **t½, plasma:** 30 min; **t½, biologic:** 8–12 hr.

Uses: Primarily used for replacement therapy in chronic cortical insufficiency. Also inflammatory or allergic disorders, but only for short-term use because the drug has a strong mineralocorticoid effect. The sterile suspension is used to treat children suffering from congenital adrenal hyperplasia.

Special Concerns: Use during pregnancy only if benefits outweigh risks.

Dosage ───────────────────
• **Tablets, Injection**
Initial or during crisis.
25–300 mg/day. Decrease gradually to lowest effective dose.
Anti-inflammatory.
25–150 mg/day, depending on severity of the disease.
Acute rheumatic fever.
200 mg b.i.d. day 1, thereafter, 200 mg/day.
Addison's disease.
Maintenance: 0.5–0.75 mg/kg/day.

RESPIRATORY CARE CONSIDERATIONS

See also *Respiratory Care Considerations* for *Corticosteroids*.
Administration/Storage: Single course of therapy should not exceed 6 weeks. Rest periods of 2–3 weeks are indicated between treatments.
Evaluate
• Replacement therapy in cortical insufficiency
• Relief of allergic manifestations
• Normal plasma cortisol levels (138–635 nmol/L at 8 a.m.)

───────────────────────────

Cromolyn sodium (Sodium cromoglycate)
(**CROH**-moh-lin)
Pregnancy Category: B
Crolom, Gastrocrom, Intal, Nalcrom ✿, Nasalcrom, Novo–Cromolyn ✿, PMS–Sodium Chromoglycate ✿, Rynacrom ✿, Vistacrom ✿ **(Rx)**
Classification: Antiasthmatic, antiallergic drug
───────────────────────────
Action/Kinetics: Cromolyn sodium appears to act locally to inhibit the degranulation of sensitized mast cells that occurs after exposure to certain antigen. The effect prevents the release of histamine, slow-reacting substance of anaphylaxis, and other endogenous substances causing hypersensitivity reactions. The drug, when effective, reduces the number and intensity of asthmatic attacks as well as decreasing allergic reactions in the eye. The drug has no antihistaminic, anti-inflammatory, or bronchodilator effects and has no role in terminating an acute attack of asthma. After inhalation, some of the drug is absorbed systemically. It is excreted about equally in urine and bile (feces). **t½:** 81 min; from lungs: 60 min. About 50% excreted unchanged through the urine and 50% through the bile. When used in the eye, approximately 0.03% is absorbed. **Onset, ophthalmic:** Several days. **Onset, nasal:** Less than 1 week. **Time to peak effect, nasal:** Up to 4 weeks.
Uses: *Inhalation:* Prophylactic and adjunct in the management of severe bronchial asthma in selected clients. Prophylaxis of exercise-induced bronchospasms and bronchospasms due to allergens, cold dry air, or environmental pollutants. *Ophthalmologic:* Conjunctivitis, including vernal keratoconjunctivitis, vernal conjunctivitis, and vernal keratitis. *Nasal:* Prophylaxis and treatment of allergic rhinitis. *PO:* Mastocytosis (improves symptoms including diarrhea, flushing, headaches, vomiting, urticaria, nausea, abdominal pain, and itching). *Investigational:* PO to treat food allergies.
Contraindications: Hypersensitivity. Acute attacks and status asthmaticus. Due to the presence of benzalkonium chloride in the product, soft contact lenses should not be worn if the drug is used in the eye. For mastocytosis in premature infants.
Special Concerns: Dosage of the ophthalmic product has not been established in children less than 4 years of age; dosage of the nasal product has not been established in children less than 6 years of age. Use with caution for long periods of time, in the presence of renal or hepatic disease, and during lactation.
Side Effects: *Respiratory:* ***Bronchospasm, laryngeal edema (rare),*** cough, eosinophilic pneumonia. *CNS:* Dizziness, drowsiness, headache. *Aller-*

───────────────────────────

gic: Urticaria, rash, angioedema, serum sickness, **anaphylaxis.** *Other:* Nausea, urinary frequency, dysuria, joint swelling and pain, lacrimation, swollen parotid gland.

Following nebulization: Sneezing, wheezing, itching, nose bleeds, burning, nasal congestion. **Following nasal solution:** Burning, stinging, irritation of nose; sneezing, nose bleeds, headache, bad taste in mouth, postnasal drip. **Following ophthalmic use:** Stinging and burning after use. Also, conjunctival injection, watery or itchy eyes, dryness around the eye, puffy eyes, eye irritation, styes.

Following PO use: *GI:* Diarrhea, taste perversion, spasm of esophagus, flatulence, dysphagia, burning of mouth and throat. *CNS:* Headache, dizziness, fatigue, migraine, paresthesia, anxiety, depression, psychosis, behavior changes, insomnia, hallucinations, lethargy, lightheadedness after eating. *Dermatologic:* Flushing, angioedema, urticaria, skin burning, skin erythema. *Musculoskeletal:* Arthralgia, stiffness and weakness in legs. *Miscellaneous:* Altered liver function test, dyspnea, dysuria, polycythemia, neutropenia.

Dosage ————————————

• **Capsules, Nebulizer Solution (2 ml) or Metered Dose Inhaler**
Prophylaxis of bronchial asthma.
Adults: 20 mg q.i.d. at regular intervals. Adjust dosage as required.
Prophylaxis of bronchospasm.
Adults: 20 mg as a single dose just prior to exposure to the precipitating factor. If used chronically, 20 mg q.i.d, up to a maximum of 160 mg/day.

• **Ophthalmic Solution**
Allergic ocular disorders.
Adults and children over 4 years: 1–2 gtt of the 4% solution in each eye 4–6 times/day at regular intervals.

• **Nasal Spray**
Allergic rhinitis.
Adults and children over 6 years: 2.6 mg in each nostril 6 times/day or 5.2 mg in each nostril 3–4 times/day at regular intervals.

• **Oral Capsules**
Mastocytosis.
Adults: 200 mg q.i.d. 30 min before meals and at bedtime. **Pediatric, term to 2 years:** 20 mg/kg/day in four divided doses; should be used in this age group only in severe incapacitating disease where benefits outweigh risks. **Pediatric, 2–12 years:** 100 mg q.i.d. 30 min before meals and at bedtime. If relief is not seen within 2–3 weeks, dose may be increased, but should not exceed 40 mg/kg/day for adults and children over 2 years of age and 30 mg/kg/day for children 6 months–2 years.

RESPIRATORY CARE CONSIDERATIONS

Administration/Storage

1. Institute only after acute episode is over, when airway is clear and client can inhale adequately.
2. Corticosteroid dosage should be continued when initiating cromolyn therapy. However, if improvement occurs, the steroid dosage may be tapered slowly. Steroid therapy may have to be reinstituted if cromolyn inhalation is impaired, in times of stress, or in adrenocortical insufficiency.
3. One drop of the ophthalmic solution contains 1.6 mg cromolyn sodium.
4. The ophthalmic solution should be protected from direct sunlight and, once opened, should be discarded after 4 weeks.
5. The ophthalmic solution contains benzylkonium chloride; therefore, soft contact lenses should not be worn during treatment.

Client/Family Teaching

1. Provide written guidelines concerning the prescribed method of medication administration and anticipated results.
2. When the medication is administered by Spinhaler, the following guidelines should be used:

• Demonstrate how to puncture and load the capsule into the Spinhaler.
• Instruct the client to inhale and exhale fully and then to introduce the mouthpiece between the lips.
• Tilt head back and inhale deeply and rapidly through the inhaler. This causes the propeller to turn rapidly and to supply more medication in one breath.
• Remove inhaler, hold breath a few seconds, and exhale slowly.
• Repeat this procedure until the powder is completely administered.
• Do not wet powder with breath while exhaling.
• Taking a sip of water or rinsing the mouth immediately before and after using the Spinhaler will diminish the throat irritation and/or cough.
• The Spinhaler should be replaced every 6 months.
3. When used in the *eye*:
• Advise client not to wear soft contacts until medically cleared.
• Drug may sting on application, but this should subside.
4. Encourage the client to continue routine self-administration of medication as ordered. It may take up to 4 weeks for frequency of asthmatic attacks to decrease.
5. With exposure bronchoconstriction, advise client to use the inhaler within 10–15 min prior to exposure of precipitating agent (i.e., exercise, antigen, environmental pollutants) for best results.
6. Provide a peak expiratory flow meter and advise client in how to monitor their asthma control and establish at what level to seek medical assistance.
7. If the client wishes to discontinue medication, stress the importance of notifying the provider. Rapid withdrawal of the drug may precipitate an asthmatic attack, and concomitant corticosteroid therapy may require adjustment.

Evaluate
• ↓ Frequency and intensity of asthmatic attacks

• Prevention of exposure-induced bronchoconstriction
• Control of symptoms of mastocytosis (↓ diarrhea, N&V, headache, flushing, and abdominal pain)
• Relief of ocular and/or nasal allergic manifestations

Cycloserine
(sye-kloh-**SEE**-reen)
Pregnancy Category: C
Seromycin **(Rx)**
Classification: Antitubercular agent for retreatment regimens

Action/Kinetics: This drug is produced by a strain of *Streptomyces orchidaceus* or *Garyphalus lavendulae.* It acts by inhibiting cell wall synthesis by interfering with the incorporation of the amino acid alanine. The drug is well absorbed from the GI tract and widely distributed in body tissues. **Time to peak plasma levels:** 3–8 hr. Cerebrospinal levels are similar to those in plasma. **t½:** 10 hr. From 60% to 70% is excreted unchanged in urine.
Uses: With other drugs to treat active pulmonary and extrapulmonary tuberculosis only when primary therapy cannot be used. Has been used to treat UTIs when other therapy has failed or if the organism has demonstrated sensitivity.
Contraindications: Hypersensitivity to cycloserine, epilepsy, depression, severe anxiety, psychosis, severe renal insufficiency, and alcoholism. Lactation.
Special Concerns: Safe use during pregnancy and in children has not been established.
Side Effects: *CNS:* Drowsiness, headache, mental confusion, tremors, vertigo, loss of memory, psychoses (possibly with *suicidal tendencies),* character changes, hyperirritability, aggression, increased reflexes, *seizures,* paresthesias, paresis, coma. Neurotoxic effects depend on blood levels of cycloserine. Hence, frequent determinations of cycloserine blood levels are indicated, especially

during the initial period of therapy. *Other:* Sudden development of CHF, skin rashes, increased transaminase.

OD   **Overdose Management:** *Symptoms:* CNS depression, including drowsiness, mental confusion, headache, vertigo, paresthesias, dysarthrias, hyperirritability, psychosis, paresis, *seizures,* and *coma.* *Treatment:* Supportive therapy. Charcoal may be more effective than emesis or gastric lavage. Hemodialysis may be used for life-threatening toxicity. Pyridoxine may treat neurotoxic effects.

Drug Interactions
Ethanol / ↑ Risk of epileptic episodes
Isoniazid / ↑ Risk of cycloserine CNS side effects (especially dizziness)

Dosage ⎯⎯⎯⎯⎯⎯⎯
• **Capsules**
Adults, initially: 250 mg q 12 hr for first 2 weeks; **then,** 0.5–1 g/day in divided doses based on blood levels. Dosage should not exceed 1 g/day. **Pediatric:** 10–20 mg/kg/day, not to exceed 0.75–1 g/day. *NOTE:* Pyridoxine, 200–300 mg/day may prevent neurotoxic effects.

RESPIRATORY CARE CONSIDERATIONS

See also *General Respiratory Care Considerations for All Anti-Infectives.*
Assessment
1. Obtain a thorough history.
2. Note any evidence of depression, anxiety, seizures, or excessive use of alcohol.
3. Obtain baseline parameters and monitor liver and renal function studies throughout therapy.
Interventions
1. Monitor I&O and observe for any sudden development of CHF in clients receiving high doses of cycloserine.
2. Report any psychotic or neurologic reactions that will necessitate withdrawing the drug, at least for a short period of time.
3. Monitor serum cycloserine levels

throughout therapy (less than 25–30 mcg/mL).
Evaluate
• Resolution of infection
• Negative sputum cultures for acid-fast bacilli
• Improved CXR and pulmonary function studies

Cyproheptadine hydrochloride
(sye-proh-**HEP**-tah-deen)
Pregnancy Category: B
Periactin, PMS–Cyproheptadine ✤ **(Rx)**
Classification: Antihistamine, piperidine-type

See also *Antihistamines.*
Action/Kinetics: Cyproheptadine also possesses antiserotonin activity.
Duration: 8 hr.
Additional Use: Cold urticaria. *Investigational:* Cluster headaches, appetite stimulant in underweight clients and those with anorexia nervosa.
Additional Contraindications: Glaucoma, urinary retention.
Special Concerns: Geriatric clients may be more sensitive to the usual adult dose.
Additional Side Effects: Increased appetite.
Laboratory Test Interferences: ↑ Serum amylase and prolactin if given with thyroid-releasing hormone.

Dosage ⎯⎯⎯⎯⎯⎯⎯
• **Syrup, Tablets**
Antihistaminic.
Adults, initial: 4 mg q 8 hr; **then,** 4–20 mg/day, not to exceed 0.5 mg/kg/day. **Pediatric, 2–6 years:** 2 mg q 8–12 hr, not to exceed 12 mg/day; **6–14 years:** 4 mg q 8–12 hr, not to exceed 16 mg/day.
Appetite stimulant.
Adults: 4 mg t.i.d. with meals. **Pediatric, 6–14 years, initial:** 2 mg t.i.d.–q.i.d. with meals; **then,** reduce dose to 4 mg t.i.d. **Pediatric, 2–6 years, initial:** 2 mg t.i.d. with meals; **then,** dose may be increased to a total of 8 mg/day.

RESPIRATORY CARE CONSIDERATIONS

See also *Respiratory Care Considerations* for *Antihistamines*.
Administration/Storage
1. Drug should not be given more than 6 months to adults and 3 months to children for appetite stimulation.

2. Anticipate the onset of action to occur within 15–30 min and to last from 3 to 6 hr.
Evaluate
• ↓ Allergic manifestations
• Weight gain
• Relief of cluster headaches

Dexamethasone

(dex-ah-**METH**-ah-zohn)
Oral: Decadron, Deronil ✦, Dexameth, Dexamethasone Intensol, Dexasone ✦, Dexone, Hexadrol **(Rx)**., PMS-Dexamethasone ✦, **Topical:** Aeroseb-Dex, Decaderm **(Rx)**. **Ophthalmic:** Maxidex Ophthalmic **(Rx)**
Classification: Glucocorticoid, synthetic

See also *Corticosteroids*.
Action/Kinetics: Long-acting. Low degree of sodium and water retention. Diuresis may ensue when clients are transferred from other corticosteroids to dexamethasone. Not recommended for replacement therapy in adrenal cortical insufficiency. **t½:** 110–210 min.
Additional Use: In acute allergic disorders, PO dexamethasone may be combined with dexamethasone sodium phosphate injection. This combination is used for 6 days. Used to test for adrenal cortical hyperfunction. Cerebral edema due to brain tumor, craniotomy, or head injury. *Investigational:* Diagnosis of depression. Antiemetic in cisplatin-induced vomiting. Prophylaxis or treatment of acute mountain sickness. Decrease hearing loss in bacterial meningitis. Bronchopulmonary dysplasia in preterm infants. Hirsutism.
Special Concerns: Use during pregnancy only if benefits outweigh risks.

Additional Drug Interactions: Ephedrine ↓ effect of dexamethasone due to ↑ breakdown by the liver.

Dosage

• **Oral Concentrate Tablets, Elixir**
Most uses.
Initial: 0.75–9 mg/day; **maintenance:** gradually reduce to minimum effective dose (0.5–3 mg/day).
Suppression test for Cushing's syndrome.
0.5 mg q 6 hr for 2 days for 24-hr urine collection (or 1 mg at 11 p.m. with blood withdrawn at 8 a.m. for blood cortisol determination).
Suppression test to determine cause of pituitary ACTH excess.
2 mg q 6 hr for 2 days (for 24-hr urine collection).
Acute allergic disorders or acute worsening of chronic allergic disorders.
Day 1: Dexamethasone sodium phosphate injection, 4–8 mg IM. **Days 2 and 3:** Two 0.75-mg dexamethasone tablets b.i.d. **Day 4:** One 0.75-mg dexamethasone tablet b.i.d. **Days 5 and 6:** One 0.75-mg dexamethasone tablet. **Day 7:** No treatment. **Day 8:** Follow-up visit to physician.
• **Topical Aerosol, Cream**
Apply sparingly as a light film to affected area b.i.d.–t.i.d.
• **Ophthalmic Suspension**

1–2 gtt in the conjunctival sac q hr during day and q 2 hr during night until a satisfactory response obtained; **then,** 1 gtt q 4 hr and finally 1 gtt q 6–8 hr.

RESPIRATORY CARE CONSIDERATIONS

See also *Respiratory Care Considerations* for *Corticosteroids*.

Evaluate
• Status of adrenal cortical function
• ↓ Symptoms of allergic response
• ↓ Cerebral edema
• Control of cisplatin-induced vomiting
• Prevention of mountain sickness

Dexamethasone acetate
(dex-ah-**METH**-ah-zohn)

Dalalone D.P., Dalalone L.A., Decadron-LA, Decaject-L.A., Dexasone L.A., Dexone LA, Solurex LA **(Rx)**
Classification: Glucocorticoid, synthetic

See also *Corticosteroids*.

Action/Kinetics: This ester of dexamethasone is practically insoluble and provides the prolonged activity suitable for repository injections, although it has a prompt onset of action. Not for IV use.

Special Concerns: Use during pregnancy only if benefits outweigh risks.

Dosage ———————————
• **Repository Injection, IM**
8–16 mg q 1–3 weeks, if necessary.
• **Intralesional**
0.8–1.6 mg.
• **Soft Tissue and Intra-articular**
4–16 mg repeated at 1–3-week intervals.

RESPIRATORY CARE CONSIDERATIONS

See Respiratory Care Considerations for Corticosteroids.

Evaluate
• ↓ Inflammation
• Reports of symptomatic improvement

Dexamethasone sodium phosphate
(dex-ah-**METH**-ah-zohn)

Systemic: Dalalone, Decadron Phosphate, Decaject, Dexasone, Dexone, Hexadrol Phosphate, R.O.-Dexone ✦, Solurex **(Rx)**. **Inhaler:** Decadron Phosphate Respihaler **(Rx)**. **Nasal:** Decadron Phosphate Turbinaire **(Rx)**. **Ophthalmic:** AK-Dex, Decadron Phosphate Ophthalmic, Diodex ✦, Maxidex, PMS-Dexamethasone Sodium Phosphate ✦, Spersadex ✦ **(Rx)**. **Otic:** AK-Dex, Decadron, I-Methasone **(Rx)**. **Topical:** Decadron Phosphate **(Rx)**
Classification: Glucocorticoid, synthetic

See also *Corticosteroids*.

Additional Use: For IV or IM use in emergency situations when dexamethasone cannot be given PO. Has a rapid onset and a short duration of action. Routes of administration include inhalation (especially for bronchial asthma), ophthalmic, topical, intrasynovial, and intra-articular. Intranasally for nasal polyps, allergic or inflammatory nasal conditions.

Contraindications: Acute infections, persistent positive sputum cultures of *Candida albicans*. Lactation.

Special Concerns: Use during pregnancy only if benefits outweigh risks.

Side Effects: *Following inhalation:* Nasal and nasopharyngeal irritation, burning, dryness, stinging, headache.

Dosage ———————————
• **IM, IV**
Most uses.
Range: 0.5–9 mg/day (⅓–½ the PO dose q 12 hr).
Cerebral edema.
Adults, initial: 10 mg IV; **then,** 4 mg IM q 6 hr until maximum effect obtained (usually within 12–24 hr). Switch to PO therapy (1–3 mg t.i.d.) as soon as feasible and then slowly withdraw over 5–7 days.
Shock, unresponsive.

Initial: either 1–6 mg/kg IV or 40 mg IV; **then,** repeat IV dose q 2–6 hr as long as necessary.
• **Intralesional, Intra-articular, Soft Tissue Injections**
0.4–6 mg, depending on the site (e.g., small joints: 0.8–1 mg; large joints: 2–4 mg; soft tissue infiltration: 2–6 mg; ganglia: 1–2 mg; bursae: 2–3 mg; tendon sheaths: 0.4–1 mg.
• **Metered Dose Inhaler**
Bronchial asthma.
Adults, initial: 3 inhalations (84 mcg dexamethasone/inhalation) t.i.d.–q.i.d.; **maximum:** 3 inhalations/dose; 12 inhalations/day. **Pediatric: initial,** 2 inhalations t.i.d.–q.i.d.; **maximum:** 2 inhalations/dose; 8 inhalations/day.
• **Intranasal**
Allergies, nasal polyps.
Adults: 2 sprays (total of 168 mcg dexamethasone) in each nostril b.i.d.–t.i.d. (maximum: 12 sprays/day); **pediatric, 6–12 years:** 1–2 sprays (total of 84–168 mcg dexamethasone) in each nostril b.i.d. (maximum: 8 sprays/day).
• **Ophthalmic Ointment**
Instill a small amount of the ointment into the conjunctival sac t.i.d.–q.i.d. As response is obtained, reduce the number of applications.
• **Ophthalmic Solution**
Instill 1–2 gtt into the conjunctival sac q hr during the day and q 2 hr at night until response obtained; **then,** reduce to 1 gtt q 4 hr and later 1 gtt t.i.d.–q.i.d. may control symptoms.
• **Otic Solution**
3–4 gtt into the ear canal b.i.d.–t.i.d.
• **Topical Cream**
Apply sparingly to affected areas and rub in.

RESPIRATORY CARE CONSIDERATIONS

See also *Respiratory Care Considerations* for *Corticosteroids.*
Administration/Storage
1. Do not use preparation containing lidocaine IV.
2. For IV administration may give undiluted over 1 min.

3. For intranasal use, some clients are controlled using 1 spray in each nostril b.i.d.
Evaluate
• Improvement in pulmonary function
• Relief of allergic manifestations
• Suppression of inflammatory and immune response
• Reversal of symptoms of shock; enhanced tissue perfusion

Dexchlorpheniramine maleate
(dex-klor-fen-**EAR**-ah-meen)
Pregnancy Category: B
Dexchlor, Poladex T.D., Polaramine **(Rx)**
Classification: Antihistamine, alkylamine type

See also *Antihistamines.*
Action/Kinetics: Less severe sedative effects. **Duration:** 8 hr.
Special Concerns: Extended-release tablets should not be used in children. Geriatric clients may be more sensitive to the usual adult dose.

Dosage
• **Syrup, Tablets**
Adults: 2 mg q 4–6 hr as needed. **Pediatric, 5–12 years:** 1 mg q 4–6 hr as needed; **2–5 years:** 0.5 mg q 4–6 hr as needed.
• **Extended-Release Tablets**
Adults: 4–6 mg q 8–12 hr as needed.

RESPIRATORY CARE CONSIDERATIONS

See also *Respiratory Care Considerations* for *Antihistamines.*
Evaluate: Symptomatic relief and ↓ allergic manifestations

Dextromethorphan hydrobromide
(dex-troh-meth-**OR**-fan)
Balminil D.M. Syrup ✿, Benylin DM, Calmylin #1 ✿, Children's Hold, Delsym, Formula 44 Adult/Pediatric ✿,

Hold DM, Koffex DM Syrup ✤, Pertussin CS, Pertussin ES, Robidex Syrup ✤, Robitussin Cough Calmers, Robitussin Pediatric, St. Joseph Cough Suppressant, Scot-Tussin DM Cough Chasers, Sucrets Cough Control, Suppress, Trocal, Vick's Formula 44, Vick's Formula 44 Pediatric Formula **(OTC)**

Classification: Nonnarcotic antitussive

Action/Kinetics: Dextromethorphan selectively depresses the cough center in the medulla. Dextromethorphan 15–30 mg is equal to 8–15 mg codeine as an antitussive. It is a common ingredient of nonprescription cough medications; it does not produce physical dependence or respiratory depression. Well absorbed from GI tract. **Onset:** 15–30 min. **Duration:** 3–6 hr. The sustained liquid contains dextromethorphan plistirex equivalent to 30 mg dextromethorphan hydrobromide per 5 mL.

Uses: Symptomatic relief of nonproductive cough due to colds or inhaled irritants.

Contraindications: Persistent or chronic cough or when cough is accompanied by excessive secretions. Use during first trimester of pregnancy unless directed otherwise by physician.

Special Concerns: Use is not recommended in children less than 2 years of age. Use with caution in clients with nausea, vomiting, high fever, rash, or persistent headache.

Side Effects: *CNS:* Dizziness, drowsiness. *GI:* N&V, stomach pain.

OD **Overdose Management:** *Symptoms:* **Adults:** Dysphoria, slurred speech, ataxia, altered sensory perception. **Children:** Ataxia, *convulsions, respiratory depression.* *Treatment:* Treat symptoms and provide support.

Drug Interactions: Use with MAO inhibitors may cause nausea, hypotension, hyperpyrexia, myoclonic leg jerks, and coma.

Dosage
• **Capsules, Liquid, Lozenges, Syrup, Concentrate, Tablets**
Antitussive.

Adults and children over 12 years: 10–30 mg q 4–8 hr, not to exceed 120 mg/day; **pediatric, 6–12 years:** either 5–10 mg q 4 hr or 15 mg q 6–8 hr, not to exceed 60 mg/day; **pediatric, 2–6 years:** either 2.5–7.5 mg q 4 hr or 7.5 mg q 6–8 hr of the syrup, not to exceed 30 mg/day.

• **Sustained-Release Suspension**
Antitussive.

Adults: 60 mg q 12 hr. **Pediatric, 6–12 years:** 30 mg q 12 hr, not to exceed 60 mg/day; **pediatric, 2–6 years:** 15 mg q 12 hr, not to exceed 30 mg/day.

RESPIRATORY CARE CONSIDERATIONS

Administration/Storage

1. Increasing the dose of dextromethorphan will not increase its effectiveness but will increase the duration of action.

2. The lozenges should not be given to children under 6 years of age.

Assessment

1. Note the length of time the client has had the cough. Document sputum production and characteristics. If the cough persists beyond a week, dextromethorphan should not be given.

2. Determine if the client has had nausea, vomiting, persistent headaches, or a high fever.

3. If the client is pregnant, determine which trimester of pregnancy. The drug is contraindicated in the first trimester.

Evaluate: Control of cough with improved sleep patterns

Dezocine

(**DEZ**-oh-seen)

Pregnancy Category: C

Dalgan **(Rx)**

Classification: Narcotic agonist-antagonist analgesic

See also *Narcotic Analgesics*.

Action/Kinetics: Dezocine is a parenteral narcotic analgesic possessing both agonist and antagonist activity. It is similar to morphine with respect to analgesic potency and onset and duration of action. However, there is less risk of abuse due to the mixed agonist-antagonist properties of the drug. The narcotic antagonist activity is greater than that of pentazocine. **Onset:** Approximately 30 min after IM and approximately 15 min after IV. **Peak effect:** 30–150 min. **Peak plasma levels:** 10–38 ng/mL after a 10-mg dose. **Duration:** 2–4 hr. **t½, after IV:** 2.4 hr. Approximately two-thirds of a dose is excreted in the urine mostly as the glucuronide conjugate.

Uses: Analgesic when use of a narcotic is desirable.

Contraindications: Lactation. Individuals dependent on narcotics. SC administration.

Special Concerns: Elderly clients are at an increased risk for altered respiratory patterns and mental changes.

Side Effects: *CNS:* Sedation (common), dizziness, vertigo, confusion, anxiety, crying, sleep disturbances, delusions, headache, depression, delirium. *Respiratory:* Respiratory depression, atelectasis. *CV:* Hypotension, irregular heart or pulse, hypertension, chest pain, pallor, thrombophlebitis. *GI:* N&V, dry mouth, constipation, abdominal pain, diarrhea. *Dermatologic:* Reactions at the injection site, pruritus, rash, erythema. *EENT:* Diplopia, blurred vision, congestion in ears, tinnitus. *GU:* Urinary frequency, retention, or hesitancy. *Miscellaneous:* Sweating, chills, edema, flushing, low hemoglobin, muscle cramps or aches, muscle pain, slurred speech.

OD **Overdose Management:** *Treatment:* Naloxone IV with appropriate supportive measures including oxygen, IV fluids, vasopressors, and assisted ventilation.

Drug Interactions: Additive depressant effect when used with general anesthetics, sedatives, antianxiety drugs, hypnotics, alcohol, and other opiate analgesics.

Dosage ———————
• **IM**

Analgesia.
Adults: 5–20 mg (usual is 10 mg) as a single dose; dose may be repeated q 3–6 hr with dosage adjusted, if necessary, depending on the status of the client.
• **IV**
Analgesia.
Adults: 2.5–10 mg (usual initial dose is 5 mg) repeated q 2–4 hr.

RESPIRATORY CARE CONSIDERATIONS

See also *Respiratory Care Considerations* for *Narcotic Analgesics.*

Administration/Storage
1. The maximum single dose should not exceed 20 mg and the maximum daily dose should not exceed 120 mg.
2. Dezocine can be stored at room temperature protected from light.
3. The solution should not be used if it contains a precipitate.

Assessment
1. Note any client sulfite sensitivity because drug contains sodium metabisulfite.
2. Determine any history or current use of opiate drugs because dezocine may precipitate an acute withdrawal syndrome.
3. Document location, onset, duration, and intensity of pain; note alleviating factors.
4. Note any evidence of impaired renal or liver function; obtain pretreatment lab values.
5. Assess for any evidence of head injury or increased ICP.

Interventions
1. Monitor for evidence of allergic reaction.
2. Record VS and assess mental status and respiratory patterns.
3. Anticipate reduced dosage in clients with renal or hepatic dysfunction.
4. Geriatric clients should receive reduced doses and be individually evaluated for subsequent dose levels.
5. If dezocine is administered with CNS depressants, anticipate the dose

of one or both agents should be reduced.

Evaluate: Satisfactory pain management as evidenced by ↑ activity, improved appetite, and reports of effective pain control

Diazoxide IV
(dye-az-**OX**-eyed)
Pregnancy Category: C
Hyperstat IV **(Rx)**
Classification: Antihypertensive, direct action on vascular smooth muscle

See also *Antihypertensive Agents* and *Diazoxide Oral*.

Action/Kinetics: Diazoxide is thought to exert a direct action on vascular smooth muscle to cause arteriolar vasodilation and decreased peripheral resistance. **Onset:** 1–5 min. **Time to peak effect:** 2–5 min. **Duration** (variable): usual, 3–12 hr. Excreted through the kidney (50% unchanged).

Uses: May be the drug of choice for hypertensive crisis (malignant and nonmalignant hypertension) in hospitalized adults and children. Often given concomitantly with a diuretic. Especially suitable for clients with impaired renal function, hypertensive encephalopathy, hypertension complicated by LV failure, and eclampsia. Ineffective for hypertension due to pheochromocytoma.

Contraindications: Hypersensitivity to drug or thiazide diuretics. Treatment of compensatory hypertension due to aortic coarctation or AV shunt. Dissecting aortic aneurysm.

Special Concerns: A decrease in dose may be necessary in geriatric clients due to age-related decreases in renal function. If given prior to delivery, fetal or neonatal hyperbilirubinemia, thrombocytopenia, or altered carbohydrate metabolism may result. Use with caution during lactation and in clients with impaired cerebral or cardiac circulation.

Side Effects: *CV:* Hypotension (may be severe enough to cause shock), sodium and water retention, especially in clients with impaired cardiac reserve, ***atrial or ventricular arrhythmias, cerebral or myocardial ischemia,*** marked ECG changes with possibility of ***MI*** , palpitations, bradycardia, SVT, chest discomfort or nonanginal chest tightness. *CNS:* Cerebral ischemia manifested by unconsciousness, ***seizures,*** paralysis, confusion, numbness of the hands. Headache, dizziness, weakness, drowsiness, lightheadedness, somnolence, lethargy, euphoria, weakness of short duration, apprehension, anxiety, malaise, blurred vision. *Respiratory:* Tightness in chest, cough, dyspnea, sensation of choking. *GI:* N&V, diarrhea, anorexia, parotid swelling, change in sense of taste, salivation, dry mouth, ileus, constipation, acute pancreatitis (rare). *Other:* Hyperglycemia (may be serious enough to require treatment), sweating, flushing, sensation of warmth, transient neurologic findings due to alteration in regional blood flow to the brain, hyperosmolar coma in infants, tinnitus, hearing loss, retention of nitrogenous wastes, acute pancreatitis, back pain, increased nocturia, lacrimation, hypersensitivity reactions, papilledema, hirsutism, decreased libido. Pain, cellulitis without sloughing, warmth or pain along injected vein, phlebitis at injection site, extravasation.

OD **Overdose Management:** *Symptoms:* Hypotension, excessive hyperglycemia. *Treatment:* Use the Trendelenburg maneuver to reverse hypotension.

Drug Interactions
Anticoagulants, oral / ↑ Effect of oral anticoagulants due to ↓ plasma protein binding
Nitrites / ↑ Hypotensive effect
Phenytoin / Diazoxide ↓ anticonvulsant effect of phenytoin
Reserpine / ↑ Hypotensive effect
Sulfonylureas / Destablization of the client resulting in hyperglycemia
Thiazide diuretics / ↑ Hyperglycemic, hyperuricemic, and antihypertensive effect of diazoxide
Vasodilators, peripheral / ↑ Hypotensive effect

Laboratory Test Interferences:
False + or ↑ uric acid.

Dosage ————————————
- **IV Push (30 sec or less)**
  Hypertensive crisis.
Adults: 1–3 mg/kg up to a maximum of 150 mg; may be repeated at 5–15-min intervals until adequate BP response obtained. Drug may then be repeated at 4–24-hr intervals for 4–5 days or until oral antihypertensive therapy can be initiated. **Pediatric:** 1–3 mg/kg (30–90 mg/m²) using the same dosing intervals as adults.

Repeated use can result in sodium and water retention; therefore, a diuretic may be needed to avoid CHF and for maximum reduction of BP.

RESPIRATORY CARE CONSIDERATIONS

See also *Respiratory Care Considerations* for *Antihypertensive Agents* and *Diazoxide oral.*
Administration/Storage
1. Do not administer IM or SC. Medication is highly alkaline.
2. Ensure patency and inject rapidly (30 sec) undiluted into a peripheral vein to maximize response.
3. Assess site for signs of irritation or extravasation. If extravasation should occur, apply ice packs.
4. Protect from light, heat, and freezing.
5. Have a sympathomimetic drug, such as norepinephrine, available to treat severe hypotension should it occur.
6. Ampules should be protected from light and stored between 2°C and 30°C (36°F and 86°F).
Assessment
1. Note client history for hypersensitivity to thiazide diuretics, sulfa drugs, or diazoxide.
2. Particularly note if client has diabetes mellitus. Diazoxide can cause serious elevations in blood sugar levels.
3. Obtain uric acid level and assess for evidence of hyperuricemia.

Interventions
1. Monitor BP frequently until it has stabilized and then every hour thereafter until hypertensive crisis is resolved. Obtain final BP upon arising, prior to ambulation.
2. Explain to client the need to remain in a recumbent position during and for 30 min after injection to avoid orthostatic hypotension.
3. Maintain the client in a recumbent position for 8–10 hr if furosemide is also administered.
4. Note client complaints of sweating, flushing, or evidence of hyperglycemia and be prepared to treat.
Evaluate: Significant reduction in BP during hypertensive crisis

Diazoxide oral
(dye-az-**OX**-eyed)
Pregnancy Category: C
Proglycem **(Rx)**
Classification: Insulin antagonist, hypotensive agent

Action/Kinetics: Diazoxide is related to the thiazide diuretics. It inhibits the release of insulin from beta islet cells of the pancreas, leading to an increase in blood glucose levels. Effect is dose related. Diazoxide causes sodium, potassium, uric acid, and water retention. Other effects include increased pulse rate, increased serum uric acid levels, increased serum free fatty acids, decreased para-aminohippuric acid clearance from the kidneys (little effect on GFR). **Onset:** 1 hr. **t½:** 28 hr (up to 53 hr in clients with anuria). **Duration:** 8 hr. The drug is over 90% bound to plasma proteins. Metabolized in the liver although 50% is excreted through the kidneys unchanged.
Uses: Management of hypoglycemia due to hyperinsulinism, including inoperable islet cell adenoma or carcinoma or extrapancreatic malignancies in adults. In children, for treatment of hyperinsulinemia due to leucine sensitivity , islet cell hyperplasia, nesidioblastosis, extrapancreatic malignancy, islet cell adenoma or

adenomatosis. The drug is used parenterally as an antihypertensive agent (see *Diazoxide*).

Contraindications: Functional hypoglycemia, hypersensitivity to diazoxide or thiazides.

Special Concerns: Infants are particularly prone to development of edema. Use with extreme caution in clients with history of gout and in those in whom edema presents a risk (cardiac disease).

Side Effects: *CV:* Sodium and fluid retention (common); precipitation of CHF in clients with compromised cardiac reserve, palpitations, increased HR, hypotension, transient hypertension, chest pain (rare). *Metabolic:* Hyperglycemia, glycosuria, *diabetic ketoacidosis, hyperosmolar nonketotic coma.* *GI:* N&V, diarrhea, transient taste loss, anorexia, ileus, abdominal pain. *CNS:* Weakness, headache, insomnia, extrapyramidal symptoms, dizziness, paresthesia, fever, malaise, anxiety, polyneuritis. *Hematologic:* Thrombocytopenia with or without purpura, eosinophilia, neutropenia, decreased hemoglobin/hematocrit, excessive bleeding, decreased IgG. *Dermatologic:* Skin rashes, hirsutism, herpes, loss of hair from scalp, monilial dermatitis, pruritus. *GU:* Hematuria, decrease in urine production, nephrotic syndrome (reversible), azotemia, albuminuria. *Ophthalmologic:* Blurred or double vision, lacrimation, transient cataracts, ring scotoma, subconjunctival hemorrhage. *Other:* Pancreatitis, *pancreatic necrosis,* galactorrhea, gout, premature aging of bone, polyneuritis, enlargement of lump in breast.

OD **Overdose Management:** *Symptoms:* Hypotension; excessive hyperglycemia. *Treatment:* Insulin to treat hyperglycemia; use Trendelenburg maneuver to reverse hypotension.

Drug Interactions
Alpha-adrenergic blocking agents / ↓ Effect of diazoxide
Anticoagulants, oral / ↑ Effect of anticoagulant due to ↓ plasma protein binding

Antihypertensives / Excessive ↓ BP due to additive effects
Phenothiazines / ↑ Effects of diazoxide, including hyperglycemia
Phenytoin / ↓ Effect of phenytoin due to ↑ breakdown by liver
Sulfonylureas / ↓ Effect of both drugs
Thiazide diuretics / ↑ Hyperglycemic and hyperuricemic effects; hypotension may occur.

Laboratory Test Interferences: ↑ Serum uric acid, AST, alkaline phosphatase; ↓ creatinine clearance.

Dosage
• **Capsules, Oral Suspension**
Diabetes.
Dosage is individualized on the basis of blood glucose level and response of client. **Adults and children, usual, initial:** 1 mg/kg q 8 hr (adjust according to response); **maintenance:** 3–8 mg/kg/day divided into two or three equal doses q 8–12 hr. **Infants and newborns, initial:** 3.3 mg/kg q 8 hr (adjust according to response); **maintenance:** 8–15 mg/kg/day divided into two or three equal doses q 8–12 hr.

RESPIRATORY CARE CONSIDERATIONS
Administration/Storage:
1. Blood glucose levels and urinary glucose and ketones must be monitored carefully until stabilized, which usually takes 1 week. The drug is discontinued if a satisfactory effect has not been established within 2–3 weeks.
2. Have available insulin and IV fluids to counteract possible ketoacidosis.
3. The drug should be taken on a regular basis with no doses skipped and no extra doses taken.
4. The suspension should be protected from light.
Assessment
1. Document indications for therapy and time frame for anticipated results.
2. Note any sensitivity to thiazides.
3. Determine any history of gout or CAD.

Interventions
1. If the client has a history of CHF, observe carefully for fluid retention, which could precipitate heart failure.
2. If currently taking an antihypertensive agent, monitor BP for potentiation of antihypertensive effect.
3. Observe for ecchymosis, petechiae, or frank bleeding. These symptoms should be reported as they may require discontinuation of the drug.
4. If the client has had an overdosage of drug, observe closely for the first 7 days until blood sugar level is again within normal limits (80–110 mg/100 mL).
5. If hirsutism develops, reassure that the condition should subside once the drug is discontinued.
6. Review list of drug side effects to determine if clinical presentations may be drug related.

Evaluate: Control of hypoglycemia with restoration of serum glucose levels

---

Dicloxacillin sodium
(dye-klox-ah-**SILL**-in)
Dycill, Dynapen, Pathocil **(Rx)**
Classification: Antibiotic, penicillin

See also *Anti-Infectives* and *Penicillins.*
Action/Kinetics: This drug is penicillinase-resistant and acid-resistant. **Peak serum levels: IM, PO,** 4–20 mcg/mL after 1 hr. **t½:** 40 min. Chiefly excreted in urine.
Uses: Resistant staphylococcal infections. To initiate therapy in any suspected staphylococcal infection. Infections due to Streptococcus pneumoniae.
Contraindications: Treatment of meningitis.

Dosage ───────────
• **Capsules, Oral Suspension**
Skin and soft tissue infections, mild to moderate URTIs.
Adults and children over 40 kg: 125 mg q 6 hr; **pediatric:** 12.5

mg/kg/day in four equal doses given q 6 hr.
Lower respiratory tract infections or disseminated infections.
Adults and children over 40 kg: 250 mg q 6 hr, up to a maximum of 4 g/day; **pediatric:** 12–25 mg/kg/day in four equal doses given q 6 hr. Dosage not established for the newborn.

RESPIRATORY CARE CONSIDERATIONS

See also *General Respiratory Care Considerations for All Anti-Infectives* and *Penicillins.*

Administration/Storage
1. To prepare PO suspension, shake container to loosen powder, measure water for reconstitution as indicated on label, add half of the water, and immediately shake vigorously because usual handling may cause lumps. Add the remainder of the water and again shake vigorously.
2. Shake well before pouring each dose.
3. The reconstituted PO solution is stable for 7 days at room temperature, 10 days if refrigerated, and 21 days if frozen.
4. Give at least 1 hr before meals or no sooner than 2–3 hr after a meal with a full glass of water.

Assessment
1. Note indications for therapy and onset and duration of symptoms.
2. Determine that lab cultures are performed prior to therapy.

Evaluate
• Reports of symptomatic relief
• Negative lab culture reports

Digitoxin
(dih-jih-**TOX**-in)
Pregnancy Category: C
Crystodigin, Digitaline ✦ **(Rx)**
Classification: Cardiac glycoside

See also *Cardiac Glycosides.*
Action/Kinetics: Most potent of the digitalis glycosides. Its slow onset of action makes it unsuitable for emer-

---

gency use. Almost completely absorbed from GI tract. **Onset: PO,** 1–4 hr; maximum effect: 8–12 hr. **t½:** 5–9 days; **Duration:** 2 weeks. Significant protein binding (over 90%). Metabolized by the liver and excreted as inactive metabolites through the urine. **Therapeutic serum levels:** 14–26 ng/mL. Withhold drug and check with physician if serum level exceeds 35 ng/mL, indicating toxicity.

Uses: Drug of choice for maintenance in CHF.

Special Concerns: Digitalis tablets may not be suitable for small children; thus, other digitalis products should be considered.

Additional Drug Interactions

Aminoglutethimide / ↓ Effect of digitoxin due to ↑ breakdown by liver

Barbiturates / ↓ Effect of digitoxin due to ↑ breakdown by liver

Diltiazem / May ↑ serum levels of digitoxin

Phenylbutazone / ↓ Effect of digitoxin due to ↑ breakdown by liver

Phenytoin / ↓ Effect of digitoxin due to ↑ breakdown by liver

Quinidine / May ↑ serum levels of digitoxin

Rifampin / ↓ Effect of digitoxin due to ↑ breakdown by liver

Verapamil / May ↑ serum levels of digitoxin

Dosage —————————
• **Tablets**
  Digitalizing (loading) dose: Rapid.
Adults: 0.6 mg followed by 0.4 mg in 4–6 hr; **then,** 0.2 mg q 4–6 hr until therapeutic effect achieved.
  Digitalizing (loading) dose: Slow.
Adults: 0.2 mg b.i.d. for 4 days.
  Digitalizing (loading) dose: children.
After the neonatal period, the doses are as follows: **Under one year:** 0.045 mg/kg/day divided into three, four, or more doses with 6 hr between doses; **one to two years:** 0.04 mg/kg/day divided into three, four, or more doses with 6 hr between doses; **over two years:** 0.03

mg/kg/day (0.75 mg/m²) divided into three, four, or more doses with 6 hr between doses.
  Maintenance dose: PO.
Adults: 0.05–0.3 mg/day (**usual:** 0.15 mg/day). **Children:** Give one-tenth of the digitalizing dose.

RESPIRATORY CARE CONSIDERATIONS

See also *Respiratory Care Considerations* for *Cardiac Glycosides.*

Administration/Storage
1. Incompatible with acids and alkali.
2. Protect from light.
3. Premature and immature infants are especially sensitive to digitoxin and require a decreased dose that must be determined carefully.

Evaluate
• Control of S&S of CHF
• Serum digitoxin level within desired range (14–26 ng/mL)

—————————————————————

Digoxin
(dih-**JOX**-in)
Pregnancy Category: A
Lanoxicaps, Lanoxin, Novo–Digoxin
★ **(Rx)**
Classification: Cardiac glycoside

—————————————————————

See also *Cardiac Glycosides.*
Action/Kinetics: Action prompter and shorter than that of digitoxin. **Onset: PO,** 0.5–2 hr; **time to peak effect:** 2–6 hr. **Duration:** Over 24 hr. **Onset, IV:** 5–30 min; **time to peak effect:** 1–4 hr. **Duration:** 6 days. **t½:** 30–40 hr. **Therapeutic serum level:** 0.5–2.0 ng/mL. From 20% to 25% is protein bound. Serum levels above 2.5 ng/mL indicate toxicity. Fifty percent to 70% is excreted unchanged by the kidneys. Bioavailability depends on the dosage form: tablets (60%–80%), capsules (90%–100%), and elixir (70%–85%). Thus, changing dosage forms may require dosage adjustments.

Uses: May be drug of choice for CHF because of rapid onset, relatively short duration, and ability to be administered PO or IV.

OD **Overdose   Management:**
Treatment: Use digoxin immune Fab
(see what follows).
Additional Drug Interactions
1. The following drugs increase serum digoxin levels, leading to possible toxicity: Aminoglycosides, amiodarone, anticholinergics, benzodiazepines,   captopril,   diltiazem,
erythromycin, esmolol, flecainide,
hydroxychloroquine, ibuprofen, indomethacin, nifedipine, quinidine,
quinine, tetracyclines, tolbutamide,
verapamil.
2. Disopyramide may alter the pharmacologic effect of digoxin.
3. Penicillamine decreases serum digoxin levels.

Dosage
• **Capsules**
   Digitalization: Rapid.
Adults: 0.4–0.6 mg initially followed
by 0.1–0.3 mg q 6–8 hr until desired
effect achieved.
   Digitalization: Slow.
Adults: A total of 0.05–0.35 mg/day
divided in two doses for a period of
7–22 days to reach steady-state serum
levels. **Pediatric.** Digitalizing dosage is divided into three or more
doses with the initial dose being
about one-half the total dose; doses
are given q 4–8 hr. **Children, 10
years and older:** 0.008–0.012
mg/kg. **5–10 years:** 0.015–0.03
mg/kg. **2–5 years:** 0.025–0.035
mg/kg. **1 month–2 years:** 0.03–0.05
mg/kg. **Neonates, full-term:**
0.02–0.03 mg/kg. **Neonates, premature:** 0.015–0.025 mg/kg.
   Maintenance.
Adults: 0.05–0.35 mg once or twice
daily. **Premature neonates:**
20%–30% of total digitalizing dose
divided and given in two to three
daily doses. **Neonates to 10 years:**
25%–35% of the total digitalizing
dose divided and given in two to
three daily doses.
• **Elixir, Tablets**
   Digitalization: Rapid.
Adults: A total of 0.75–1.25 mg divid-

ed into two or more doses each giv-
en at 6–8-hr intervals.
   Digitalization: Slow.
Adults: 0.125–0.5 mg/day for 7
days. **Pediatric.** (Digitalizing dose is
divided into two or more doses and
given at 6–8-hr intervals.) **Children,
10 years and older, rapid or slow:**
Same as adult dose. **5–10 years:**
0.02–0.035 mg/kg. **2–5 years:**
0.03–0.05 mg/kg. **1 month–2 years:**
0.035–0.06 mg/kg. **Premature and
newborn infants to 1 month:**
0.02–0.035 mg/kg.
   Maintenance.
Adults: 0.125–0.5 mg/day. **Pediatric:** One-fifth to one-third the total
digitalizing dose daily. *NOTE:* An alternate regimen (referred to as the
"small-dose" method)   is   0.017
mg/kg/day. This dose causes less
toxicity.
• **IV**
   Digitalization.
Adults: Same as tablets. **Maintenance:** 0.125–0.5 mg/day in divided
doses or as a single dose. **Pediatric:**
Same as tablets.

RESPIRATORY CARE
CONSIDERATIONS

See also *Respiratory Care Considerations* for *Cardiac Glycosides.*
Administration/Storage
1. IV injections should be given
over 5 min (or longer) either undiluted or diluted fourfold or greater with
sterile water for injection, 0.9% sodium   chloride   injection,   lactated
Ringer's injection, or 5% dextrose injection.
2. Lanoxicaps gelatin capsules are
more bioavailable than tablets. Thus,
the 0.05-mg capsule is equivalent to
the 0.0625-mg tablet; the 0.1-mg
capsule is equivalent to the 0.125-
mg tablet, and the 0.2-mg capsule is
equivalent to the 0.25-mg tablet.
3. Differences   in   bioavailability
have been noted between products;
thus, clients should be monitored
when changing from one product to
another.
4. Protect from light.

Evaluate

- Control of S&S of CHF (↑ CO, ↓ HR, ↑ urine output, ↓ rales, ↓ weight)
- Therapeutic serum digoxin level (0.5–2.0 ng/mL)

D

Digoxin Immune Fab (Ovine)

(dih-**JOX**-in)
Pregnancy Category: C
Digibind **(Rx)**
Classification: Digoxin antidote

Action/Kinetics: Digoxin immune Fab are antibodies that bind to digoxin. The antibody is produced in sheep by immunization with digoxin bound to human albumin. In cases of digoxin toxicity, the antibodies can bind to digoxin and the complex is excreted through the kidneys. As serum levels of digoxin decrease, digoxin bound to tissue is released into the serum to maintain equilibrium and this is then bound and excreted. The net result is a decrease in both tissue and serum digoxin. **Onset:** Less than 1 min. Improvement in signs of toxicity occurs within 30 min. t½: 15–20 hr (after IV administration). Each vial contains 38 mg of pure digoxin immune Fab, which will bind approximately 0.5 mg digoxin or digitoxin.

Uses: Life-threatening digoxin or digitoxin toxicity or overdosage. Symptoms of toxicity include severe sinus bradycardia, second- or third-degree heart block which does not respond to atropine, ventricular tachycardia, ventricular fibrillation.

NOTE: Cardiac arrest can be expected if a healthy adult ingests more than 10 mg digoxin or a healthy child ingests more than 4 mg. Also, steady-state serum concentrations of digoxin greater than 10 ng/mL or potassium concentrations greater than 5 mEq/L as a result of digoxin therapy require use of digoxin immune Fab.

Special Concerns: Use with caution during lactation. Use in infants only if benefits outweigh risks. Clients sensitive to products of sheep origin may also be sensitive to digoxin immune Fab. Skin testing may be appropriate for high-risk clients.

Side Effects: *CV:* Worsening of CHF or low CO, atrial fibrillation (all due to withdrawal of the effects of digoxin). *Other:* Hypokalemia. Rarely, hypersensitivity reactions occur, including fever and *anaphylaxis.*

Dosage

- **IV**

Dosage depends on the serum digoxin concentration. A large dose has a faster onset but there is an increased risk of allergic or febrile reactions. The package insert should be carefully consulted. **Adults, usual:** Six vials (228 mg) is usuallly enough to reverse most cases of toxicity. **Children, less than 20 kg:** A single vial (38 mg) should be sufficient.

RESPIRATORY CARE CONSIDERATIONS

Administration/Storage

1. The lyophilized material should be reconstituted with 4 mL of sterile water for injection to give a concentration of 10 mg/mL. If small doses are required (e.g., in infants), reconstituted antibody can be further diluted with 36 mL sterile isotonic saline to obtain a concentration of 1 mg/mL.
2. The reconstituted antibody should be used immediately. However, it may be stored for up to 4 hr at 2°C–8°C (36°F–46°F).
3. The dose should be administered over a 30-min period through a 0.22-μm membrane filter. A bolus injection may be used if there is immediate danger of cardiac arrest.
4. The total number of vials of antibody needed can be determined by dividing the total body load (in mg) by the amount of digoxin bound by each vial (0.6 mg).
5. If acute digoxin ingestion results in severe symptoms and a serum concentration is not known, 800 mg (20 vials) of digoxin immune Fab may be given. However, volume overload must be monitored in small children.

6. The dosage in infants should be administered with a tuberculin syringe.

Assessment

1. Determine amount of drug ingested and time of overdose to ensure appropriate dosing (generally a 38-mg vial will bind 0.5 mg of digoxin).

2. Document pretreatment digoxin or digitoxin levels.

3. If previous reaction suspected and in high-risk clients, consider performing skin testing. Prepare a 10-mL solution (0.1 mL of drug in 9.9 mL NSS) and perform an intradermal injection or scratch test. Administer 0.1 mL intradermally or a scratch test may be performed by placing 1 drop of solution on the skin and making a scratch through the drop with a sterile needle; assess site in 20 min. A positive reaction would consist of a urticarial wheal with erythematous surrounding skin. *Do not* use if reaction is positive.

4. Clients with known allergy to sheep proteins should be appropriately identified and this information should be documented in their records. Do not administer digoxin immune Fab to these persons.

5. Evaluate lab data for electrolyte imbalance and correct. Note the presence of hypokalemia or evidence of increased CHF and document.

Interventions

1. Monitor VS and cardiac rhythm. Have epinephrine (1:1,000) available in the event of a hypersensitivity reaction.

2. Wait several days if redigitalization is anticipated to ensure complete elimination of digibind.

3. Anticipate that serum digoxin levels will take 5–7 days to stabilize following treatment, although improvement in S&S of toxicity should be evident in 30 min.

Evaluate

• Resolution of digoxin toxicity with serum levels to within desired range

• Restoration of baseline cardiac rhythm

Diltiazem hydrochloride
(dill-**TIE**-ah-zem)
Pregnancy Category: C
Apo-Diltiaz ✦, Cardizem, Cardizem CD, Cardizem Injectable, Cardizem Lyo-Ject, Cardizem-SR, Dilacor XR, Diltiazem HCl Extended Release, Novo-Diltiazem ✦, Nu-Diltiaz ✦, Syn-Diltiazem ✦, Tiazac **(Rx)**
Classification: Calcium channel blocking agent (antianginal, antihypertensive)

See also *Calcium Channel Blocking Agents.*

Action/Kinetics: Decreases SA and AV conduction and prolongs AV node effective and functional refractory periods. The drug also decreases myocardial contractility and peripheral vascular resistance. **Tablets: Onset,** 30–60 min; **time to peak plasma levels:** 2–3 hr; **t½, first phase:** 20–30 min; **second phase:** about 3–4.5 hr (5–8 hr with high and repetitive doses); **duration:** 4–8 hr. **Extended-Release Capsules: Onset,** 2–3 hr; **time to peak plasma levels:** 6–11 hr; **t½:** 5–7 hr; **duration:** 12 hr. **Therapeutic serum levels:** 0.05–0.2 mcg/mL. Metabolized to desacetyldiltiazem, which manifests 25%–50% of the activity of diltiazem. Excreted through both the bile and urine.

Uses: Tablets: Vasospastic angina (Prinzmetal's variant). Chronic stable angina (classic effort-associated angina), especially in clients who cannot use beta-adrenergic blockers or nitrates or who remain symptomatic after clinical doses of these agents. **Sustained-Release Capsules:** Essential hypertension, angina. **Parenteral:** Atrial fibrillation or flutter. Paroxysmal SVT. Cardizem Lyo-Ject is used on an emergency basis for atrial fibrillation or atrial flutter. *Investigational:* Prophylaxis of reinfarction of nonQ wave MI; tardive dyskinesia, Raynaud's syndrome.

Contraindications: Hypotension. Second- or third-degree AV block and sick sinus syndrome except in presence of a functioning ventricular pacemaker. Acute MI, pulmonary congestion. Lactation.

Special Concerns: Safety and effectiveness in children have not been determined. The half-life may be increased in geriatric clients. Use with caution in hepatic disease and in CHF. Abrupt withdrawal may cause an increase in the frequency and duration of chest pain. Use with beta blockers or digitalis is usually well tolerated, although the effects of coadministration cannot be predicted (especially in clients with left ventricular dysfunction or cardiac conduction abnormalities).

Side Effects: *CV:* AV block, bradycardia, CHF, hypotension, syncope, palpitations, peripheral edema, *arrhythmias,* angina, tachycardia, *abnormal ECG, ventricular extrasystoles.* *GI:* N&V, diarrhea, constipation, anorexia, abdominal discomfort, cramps, dry mouth, dysgeusia. *CNS:* Weakness, nervousness, dizziness, lightheadedness, headache, depression, psychoses, hallucinations, disturbances in sleep, somnolence, insomnia, amnesia, abnormal dreams. *Dermatologic:* Rashes, dermatitis, pruritus, urticaria, erythema multiforme, *Stevens-Johnson syndrome.* *Other:* Photosensitivity, joint pain or stiffness, flushing, nasal or chest congestion, dyspnea, SOB, nocturia/polyuria, sexual difficulties, weight gain, paresthesia, tinnitus, tremor, asthenia, gynecomastia, gingival hyperplasia, petechiae, ecchymosis, purpura, bruising, hematoma, leukopenia, double vision, epistaxis, eye irritation, thirst, alopecia, *bundle branch block,* abnormal gait, hyperglycemia.

Additional Drug Interactions
Anesthetics / ↑ Risk of depression of cardiac contractility, conductivity, and automaticity as well as vascular dilation
Carbamazepine / ↑ Effect of diltiazem due to ↓ breakdown by liver

Cimetidine / ↑ Bioavailability of diltiazem
Cyclosporine / ↑ Effect of cyclosporine possibly leading to renal toxicity
Digoxin / ↑ Serum digoxin levels are possible
Lithium / ↑ Risk of neurotoxicity
Ranitidine / ↑ Bioavailability of diltiazem
Theophyllines / ↑ Risk of pharmacologic and toxicologic effects of theophyllines

Laboratory Test Interferences: ↑ Alkaline phosphatase, CPK, LDH, AST, ALT.

Dosage ——————————————
• **Tablets**
  Angina.
Adults, initial: 30 mg q.i.d. before meals and at bedtime; **then,** increase gradually to total daily dose of 180–360 mg (given in three to four divided doses). Increments may be made q 1–2 days until the optimum response is attained.
• **Capsules, Sustained-Release**
  Angina.
Cardizem CD: Adults, initial: 120 or 180 mg once daily. Up to 480 mg/day may be required. Dosage adjustments should be carried out over a 7–14-day period.
Dilacor XR: Adults, initial: 120 mg once daily; **then,** dose may be titrated, depending on the needs of the client, up to 480 mg once daily. Titration may be carried out over a 7–14-day period.
  Hypertension.
Cardizem CD: Adults, initial: 180–240 mg once daily. Maximum antihypertensive effect usually reached within 14 days. Usual range is 240–360 mg once daily.
Cardizem SR: Adults, initial: 60–120 mg b.i.d.; **then,** when maximum antihypertensive effect is reached (approximately 14 days), adjust dosage to a range of 240–360 mg/day.
Dilacor XR: Adults, initial: 180–240 mg once daily. Usual range is 180–480 mg once daily. The dose may be increased to 540 mg/day

with little or no increased risk of side effects.

Tiazac: Adults, initial: 120–240 mg once daily. Usual range is 120–360 mg once daily, although doses up to 540 mg once daily have been used.

- **IV Bolus**

    Atrial fibrillation/flutter; paroxysmal SVT.

Adults, initial: 0.25 mg/kg (average 20 mg) given over 2 min; **then,** if response is inadequate, a second dose may be given after 15 min. The second bolus dose is 0.35 mg/kg (average 25 mg) given over 2 min. Subsequent doses should be individualized. Some clients may respond to an initial dose of 0.15 mg/kg (duration of action may be shorter).

- **IV Infusion**

    Atrial fibrillation/flutter.

Adults: 10 mg/hr following IV bolus dose(s) of 0.25 mg/kg or 0.35 mg/kg. Some clients may require 5 mg/hr while others may require 15 mg/hr. Infusion may be maintained for 24 hr.

- **Cardizem Lyo-Ject**

    Atrial fibrillation/atrial flutter.

Delivery system consists of a dual-chamber, prefilled, calibrated syringe containing 25 mg of diltiazem hydrochloride in one chamber and 5 mL of diluent in the other chamber.

RESPIRATORY CARE CONSIDERATIONS

See also *Respiratory Care Considerations* for *Calcium Channel Blocking Agents.*

Administration/Storage

1. Sublingual nitroglycerin may be taken concomitantly for acute angina.
2. Diltiazem may be taken together with long-acting nitrates.
3. The sustained-release capsules should be taken on an empty stomach.
4. Sustained-release capsules should not be opened, chewed, or crushed and should be swallowed whole.
5. Clients taking other forms of diltiazem can be safely switched to Dilacor XR at the nearest equivalent to-

tal daily dose. Titration to larger or smaller doses may be necessary.

6. Use with beta blockers or digitalis is usually well tolerated, but the combined effects cannot be predicted, especially in clients with cardiac conduction abnormalities or LV dysfunction.
7. The infusion may be maintained for up to 24 hr. Use for more than 24 hr is not recommended.
8. May be administered by direct IV over 2 min or as an infusion (see *Dosage*). For IV infusion, the drug may be mixed with NSS, 5% dextrose, or 5% dextrose and 0.45% NaCl.
9. The injection should be refrigerated at 2°C–8°C (36°F–46°F). The solution may be stored at room temperature for 1 month, after which any remaining solution should be destroyed.

Assessment

1. Document indications for therapy, onset of symptoms, and previous treatment modalities.
2. Note any evidence of peripheral edema or CHF.
3. Review ECG for any evidence of AV block.
4. Obtain baseline lab studies and note any evidence of hepatic and/or renal dysfunction.
5. Anticipate reduced dosage of diltiazem in clients with impaired renal or hepatic function.
6. The plasma half-life of the drug may be prolonged in elderly clients. Therefore, monitor these clients closely.

Evaluate

- ↓ Frequency and intensity of vasospastic anginal attacks
- ↓ BP
- Restoration of stable cardiac rhythm

Diphenhydramine hydrochloride

(dye-fen-**HY**-drah-meen)

Pregnancy Category: B

Allerdryl ✿, AllerMax, Allernix ✿, Beldin Cough, Belix, Bena-D 50, Benadryl, Benadryl Complete Allergy, Benadryl Dye-Free Allergy Medication, Ben-Allergin-50, Benylin Cough, Benaphen, Bydramine Cough, Diahist, Dihydrex, Diphenacen-10, Diphenadryl, Diphen Cough, Fenylhist, Fynex, Hydril, Hyrexin-50, Nauzene Maximum Strength, Noradryl, Nordryl, Nordryl Cough, Nytol ✿, Nytol Extra Strength ✿, PMS-Diphenhydramine ✿, Sleep-Eze D ✿, Sleep-Eze D Extra Strength ✿, Tusstat, Valdrene (OTC and Rx). **Sleep-Aids:** Dormin, Miles Nervine, Nytol, Sleep-eze 3, Sleep-Eze D ✿, Sleepwell 2-nite, Sominex **(OTC)**

Classification: Antihistamine, ethanolamine-type; antiemetic

See also *Antihistamines*.

Additional Use: Treatment of parkinsonism in geriatric clients unable to tolerate more potent drugs. Also for mild parkinsonism in other age groups. Drug-induced extrapyramidal symptoms. Motion sickness, antiemetic, as a sleep-aid. Coughs, including those due to allergy.

Dosage _____

• **Capsules, Chewable Tablets, Elixir, Syrup, Tablets**

Antihistamine, antiemetic, antimotion sickness, parkinsonism.

Adults: 25–50 mg t.i.d.–q.i.d.; **pediatric, over 9.1 kg:** 12.5–25 mg t.i.d.–q.i.d. (or 5 mg/kg/day not to exceed 300 mg/day or 150 mg/m²/day).

Sleep aid.

Adults: 50 mg at bedtime.

Antitussive.

Adults: 25 mg q 4 hr, not to exceed 150 mg/day; **pediatric, 6–12 years:** 12.5–25 mg q 4–6 hr, not to exceed 75 mg/day; **pediatric, 2–6 years:** 6.25 mg q 4–6 hr, not to exceed 25 mg/day.

• **IV, Deep IM**

Parkinsonism.

Adults: 10–50 mg up to 100 mg if needed (not to exceed 400 mg/day); **pediatric:** 1.25 mg/kg (or 37.5 mg/m²) q.i.d., not to exceed a total of 300 mg/day.

RESPIRATORY CARE CONSIDERATIONS

See also *Respiratory Care Considerations* for *Antihistamines*

Administration/Storage

1. When using for motion sickness, the full prophylactic dose should be administered 30 min prior to travel and preferably 1–2 hr before exposures that precipitate sickness.

2. Similar doses should also be taken with meals and at bedtime.

3. Determine client symptoms that necessitate drug administration and note as drug has multiple indications.

4. Should not be used for more than 2 weeks to treat insomnia.

5. For IV administration, may give undiluted with each 25 mg over at least 1 min.

Evaluate

• ↓ Allergic manifestations
• Relief of nausea in motion sickness
• Control of cough
• Promotion of sleep
• Relief of dyskinesias and extrapyramidal symptoms with parkinsonism

Dirithromycin

(die-**rih**-throw-**MY**- sin)
Pregnancy Category: C
Dynabac **(Rx)**
Classification: Antibiotic, macrolide

Action/Kinetics: Dirithromycin is a semisynthetic macrolide antibiotic that is actually a prodrug; it is rapidly absorbed and converted during intestinal absorption to the active erythromycylamine. The drug is distributed throughout the body, including the lungs, GI tract, skin, soft tissues, and GU tract. Erythromycylamine acts by binding to the 50S ribosomal subunits of microorganisms, resulting in inhibition of protein synthesis. t½: 2–36 hr. From 81% to 97% of erythromycylamine is excreted in the feces via the bile.

Uses: Acute bacterial exacerbations of chronic bronchitis due to *Moraxella catarrhalis* or *Streptococcus pneu-*

moniae. Secondary bacterial infections of acute bronchitis due to *M. catarrhalis* or *S. pneumoniae.* Community-acquired pneumonia due to *Legionella pneumophila, Mycoplasma pneumoniae,* or *S. pneumoniae.* Pharyngitis or tonsillitis due to *Streptococcus pyogenes.* Uncomplicated infections of the skin and skin structures due to Staphylococcus aureus.

Contraindications: Hypersensitivity to erythromycin or any other macrolide antibiotic. Use in children less than 12 years of age. Use in clients with known, suspected, or potential bacteremias since serum levels of the drug are not high enough in the serum to be effective. Use for the empiric treatment of acute bacterial exacerbations of chronic or secondary bacterial infections of acute bronchitis or for empiric treatment of uncomplicated skin and skin structure infections.

Special Concerns: Although dirithromycin eradicates *S. pyogenes* from the nasopharynx, data are lacking as to its effectiveness in preventing rheumatic fever. Use with caution during lactation. Safety and efficacy have not been determined in children less than 12 years of age.

Side Effects: *GI:* ***Pseudomembranous colitis,*** abdominal pain, nausea, diarrhea, vomiting, dyspepsia, GI disorder, flatulence, abnormal stools, constipation, dry mouth, gastritis, gastroenteritis, mouth ulceration, taste perversion, thirst. *CNS:* Headache, dizziness, vertigo, insomnia, anxiety, depression, nervousness, paresthesia, somnolence. *CV:* Palpitation, vasodilation, syncope. *GU:* Dysmenorrhea, urinary frequency, vaginal moniliasis, vaginitis. *Dermatologic:* Rash, pruritus, urticaria, sweating. *Respiratory:* Increased cough, dyspnea, hyperventilation. *Miscellaneous:* Nonspecific pain, asthenia, anorexia, dehydration, edema, epistaxis, eye disorder, fever, flu syndrome, hemoptysis, malaise, peripheral edema, ***allergic reaction,*** amblyopia, eye disorder, myalgia, neck pain, tinnitus, tremor.

OD **Overdose Management:** *Symptoms:* N&V, epigastric distress, diarrhea. *Treatment:* Treat symptoms.

Drug Interactions: The absorption of dirithromycin is slightly enhanced when the drug is given with either antacids or H-2 antagonists.

Laboratory Test Interferences: ↑ ALT, AST, alkaline phosphatase, potassium, CPK, bands, segs, basophils, eosinophils, platelet count, total bilirubin, creatinine, GGT, leukocyte count, lymphocytes, monocytes, phosphorus, uric acid. ↓ Bicarbonate, albumin, chloride, hematocrit, hemoglobin, neutrophils, phosphorus, platelet count, total protein.

Dosage ⎯⎯⎯⎯⎯⎯⎯
• **Tablets, Enteric-Coated**
   Acute bacterial exacerbations of chronic bronchitis.
Adults and children over 12 years of age: 500 mg once a day for 7 days.
   Secondary bacterial infection of acute bronchitis.
Adults and children over 12 years of age: 500 mg once a day for 7 days.
   Community-acquired pneumonia.
Adults and children over 12 years of age: 500 mg once a day for 14 days.
   Pharyngitis or tonsillitis.
Adults and children over 12 years of age: 500 mg once a day for 10 days.
   Uncomplicated skin and skin structure infections.
Adults and children over 12 years of age: 500 mg once a day for 7 days.

RESPIRATORY CARE CONSIDERATIONS

See also *General Respiratory Care Considerations for All Anti-infectives and erythromycins.*

Administration/Storage

1. Dirithromycin should be given with food or within 1 hr of having eaten.

2. The enteric-coated tablets should not be cut, chewed, or crushed.

Assessment

1. Document indications for therapy and type, onset, and duration of symptoms.

2. Ensure that appropriate cultures have been obtained for C&S prior to initiating therapy and assess carefully for development of superinfection.

3. Although dirithromycin does not appear to cause cardiovascular problems when taken with certain antihistamines (e.g., terfenadine), caution should still be exercised.

Evaluate

- Resolution of infection
- Negative lab culture reports

Disopyramide phosphate

(dye-so-**PEER**-ah-myd)

Pregnancy Category: C

Norpace, Norpace CR, Rythmodan ✽, Rythmodan-LA ✽ **(Rx)**

Classification: Antiarrhythmic, class IA

Action/Kinetics: Disopyramide decreases the rate of diastolic depolarization (phase 4), decreases the upstroke velocity (phase 0), increases the action potential duration (of normal cardiac cells), and prolongs the refractory period (phases 2 and 3). It manifests weak anticholinergic effects although it has fewer side effects than quinidine. The drug does not affect BP significantly, and it can be used in digitalized and nondigitalized clients. **Onset:** 30 min. **Peak plasma levels:** 2 hr. **Duration:** average of 6 hr (range 1.5–8 hr). **t½:** 4–10 hr. **Therapeutic serum levels:** 2–4 mcg/mL. Serum levels should not be used to adjust the dose because of variance in protein binding and potential toxicity of unbound drug. **Protein binding:** 40%–60%. The bioavailability of the controlled-release capsules appears to be similar to that of the immediate-release capsules.

Both unchanged drug (50%) and metabolites (30%) are excreted through the urine. Approximately 15% is excreted through the bile.

Uses: Life-threatening ventricular arrhythmias (e.g., sustained ventricular tachycardia). Disopyramide has not been shown to improve survival in clients with ventricular arrhythmias. *Investigational:* Paroxysmal SVT.

Contraindications: Hypersensitivity to drug. Cardiogenic shock, heart failure, heart block (especially preexisting second- and third-degree AV block if no pacemaker is present), congenital QT prolongation, asymptomatic ventricular premature contractions, sick sinus syndrome, glaucoma, urinary retention, myasthenia gravis. Use of controlled-release capsules in clients with severe renal insufficiency. Lactation.

Special Concerns: Safe use during childhood, labor, and delivery has not been established. Use with caution in Wolff-Parkinson-White syndrome or bundle branch block. Dosage should be decreased in impaired hepatic function. Geriatric clients may be more sensitive to the anticholinergic effects of this drug. The drug may be ineffective in hypokalemia and toxic in hyperkalemia.

Side Effects: *Increased risk of death when used in clients with non-life-threatening cardiac arrhythmias.* CV: Hypotension, CHF, *worsening of arrhythmias,* edema, weight gain, cardiac conduction disturbances, SOB, syncope, chest pain, AV block, *severe myocardial depression (with hypotension and increased venous pressure).* Anticholinergic: Dry mouth, urinary retention, constipation, blurred vision, dry nose, eyes, and throat. GU: Urinary frequency and urgency, urinary retention, impotence, dysuria. GI: Nausea, pain, flatulence, anorexia, diarrhea, vomiting, severe epigastric pain. CNS: Headache, nervousness, dizziness, fatigue, depression, insomnia, psychoses. Dermatologic: Rash, dermatoses, itching. Other: Fever, respiratory problems, gynecomastia, *anaphylaxis,* malaise, muscle weakness, numbness, tingling, angle-closure glaucoma, hypoglyce-mia, reversible cholestatic jaundice, symptoms of lupus erythematosus (usually in clients switched to dis-opyramide from procainamide).

OD **Overdose Management:** *Symptoms:* Apnea, loss of conscious-ness, **cardiac arrhythmias** (widening of QRS complex and QT interval, con-duction disturbances), hypotension, bradycardia, anticholinergic symp-toms, **loss of spontaneous respiration, death.** *Treatment:* Induction of vom-iting, gastric lavage, or a cathartic followed by activated charcoal. Monitor ECG. IV isoproterenol, IV dopamine, cardiac glycosides, diu-retics, intra-aortic balloon counter-pulsation, assisted ventilation, he-modialysis. Use endocardial pacing to treat AV block and neostigmine to treat anticholinergic symptoms.

Drug Interactions
Anticoagulants / ↓ PT after discon-tinuing disopyramide
Beta-adrenergic blockers / Possible ↓ clearance of disopyramide; sinus bradycardia, hypotension
Digoxin / ↑ Serum digoxin levels (may be beneficial)
Erythromycin / ↑ Disopyramide lev-els → arrhythmias and ↑ QTc inter-vals
Phenytoin / ↓ Effect due to ↑ breakdown by liver; ↑ anticholiner-gic effects
Quinidine / ↑ Disopyramide serum levels or ↓ quinidine levels
Rifampin / ↓ Effect due to ↑ break-down by liver
Laboratory Test Interferences: ↑ Creatinine, BUN, cholesterol, triglyce-rides, and liver enzymes.

Dosage ———————————
• **Immediate-Release Capsules**
    Antiarrhythmic.
Adults, initial loading dose: 300 mg of immediate-release capsule (200 mg if client weighs less than 50 kg); **maintenance:** 400–800 mg/day in four divided doses (usual: 150 mg q 6 hr). **For clients less than 50 kg, maintenance:** 100 mg q 6 hr.

Children, less than 1 year: 10–30 mg/kg/day in divided doses q 6 hr; **1–4 years of age:** 10–20 mg/kg/day in divided doses q 6 hr; **4–12 years of age:** 10–15 mg/kg/day in divided doses q 6 hr; **12–18 years of age:** 6–15 mg/kg/day in divided doses q 6 hr.
    Severe refractory tachycardia.
Up to 400 mg q 6 hr may be re-quired.
    Cardiomyopathy.
Do not administer a loading dose; give 100 mg q 6 hr of immediate-re-lease or 200 mg q 12 hr for con-trolled-release.
• **Extended-Release Capsules**
    Antiarrhythmic, *maintenance only.*
Adults: 300 mg q 12 hr (200 mg q 12 hr for body weight less than 50 kg).
    NOTE: For all uses, dosage must be decreased in clients with renal or hepatic insufficiency.
    Moderate renal failure or hepatic failure.
100 mg q 6 hr (or 200 mg/12 hr of sustained-release form).
    Severe renal failure.
100 mg q 8–24 hr depending on se-verity (with or without an initial loading dose of 150 mg).

RESPIRATORY CARE CONSIDERATIONS

See also *Respiratory Care Considera-tions* for *Antiarrhythmic Agents.*
Administration/Storage
1. Administer drug only after ECG assessment has been done.
2. Use with other antiarrhythmics (e.g., class IA or propranolol) should be reserved for life-threatening ar-rhythmias unresponsive to a single agent.
3. The controlled-release capsule should not be used for initial dos-age. These are intended for mainte-nance therapy.
4. When the client is being trans-ferred from the regular PO capsule, the first controlled-release capsule should be given 6 hr after the last regular dose.

5. For children, a 1–10-mg/mL suspension may be made by adding the contents of the immediate-release capsule (the controlled-release capsule should not be used) to cherry syrup. The syrup is stable for 1 month if refrigerated. The syrup should be shaken thoroughly before use and dispensed in an amber bottle.

Assessment

1. Document indications for therapy and type and onset of symptoms.
2. If client has been taking other antiarrhythmic agents, identify and document response to that therapy.
3. Assess for any evidence of hypersensitivity to the drug.
4. Note any client complaint of dribbling urine, frequency of voiding, or sensation of bladder fullness. The condition may worsen once the client begins taking disopyramide.
5. Determine serum potassium levels and, if low, take corrective measures before initiating therapy.
6. Ensure that baseline ECG is available for comparison.

Interventions

1. Clients who have been receiving other antiarrhythmic agents and who are now being placed on disopyramide therapy need to be monitored closely for anticholinergic side effects.
2. Monitor BP frequently for hypotensive effect. Clients with poor LV function are more likely to develop hypotension and require close monitoring.
3. If the client is receiving the drug in the hospital, monitor ECG for QRS widening and QT prolongation. If this occurs, the drug should be discontinued.
4. Report symptoms of CHF, such as cough, dyspnea, moist rales, and cyanosis.
5. Monitor serum potassium levels to ensure effective response to disopyramide. Hyperkalemia increases drug toxicity.
6. Assess I&O and weights. Question clients about urinary hesitancy, difficulty voiding, or a sense of not completely emptying the bladder. This is particularly important in men

with prostatic hypertrophy and in elderly clients who have had prior urinary tract problems; palpate bladder if hesitancy is severe.
7. If the ECG shows a new onset of first-degree heart block, do not administer the drug. Report and anticipate the dosage of drug will be reduced.

Evaluate

• Termination and control of ventricular arrhythmias
• Restoration of stable cardiac rhythm

Disulfiram

(dye-**SUL**-fih-ram)
Antabuse **(Rx)**
Classification: Treatment of alcoholism

Action/Kinetics: Disulfiram produces severe hypersensitivity to alcohol. It is used as an adjunct in the treatment of alcoholism. The toxic reaction to disulfiram appears to be due to the inhibition of liver enzymes that participate in the normal degradation of alcohol. When alcohol and disulfiram are both present, acetaldehyde accumulates in the blood. High levels of acetaldehyde produce a series of symptoms referred to as the disulfiram-alcohol reaction or syndrome. The specific symptoms are listed under *Side Effects*. The symptoms vary individually, are dose-dependent with respect to both alcohol and disulfiram, and persist for periods ranging from 30 min to several hours. A single dose of disulfiram may be effective for 1–2 weeks. **Onset:** May be delayed up to 12 hr because disulfiram is initially localized in fat stores.

Uses: To prevent further ingestion of alcohol in chronic alcoholics. Disulfiram should be given only to cooperating clients fully aware of the consequences of alcohol ingestion.

Contraindications: Alcohol intoxication. Severe myocardial or occlusive coronary disease. Use of paraldehyde or alcohol-containing products such as cough syrups. If client is exposed to ethylene dibromide.

Special Concerns: Use in pregnancy only if benefits outweigh risks. Use with caution in narcotic addicts or clients with diabetes, goiter, epilepsy, psychosis, hypothyroidism, hepatic cirrhosis, or nephritis.

Side Effects: In the absence of alcohol, the following symptoms have been reported: Drowsiness (most common), headache, restlessness, fatigue, psychoses, peripheral neuropathy, dermatoses, hepatotoxicity, metallic or garlic taste, arthropathy, impotence. **In the presence of alcohol,** the following symptoms may be manifested. *CV:* Flushing, chest pain, palpitations, tachycardia, hypotension, syncope, arrhythmias, *CV collapse, MI, acute CHF. CNS:* Throbbing headaches, vertigo, weakness, uneasiness, confusion, unconsciousness, *seizures, death. GI:* Nausea, severe vomiting, thirst. *Respiratory:* Respiratory difficulties, dyspnea, hyperventilation, *respiratory depression. Other:* Throbbing in head and neck, sweating. In the event of an Antabuse-alcohol interaction, measures should be undertaken to maintain BP and treat shock. Oxygen, antihistamines, ephedrine, and/or vitamin C may also be used.

Drug Interactions
Anticoagulants, oral / ↑ Effect of anticoagulants by ↑ hypoprothrombinemia
Barbiturates / ↑ Effect of barbiturates due to ↓ breakdown by liver
Chlordiazepoxide, diazepam / ↑ Effect of chlordiazepoxide or diazepam due to ↓ plasma clearance
Isoniazid / ↑ Side effects of isoniazid (especially CNS)
Metronidazole / Acute toxic psychosis or confusional state
Paraldehyde / Concomitant use produces Antabuse-like effect
Phenytoin / ↑ Effect of phenytoin due to ↓ breakdown by liver
Tricyclic antidepressants / Acute organic brain syndrome

Dosage
• **Tablets**
  Alcoholism.

Adults, initial (after alcohol-free interval of 12–48 hr): 500 mg/day for 1–2 weeks; **maintenance: usual,** 250 mg/day (range: 120–500 mg/day). Dose should not exceed 500 mg/day.

RESPIRATORY CARE CONSIDERATIONS

Administration/Storage
1. Tablets can be crushed or mixed with liquid.
2. Clients should always carry appropriate identification indicating disulfiram is being taken.
3. Have oxygen, pressor agents, and antihistamines available to treat disulfiram-alcohol reactions.

Client/Family Teaching
1. Emphasize to the family that disulfiram should never be given to the client without client's knowledge.
2. Explain the effects of disulfiram and emphasize the need for close medical and psychiatric supervision.
3. If the client experiences CNS side effects, explain that these will lessen as the drug is continued.
4. Ingesting as little as 30 mL of 100-proof alcohol (e.g., one shot) while on disulfiram therapy may cause severe symptoms (within 15 min and last for several hours) and possibly death.
5. Avoid alcohol in any form, in foods, sauces, or other medications, such as cough syrups or tonics. Clients should also be advised to avoid vinegar, paregoric, skin products, liniments, or lotions containing alcohol.
6. Instruct to read carefully all labels on foods before consuming them to avoid those that may contain some form of alcohol.
7. Discuss with clients the fact that they may feel tired, experience drowsiness and headaches, and develop a metallic or garlic-like taste. These side effects tend to subside after about 2 weeks of therapy.
8. Explain to male clients that they may have occasional impotence. This is usually transient. Remind clients that they should discuss this

problem with the provider before discontinuing the medication.

9. If skin eruptions occur, advise client to report since an antihistamine may be prescribed.

10. Advise clients to carry an identification card stating that they are taking disulfiram and describing the symptoms and treatment if clients have a disulfiram reaction. Included should be the name of the person treating the client and a telephone number where the provider may be reached. (Cards may be obtained from the Wyeth-Ayerst Laboratories, P.O. Box 8299, Philadelphia, PA 19101-1245; attention: Professional Services.)

11. Advise client and family to attend meetings of local support groups such as Alcoholics Anonymous (AA) and Al-Anon to gain a better understanding of the disease. These groups offer the support, structure, referral, and encouragement that may help the client in the quest for an alcohol-free life.

Evaluate: Freedom from alcohol and its effects with resultant sobriety

Dobutamine hydrochloride

(doh-**BYOU**-tah-meen)
Pregnancy Category: B
Dobutrex **(Rx)**
Classification: Sympathomimetic drug, direct-acting; cardiac stimulant

See also *Sympathomimetic Drugs.*

Action/Kinetics: Stimulates beta-1 receptors (in the heart), increasing cardiac function, CO, and SV, with minor effects on HR. The drug decreases after load reduction although SBP and pulse pressure may remain unchanged or increase (due to increased CO). Dobutamine also decreases elevated ventricular filling pressure and helps AV node conduction. **Onset:** 1–2 min. **Peak effect:** 10 min. **t½:** 2 min. **Therapeutic plasma levels:** 40–190 ng/mL. Metabolized by the liver and excreted in urine.

Uses: Short-term treatment of cardiac decompensation in adults secondary to depressed contractility due to organic heart disease or cardiac surgical procedures. *Investigational:* Congenital heart disease in children undergoing diagnostic cardiac catheterization.

Contraindications: Idiopathic hypertrophic subaortic stenosis.

Special Concerns: Safe use during childhood or after AMI not established.

Side Effects: *CV:* Marked increase in HR, BP, and *ventricular ectopic activity,* precipitous drop in BP, premature ventricular beats, anginal and nonspecific chest pain, palpitations. *Hypersensitivity:* Skin rash, pruritus of the scalp, fever, eosinophilia, *bronchospasm.* *Other:* Nausea, headache, SOB, fever, phlebitis, and local inflammatory changes at the injection site.

OD **Overdose Management:** *Symptoms:* Excessive alteration of BP, anorexia N&V, tremor, anxiety, palpitations, headache, SOB, anginal and nonspecific chest pain, *myocardial ischemia, ventricular fibrillation or tachycardia.* *Treatment:* Reduce the rate of administration or discontinue temporarily until the condition stabilizes. Establish an airway, ensuring oxygenation and ventilation. Initiate resuscitative measures immediately. Treat severe ventricular tachyarrhythmias with propranolol or lidocaine.

Additional Drug Interactions: Concomitant use with nitroprusside causes ↑ CO and ↓ pulmonary wedge pressure.

Dosage
• **IV Infusion**
Adults, individualized, usual: 2.5–15 mcg/kg/min (up to 40 mcg/kg/min). Rate of administration and duration of therapy depend on response of client, as determined by HR, presence of ectopic activity, BP, and urine flow.

RESPIRATORY CARE CONSIDERATIONS

See also *Respiratory Care Considerations* for *Sympathomimetic Drugs*.

Administration/Storage

1. Reconstitute solution according to directions provided by manufacturer. Dilution process takes place in two stages.

2. The more concentrated solution may be stored in refrigerator for 48 hr and at room temperature for 6 hr. After dilution (in glass or Viaflex containers), the solution is stable for 24 hr at room temperature.

3. Before administration, the solution is diluted further according to the fluid needs of the client. This more dilute solution should be used within 24 hr. Solutions that can be used for further dilution include 5% dextrose injection, 5% dextrose and 0.45% sodium chloride injection, 5% dextrose and 0.9% sodium chloride injection, 10% dextrose injection, Isolyte M 5% dextrose injection, lactated Ringer's injection, 5% dextrose in lactated Ringer's injection, Normosol-M in D5W, 20% Osmitrol in water for injection, 0.9% sodium chloride injection, and sodium lactate injection.

4. Dilute solutions of dobutamine may darken. This does not affect the potency of the drug when used within the time spans detailed above.

5. The drug is incompatible with alkaline solutions. Dobutamine should not be given with agents or diluents containing both sodium bisulfite and ethanol. Dobutamine is physically incompatible with hydrocortisone sodium succinate, cefazolin, cefamandole, neutral cephalothin, penicillin, sodium ethacrynate, and heparin sodium.

6. Dobutamine is compatible when given through common tubing with dopamine, lidocaine, tobramycin, verapamil, nitroprusside, potassium chloride, and protamine sulfate.

7. Have available IV equipment to infuse volume expanders before therapy with dobutamine is started.

8. Medication should be administered using an electronic infusion device. Carefully reconstitute and calculate dosage according to the client's weight and the desired response.

Assessment

1. Document indications for therapy and onset of symptoms.

2. Note other agents prescribed and the outcome.

3. Determine that client is adequately hydrated prior to infusion.

Interventions

1. Be prepared to monitor CVP to assess vascular volume and right-sided cardiac pumping efficiency. The normal range is 5–10 cm water (1–7 mm Hg).

2. An elevated CVP generally indicates disruption of CO, as in pump failure or pulmonary edema. A low CVP may indicate hypovolemia.

3. Be prepared to monitor PAWP to assess the pressures in the left atrium and left ventricle and to measure the efficiency of CO. The usual PAWP range is 6–12 mm Hg.

4. Monitor ECG and BP continuously during drug administration.

5. Obtain written parameters for SBP and titrate infusion as ordered.

6. Monitor and record I&O.

7. Monitor blood sugar in clients with diabetes as an increased insulin dose may be necessary.

Evaluate

• Improved CO and coronary blood flow

• SBP > 90 mm Hg

• ↑ Urinary output

Dopamine hydrochloride

(**DOH**-pah-meen)

Pregnancy Category: C

Intropin, Revimine ✹ **(Rx)**

Classification: Sympathomimetic, direct- and indirect-acting; cardiac stimulant and vasopressor

See also *Sympathomimetic Drugs*.

D

Action/Kinetics: Dopamine is the immediate precursor of epinephrine in the body. Exogenously administered, dopamine produces direct stimulation of beta-1 receptors and variable (dose-dependent) stimulation of alpha receptors (peripheral vasoconstriction). Also, dopamine will cause a release of norepinephrine from its storage sites . These actions result in increased myocardial contraction, CO, and SV, as well as increased renal blood flow and sodium excretion. Exerts little effect on DBP and induces fewer arrhythmias than are seen with isoproterenol. **Onset:** 5 min. **Duration:** 10 min. t½: 2 min. The drug does not cross the blood-brain barrier. Metabolized in liver and excreted in urine.

Uses: Cardiogenic shock due to MI, trauma, endotoxic septicemia, open heart surgery, renal failure, and chronic cardiac decompensation (as in CHF). Clients most likely to respond include those in whom urine flow, myocardial function, and BP have not deteriorated significantly. Best responses are observed when the time is short between onset of symptoms of shock and initiation of dopamine and volume correction. *Investigational:* COPD, CHF, respiratory distress syndrome in infants.

Additional Contraindications: Pheochromocytoma, uncorrected tachycardia or arrhythmias. Pediatric clients.

Special Concerns: Use with caution during lactation. Safety and efficacy have not been established in children. Dosage may have to be adjusted in geriatric clients with occlusive vascular disease.

Additional Side Effects: *CV:* Ectopic heartbeats, tachycardia, anginal pain, palpitations, vasoconstriction, hypotension, hypertension. Infrequently: aberrant conduction, bradycardia, widened QRS complex. *Other:* Dyspnea, headache, mydriasis. Infrequently, piloerection, azotemia, polyuria. High doses may cause mydriasis and ventricular arrhythmia. Extravasation may result in necrosis and sloughing of surrounding tissue.

OD **Overdose Management:** *Symptoms:* Extravasation. *Treatment:* To prevent sloughing and necrosis, infiltrate as soon as possible with 10–15 mL of 0.9 NaCl solution containing 5–10 mg phentolamine using a syringe with a fine needle. Infiltrate liberally throughout the ischemic area.

Additional Drug Interactions
Diuretics / Additive or potentiating effect
Phenytoin / Hypotension and bradycardia
Propranolol / ↓ Effect of dopamine

Dosage —————————
• **IV Infusion**
  Shock.
Initial: 2–5 mcg/kg/min; **then,** increase in increments of 1–4 mcg/kg/min at 10–30-min intervals until desired response is obtained.
  Severely ill clients.
Initial: 5 mcg/kg/min; **then,** increase rate in increments of 5–10 mcg/kg/min up to 20–50 mcg/kg/min as needed.
NOTE: Dopamine is a potent drug. Be sure to dilute the drug before administration. The drug should not be given as a bolus dose.

RESPIRATORY CARE CONSIDERATIONS

See also *Respiratory Care Considerations* for *Sympathomimetic Drugs.*

Administration/Storage
1. Drug must be diluted before use—see package insert.
2. For reconstitution use dextrose or saline solutions: 200 mg/250 mL for a concentration of 0.8 mg/mL or 800 mcg/mL; 400 mg/250 mL for a concentration of 1.6 mg/mL or 1,600 mcg/mL. Alkaline solutions such as 5% sodium bicarbonate, oxidizing agents, or iron salts will inactivate dopamine.
3. Dilute solution is stable for 24 hr at room temperature, although dilution just prior to administration is recommended. Protect from light.
4. To prevent overloading system with excess fluid, clients receiving high doses of dopamine may receive

more concentrated solutions than average.

5. Medication should be administered using an electronic infusion device. Carefully reconstitute and calculate dosage according to the client's weight.

6. When discontinuing the infusion, gradually decrease the dose since sudden cessation may cause marked hypotension.

Assessment

1. Document indications for therapy and onset of symptoms.

2. Determine that client is hydrated prior to initiating infusion.

Interventions

1. Monitor VS and ECG during drug administration.

2. Obtain written parameters for SBP and titrate the infusion as ordered.

3. Monitor I&O. If medication is being administered for renal perfusion, infuse as ordered, usually less than 5 mcg/kg/min.

4. Be prepared to monitor CVP and pulmonary artery wedge pressures.

5. Monitor for ectopic heart beats, palpitations, anginal pain, or vasoconstriction. If these side effects occur, document and report.

Evaluate

• SBP > 90 mm Hg

• Improved organ perfusion and hemodynamics (e.g., ↑ CO, ↑ SV)

• ↑ Urine output

Dornase alfa recombinant

(**DOR**-nace **AL**-fah)
Pregnancy Category: B
Pulmozyme **(Rx)**
Classification: Drug for cystic fibrosis

Action/Kinetics: This drug is a highly purified solution of recombinant human deoxyribonuclease I (rhDNase), an enzyme that selectively cleaves DNA. It is produced by genetically engineered Chinese hamster ovary cells that contain DNA encoded for the native human protein, deoxyribonuclease. The amino acid sequence is identical to that of the native human enzyme. Cystic fibrosis clients have viscous purulent secretions in the airways that contribute to reduced pulmonary function and worsening of infection. These secretions contain high concentrations of extracellular DNA released by degenerating leukocytes that accumulate as a result of infection. Dornase alfa hydrolyzes the DNA in sputum of cystic fibrosis clients, thereby reducing sputum viscoelasticity and reducing infections.

Uses: In cystic fibrosis clients in conjunction with standard therapy to decrease the frequency of respiratory infections that require parenteral antibiotics and to improve pulmonary function.

Contraindications: Use in clients with known sensitivity to dornase alfa or products from Chinese hamster ovary cells.

Special Concerns: Safety and effectiveness of daily use have not been demonstrated in clients less than 5 years of age, in clients with forced vital capacity (FVC) of less than 40% of predicted or for longer than 12 months. Use with caution during lactation.

Side Effects: *Respiratory:* Pharyngitis, voice alteration, and laryngitis are the most common. Also, *apnea,* bronchiectasis, bronchitis, change in sputum, cough increase, dyspnea, hemoptysis, lung function decrease, nasal polyps, pneumonia, pneumothorax, rhinitis, sinusitis, sputum increase, wheezing. *Body as a whole:* Abdominal pain, asthenia, fever, flu syndrome, malaise, sepsis, weight loss. *GI:* Intestinal obstruction, gall bladder disease, liver disease, pancreatic disease. *Miscellaneous:* Rash, urticaria, chest pain, conjunctivitis, diabetes mellitus, hypoxia.

Dosage —————————————

• **Inhalation Solution**

Cystic fibrosis.

One 2.5-mg single-dose ampule inhaled once daily using a recommended nebulizer (see what fol-

D

lows). Older clients and clients with baseline FVC above 85% may benefit from twice daily dosing.

RESPIRATORY CARE CONSIDERATIONS
Administration/Storage
1. Approved nebulizers include the disposable jet nebulizer Hudson T U-draft II, disposable jet nebulizer Marquest Acorn II in conjunction with a Pulmo-Aide compressor, and the reusable PARI LC Jet+ nebulizer in conjunction with the PARI PRONEB compressor. Safety and efficacy have been demonstrated with only these nebulizers.
2. The drug should not be diluted or mixed with other drugs in the nebulizer. Mixing with other drugs could lead to adverse physicochemical or functional changes in dornase alfa.
3. The drug must be stored in the refrigerator at 2°C–8°C (36°F–46°F) in the protective foil pouch and protected from strong light.
4. The product should be refrigerated when transported and should not be exposed to room temperature for a total time of 24 hr.
5. The solution should be discarded if it is cloudy or discolored.
6. The product does not contain a preservative; thus, once opened, the entire ampule must be used or discarded.

Assessment
1. Document age of symptom onset of cystic fibrosis, other therapies prescribed, and the outcome.
2. Drug is produced by genetically engineered Chinese hamster ovary cells; assess for sensitivity.
3. Obtain baseline pulmonary function parameters. Drug is for children over 5 years old with baseline FVC above 40%.

Client/Family Teaching
1. Review the dose, frequency, and proper method for inhalation administration. Explain that drug is administered by inhalation of an aerosol mist generated by a compressed air-driven nebulizer system.
2. Ensure that client/family are familiar with the goals of therapy and the use, care, and storage of inhalation equipment. Observe their technique and provide written guidelines.
3. Stress that treatments must be performed on a daily schedule to obtain full pharmacologic benefits.
4. Advise that standard prescribed therapies for cystic fibrosis such as chest PT, antibiotics, bronchodilators, oral and inhaled corticosteroids, enzyme supplements, vitamins, and analgesics should be continued during treatment with dornase alfa.
5. Review symptoms that require immediate medical intervention: severe rashes, itching, respiratory distress, fever, etc.
6. Advise family members caring for client with cystic fibrosis to learn CPR.
7. Identify support groups that may assist family to adjust and cope with this chronic disease.

Evaluate
• ↓ Frequency of respiratory tract infectious exacerbations and ↓ sputum viscosity in clients with cystic fibrosis
• Clinical evidence of improved pulmonary function studies

Doxacurium chloride
(dox-ah-**KYOUR**-ee-um **KLOR**-ide)
Pregnancy Category: C
Neuromax, Nuromax ✽ **(Rx)**
Classification: Neuromuscular blocking agent

See also *Neuromuscular Blocking Agents*.

Action/Kinetics: Doxacurium binds to cholinergic receptors on the motor end-plate to block the action of acetylcholine; this results in a blockade of neuromuscular transmission. Doxacurium is up to 3 times more potent than pancuronium and up to 12 times more potent than metocurine. The time to maximum neuromuscular blockade during balanced anesthesia is dose-dependent and ranges from 9.3 min (following doses of 0.025 mg/kg) to 3.5 min (following doses of 0.08 mg/kg). The time to 25% recovery from blockade following balanced anesthesia ranges from 55 min for doses of 0.025 mg/kg to 160 min for doses of 0.08 mg/kg. **t½, elimination:** Dose-dependent, ranging from 86 to 123 min. The half-life is prolonged in kidney transplant clients. Children require higher doses on a mg/kg basis than adults to achieve the same level of blockade. Also, the onset, time, and duration of block are shorter in children than adults. The blockade may be reversed by anticholinesterase agents. The drug is excreted unchanged through the urine and bile. **Uses:** Adjunct to general anesthesia to provide skeletal muscle relaxation during surgery. Skeletal muscle relaxation for ET intubation or to facilitate mechanical ventilation.

Special Concerns: Use with caution during lactation. Safety and effectiveness have not been determined in children less than 2 years of age. The duration of action may be up to twice as long for clients over 60 years of age and those who are obese (more than 30% more than ideal body weight for height). Malignant hyperthermia may occur in any client receiving a general anesthetic. A profound effect may be noted in clients with neuromuscular diseases such as myasthenia gravis and the myasthenic syndrome.

Side Effects: *Neuromuscular:* Skeletal muscle weakness, **profound and prolonged skeletal muscle paralysis causing respiratory insufficiency and apnea;** difficulty in reversing the neuromuscular blockade. *CV:* Hypotension, flushing, **ventricular fibrillation, MI.** *Respiratory:* Wheezing, **bronchospasm.** *Dermatologic:* Urticaria, reaction at injection site. *Miscellaneous:* Fever, diplopia.

OD **Overdose Management:** *Symptoms:* Prolonged neuromuscular block. *Treatment:* Maintain a patent airway and use controlled ventilation if necessary until recovery of normal neuromuscular function. Once recovery begins, it can be facil-

itated by giving neostigmine, 0.06 mg/kg.

Drug Interactions
Aminoglycosides / ↑ Effect of doxacurium
Bacitracin / ↑ Effect of doxacurium
Carbamazepine / ↑ Onset of effects and ↓ the duration of action of doxacurium
Clindamycin / ↑ Effect of doxacurium
Colistin / ↑ Effect of doxacurium
Enflurane / ↓ Amount of doxacurium necessary to cause blockade and ↑ the duration of action
Halothane / ↓ Amount of doxacurium necessary to cause blockade and ↑ the duration of action
Isoflurane / ↓ Amount of doxacurium necessary to cause blockade and ↑ the duration of action
Lincomycin / ↑ Effect of doxacurium
Lithium / ↑ Effect of doxacurium
Local anesthetics / ↑ Effect of doxacurium
Magnesium salts / ↑ Effect of doxacurium
Phenytoin / ↑ Onset of effects and ↓ the duration of action of doxacurium
Polymyxins / ↑ Effect of doxacurium
Procainamide / ↑ Effect of doxacurium
Quinidine / ↑ Effect of doxacurium
Sodium colistimethate / ↑ Effect of doxacurium
Tetracyclines / ↑ Effect of doxacurium

Dosage
• **IV Only**

As a component of thiopental/narcotic induction-intubation, to produce neuromuscular blockade of long duration.
Adults, initial: 0.05 mg/kg.

If administered during steady-state enflurane, halothane, or isoflurane anesthesia.
Reduce dose by one-third. **Children:** 0.03 mg/kg for blockade lasting about 30 min or 0.05 mg/kg for

blockade lasting about 45 min when used during halothane anesthesia. Maintenance doses are required more frequently in children.

Used with succinylcholine to facilitate ET intubation.

Initial: 0.025 mg/kg will provide approximately 60 min of effective blockade. **Maintenance doses:** Required about 60 min after an initial dose of 0.025 mg/kg or 100 min after an initial dose of 0.05 mg/kg during balanced anesthesia. Maintenance doses between 0.005–0.01 mg/kg provide an average of 30 min and 45 min, respectively, of additional neuromuscular blockade.

RESPIRATORY CARE CONSIDERATIONS

See also *Respiratory Care Considerations* for *Neuromuscular Blocking Agents.*

Administration/Storage

1. The dose is individualized for each client.

2. The dose should be reduced in debilitated clients, in clients with neuromuscular disease, severe electrolyte abnormalities, and carcinomatosis.

3. The dose may need to be increased in burn clients.

4. The dose for obese clients is determined using the ideal body weight (IBW) calculated as follows:

• For men: IBW (kg) = (106 + [6 × inches in height above 5 feet])/2.2

• For women: IBW (kg) = (106 + [5 × inches in height above 5 feet])/2.2

5. Doxacurium may not be compatible with alkaline solutions with a pH more than 8 (e.g., barbiturates).

6. Doxacurium may be mixed with 5% dextrose injection, 5% dextrose and 0.9% sodium chloride injection, 0.9% sodium chloride injection, lactated Ringer's injection, and 5% dextrose and lactated Ringer's injection. The drug is also compatible with alfentanil, fentanyl, and sufentanil.

7. Doxacurium diluted 1:10 with 5% dextrose injection or 0.9% sodium chloride injection is stable for 24 hr if stored in polypropylene syringes at

5°C–25°C (41°F–77°F). However, immediate use of the drug, if diluted, is preferable.

8. Any unused portion of diluted doxacurium should be discarded after 8 hr at room temperature.

Assessment

1. Determine any history of neuromuscular disease (e.g., myasthenia gravis) as doxacurium may have profound effects in these clients.

2. Note any drugs client is currently prescribed that may interact unfavorably with doxacurium.

3. Identify burn victims and anticipate altered requirements of drug as these clients tend to develop a resistance to doxacurium.

4. Obtain baseline weight, VS, and serum electrolyte levels.

Interventions

1. The drug should only be given if there are facilities for intubation, assisted ventilation, and oxygen therapy, and the availability of an antagonist.

2. The drug should be administered only by those experienced with skeletal muscle relaxants.

3. A peripheral nerve stimulator should be used to monitor drug response and recovery.

4. Since doxacurium has no effect on consciousness, pain threshold, or cerebration, it generally should not be administered before unconsciousness (to avoid client stress).

5. Determine need for additional medication for anxiety and for sedation and administer as needed.

6. Explain all procedures and provide emotional support. Reassure clients that they will be able to talk and move once the drug effects are reversed.

7. Position the client for comfort and so that the body is in proper alignment. Turn client and perform mouth care and eye care frequently.

8. Provide continuous ventilatory support. Make certain that the ventilator alarms are set and on at all times. Assess airway at frequent intervals and have a suction machine readily available.

9. Monitor and record VS, I&O.

Client/Family Teaching

1. Explain all procedures and provide emotional support. Reassure clients that they will be able to talk and move once the drug effects are reversed.

2. Explain the direction of recovery, i.e., facial muscles, diaphragm, legs, arms, and torso.

3. Advise that residual weakness and respiratory difficulty may slow recovery.

Evaluate

• Desired level of skeletal muscle relaxation/paralysis

• Facilitation of ET intubation and tolerance of mechanical ventilation

• Suppression of the twitch response when tested with a peripheral nerve stimulator

---

Doxazosin mesylate

(dox-**AYZ**-oh-sin)
Pregnancy Category: B
Cardura **(Rx)**
Classification: Antihypertensive

Action/Kinetics: Doxazosin is a quinazoline compound that blocks the alpha-1 (postjunctional) adrenergic receptors resulting in a decrease in systemic vascular resistance and a corresponding decrease in BP. **Peak plasma levels:** 2–3 hr. **Peak effect:** 2–6 hr. Significantly bound (98%) to plasma proteins. Metabolized in the liver to active and inactive metabolites, which are excreted through the feces and urine. **t½:** 22 hr.

Uses: Alone or in combination with diuretics or beta-adrenergic blocking drugs for the treatment of hypertension. Treatment of benign prostatic hyperplasia.

Contraindications: Use in clients allergic to prazosin or terazosin.

Special Concerns: Use with caution during lactation. Safety and effectiveness have not been demonstrated in children. Due to the possibility of severe hypotension, the 2-, 4-, and 8-mg tablets are not to be used for initial therapy. Use with caution in clients with impaired hepatic function or

in those who are taking drugs known to influence hepatic metabolism.

Side Effects: *CV:* Dizziness (most frequent), syncope, vertigo, lightheadedness, edema, palpitation, arrhythmia, postural hypotension, tachycardia, peripheral ischemia. *CNS:* Fatigue, headache, paresthesia, kinetic disorders, ataxia, somnolence, nervousness, depression, insomnia. *Musculoskeletal:* Arthralgia, arthritis, muscle weakness, muscle cramps, myalgia, hypertonia. *GU:* Polyuria, sexual dysfunction, urinary incontinence, urinary frequency. *GI:* Nausea, diarrhea, dry mouth, constipation, dyspepsia, flatulence, abdominal pain, vomiting. *Respiratory:* Fatigue or malaise, rhinitis, epistaxis, dyspnea. *Miscellaneous:* Rash, pruritus, flushing, abnormal vision, conjunctivitis, eye pain, tinnitus, chest pain, asthenia, facial edema, generalized pain, slight weight gain.

OD **Overdose Management:** *Symptoms:* Hypotension. *Treatment:* IV fluids.

Dosage

• **Tablets**

Hypertension.

Adults: initial, 1 mg once daily at bedtime; **then,** depending on the response (client's standing BP both 2–6 hr and 24 hr after a dose), the dose may be increased to 2 mg/day. A maximum of 16 mg/day may be required to control BP.

Benign prostatic hyperplasia.

Initial: 1 mg once daily. **Maintenance:** Depending on the urodynamics and symptoms, dose may be increased to 2 mg daily and then 4–8 mg once daily (maximum recommended dose). The recommended titration interval is 1–2 weeks.

RESPIRATORY CARE CONSIDERATIONS

Administration/Storage

1. To minimize the possibility of severe hypotension, initial dosage should be limited to 1 mg/day.

2. The drug should be given once daily at bedtime.

3. Increasing the dose higher than 4 mg/day increases the possibility of severe syncope, postural dizziness, vertigo, and postural hypotension.

Assessment

1. Document indications for therapy, other agents used, and the outcome.

2. Note any allergy to prazosin or terazosin as drug is a quinazoline derivative.

3. Determine hepatic function and note any history of liver failure.

4. List drugs client prescribed to ensure there will be no drug interactions.

5. Anticipate that it may take 4–5 days to achieve desired response.

6. When used for BPH, the BP should be evaluated routinely.

Evaluate

• Control of hypertension (e.g., maintaining SBP < 140 and DBP < 90 mm Hg)

• Improvement in symptoms of BPH with ↓ nocturnal dysuria

Doxycycline calcium
(dox-ih-**SYE**-kleen)
Pregnancy Category: D
Vibramycin **(Rx)**

Doxycycline hyclate
(dox-ih-**SYE**-kleen)
Pregnancy Category: D
Apo-Doxy ✽, Doryx, Doxy 100 and 200, Doxy-Caps, Doxycin ✽, Doxychel Hyclate, Doxytec ✽, Novo-Doxylin ✽, Nu-Doxycycline ✽, Vibramycin, Vibramycin IV, Vibra-Tabs, Vivox **(Rx)**

Doxycycline monohydrate
(dox-ih-**SYE**-kleen)
Pregnancy Category: D
Monodox, Vibramycin **(Rx)**
Classification: Antibiotic, tetracycline

See also *Anti-Infectives* and *Tetracyclines*.

Action/Kinetics: More slowly absorbed, and thus more persistent, than other tetracyclines. Preferred for clients with impaired renal function for treating infections outside the urinary tract. From 80% to 95% is bound to serum proteins. **t½:** 14.5–22 hr; 30%–40% excreted unchanged in urine.

Additional Use: Orally for uncomplicated gonococcal infections in adults (except anorectal infections in males); acute epididymo-orchitis caused by *Neisseria gonorrhoeae* and *Chlamydia trachomatis;* gonococcal arthritis-dermatitis syndrome; nongonococcal urethritis caused by *C. trachomatis* and *Ureaplasma urealyticum.* Prophylaxis of malaria due to *Plasmodium falciparum* in shortterm travelers (< 4 months) to areas with chloroquine- or pyrethamine-sulfadoxine-resistant strains.

Contraindications: Prophylaxis of malaria in pregnant individuals and in children less than 8 years old. Use during the last half of pregnancy and in children up to 8 years of age (tetracycline may cause permanent discoloration of the teeth). Lactation.

Special Concerns: Safety for IV use in children less than 8 years of age has not been established.

Additional Drug Interactions: Carbamazepine, phenytoin, and barbiturates ↓ effect of doxycycline by ↑ breakdown of doxycycline by the liver.

Dosage
• **Capsules, Delayed-Release Capsules, Oral Suspension, Syrup, Tablets, IV**
Infections.
Adult: First day, 100 mg q 12 hr; **maintenance:** 100–200 mg/day, depending on severity of infection. **Children, over 8 years (45 kg or less): First day,** 4.4 mg/kg in 1–2 doses; **then,** 2.2–4.4 mg/kg/day in divided doses depending on severity of infection. Children over 45 kg should receive the adult dose.
Acute gonorrhea.
200 mg at once given PO; **then,** 100 mg at bedtime on first day, followed by 100 mg b.i.d. for 3 days. Alternatively, 300 mg immediately followed in 1 hr with 300 mg.

Syphilis (primary/secondary).
300 mg/day in divided PO doses for 10 days.

C. trachomatis infections.
100 mg b.i.d. PO for minimum of 7 days.

Prophylaxis of "traveler's diarrhea."
100 mg/day given PO.

Prophylaxis of malaria.
Adults: 100 mg PO once daily; **children, over 8 years of age:** 2 mg/kg/day up to 100 mg/day.

• **IV**

Endometritis, parametritis, peritonitis, salpingitis.
100 mg b.i.d. with 2 g cefoxitin, IV, q.i.d. continued for at least 4 days or 2 days after improvement observed. This is followed by doxycycline, PO, 100 mg b.i.d. for 10–14 days of total therapy.

NOTE: The Centers for Disease Control have established treatment schedules for STDs.

RESPIRATORY CARE CONSIDERATIONS

See also *General Respiratory Care*

Considerations for All Anti-Infectives and for *Tetracyclines.*

Administration/Storage

1. The powder for suspension has an expiration date of 12 months from date of issue.
2. Solution is stable for 2 weeks when stored in refrigerator.
3. Follow directions on vial for dilution. Concentrations should be no lower than 0.1 mg/mL and no higher than 1.0 mg/mL.
4. During infusion protect solution from light.
5. Complete administration of solutions diluted with NaCl injection, D5W, Ringer's injection, and 10% invert sugar within 12 hr.
6. Complete administration of solutions diluted with lactated Ringer's injection or 5% dextrose in lactated Ringer's injection within 6 hr.
7. Prophylaxis for malaria can begin 1–2 days before travel begins, during travel, and for 4 weeks after leaving the malarious area.

Evaluate

• Resolution of infection and reports of symptomatic improvement
• Negative lab culture reports

E

Edrophonium chloride
(ed-roh-**FOH**-nee-um)
Pregnancy Category: C
Enlon, Reversol, Tensilon **(Rx)**

————*COMBINATION DRUG*————

Edrophonium chloride and Atropine sulfate
(ed-roh-**FOH**-nee-um)
Pregnancy Category: C
Enlon-Plus **(Rx)**
Classification: Cholinesterase inhibitor, indirectly-acting

See also *Neostigmine* and *Atropine Sulfate.*

Action/Kinetics: Edrophonium is a short-acting agent mostly used for diagnosis and not for maintenance therapy. By increasing the duration of action at the motor end plate, edrophonium causes a transient increase in muscle strength in myasthenia gravis clients and either no change or a slight weakness in muscle strength in clients with other disorders. Atropine has been added to edrophonium to counteract the muscarinic side effects that will occur due to edrophonium (e.g., increased secretions, bradycardia, bronchoconstriction).
Onset: IM, 2–10 min; **IV, <1 min.**
Duration: IM, 5–30 min; IV, 10

min. Eliminated through the kidneys.

Uses: *Edrophonium.* Differential diagnosis of myasthenia gravis. Adjunct to evaluate requirements for treating myasthenia gravis. Adjunct to treat respiratory depression due to curare and similar nondepolarizing agents such as gallamine, pancuronium, and tubocurarine.

Edrophonium and Atropine. To antagonize or reverse nondepolarizing neuromuscular blocking agents. Adjunct to treat respiratory depression caused by overdosage of curare.

Contraindications: Edrophonium combined with atropine is not recommended for use in the differential diagnosis of myasthenia gravis.

Special Concerns: Edrophonium combined with atropine is not effective against depolarizing neuromuscular blocking agents.

Dosage ————————————
• **Edrophonium, IV**
Differential diagnosis of myasthenia gravis.
IV, Adults: 2 mg initially over 15–30 sec; with needle in place, wait 45 sec; if no response occurs after 45 sec inject an additional 8 mg. If a cholinergic reaction is obtained following 2 mg (muscarinic side effects, skeletal muscle fasciculations, increased muscle weakness), test is discontinued and atropine, 0.4–0.5 mg, is given IV. The test may be repeated in 30 min. **Pediatric, up to 34 kg, IV:** 1 mg; if no response after 45 sec, can give up to 5 mg. **Pediatric, over 34 kg, IV:** 2 mg; if no response after 45 sec, can give up to 10 mg in 1-mg increments q 30–45 sec. **Infants:** 0.5 mg. If IV injection is not feasible, IM can be used.

To evaluate treatment needs in myasthenic clients.
1 hr after PO administration of drug used to treat myasthenia, give edrophonium IV, 1–2 mg. (*NOTE:* Response will be myasthenic in undertreated clients, adequate in controlled clients, and cholinergic in overtreated clients.)

Curare antagonist.

Slow IV: 10 mg over 30–45 sec to detect onset of cholinergic reaction; repeat if necessary to maximum of 40 mg. Should not be given before use of curare, gallamine, or tubocurarine.
• **Edrophonium, IM**
Differential diagnosis of myasthenia gravis.
Adults: 10 mg; if hyperreactivity occurs, retest after 30 min with 2 mg IM to rule out false negative. **Pediatric, up to 34 kg:** 2 mg; **more than 34 kg:** 5 mg. (There is a 2–10-min delay in reaction with IM route.)
• **Edrophonium and Atropine, IV**
Adults: 0.5–1 mg/kg edrophonium and 0.007–0.014 mg/kg atropine.

RESPIRATORY CARE CONSIDERATIONS

See also *Respiratory Care Considerations* for *Neostigmine* and *Atropine Sulfate.*

Administration/Storage
1. Edrophonium should not be given before curare or curare-like drugs.
2. Have IV atropine sulfate available to use as an antagonist.
3. When atropine is combined with edrophonium, the response should be monitored carefully and assisted or controlled ventilation should be undertaken.
4. Recurarization has not been noted following satisfactory reversal with edrophonium and atropine.

Assessment
1. Document indications for therapy.
2. List drugs client currently prescribed.
3. Note any history of asthma, seizures, CAD, or hyperthyroidism.

Interventions
1. Observe closely in a monitored environment during drug administration; drug effects last up to 30 min.
2. Monitor VS and I&O at least q 4 hr.
3. Document and report side effects such as increased salivation, bronchial spasm, bradycardia, and cardiac arrhythmia. This is particularly

important when working with elderly clients.

4. When the drug is being administered as an antidote for curare, assess client for the effects of each dose of drug. Do not administer the next dose of drug unless the prior effects have been observed and recorded. Larger doses of medication may potentiate effects.

5. Evaluate respiratory effort and provide assisted ventilation as needed.

6. During cholinergic crisis, monitor state of consciousness closely.

Evaluate
• With myasthenia gravis (transient ↑ muscle strength, improved gait)
• Curare antagonist
• Reversal of respiratory depression R/T nondepolarizing neuromuscular blocking agents
• Differentiation of myasthenic from cholinergic crisis

Enalapril maleate
(en-**AL**-ah-prill)
Pregnancy Category: D
Apo-Enalapril ✦, Vasotec, Vasotec I.V., Vasotec Oral ✦ **(Rx)**
Classification: Angiotensin-converting enzyme inhibitor

See also *Angiotensin-Converting Enzyme Inhibitors.*

Action/Kinetics: Enalapril is converted in the liver by hydrolysis to the active metabolite, enalaprilat. The parenteral product is enalaprilat injection. **Onset, PO:** 1 hr; **IV,** 15 min. **Time to peak action, PO:** 4–6 hr; **IV,** 1–4 hr. **Duration, PO:** 24 hr; **IV,** About 6 hr. Approximately 50%–60% is protein bound. **t½, enalapril, PO:** 1.3 hr; **IV,** 15 min. **t½, enalaprilat, PO:** 11 hr. Enalapril is excreted through the urine (half unchanged) and feces; over 90% of enalaprilat is excreted through the urine.

Uses: Alone or in combination with a thiazide diuretic for the treatment of hypertension (step I therapy). As adjunct with digitalis and diuretic in acute and chronic CHF. *Investiga-*

tional: Hypertension in children, hypertension related to scleroderma renal crisis, diabetic nephropathy, asymptomatic left ventricular dysfunction following MI. Enalaprilat may be used for hypertensive emergencies (effect is variable).

Special Concerns: Use with caution during lactation. Safety and effectiveness have not been determined in children.

Side Effects: *CV:* Palpitations, hypotension, chest pain, angina, *CVA, MI,* orthostatic hypotension, disturbances in rhythm, tachycardia, *cardiac arrest,* orthostatic effects, atrial fibrillation, bradycardia. *GI:* N&V, diarrhea, abdominal pain, alterations in taste, anorexia, dry mouth, constipation, dyspepsia, glossitis, ileus, melena, stomatitis. *CNS:* Insomnia, headache, fatigue, dizziness, paresthesias, nervousness, sleepiness, ataxia, confusion, depression, vertigo. *Hepatic:* Hepatitis, hepatocellular or cholestatic jaundice, pancreatitis, elevated liver enzymes, hepatic failure. *Respiratory:* Bronchitis, cough, dyspnea, bronchospasm, upper respiratory infection, pneumonia, pulmonary infiltrates, asthma, *pulmonary embolism and infarction, pulmonary edema. Renal:* Renal dysfunction, oliguria, UTI, transient increases in creatinine and BUN. *Hematologic:* Rarely, neutropenia, thrombocytopenia, bone marrow depression, decreased H&H in hypertensive and CHF clients. Hemolytic anemia, including hemolysis, in clients with G6PD deficiency. *Dermatologic:* Rash, pruritus, alopecia, flushing, erythema multiforme, exfoliative dermatitis, photosensitivity, urticaria, increased sweating, pemphigus, *Stevens-Johnson syndrome,* herpes zoster, toxic epidermal necrolysis. *Other:* Angioedema, asthenia, impotence, blurred vision, fever, arthralgia, arthritis, vasculitis, eosinophilia, tinnitus, syncope, myalgia, rhinorrhea, sore throat, hoarseness, conjunctivitis, tearing, dry eyes, loss of sense of smell, hearing loss, peripheral neuropathy, anosmia, myositis, flank pain, gynecomastia.

Additional Drug Interactions: Rifampin may ↓ the effects of enalapril. Explain that drug should not be discontinued without first reporting this side effect to the physician.

Dosage

• **Tablets (Enalapril)**

Antihypertensive in clients not taking diuretics.

Initial: 5 mg/day; **then,** adjust dosage according to response (range: 10–40 mg/day in one to two doses).

Antihypertensive in clients taking diuretics.

Initial: 2.5 mg. Since hypotension may occur following the initiation of enalapril, the diuretic should be discontinued, if possible, for 2–3 days before initiating enalapril. If BP is not maintained with enalapril alone, diuretic therapy may be resumed.

Adjunct with diuretics and digitalis in heart failure.

Initial: 2.5 mg 1–2 times/day; **then,** depending on the response, 5–20 mg/day in two divided doses. Dose should not exceed 40 mg/day. Dosage must be adjusted in clients with renal impairment or hyponatremia.

In clients with impaired renal function.

Initial: 5 mg/day if C_{CR} ranges between 30 and 80 mL/min and serum creatinine is less than 3 mg/dL; 2.5 mg/day if C_{CR} is less than 30 mL/min and serum creatinine is more than 3 mg/dL and in dialysis clients on dialysis days.

Renal impairment or hyponatremia.

Initial: 2.5 mg/day if serum sodium is less than 130 mEq/L and serum creatinine is more than 1.6 mg/dL. The dose may be increased to 2.5 mg b.i.d. and then 5 mg b.i.d. or higher if required; dose is given at intervals of 4 or more days. Maximum daily dose is 40 mg.

Asymptomatic LV dysfunction following MI.

2.5–20 mg/day beginning 72 hr or longer after onset of MI. Therapy is continued for 1 yr or longer.

NOTE: Dosage should be decreased in clients with a C_{CR} less than 30 mL/min and a serum creatinine level greater than 3 mg/dL.

• **IV (Enalaprilat)**

Hypertension.

1.25 mg over a 5-min period; repeat q 6 hr.

Antihypertensive in clients taking diuretics.

Initial: 0.625 mg over 5 min; if an adequate response is seen after 1 hr, administer another 0.625-mg dose. Thereafter, 1.25 mg q 6 hr.

Clients with impaired renal function.

Give enalapril, 1.25 mg q 6 hr for clients with a C_{CR} more than 30 mL/min and an initial dose of 0.625 mg for clients with a C_{CR} less than 30 mL/min. If there is an adequate response, an additional 0.625 mg may be given after 1 hr; thereafter, additional 1.25-mg doses can be given q 6 hr. For dialysis clients, the initial dose is 0.625 mg q 6 hr.

RESPIRATORY CARE CONSIDERATIONS

See also *Respiratory Care Considerations* for *Angiotensin-Converting Enzyme Inhibitors* and *Antihypertensive Agents.*

Administration/Storage

1. Following IV administration, the peak effect after the first dose may not be observed for 4 hr (whether or not the client is on a diuretic). For subsequent doses, the peak effect is usually within 15 min.

2. Enalapril should be given as a slow IV infusion (over 5 min) either alone or diluted up to 50 mL with an appropriate diluent. Any of the following can be used: 5% dextrose injection, 5% dextrose in lactated Ringer's injection, Isolyte E, 0.9% sodium chloride injection, or 0.9% sodium chloride injection in 5% dextrose.

3. When used initially for heart failure, observe the client for at least 2 hr after the initial dose and until the BP has stabilized for an additional hour. If possible, the dose of diuretic should be reduced.

4. To convert from IV to PO therapy in clients on a diuretic, begin with 2.5 mg/day for clients responding to a 0.625-mg IV dose. Thereafter, 2.5 mg/day may be given.

5. To convert from PO to IV enalapril therapy in clients not on a diuretic, use the recommended IV dose (i.e., 1.25 mg/6 hr). To convert from IV to PO therapy, begin with 5 mg/day.

6. Anticipate lowered dosage for clients receiving diuretics and in those with impaired renal function.

Assessment

1. Document indications for therapy, presenting symptoms, and other agents used and the outcome.

2. List any prescribed drugs that may interact unfavorably with enalapril.

3. Record baseline ECG, VS, and weight.

4. Obtain CBC, serum electrolytes, and liver and renal function studies as baseline data and monitor.

Evaluate

• ↓ BP with HTN

• ↓ Preload and afterload with CHF

Ephedrine sulfate
(eh-**FED**-rin)

Pregnancy Category: C

Nasal decongestants: Kondon's Nasal, Pretz-D, Vatronol Nose Drops **(OTC). Systemic:** Ephed II (Rx: Injection; OTC: Oral dosage forms)

Classification: Adrenergic agent, direct- and indirect-acting

See also *Sympathomimetic Drugs* and *Nasal Decongestants*.

Action/Kinetics: Releases norepinephrine from synaptic storage sites. Has direct effects on alpha, beta-1, and beta-2 receptors, causing increased BP due to arteriolar constriction and cardiac stimulation, bronchodilation, relaxation of GI tract smooth muscle, nasal decongestion, mydriasis, and increased tone of the bladder trigone and vesicle sphincter. It may also increase skeletal muscle strength, especially in myasthenia clients. Significant CNS effects in-

clude stimulation of the cerebral cortex and subcortical centers. Hepatic glycogenolysis is increased, but not as much as with epinephrine. Ephedrine is more stable and longer-lasting than epinephrine. It is rapidly and completely absorbed following parenteral use. **Onset, IM:** 10–20 min; **PO:** 15–60 min; **SC: < 20 min. Duration, IM, SC:** 30–60 min; **PO: 3–5 hr. t½, elimination:** About 3 hr when urine is at a pH of 5 and about 6 hr when urinary pH is 6.3. Excreted mostly unchanged through the urine (rate dependent on urinary pH—increased in acid urine).

Uses: Bronchial asthma and reversible bronchospasms associated with obstructive pulmonary diseases. Nasal congestion in vasomotor rhinitis, acute sinusitis, hay fever, and acute coryza. Parenterally to treat narcolepsy and depression. Parenterally as a vasopressor to treat shock. In acute hypotension states, especially that associated with spinal anesthesia and Stokes-Adams syndrome with complete heart block.

NOTE: Tolerance may develop; however, temporary cessation of therapy restores the client's original response to the drug.

Additional   Contraindications: Angle closure glaucoma, anesthesia with cyclopropane or halothane, thyrotoxicosis, diabetes, obstetrics where maternal BP is greater than 130/80. Lactation.

Special Concerns: Geriatric clients may be at higher risk to develop prostatic hypertrophy. The drug may cause hypertension resulting in intracranial hemorrhage; it may also cause anginal pain in clients with coronary insufficiency or ischemic heart disease.

Additional Side Effects: *CNS:* Nervousness, shakiness, confusion, delirium, hallucinations. Anxiety and nervousness following prolonged use. *CV:* Precordial pain, *excessive doses may cause hypertension sufficient to result in cerebral hemorrhage. GU:* Difficult and painful urination, urinary retention in males with prostatism, decrease in urine formation. *Miscellaneous:* Pallor, respiratory difficulty, hypersensitivity reactions. *Abuse:* Prolonged abuse can cause an anxiety state, including symptoms of paranoid schizophrenia, tachycardia, poor nutrition and hygiene, dilated pupils, cold sweat, and fever.

Additional Drug Interactions

Dexamethasone / Ephedrine effect of dexamethasone

Diuretics / Diuretics response to sympathomimetics

Furazolidone / Pressor effect possible hypertensive crisis and intracranial hemorrhage

Guanethidine / Effect of guanethidine by displacement from its site of action

Halothane / Serious arrhythmias due to sensitization of the myocardium to sympathomimetics by halothane

MAO Inhibitors / Pressor effect possible hypertensive crisis and intracranial hemorrhage

Methyldopa / Effect of ephedrine in methyldopa-treated clients

Oxytocic drugs / Severe persistent hypertension

Dosage ————————

• **Capsules**

Bronchodilator, systemic nasal decongestant, CNS stimulant.

Adults: 25–50 mg q 3–4 hr. **Pediatric:** 3 mg/kg (100 mg/m²) daily in four to six divided doses.

• **SC, IM, Slow IV**

Bronchodilator.

Adults: 12.5–25 mg; subsequent doses determined by client response. **Pediatric:** 3 mg/kg (100 mg/m²) daily divided into four to six doses SC or IV.

Vasopressor.

Adults: 25–50 mg (IM or SC) or 5–25 mg (by slow IV push) repeated at 5- to 10-min intervals, if necessary. Absorption following IM is more rapid than following SC use. **Pediatric (IM):** 16.7 mg/m² q 4–6 hr.

• **Topical (0.25% Spray)**

Nasal decongestant.

Adults and children over 6 years: 2–3 gtt of solution or small amount of jelly in each nostril q 4 hr. Should not be used topically for more than 3 or 4 consecutive days. Not to be used in children under 6 years of age unless so ordered by physician.

RESPIRATORY CARE CONSIDERATIONS

See also *Respiratory Care Considerations* for *Sympathomimetic Drugs* and *Nasal Decongestants.*

Administration/Storage

1. May administer 10 mg IV undiluted over at least 1 min.

2. Use only clear solutions and discard any unused solution with IV therapy. Protect against exposure to light, as the drug is subject to oxidation.

Assessment

1. Document indications for therapy and onset and type of symptoms.

2. Obtain a thorough history, noting any disorders that may preclude therapy with ephedrine.

3. Assess mental status prior to beginning drug therapy.

4. Obtain baseline ECG and VS. If the drug is being administered for hypotension, monitor BP frequently until stabilized.

5. Assess pulmonary function and document findings.

Interventions

1. If the client has used ephedrine for prolonged periods of time, observe for drug resistance. Allow the client to rest without medication for 3–4 days, then resume therapy. The client will usually respond to the drug again. Report if there is no further response.

2. Monitor mental status regularly. Report any signs of depression, lack of interest in personal appearance, or complaints of insomnia or anorexia.

3. Monitor I&O. Elderly men may have difficulty and pain on urination. Be alert for urinary retention and report any difficulty in voiding.

Client/Family Teaching

1. Teach the client and family how to

take and maintain a written record of radial pulse readings. Report an elevated or irregular pulse rate.

2. Notify provider if SOB is unrelieved by medication and accompanied by chest pain, dizziness, or palpitations.

3. Advise male clients to report any difficulty with voiding. This may be caused by drug-induced urinary retention.

4. Avoid any OTC drugs or alcohol.

Evaluate

- Improved airway exchange
- ↓ Nasal congestion and mucous production
- ↑ BP
- Control of narcolepsy

Epinephrine

(ep-ih-**NEF**-rin)
Pregnancy Category: C
Adrenalin Chloride Solution, Bronkaid Mist, Bronkaid Mistometer ✦, EpiE-Z Pen, EpiE-Z Pen Jr., Epipen, Epipen Jr., Primatene Mist Solution, Sus-Phrine (Both Rx and OTC)

Epinephrine bitartrate

(ep-ih-**NEF**-rin)
Pregnancy Category: C
Asthmahaler Mist, Bronitin Mist, Bronkaid Mist Suspension, Epitrate, Primatene Mist Suspension **(OTC)**

Epinephrine borate

(ep-ih-**NEF**-rin)
Pregnancy Category: C
Epinal Ophthalmic Solution **(Rx)**

Epinephrine hydrochloride

(ep-ih-**NEF**-rin)
Pregnancy Category: C
Adrenalin Chloride, AsthmaNefrin, Epifrin, Glaucon, microNefrin, Nephron, S-2 Inhalant, Vaponefrin (Both Rx and OTC)
Classification: Adrenergic agent, direct-acting

See also *Sympathomimetic Drugs* and *Nasal Decongestants.*

Action/Kinetics: Epinephrine, a natural hormone produced by the adrenal medulla, induces marked stimulation of alpha, beta-1, and beta-2 receptors, causing sympathomimetic stimulation, pressor effects, cardiac stimulation, bronchodilation, and decongestion. Epinephrine crosses the placenta but not the blood-brain barrier. **Extreme caution must be taken never to inject 1:100 solution intended for inhalation—injection of this concentration has caused death. SC: Onset,** 6–15 min; **duration: <1–4 hr. Inhalation: Onset, 1–5 min; duration: 1–3 hr. IM, Onset:** variable; duration: <1–4 hr. Epinephrine is ineffective when given PO.

Uses: Cardiac arrest, Stokes-Adams syndrome, low CO following ECB. To prolong the action of local anesthetics. As a hemostatic during ocular surgery; treatment of conjunctival congestion during surgery; to induce mydriasis during surgery; treat ocular hypertension during surgery. Topically to control bleeding. Acute bronchial asthma, bronchospasms due to emphysema, chronic bronchitis, or other pulmonary diseases. Treatment of anaphylaxis, angioedema, anaphylactic shock, drug-induced allergic reactions, transfusion reactions, insect bites or stings. As an adjunct in the treatment of open-angle glaucoma (may be used with miotics, beta blockers, hyperosmotic agents, or carbonic anhydrase inhibitors). To produce mydriasis; to treat conjunctivitis. *NOTE:* Autoinjectors are available for emergency self-administration of first aid for anaphylactic reactions due to insect stings or bites, foods, drugs, and other allergens as well as idiopathic or exercise-induced anaphylaxis.

Additional Contraindications: Narrow-angle glaucoma. Use when wearing soft contact lenses (may discolor lenses). Aphakia. Lactation.

Special Concerns: May cause anoxia in the fetus. Administer parenteral epinephrine to children with caution. Syncope may occur if epinephrine is given to asthmatic children. Administration of the SC injection by the IV route may cause severe or fatal hypertension or cerebrovascular hemorrhage. Epinephrine may temporarily increase the rigidity and tremor of parkinsonism. Use with caution and in small quantities in the toes, fingers, nose, ears, and genitals or in the presence of peripheral vascular disease as vasoconstriction-induced tissue sloughing may occur. Safety and efficacy of ophthalmic products have not been determined in children.

Additional Side Effects: *CV: Fatal ventricular fibrillation, cerebral or subarachnoid hemorrhage,* obstruction of central retinal artery. *A rapid and large increase in BP may cause aortic rupture, cerebral hemorrhage, or angina pectoris. GU:* Decreased urine formation, urinary retention, painful urination. *CNS:* Anxiety, fear, pallor. Parenteral use may cause or aggravate disorientation, memory impairment, psychomotor agitation, panic, hallucinations, *suicidal or homicidal tendencies,* schizophrenic-type behavior. *Miscellaneous:* Prolonged use or overdose may cause elevated serum lactic acid with severe metabolic acidosis. *At injection site:* Bleeding, urticaria, wheal formation, pain. Repeated injections at the same site may cause necrosis from vascular constriction. *Ophthalmic:* Transient stinging or burning when administered, conjunctival hyperemia, brow ache, headache, blurred vision, photophobia, allergic lid reaction, ocular hypersensitivity, poor night vision, eye ache, eye pain. Prolonged ophthalmic use may cause deposits of pigment in the cornea, lids, or conjunctiva. When used for glaucoma in aphakic clients, reversible cystoid macular edema.

Additional Drug Interactions
Beta-adrenergic blocking agents / Initial effectiveness in treating glaucoma of this combination may ↓ over time

Chymotrypsin / Epinephrine, 1:100, will inactivate chymotrypsin in 60 min

Laboratory Test Interferences: False + or ↑ BUN, fasting glucose, lactic acid, urinary catecholamines, glucose (Benedict's). ↓ Coagulation time. The drug may affect electrolyte balance.

Dosage ———————————
- **Metered Dose Inhaler**
  Bronchodilation.

Adults and children over 4 years of age: 0.2–0.275 mg (1 inhalation) of the Aerosol or 0.16 mg (1 inhalation) of the Bitartrate Aerosol; may be repeated after 1–2 min if needed. At least 3 hr should elapse before subsequent doses. Dosage not established in children less than 4 years of age.

- **Inhalation Solution**
  Bronchodilation.

Adults and children over 6 years of age: 1 inhalation of the 1% solution (of the base); may be repeated after 1–2 min.

- **IM, IV, SC**
  Bronchodilation using the solution (1:1,000).

Adults: 0.3–0.5 mg SC or IM repeated q 20 min–4 hr as needed; dose may be increased to 1 mg/dose. **Infants and children (except premature infants and full-term newborns):** 0.01 mg/kg (0.3 mg/m²) SC up to a maximum of 0.5 mg/dose; may be repeated q 15 min for two doses and then q 4 hr as needed.

Bronchodilation using the sterile suspension (1:200).

Adults: 0.5–1.5 mg SC. **Infants and children, 1 month–12 years:** 0.025 mg/kg SC; **children less than 30 kg:** 0.75 mg as a single dose.

Anaphylaxis.

Adults: 0.2–0.5 mg SC q 10–15 min as needed, up to a maximum of 1 mg/dose if needed. **Pediatric:** 0.01 mg/kg (0.3 mg/m²) up to a maximum of 0.5 mg/dose; may be repeated q 15 min for two doses and then q 4 hr as needed.

- **Autoinjector, IM**
  First aid for anaphylaxis.

The autoinjectors deliver a single dose of either 0.3 mg or 0.15 mg (for children) of epinephrine. In cases of a severe reaction, repeat injections may be necessary.

Vasopressor.
Adults, IM or SC, initial: 0.5 mg repeated q 5 min if needed; **then,** give 0.025–0.050 mg IV q 5–15 min as needed. **Adults, IV, initial:** 0.1–0.25 mg given slowly. May be repeated q 5–15 min as needed. Or, use IV infusion beginning with 0.001 mg/min and increasing the dose to 0.004 mg/min if needed. **Pediatric, IM, SC:** 0.01 mg/kg, up to a maximum of 0.3 mg repeated q 5 min if needed. **Pediatric, IV:** 0.01 mg/kg/5–15 min if an inadequate response to IM or SC administration is observed.

Cardiac stimulant.
Adults, intracardiac or IV: 0.1–1 mg repeated q 5 min if needed. **Pediatric, intracardiac or IV:** 0.005–0.01 mg/kg (0.15–0.3 mg/m²) repeated q 5 min if needed; this may be followed by IV infusion beginning at 0.0001 mg/kg/min and increased in increments of 0.0001 mg/kg/min up to a maximum of 0.0015 mg/kg/min.

Adjunct to local anesthesia.
Adults and children: 0.1–0.2 mg in a 1:200,000–1:20,000 solution.

Adjunct with intraspinal anesthetics.
Adults: 0.2–0.4 mg added to the anesthetic spinal fluid.
• **Solution**

Antihemorrhagic, mydriatic.
Adults and children, intracameral or subconjunctival: 0.01%–0.1% solution.

Topical antihemorrhagic.
Adults and children: 0.002%–0.1% solution.

Nasal decongestant.
Adults and children over 6 years of age: Apply 0.1% solution as drops or spray or with a sterile swab as needed.
• **Borate Ophthalmic Solution, Hydrochloride Ophthalmic Solution**

Glaucoma.
Adults: 1–2 gtt into affected eye(s) 1–2 times/day. Determine frequency of use by tonometry. Dosage has not been established in children.

RESPIRATORY CARE CONSIDERATIONS

See also *Respiratory Care Considerations* for *Sympathomimetic Drugs* and *Nasal Decongestants*.

Administration/Storage
1. *Never administer* 1:100 solution IV. Use 1:1,000 solution for IV administration.
2. Preferably use a tuberculin syringe to measure epinephrine, as the parenteral doses are small and the drug is potent. An error in measurement may be disastrous.
3. For direct IV administration to adults, the drug must be well diluted as a 1:1,000 solution and quantities of 0.05–0.1 mL of solution should be injected cautiously and slowly, taking about 1 min for each injection, noting the response of the client (BP and pulse). Dose may be repeated several times if necessary.
4. May be further diluted in D5%/W or NSS and infused with an electronic infusion device for safety and accuracy.
5. Briskly massage site of SC or IM injection to hasten the action of the drug. Do not expose epinephrine to heat, light, or air, as this causes deterioration of the drug.
6. Discard if solution is reddish brown and after expiration date.
7. Because of the presence of sodium bisulfite as a preservative in the topical preparation, there may be slight stinging after administration.
8. The topical preparation should not be used in children under 6 years of age.
9. Ophthalmic use may result in discomfort, which decreases over time.
10. The ophthalmic preparation is not for injection or intraocular use.
11. If the ophthalmic product for glaucoma is used with a miotic, the miotic should be instilled first.

12. The ophthalmic product should be kept tightly sealed and protected from light. It should be stored at 2°C–4°C (36°F–75°F). The solution should be discarded if it becomes discolored or contains a precipitate.

Assessment

1. Note any history of sulfite sensitivity.

2. Document indications for therapy and describe type and onset of symptoms and anticipated results.

3. Assess cardiopulmonary function and document findings.

Interventions

1. Closely monitor the client receiving solutions of IV epinephrine. Keep the environment as peaceful as possible and monitor ECG continuously.

2. Monitor BP and pulse every minute until the desired effect from the drug has been achieved. Then take it every 2–5 min until condition has stabilized. Once stable, monitor BP q 15–30 min as indicated.

3. Note any symptoms of shock such as cold, clammy skin, cyanosis, and loss of consciousness. If the client goes into hypovolemic shock, be prepared to assist with administering additional IV fluids.

Client/Family Teaching

1. Review appropriate indications, methods, and time frames for medication administration.

2. Explain method for administration carefully. When prescribed for anaphylaxis, advise to administer autoinjector immediately and then to seek further medical evaluation and follow-up.

3. Report any increased restlessness, chest pain, or insomnia as dosage adjustment may be necessary.

4. Limit intake of caffeine, as with colas, coffee, tea, and chocolate.

5. Do not take any OTC drugs without provider approval.

6. Advise that the ophthalmic solution may burn on administration but should subside. Caution that these preparations may stain contact lens.

7. Use caution when performing activities that require careful vision as ophthalmic solution may diminish visual fields, cause double vision, and alter night vision.

8. Stress the importance of ophthalmic evaluations to determine dosage requirements and response to therapy.

9. Advise to rinse mouth after MDI use.

Evaluate

• Return of cardiac activity following cardiac arrest

• Improved CO following EC bypass

• ↓ Intraocular pressures

• Reversal of S&S of anaphylaxis

• Improved airway exchange with acute bronchospasms

• Promotion of hemostasis during ocular surgery

Epoprostenol sodium
(eh-poh-**PROST**-en-ohl)
Pregnancy Category: B
Flolan **(Rx)**
Classification: Antihypertensive, miscellaneous

See also *Antihypertensive Agents*.

Action/Kinetics: Epoprostenol acts by direct vasodilation of pulmonary and systemic arterial vascular beds and by inhibition of platelet aggregation. IV infusion in clients with pulmonary hypertension results in increases in cardiac index and SV and decreases in pulmonary vascular resistance, total pulmonary resistance, and mean systemic arterial pressure. The drug is rapidly hydrolyzed at the neutral pH of the blood as well as by enzymatic degradation. Metabolites are less active than the parent compound. **t½:** 6 min.

Uses: Long-term IV treatment of primary pulmonary hypertension in New York Heart Association Class III and Class IV clients.

Contraindications: Chronic use in those with CHF due to severe LV systolic dysfunction. Chronic use in clients who develop pulmonary edema during dose ranging.

Special Concerns: Abrupt withdrawal or sudden large decreases in the dose may cause rebound pulmonary hypertension. Dose selection in the elderly should be cautious due to the greater frequency of decreased hepatic, renal, or cardiac function as well as concomitant disease or other drug therapy. Use with caution during lactation. Safety and efficacy have not been determined in children.

Side Effects: Side effects have been classified as those occurring during acute dose ranging, those as a result of the drug delivery system, and those occurring during chronic dosing.

Those occurring during acute dose ranging. *CV:* Flushing, hypotension, bradycardia, tachycardia. *GI:* N&V, abdominal pain, dyspepsia. *CNS:* Headache, anxiety, nervousness, agitation, dizziness, hypesthesia, paresthesia. *Miscellaneous:* Chest pain, musculoskeletal pain, dyspnea, back pain, sweating.

Those occurring as a result of the drug delivery system. *Due to the chronic indwelling catheter:* Local infection, pain at the injection site, sepsis, infections.

Those occurring during chronic dosing. *CV:* Flushing, tachycardia. *GI:* N&V, diarrhea. *CNS:* Headache, anxiety, nervousness, tremor, dizziness, hypesthesia, hyperesthesia, paresthesia. *Musculoskeletal:* Jaw pain, myalgia, nonspecific musculoskeletal pain. *Miscellaneous:* Flu-like symptoms, chills, fever, sepsis.

OD **Overdose Management:** *Symptoms:* Flushing, headache, hypotension, tachycardia, nausea, vomiting, diarrhea. *Treatment:* Reduce dose of epoprostenol.

Drug Interactions
Anticoagulants / Possible ↑ risk of bleeding
Antiplatelet drugs / Possible ↑ risk of bleeding
Diuretics / Additional ↓ in BP
Vasodilators / Additional ↓ in BP

Dosage —————————
• **Chronic IV Infusion**
  Pulmonary hypertension.
Acute dose ranging: The initial

chronic infusion rate is first determined. The mean maximum dose that did not elicit dose-limiting pharmacologic effects was 8.6 ng/kg/min. **Continuous chronic infusion, initial:** 4 ng/kg/min less than the maximum-tolerated infusion rate determined during acute dose ranging. If the maximum-tolerated infusion rate is less than 5 ng/kg/min, start the chronic infusion at one-half the maximum-tolerated infusion rate. **Dosage adjustments:** Changes in the chronic infusion rate are based on persistence, recurrence, or worsening of the symptoms of primary pulmonary hypertension. If symptoms require an increase in infusion rate, increase by 1–2 ng/kg/min at intervals (at least 15 min) sufficient to allow assessment of the clinical response. If a decrease in infusion rate is necessary, gradually make 2-ng/kg/min decrements every 15 min or longer until the dose-limiting effects resolve. Abrupt withdrawal or sudden large reductions in infusion rates are to be avoided.

RESPIRATORY CARE CONSIDERATIONS

See also *Respiratory Care Considerations* for *Antihypertensive Agents.*

Administration/Storage
1. Chronic administration is delivered continuously by a permanent indwelling central venous catheter and an ambulatory infusion pump (see package insert for requirements for the infusion pump). Unless contraindicated, the client should receive anticoagulant therapy to decrease the risk of pulmonary thromboembolism or systemic embolism.
2. Reconstituted solutions are not to be diluted or administered with other parenteral solutions or medications.
3. Check the package insert carefully for instructions to make 100 mL of a solution with the appropriate final concentration of drug and for infusion delivery rates for doses equal to or

less than 16 ng/kg/min based on client weight, drug delivery rate, and concentration of solution to be used.

4. Unopened vials are to be protected from light and stored at 15°C–25°C (59°F–77°F). Reconstituted solutions are to be protected from light and refrigerated at 2°C–8°C (36°F–46°F) for no more than 40 hr.

5. Reconstituted solutions are not to be frozen. Any solution refrigerated for more than 48 hr should be discarded.

6. A single reservoir of reconstituted solution can be given at room temperature for 8 hr; alternatively, it can be used with a cold pouch and given for up to 24 hr. The solution should not be exposed to sunlight.

Assessment

1. Perform a full cardiopulmonary assessment and note findings.

2. Based on client symptoms, determine in which New York Heart Association functional class client qualifies (III or IV). Note agents previously used and the outcome.

3. List other drugs prescribed to ensure that none interact unfavorably.

4. Determine mental status and ability to handle medication preparation and IV administration; or identify someone in the home that can and is willing to perform this function on a regular basis and/or initiate home infusion referral.

5. Determine that a permanent indwelling central venous catheter is available for continuous ambulatory delivery once dose ranging has been completed.

6. Assess central venous access site for any evidence of infection, discharge, odor, erythema, or swelling.

7. Consult manufacturer's guidelines for dosage and delivery rate based on client weight for acute dose ranging.

Evaluate: Improvement in exercise capacity with reports of less dyspnea and less fatigue

---

Erythromycin base
(eh-**rih**-throw-**MY**-sin)
Pregnancy Category: B (A/T/S,

Erymax, Staticin, and T-Stat are C)
Capsules/Tablets: Apo-Erythro Base ✿, Apo-Erythro-EC ✿, Diomycin ✿, E-Base Caplets, E-Base Tablets, E-Mycin, Erybid ✿, Eryc, Ery-Tab, Erythro-Base ✿, Erythromid ✿, Erythromycin Base Film-Tabs, Novo–Rythro EnCap ✿, PCE Dispertab, PMS-Erythromycin, Robimycin Robitabs. **Gel, topical:**A/T/S, Erygel. **Ointment, topical:** Akne-mycin. **Ointment,, ophthalmic:** Ilotycine Ophthalmic, **Pledgets:** Erycette, T-Stat. **Solution,** Del-Mycin, Eryderm 2%, Erymax, Erytha-Derm, Staticin, Theramycin Z, T-Stat **(Rx)**

Classification: Antibiotic, erythromycin

See also *Erythromycins* and *Anti-Infective Agents.*

Uses: See *Erythromycins, . Ophthalmic solution:* Treatment of ocular infections (along with PO therapy) due to *Streptococcus pneumoniae, Staphylococcus aureus, S. pyogenes, Corynebacterium* species, *Haemophilus influenzae,* and *Bacteroides* infections. Also prophylaxis of ocular infections due to *Neisseria gonorrhoeae* and *Chlamydia trachomatis. Topical solution:* Acne vulgaris. *Topical ointment:* Prophylaxis of infection in minor skin abrasions; treatment of superficial infections of the skin. Acne vulgaris.

Contraindications: Use of topical preparations in the eye or near the nose, mouth, or any mucous membrane. Ophthalmic use in dendritic keratitis, vaccinia, varicella, myobacterial infections of the eye, fungal diseases of the eye. Use with steroid combinations following uncomplicated removal of a corneal foreign body.

Special Concerns: Use of other drugs for acne may result in a cumulative irritant effect.

Additional Side Effects: *When used topically:* Erythema, desquamation, burning sensation, eye irritation, tenderness, dryness, pruritus, oily skin, generalized urticaria.

Drug Interactions: Antagonism has been observed when topical erythromycin is used with clindamycin.

Dosage
• **Delayed-Release Capsules, Enteric-Coated Tablets, Delayed-Release Tablets, Film-Coated Tablets, Suspension**

Respiratory tract infections due to Mycoplasma pneumoniae.
500 mg q 6 hr for 5–10 days (up to 3 weeks for severe infections).

Upper respiratory tract infections (mild to moderate) due to S. pyogenes and S. pneumoniae.
250–500 mg q.i.d. (or 20–50 mg/kg/day in divided doses) for 10 days.

Upper respiratory tract infections due to H. influenzae.
Erythromycin ethylsuccinate, 50 mg/kg/day, plus sulfisoxazole, 150 mg/kg/day, given together for 10 days.

Lower respiratory tract infections (mild to moderate) due to S. pyogenes and S. pneumoniae.
250–500 mg q.i.d. (or 20–50 mg/kg/day in divided doses) for 10 days.

Intestinal amebiasis due to Entamoeba histolytica.
Adults: 250 mg q.i.d. for 10–14 days; **pediatric:** 30–50 mg/kg/day in divided doses for 10–14 days.

Legionnaire's disease.
500–1,000 mg q.i.d. for 3 weeks (or 1–4 g/day in divided doses).

Bordetella pertussis.
500 mg q.i.d. for 10 days (or 40–50 mg/kg/day in divided doses for 5–14 days).

Infections due to Corynebacterium diphtheriae.
500 mg q.i.d. for 10 days.

Erythrasma.
250 mg t.i.d. for 3 weeks.

Primary syphilis.
20 g in divided doses over 10 days.

Chlamydial infections.
Infants: 50 mg/kg/day in four divided doses for 14 (conjunctivitis) to 21 (pneumonia) days; **adults:** 500 mg q.i.d. for 7 days or 250 mg q.i.d. for 14 days for urogenital infections.

Mild to moderate skin and skin structure infections due to S. pyogenes and S. aureus.
250–500 mg q 6 hr (or 50 mg/kg/day in divided doses—to a maximum of 4 g/day) for 10 days.

Listeria monocytogenes infections.
500 mg q 12 hr (or 250 mg q 6 hr), up to maximum of 4 g/day.

Pelvic inflammatory disease, acute N. gonorrhoeae.
Erythromycin lactobionate, 500 mg IV q 6 hr for 3 days; **then,** 250 mg erythromycin base q 6 hr for 7 days. Alternatively for pelvic inflammatory disease, 500 mg PO q.i.d. for 10–14 days.

Prophylaxis of initial or recurrent rheumatic fever.
250 mg b.i.d.

Bacterial endocarditis due to alpha-hemolytic streptococcus.
Adults: 1 g 2 hr prior to the procedure; **then,** 500 mg 6 hr after the initial dose. **Pediatric,** 20 mg/kg 2 hr prior to the procedure; **then,** 10 mg/kg 6 hr after the initial dose.

Pneumonia of infancy, conjunctivitis of the newborn, and urogenital infections during pregnancy due to C. trachomatis.
500 mg q.i.d. for 7 days (or 250 mg q.i.d. for 14 days).

Nongonococcal urethritis due to Ureaplasma urealyticum.
500 mg q.i.d. for at least 7 days.

Erythrasma due to Corynebacterium minutissimum.
250 mg t.i.d. for 21 days.

• **Ophthalmic Ointment**
Mild to moderate infections.
0.5-in. ribbon b.i.d.–t.i.d.

Acute infections.
0.5 in. q 3–4 hr until improvement is noted.

Prophylaxis of neonatal gonococcal or chlamydial conjunctivitis.
0.2–0.4 in. into each conjunctival sac.

• **Topical Gel (2%), Ointment (2%), Solution (2%)**
Clean the affected area and apply, using fingertips or applicator, morning and evening, to affected areas. If no improvement is seen after 6 to 8

E

---

weeks, therapy should be discontinued.

RESPIRATORY CARE CONSIDERATIONS

See also *Respiratory Care Considerations* for *Erythromycins*.

Administration/Storage

1. The ophthalmic ointment should not be washed from the eyes.

2. Before applying the topical solution, the affected areas should be washed, rinsed, and dried. The hands should be washed after application of erythromycin.

3. A sterile bandage may be used with the topical ointment.

4. The topical solution and ophthalmic products are for external use only.

5. Should be taken on an empty stomach, although the delayed-release forms of the base can be taken without regard for meals.

6. The topical gel is prepared by adding 3 mL of ethyl alcohol to the vial and immediately shaking to dissolve erythromycin. This solution is added to the gel and stirred until it appears homogenous in appearance (1–1.5 min). The gel should be refrigerated.

Assessment

1. Document indications for therapy and type and onset of symptoms.

2. Assess for any previous sensitivity reactions.

3. Determine that cultures, CBC, documentation, and appropriate diagnostic studies have been performed prior to initiating therapy.

Evaluate

• Negative C&S results
• Reports of symptomatic relief
• Desired infection prophylaxis

Erythromycin estolate
(eh-**rih**-throw-**MY**-sin)
Pregnancy Category: B
Ilosone, Novo-Rythro Estolate ✿ **(Rx)**
Classification: Antibiotic, erythromycin

See also *Erythromycins*.

Action/Kinetics: Most active form of erythromycin, with relatively long-lasting activity.

Uses: See *Erythromycins*.

Additional Contraindications: Cholestatic jaundice or preexisting liver dysfunction. Not recommended for treatment of chronic disorders such as acne or furunculosis or for prophylaxis of rheumatic fever.

Additional Side Effects: Hepatotoxicity.

Dosage

• **Capsules, Suspension, Tablets**

See *Erythromycin base*. Similar blood levels are achieved using erythromycin base, estolate, or stearate.

RESPIRATORY CARE CONSIDERATIONS

See also *Respiratory Care Considerations* for *Erythromycins*.

Administration/Storage

1. Shake oral suspension well before pouring.

2. Do not store suspension longer than 2 weeks at room temperature.

3. Chewable tablets must be chewed or crushed.

4. Can be taken without regard for meals.

Assessment

1. Document indications for therapy and duration and onset of symptoms.

2. Note any evidence of liver dysfunction.

Evaluate: Resolution of infection

Erythromycin ethylsuccinate
(eh-**rih**-throw-**MY**-sin)
Pregnancy Category: B
Apo-Erythro-ES, E.E.S. 200 and 400, E.E.S. Granules, EryPed, EryPed 200, EryPed 400, EryPed Drops, Erythro-ES ✿, Novo-Rythro Ethylsuccinate ✿ **(Rx)**
Classification: Antibiotic, erythromycin

See also *Erythromycins*.
Uses: See *Erythromycins*.

Additional   Contraindications: Preexisting liver disease.

Dosage
• **Oral   Suspension,   Tablets, Chewable Tablets**
See *Erythromycin base. NOTE:* 400 mg of erythromycin ethylsuccinate will achieve the same blood levels of erythromycin as 250 mg of the base, estolate, or stearate forms.

Hemophilus influenzae infections. Erythromycin   ethylsuccinate,   50 mg/kg/day with sulfisoxazole, 150 mg/kg/day, both for a total of 10 days.

RESPIRATORY CARE CONSIDERATIONS

See also *Respiratory Care Considerations* for *Erythromycins.*
Administration/Storage
1. Refrigerate aqueous suspension, and store for maximum of 1 week.
2. Chewable   tablets   must   be chewed or crushed.
3. Can be taken without regard to meals.
Evaluate: Resolution of infection

Erythromycin lactobionate
(eh-**rih**-throw-**MY**-sin)
Pregnancy Category: B
Erythrocin Lactobionate IV **(Rx)**
Classification: Antibiotic, erythromycin

See also *Erythromycins.*
Uses: For seriously ill or vomiting clients with infections caused by susceptible organisms; acute pelvic inflammatory disease due to gonorrhea. Legionnaire's disease.
Additional Side Effects: Transient deafness.
Additional   Drug   Interactions: Some physicians recommend that no drugs be added to IV solutions of erythromycin lactobionate.

Dosage
• **IV**

Adults and children: 15–20 mg/kg/day up to 4 g/day in severe infections.

Acute pelvic inflammatory disease caused by gonorrhea.
500 mg q 6 hr for 3 days followed by 250 mg erythromycin stearate, **PO,** q 6 hr for 7 days.

Legionnaire's disease.
1–4 g/day in divided doses. Change to PO therapy as soon as possible.

RESPIRATORY CARE CONSIDERATIONS

See also *Respiratory Care Considerations* for *Erythromycins.*
Administration/Storage
1. Sterile water for injection is the preferred diluent. However, 5% dextrose injection or 5% dextrose and lactated Ringer's injection may also be used provided that they are first buffered with 4% sodium bicarbonate injection.
2. For intermittent IV administration, solution may be further diluted in 100 to 250 mL of D5%/W or NSS and infused over 20–60 min.
3. The initial reconstituted solution is stable for 2 weeks if refrigerated or for 24 hr at room temperature. However,   the   final   diluted   solution should be given within 8 hr. The reconstituted piggyback vial should be used within 24 hr if stored in the refrigerator or 8 hr if stored at room temperature.
4. If the reconstituted solution is frozen, it can be stored for 30 days. Once thawed, it should be used within 8 hr. A thawed solution should not be refrozen.
Assessment
1. Document indications for therapy, noting type and onset of symptoms.
2. Obtain baseline CBC and C&S studies.
3. Assess for any hearing deficits.
Evaluate
• Resolution of infection
• Negative follow-up C&S reports

E

Erythromycin stearate
(eh-**rih**-throw-**MY**-sin)
Pregnancy Category: B
Apo-Erythro-S ✤, Eramycin, Novo-Rythro Stearate ✤, Nu-Erythromycin-S ✤ **(Rx)**
Classification: Antibiotic, erythromycin

See also *Erythromycins*.
Uses: See *Erythromycins*.
Additional Side Effects: Drug causes more allergic reactions (e.g., skin rash and urticaria) than other erythromycins. Hepatotoxicity.

Dosage ————————
• **Tablets, Film Coated**
See *Erythromycin base*. Similar blood levels are achieved using erythromycin base, estolate, or stearate forms.

RESPIRATORY CARE CONSIDERATIONS

See also *Respiratory Care Considerations* for *Erythromycins*.
Administration/Storage: Should be taken on an empty stomach.
Client/Family Teaching
1. Do not administer with meals because food decreases absorption.
2. Report any evidence of allergic reaction such as rash or itching.
Evaluate: Resolution of infection with symptomatic relief

Esmolol hydrochloride
(**EZ**-moh-lohl)
Pregnancy Category: C
Brevibloc **(Rx)**
Classification: Beta-adrenergic blocking agent

See also *Beta-Adrenergic Blocking Agents*.
Action/Kinetics: Esmolol preferentially inhibits beta-1 receptors. It has a rapid onset (<5 min) and a short duration of action. It has no membrane stabilizing or intrinsic sympathomimetic activity. Low lipid solubility. **t½:** 9 min. Is rapidly metabolized by esterases in RBCs.
Uses: Supraventricular tachycardia or arrhythmias, sinus tachycardia.

Special Concerns: Dosage has not been established in children.
Additional Side Effects: *Dermatologic:* Inflammation at site of infusion, flushing, pallor, induration, erythema, burning, skin discoloration, edema. *Other:* Urinary retention, midscapular pain, asthenia, changes in taste.
Additional Drug Interactions
Digoxin / Esmolol ↑ digoxin blood levels
Morphine / Morphine ↑ esmolol blood levels

Dosage ————————
• **IV Infusion**
SVT.
Initial: 500 mcg/kg/min for 1 min; **then,** 50 mcg/kg/min for 4 min. If after 5 min an adequate effect is not achieved, repeat the loading dose followed by a maintenance infusion of 100 mcg/kg/min for 4 min. This procedure may be repeated, increasing the maintenance infusion by 50 mcg/kg/min increments (for 4 min) until the desired HR or lowered BP is approached. **Then,** omit the loading infusion and reduce incremental infusion rate from 50 to 25 mcg/kg/min or less. The interval between titrations may be increased from 5 to 10 min.

Once the HR has been controlled, the client may be transferred to another antiarrhythmic agent. The infusion rate of esmolol should be reduced by 50% 30 min after the first dose of the alternative antiarrhythmic agent. If satisfactory control is observed for 1 hr after the second dose of the alternative agent, the esmolol infusion may be stopped.

RESPIRATORY CARE CONSIDERATIONS

See also *Respiratory Care Considerations* for *Beta-Adrenergic Blocking Agents*.
Administration/Storage
1. Infusions of esmolol may be necessary for 24–48 hr.
2. Esmolol HCl is not intended for direct IV push administration.
3. The concentrate should not be diluted with sodium bicarbonate.

4. To minimize venous irritation and thrombophlebitis, infusion concentrations should not be greater than 10 mg/mL.

5. Diluted esmolol (concentration of 10 mg/mL) is compatible with 5% dextrose injection, 5% dextrose in lactated Ringer's injection, 5% dextrose in Ringer's injection, 5% dextrose and 0.9% sodium chloride injection, 5% dextrose and 0.45% sodium chloride injection, 0.45% sodium chloride injection, lactated Ringer's injection, potassium chloride (40 mEq/L) in 5% dextrose injection, 0.9% sodium chloride injection, and 0.45% sodium chloride injection.

Assessment
1. Note indications for therapy and type, onset, and duration of symptoms.
2. Document baseline cardiopulmonary assessment; include ECG.

Interventions
1. Monitor client closely for evidence of hypotension and/or bradycardia. Request written parameters for withholding drug.
2. Infusions should be administered in a monitored environment with an electronic infusion device. Wean according to guidelines.
3. Monitor ECG and VS. Ensure that BP and HR are within desired range.
4. Have emergency drugs and equipment readily available.

Evaluate
• Suppression of supraventricular tachyarrhythmias
• Restoration of stable cardiac rhythm

Ethacrynate sodium
(eth-ah-**KRIH**-nayt)
Pregnancy Category: B
Sodium Edecrin **(Rx)**

Ethacrynic acid
(eth-ah-**KRIH**-nik **AH**-sid)
Pregnancy Category: B
Edecrin **(Rx)**
Classification: Diuretics, loop

See also *Loop Diuretics.*

Action/Kinetics: Ethacrynic acid inhibits the reabsorption of sodium and chloride in the loop of Henle; the drug also decreases reabsorption of sodium and chloride and increases potassium excretion in the distal tubule. It also acts directly on the proximal tubule to enhance excretion of electrolytes. Large quantities of sodium and chloride and smaller amounts of potassium and bicarbonate ion are excreted during diuresis. **Onset: PO,** 30 min; **IV,** Within 5 min. **Peak: PO,** 2 hr; **IV,** 15–30 min. **Duration: PO,** 6–8 hr. **IV,** 2 hr. **t½, after PO:** 60 min. Metabolites are excreted through the urine. Diuresis and electrolyte loss are more pronounced with ethacrynic acid than with thiazide diuretics. Ethacrynic acid is often effective in clients refractory to other diuretics. Careful monitoring of the diuretic effects is necessary.

Uses: Of value in clients resistant to less potent diuretics. CHF, acute pulmonary edema, edema associated with nephrotic syndrome, ascites due to idiopathic edema, lymphedema, malignancy. Short-term use for ascites as a result of malignancy, lymphedema, or idiopathic edema; also, for short-term use in pediatric clients (except infants) with congenital heart disease. *Investigational.* **Ethacrynic acid:** Single injection into the eye to treat glaucoma (effective for a week or more). **Ethacrynate sodium:** Hypercalcemia, bromide intoxication, and with mannitol in ethylene glycol poisoning.

Contraindications: Usually not recommended during pregnancy. Lactation. Not recommended for use in neonates. Anuria and severe renal damage. Clients with history of gout should be watched closely.

Special Concerns: Geriatric clients may be more sensitive to the usual adult dose. To be used with caution in diabetic clients and those with hepatic cirrhosis (who are particularly susceptible to electrolyte imbalance). Safety and efficacy of oral use in infants and IV use in children have not been established.

Side Effects: *Electrolyte imbalance:* Hypokalemia, hyponatremia, hypochloremic alkalosis, hypomagnesemia, hypocalcemia. *GI:* Anorexia, nausea, vomiting, diarrhea (may be sudden watery, profuse diarrhea), acute pancreatitis, abdominal discomfort or pain, jaundice, *GI bleeding or hemorrhage,* dysphagia. *Hematologic:* Severe neutropenia, thrombocytopenia, **agranulocytosis,** rarely Henoch-Schoenlein purpura in clients with rheumatic heart disease. *CNS:* Apprehension, confusion, vertigo, headache. *Body as a whole:* Fever, chills, fatigue, malaise. *Otic:* Sense of fullness in the ears, tinnitus, irreversible hearing loss. *Miscellaneous:* Hematuria, acute gout, abnormal liver function tests in seriously ill clients on multiple drug therapy including ethacrynic acid, blurred vision, rash, local irritation and pain following parenteral use, hyperuricemia, hyperglycemia.

Ethacrynic acid may cause death in critically ill clients refractory to other diuretics. These include (a) clients with severe myocardial disease who also received digitalis and who developed acute hypokalemia with fatal arrhythmias and (b) those with severely decompensated hepatic cirrhosis with ascites, with or without encephalopathy, who had electrolyte imbalances with death due to intensification of the electrolyte effect.

OD **Overdose Management:** *Symptoms:* Profound water loss, electrolyte depletion (causes dizziness, weakness, mental confusion, vomiting, anorexia, lethargy, cramps), dehydration, reduction of blood volume, *circulatory collapse (possibility of vascular thrombosis and embolism). Treatment:* Replace electrolytes and fluid and monitor urine output and serum electrolyte levels. Induce emesis or perform gastric lavage. Artificial respiration and oxygen may be needed. Treat other symptoms.

Dosage
ETHACRYNATE SODIUM
• **IV**
Adults: 50 mg (base) (or 0.5–1 mg/kg); may be repeated in 2–4 hr, although only one dose is usually needed. A single 100-mg dose IV has also been used.
ETHACRYNIC ACID
• **Tablets**
Adults, initial: 50–200 mg/day in single or divided doses to produce a gradual weight loss of 2.2–4.4 kg/day (1–2 lb/day). The dose can be increased by 25–50 mg/day if needed. **Maintenance:** Usually 50–200 mg (up to a maximum of 400 mg) daily may be required in severe, refractory edema. If used with other diuretics, the initial dose should be 25 mg with increments of 25 mg. **Pediatric, initial:** 25 mg/day; can increase by 25 mg/day if needed. **Maintenance:** Adjust dose to needs of client. Dosage for infants has not been determined.

RESPIRATORY CARE CONSIDERATIONS

See also *Respiratory Care Considerations* for *Diuretics, Loop.*

Administration/Storage
1. When used PO, administer after meals.
2. Due to local pain and irritation, the drug should not be given SC or IM.
3. Reconstitute the powder for injection by adding 50 mL of 5% dextrose injection or sodium chloride injection.
4. Intermittent IV administration should be at a slow rate over a 30-min period given either directly or through IV tubing. For direct IV, may give at a rate of 10 mg/min.
5. When reconstituted with 5% dextrose injection, the resulting solution may be hazy or opalescent. Such solutions should not be used. Also, this solution should not be mixed with whole blood or its derivatives.
6. If a second IV injection is necessary, a different site should be used to prevent thrombophlebitis.

7. Use reconstituted solutions within 24 hr after which any unused solution should be discarded.

8. Ammonium chloride or arginine chloride may be prescribed for clients who are at a higher risk of developing metabolic acidosis.

Assessment

1. Document indications for therapy, any other agents trialed, and the outcome.

2. Note any history of diabetes or cirrhosis.

3. Determine that anuria is not present.

4. List drugs the client is taking to identify any with which the drug may interact unfavorably.

5. Obtain baseline electrolytes, CBC, and liver function studies.

6. If prolonged therapy is anticipated, obtain audiometric assessment.

Interventions

1. Monitor VS, I&O, and weight. Observe for excessive diuresis or weight loss because electrolyte imbalance may develop quickly.

2. Assess clients with rapid excessive diuresis for pain in their calves, in the pelvic area, or in the chest. Rapid hemoconcentration may cause thromboembolic effects.

3. Observe for GI effects that may necessitate discontinuing the drug. The drug should be withdrawn if the client manifests severe, watery diarrhea.

4. Test for occult blood in the urine and the stools.

5. Observe the client for vestibular disturbances. Do not administer the drug IV concomitantly with any other ototoxic agent. Hearing loss is most common following high dosing or rapid IV administration.

6. Monitor serum potassium levels and determine the need for supplementary potassium.

7. Since ethacrynic acid has such a profound effect on sodium excretion, dietary salt restriction is not necessary; if sodium is restricted, hyponatremia may result.

Evaluate

• Enhanced diuresis
• ↓ Edema (↑ weight loss R/T edema)
• ↓ Abdominal girth R/T ascites

Ethambutol hydrochloride

(eh-**THAM**-byou-tohl)
Etibi ♣, Myambutol **(Rx)**
Classification: Primary antitubercular agent

Action/Kinetics: Tuberculostatic. Inhibits the synthesis of metabolites resulting in impairment of cell metabolism, arrest of multiplication, and ultimately cell death. The drug is active against *Mycobacterium tuberculosis,* but not against fungi, other bacteria, or viruses. Readily absorbed after PO administration. Widely distributed in body tissues except CSF. **Peak plasma concentration:** 2–5 mcg/mL after 2–4 hr. **t½:** 3–4 hr. About 65% of metabolized and unchanged drug excreted in urine and 20%–25% unchanged drug excreted in feces. Drug accumulates in clients with renal insufficiency.

Uses: Pulmonary tuberculosis in combination with other tuberculostatic drugs.

Contraindications: Hypersensitivity to ethambutol, preexisting optic neuritis, and in children under 13 years of age.

Special Concerns: Should be used with caution and in reduced dosage in clients with gout and impaired renal function and in pregnant women.

Side Effects: *Ophthalmologic:* Optic neuritis, decreased visual acuity, loss of color (green) discrimination, temporary loss of vision or blurred vision. *GI:* N&V, anorexia, abdominal pain. *CNS:* Fever, headache, dizziness, confusion, disorientation, malaise, hallucinations. *Allergic:* Pruritus, dermatitis, **anaphylaxis.** *Miscellaneous:* Peripheral neuropathy (numbness, tingling), precipitation of gout, thrombocytopenia, joint pain, toxic epidermal necrolysis. Renal damage. Also **anaphylactic shock,** peripheral

E

---

neuritis (rare), hyperuricemia, and decreased liver function. Adverse symptoms usually appear during the early months of therapy and disappear thereafter. Periodic renal and hepatic function tests as well as uric acid determinations are recommended.

Drug Interactions: Aluminum may delay and decrease the absorption of ethambutol.

Dosage ————————
• **Tablets**
Adults, initial treatment: 15 mg/kg/day until maximal improvement noted; **for retreatment:** 25 mg/kg/day as a single dose with at least one other tuberculostatic drug; **after 60 days:** 15 mg/kg/day.

RESPIRATORY CARE CONSIDERATIONS

See also *General Respiratory Care Considerations for All Anti-Infectives.*
Administration/Storage: Ethambutol should only be used in conjunction with at least one other antituberculosis drug.
Assessment
1. Note indications for therapy, onset and duration of symptoms, other treatments prescribed, and the outcomes.
2. Ascertain that client has had a visual acuity test before ethambutol therapy. Document no preexisting visual problems (especially if dose exceeds 15 mg/kg/day).
3. Obtain baseline CBC, cultures, and liver and renal function studies and monitor throughout therapy.
4. With positive AFB cultures, assist client to identify close contacts and advise them to seek treatment.
Evaluate
• Negative sputum cultures for acid-fast bacilli
• Resolution of infection (↓ fever, ↓ WBC, ↓ sputum production and improved CXR)

Etomidate
(eh-**TOM**-ih-dayt)
Pregnancy Category: C

Amidate **(Rx)**
Classification: General anesthetic and adjunct to general anesthesia

Action/Kinetics: Etomidate is actually a hypnotic without any analgesic activity. The drug seems to act like GABA and is thought to exert its mechanism by depressing the activity of the brain stem reticular system. It has minimal CV and respiratory depressant effects. **Onset:** 1 min. **Duration:** 3–5 min. **t½:** 75 min. Rapidly metabolized in the liver with inactive metabolites excreted mainly through the urine.

Uses: Induction of general anesthesia. As a supplement to nitrous oxide during short surgical procedures.

Special Concerns: Use with caution during lactation. Safety and efficacy have not been established in children less than 10 years of age.

Side Effects: *Skeletal muscle:* Myoclonic skeletal muscle movements, tonic movements. *Respiratory:* Apnea, hyperventilation or hypoventilation, **laryngospasm.** *CV:* Either hypertension or hypotension; tachycardia or bradycardia; arrhythmias. *GI:* N&V. *Miscellaneous:* Eye movements (common), hiccoughs, snoring.

Dosage ————————
• **IV Only**
Induction of anesthesia.
Adults and children over 10 years of age: 0.2–0.6 mg/kg (usual: 0.3 mg/kg) injected over 30–60 sec.

RESPIRATORY CARE CONSIDERATIONS
Administration/Storage
1. Lower doses of etomidate may be used as adjuncts to supplement less potent general anesthetics such as nitrous oxide.
2. Etomidate may be used following preanesthetic medications.
3. The drug should be protected from extreme heat and freezing.
Interventions
1. Nausea and vomiting are likely to occur postoperatively. Have essential equipment (suction, emesis basins,

washcloths, etc.) available to manage this problem.

2. Monitor client during the immediate postoperative period for hypotension, hypertension, tachycardia, and/or bradycardia and treat symptomatically.

Evaluate: Desired anesthetic level

F

Felodipine
(feh-**LOHD**-ih-peen)
Pregnancy Category: C
Plendil, Renedil ✦ **(Rx)**
Classification: Calcium channel blocking agent

See also *Calcium Channel Blocking Agents.*

Action/Kinetics: Onset after PO: 120–300 min. **Peak plasma levels:** 2.5–5 hr. Over 99% bound to plasma protein. t½, **elimination:** 11–16 hr. Metabolized in the liver.

Uses: Treatment of mild to moderate hypertension, alone or with other antihypertensives.

Contraindications: Use during lactation.

Special Concerns: Use with caution in clients with CHF or compromised ventricular function, especially in combination with a beta-adrenergic blocking agent. Use with caution in impaired hepatic function or reduced hepatic blood flow. Felodipine may cause a greater hypotensive effect in geriatric clients. Safety and effectiveness have not been determined in children.

Side Effects: *CV:* Significant hypotension, syncope, angina pectoris, peripheral edema, palpitations, AV block, *MI, arrhythmias,* tachycardia. *CNS:* Dizziness, lightheadedness, headache, nervousness, sleepiness, irritability, anxiety, insomnia, paresthesia, depression, amnesia, paranoia, psychosis, hallucinations. *Body as a whole:* Asthenia, flushing, muscle cramps, pain, inflammation, warm feeling, influenza. *GI:* Nausea, abdominal discomfort, cramps, dyspepsia, diarrhea, constipation, vomiting, dry mouth, flatulence. *Dermatologic:* Rash, dermatitis, urticaria, pruritus. *Respiratory:* Rhinitis, rhinorrhea, pharyngitis, sinusitis, nasal and chest congestion, SOB, wheezing, dyspnea, cough, bronchitis, sneezing, respiratory infection. *Miscellaneous:* Anemia, gingival hyperplasia, sexual difficulties, epistaxis, back pain, facial edema, erythema, urinary frequency or urgency, dysuria.

Additional Drug Interactions
Cimetidine / ↑ Bioavailability of felodipine
Digoxin / ↑ Peak plasma levels of digoxin
Fentanyl / Possible severe hypotension or ↑ fluid volume
Ranitidine / ↑ Bioavailability of felodipine

Dosage
• **Tablets, Extended Release**
Hypertension.
Initial: 5 mg once daily (2.5 mg in clients over 65 years of age and in those with impaired liver function); **then:** adjust dose according to response, usually at 2-week intervals with the usual dosage range being 2.5–10 mg once daily. Doses greater than 10 mg increase the rate of peripheral edema and other vasodilatory side effects.

RESPIRATORY CARE CONSIDERATIONS

See also *Respiratory Care Considerations* for *Calcium Channel Blocking Agents.*

Administration/Storage
1. Tablets should be swallowed whole and not chewed or crushed.
2. The bioavailability is not affected

✦ = Available in Canada   ***bold italic*** = life threatening side effect

by food although it is increased more than twofold when taken with doubly concentrated grapefruit juice when compared with water or orange juice.

Assessment

1. Document onset of symptoms and any other agents previously used and the outcome.

2. Note any history of heart failure or compromised ventricular function.

3. List drugs currently prescribed and note any potential interactions.

4. During any adjustment of dosage, BP should be closely monitored in clients over 65 years of age and in clients with impaired hepatic function.

Evaluate: Control of hypertension

Fentanyl citrate

(**FEN**-tah-nil)

Pregnancy Category: C

Fentanyl Oralet, Sublimaze **(C-II) (Rx)**

Classification: Narcotic analgesic, morphine type

See also *Narcotic Analgesics*.

Action/Kinetics: Similar to those of morphine and meperidine. **IV. Onset:** 7–8 min. **Peak effect:** Approximately 30 min. **Duration:** 1–2 hr. **t½:** 1.5–6 hr. When the oral lozenge (transmucosal administration) is sucked, fentanyl citrate is absorbed through the mucosal tissues of the mouth and GI tract. **Peak effect, transmucosal:** 20–30 min. The drug is faster-acting and of shorter duration than morphine or meperidine.

Uses: Parenteral. Preanesthetic medication, induction, and maintenance of anesthesia of short duration and immediate postoperative period. Supplement in general or regional anesthesia. Combined with droperidol for preanesthetic medication, induction of anesthesia, or as adjunct in maintenance of general or regional anesthesia. Combined with oxygen for anesthesia in high-risk clients undergoing open heart surgery, orthopedic procedures, or complicated neurologic procedures.

Oral (transmucosal). Anesthetic premedication in children and adults in an operating room setting. To induce conscious sedation before diagnostic or medical procedures (use only in closely monitored situations due to the risk of hypoventilation).

Contraindications: Fentanyl transmucosal is contraindicated in children who weigh less than 10 kg (22 lb), in the treatment of acute or chronic pain, and in use of doses greater than 15 mcg/kg in children and 5 mcg/kg in adults. Myasthenia gravis and other conditions in which muscle relaxants should not be used. Clients particularly sensitive to respiratory depression. Use during labor.

The transmucosal form is contraindicated in children who weigh less than 15 kg, for the treatment of acute or chronic pain (safety for this use not established), and for doses in excess of 15 mcg/kg in children and in excess of 5 mcg/kg in adults. Use outside the hospital setting is contraindicated.

Special Concerns: Safety and effectiveness have not been determined in children less than 2 years of age. Use with caution and at reduced dosage in poor-risk clients, children, the elderly, and when other CNS depressants are used. Use of the transmucosal form carries a risk of hypoventilation that may result in death.

Additional Side Effects: Skeletal and thoracic muscle rigidity, especially after rapid IV administration. Bradycardia, *seizures,* diaphoresis.

Additional Drug Interactions: ↑ Risk of CV depression when high doses of fentanyl are combined with nitrous oxide or diazepam.

Dosage

• **IM, IV**

Preoperatively.

Adults: 0.05–0.1 mg IM 30–60 min before surgery.

Adjunct to anesthesia, induction.

Adults: 0.002–0.05 mg/kg IV, depending on length and depth of anesthesia desired; **maintenance:** 0.025–0.1 mg/kg when indicated.

Adjunct to regional anesthesia.

Adults: 0.05–0.1 mg IM or IV over 1–2 min when indicated.

Postoperatively.
Adults: 0.05–0.1 mg IM q 1–2 hr for control of pain.

As general anesthetic with oxygen and a muscle relaxant.
0.05–0.1 mg/kg (up to 0.15 mg/kg may be required).

Children, induction and maintenance of anesthesia.
Pediatric, 2–12 years: 2–3 mcg/kg.

Children, general anesthetic.
0.05–0.1 mg/kg with oxygen and a muscle relaxant when attenuation of the responses to surgical stress is important (e.g., open heart surgery).

• **Transmucosal (Oral Lozenge)**
Individualize according to weight, age, physical status, general condition and medical status, underlying pathology, use of other drugs, type of anesthetic to be used, and the type and length of the surgical procedure. Doses of 5 mcg/kg are equivalent to IM fentanyl, 0.75–1.25 mcg/kg. Clients receiving more than 5 mcg/kg should be under the direct observation of medical personnel. Children may require up to 15 mcg/kg, provided their body weight is not less than 10 kg. Clients over 65 years of age should receive a dose from 2.5 to 5 mcg/kg. The maximum dose for adults and children, regardless of weight, is 400 mcg.

RESPIRATORY CARE CONSIDERATIONS

See also *Respiratory Care Considerations* for *Narcotic Analgesics.*
Administration/Storage
1. Direct IV infusions may be given, undiluted, over a period of 2–3 min.
2. After an IV injection, onset of action should occur within a few minutes and should last for 30–60 min.
3. Clients receiving an IM injection of drug can expect to have relief within 15 min and expect a duration of 1–2 hr.
4. Protect drug from light. The transmucosal product should be protected from freezing and mois-

ture; it should be stored below 30°C (86°F).
5. Oral form is supplied as a raspberry-flavored lozenge mounted on a handle and comes in strengths of 200, 300, and 400 mcg.
6. The foil overwrap of the oral form is to be removed just prior to administration. After removing the plastic overcap, the client should be instructed to place the transmucosal unit in the mouth and to suck (not chew) it. After the drug is consumed or the client shows signs of respiratory depression, the unit is removed from the mouth by the handle. If any of the medication remains, the matrix should be separated from the handle using a twisting motion. The drug matrix is then flushed down the toilet. If any drug matrix remains on the handle, it may be removed by running the handle under warm water. The drug-free handle should be disposed of according to institutional protocol. During the disposal process, the drug matrix should not come in contact with the skin, eyes, or mucous membranes. Hands should be washed thoroughly when finished.
7. The transmucosal product should be given 20–40 min prior to time for the desired effect.
8. Lower doses of the transmucosal form should be considered in clients with head injury, cardiovascular or pulmonary disease, liver dysfunction, or hepatic disease.
9. When using the transmucosal form, the client must be attended to at all times by an individual skilled in airway management and resuscitative techniques.
10. Have naloxone available in the event of an overdose.
11. Due to excessive hypoventilation at higher doses, greater than 5 mcg/kg (maximum of 400 mcg) of the transmucosal product is contraindicated.

Assessment
1. Document indications for therapy, anticipated time frame for use,

and any previous experience with this agent.

2. Note any history of neurovascular disease.

3. Document any evidence of pulmonary disease.

Client/Family Teaching

1. Caution to rise slowly as they may experience orthostatic hypotension.

2. Drug causes dizziness and drowsiness.

3. Avoid alcohol and any other CNS depressant for at least 24 hr.

4. Reinforce that transmucosal agent is not candy with children, that it is a very potent medication.

5. Advise that recall or memory may be suppressed during drug therapy; therefore client may not fully recall events surrounding procedure. Assure that procedure was done and attempt to answer any questions they may have. Explain that this is normal with this medication.

Evaluate

• Desired level of analgesia and relaxation

• Conscious sedation during procedures

Fentanyl Transdermal System

(**FEN**-tah-nil)

Pregnancy Category: C

Duragesic-25, -50, -75, and -100 **(C-II) (Rx)**

Classification: Narcotic analgesic, morphine type

See also *Narcotic Analgesics* and *Fentanyl citrate.*

Action/Kinetics: The system provides continuous delivery of fentanyl for up to 72 hr. The amount of fentanyl released from each system each hour depends on the surface area (25 mcg/hr is released from each 10 cm²). Each system also contains 0.1 mL of alcohol/10 cm²; the alcohol enhances the rate of drug flux through the copolymer membrane and also increases the permeability of the skin to fentanyl. Following application of the system, the skin under the system absorbs fentanyl, resulting in a depot of the drug in the upper skin layers, which is then available to the general circulation. After the system is removed, the residual drug in the skin continues to be absorbed so that serum levels fall 50% in about 17 hr. The drug is metabolized in the liver and excreted mainly in the urine.

Uses: Use should be restricted for the management of severe chronic pain that cannot be managed with less powerful drugs. The patch should only be used on clients who are already on and tolerant to narcotic analgesics and who require continuous narcotic administration.

Contraindications: Use for acute or postoperative pain (including out-patient surgeries). To manage mild or intermittent pain that can be managed by acetaminophen-opioid combinations, NSAIDs, or short-acting opioids. Hypersensitivity to fentanyl or adhesives. ICP, impaired consciousness, coma, medical conditions causing hypoventilation. Use during labor and delivery. Use of initial doses exceeding 25 mcg/hr, use in children less than 12 years of age and clients under 18 years of age who weigh less than 50 kg. Lactation.

Special Concerns: Use with caution in clients with brain tumors and bradyarrhythmias, as well as in elderly, cachectic, or debilitated individuals. Safety and efficacy have not been determined in children. The systems should be kept out of the reach of children; used systems should be disposed of properly.

Additional Side Effects: Sustained hypoventilation.

Dosage

• **Transdermal System**

Analgesia.

Adults, usual initial: 25 mcg/hr unless the client is tolerant to opioids (Duragesic-50, -75, and -100 are intended for use only in clients tolerant to opioids). Initial dose should be based on (1) the daily dose, potency, and characteristics (i.e., pure agonist, mixed agonist/antagonist) of the drug the client has been taking; (2) the reliability of the relative potency estimates used to calculate the dose as estimates vary depending on the route of administration; (3) the degree, if any, of tolerance to narcotics; and (4) the general condition and status of the client.

To convert clients from PO or parenteral opioids to the transdermal system, the following method should be used: (1) the previous 24-hr analgesic requirement should be calculated; (2) convert this amount to the equianalgesic PO morphine dose; (3) find the calculated 24-hr morphine dose and the corresponding transdermal fentanyl dose using the table provided with the product; and (4) initiate treatment using the recommended fentanyl dose. The dose may be increased no more frequently than 3 days after the initial dose or q 6 days thereafter. The ratio of 90 mg/24 hr of PO morphine to 25 mcg/hr increase in transdermal fentanyl dose should be used to base appropriate dosage increments on the daily dose of supplementary opioids.

If the dose of the fentanyl transdermal system exceeds 300 mcg/hr, it may be necessary to change clients to another narcotic analgesic. In such cases, the transdermal system should be removed and treatment initiated with one-half the equianalgesic dose of the new opioid 12–18 hr later. The dose of the new analgesic should be titrated based on the level of pain reported by the client.

RESPIRATORY CARE CONSIDERATIONS

See also *Respiratory Care Considerations* for *Narcotic Analgesics* and *Fentanyl citrate.*

Administration/Storage

1. The system should be applied to a nonirritated and nonirradiated fatty, flat surface of the skin, preferably on the upper torso. If needed, hair should be clipped (not shaved) from the site prior to application.

2. Only clear water, if needed, should be used to cleanse the site prior to application. Soaps, oils, lotions, alcohol, or other agents that might irritate the skin should not be used. The skin should be allowed to dry completely prior to applying the system. If liquid comes in contact with the skin, use clear water only to remove.

3. The system should be removed from the sealed package and applied immediately by pressing firmly in place (for 10–20 sec) with the palm of the hand. **Never cut the system.** Ensure that contact of the system is complete, especially around the edges. Tape the patch to prevent dislodgement.

4. Each system should remain in place for 72 hr; if additional analgesia is required, a new system can be applied to a different skin site after removal of the previous system.

5. Systems removed from a skin site should be folded so that the adhesive side adheres to itself; it should then be flushed down the toilet immediately after removal.

6. Any unused systems should be disposed of as soon as they are no longer needed by removing them from their package and flushing down the toilet. During hospitalization, appropriate institutional guidelines for disposing of controlled substances should be followed.

7. Multiple systems may be used if the delivery rate needs to exceed 100 mcg/hr.

8. The initial evaluation of the maximum analgesic effect should not be undertaken until 24 hr after the system is applied.

9. If required, clients can use a short-acting analgesic for the first 24 hr (i.e., until analgesic efficacy is reached with the transdermal system).

10. Clients may continue to require periodic supplemental doses of a

short-acting analgesic to treat break-through pain.

11. If opioid therapy is to be discontinued, a gradual decrease in dose is recommended to minimize S&S of abrupt narcotic withdrawal.

Assessment

1. Document indications for therapy, noting onset of symptoms, previous agents used, and the outcome.

2. Rate pain level at various times throughout the day to ensure adequate dosing. Determine that dose required is based on conversion guidelines provided by manufacturer.

3. Note any history or evidence of increased ICP or brain tumors.

Evaluate

• Reports of symptomatic improvement R/T pain management

• Relief of pain as evidenced by improved appetite, ↑ activity, and ↑ socialization

Fexofenadine hydrochloride

(fex-oh-**FEN**-ah-deen)
Pregnancy Category: C
Allegra **(Rx)**
Classification: Antihistamine

See also *Antihistamines*.

Action/Kinetics: Fexofenadine, a metabolite of terfenadine, is an H_1-histamine receptor blocker. The drug is rapidly absorbed. **Peak plasma levels:** 2.6 hr. **t½, terminal:** 14.4 hr. Approximately 90% of the drug is excreted through the feces (80%) and urine (10%) unchanged.

Uses: Relief of symptoms associated with seasonal allergic rhinitis in adults and children 12 years of age and older.

Special Concerns: Use with care during lactation. Safety and efficacy have not been determined in children less than 12 years of age.

Side Effects: *CNS:* Drowsiness, fatigue. *GI:* Nausea, dyspepsia. *Miscellaneous:* Viral infection (flu, colds), dysmenorrhea, sinusitis, throat irritation.

Drug Interactions: No differences in side effects or the QTc interval were observed when fexofenadine was given with either erythromycin or ketoconazole.

Dosage —————
• **Capsules**
  Seasonal allergic rhinitis.
Adults and children over 12 years of age: 60 mg b.i.d. In clients with decreased renal function, the initial dose should be 60 mg once daily.

RESPIRATORY CARE CONSIDERATIONS

See also *Respiratory Care Considerations* for *Antihistamines*.

Assessment

1. Document onset, duration, and characteristics of symptoms; identify triggers if known.

2. Note other agents trialed, length of use, and the outcome.

3. Determine any history or evidence of renal dysfunction and anticipate reduced dosage when evident.

Evaluate: Control of symptoms of seasonal allergic rhinitis

Flecainide acetate

(fleh-**KAY**-nyd)
Pregnancy Category: C
Tambocor **(Rx)**
Classification: Antiarrhythmic, class IC

See also *Antiarrhythmic Agents*.

Action/Kinetics: Flecainide produces its antiarrhythmic effect by a local anesthetic action, especially on the His-Purkinje system in the ventricle. The drug decreases single and multiple PVCs and reduces the incidence of ventricular tachycardia. **Peak plasma levels:** 3 hr.; **steady state levels:** 3–5 days. **Effective plasma levels:** 0.2–1 mcg/mL (trough levels). **t½:** 20 hr (12–27 hr). Forty percent is bound to plasma protein. Approximately 30% is excreted in urine unchanged. Impaired renal function decreases rate of elimination of unchanged drug. Food or antacids do not affect absorption.

Uses: Life-threatening arrhythmias

manifested as sustained ventricular tachycardia. Prevention of paroxysmal supraventricular tachycardias (PSVT) and paroxysmal atrial fibrillation or flutter (PAF) associated with disabling symptoms but not structural heart disease. Antiarrhythmic drugs have not been shown to improve survival in clients with ventricular arrhythmias.

Contraindications: Cardiogenic shock, preexisting second- or third-degree AV block, right bundle branch block when associated with bifascicular block (unless pacemaker is present to maintain cardiac rhythm). Recent MI. Cardiogenic shock. Chronic atrial fibrillation. Frequent premature ventricular complexes and symptomatic nonsustained ventricular arrhythmias. Lactation.

Special Concerns: Use with caution in sick sinus syndrome, in clients with a history of CHF or MI, in disturbances of potassium levels, in clients with permanent pacemakers or temporary pacing electrodes, renal and liver impairment. Safety and efficacy in children less than 18 years of age are not established. The incidence of proarrhythmic effects may be increased in geriatric clients.

Side Effects: *CV: New or worsened ventricular arrhythmias, increased risk of death in clients with non-life-threatening cardiac arrhythmias,* new or worsened CHF, palpitations, chest pain, sinus bradycardia, sinus pause, sinus arrest, *ventricular fibrillation, ventricular tachycardia that cannot be resuscitated,* second- or third-degree AV block, tachycardia, hypertension, hypotension, bradycardia, angina pectoris. *CNS:* Dizziness, faintness, syncope, lightheadedness, neuropathy, unsteadiness, headache, fatigue, paresthesia, paresis, hypoesthesia, insomnia, anxiety, malaise, vertigo, depression, *seizures,* euphoria, confusion, depersonalization, apathy, morbid dreams, speech disorders, stupor, amnesia, weakness, somnolence. *GI:* Nausea, constipation, abdominal pain, vomiting, anorexia, dyspepsia, dry mouth, diarrhea, flatulence, change in taste. *Ophthalmic:* Blurred vision, difficulty in focusing, spots before eyes, diplopia, photophobia, eye pain, nystagmus, eye irritation, photophobia. *Hematologic:* Leukopenia, thrombocytopenia. *GU:* Decreased libido, impotence, urinary retention, polyuria. *Musculoskeletal:* Asthenia, tremor, ataxia, arthralgia, myalgia. *Dermatologic:* Skin rashes, urticaria, exfoliative dermatitis, pruritus, alopecia. *Other:* Edema, dyspnea, fever, ***bronchospasm,*** flushing, sweating, tinnitus, swollen mouth, lips, and tongue.

OD **Overdose Management:** *Symptoms:* Lengthening of PR interval; increase in QRS duration, QT interval, and amplitude of T wave; decrease in HR and contractility; conduction disturbances; hypotension; ***respiratory failure*** or asystole. *Treatment:* Charcoal will remove unabsorbed drug up to 90 min after drug ingestion. Administration of dopamine, dobutamine, or isoproterenol. Artificial respiration. Intra-aortic balloon pumping, transvenous pacing (to correct conduction block). Acidification of the urine may be beneficial, especially in those with an alkaline urine. Due to the long duration of action of the drug, treatment measures may have to be continued for a prolonged period of time.

Drug Interactions
Acidifying agents / ↑ Renal excretion of flecainide
Alkalinizing agents / ↓ Renal excretion of flecainide
Amiodarone / ↑ Plasma levels of flecainide
Cimetidine / ↑ Bioavailability and renal excretion of flecainide
Digoxin / ↑ Digoxin plasma levels
Disopyramide / Additive negative inotropic effects
Propranolol / Additive negative inotropic effects; also, ↑ plasma levels of both drugs
Smoking (Tobacco) / ↑ Plasma clearance of flecainide

Verapamil / Additive negative inotropic effects

Dosage
- **Tablets**
  Sustained ventricular tachycar-dia.
  Initial: 100 mg q 12 hr; **then,** in-crease by 50 mg b.i.d. q 4 days until effective dose reached. **Usual effective dose:** 150 mg q 12 hr; dose should not exceed 400 mg/day.
  PSVT, PAF.
  Initial: 50 mg q 12 hr; **then,** dose may be increased in increments of 50 mg b.i.d. q 4 days until effective dose reached. Maximum recom-mended dose: 300 mg/day. *NOTE:* For PAF clients, increasing the dose from 50 to 100 mg b.i.d. may in-crease efficacy without a significant in-crease in side effects.
  NOTE: For clients with a creati-nine clearance less than 35 mL/min/1.73 m², the starting dose is 100 mg once daily (or 50 mg b.i.d.). For less severe renal disease, the in-itial dose may be 100 mg q 12 hr.

RESPIRATORY CARE CONSIDERATIONS

See also *Respiratory Care Considera-tions* for *Antiarrhythmic Agents.*

Administration/Storage
1. For most situations, therapy should be started in a hospital setting (especially in clients with sympto-matic CHF, sustained ventricular ar-rhythmias, compensated clients with significant myocardial dysfunction, or sinus node dysfunction).
2. For clients with renal impairment, the dosage should be increased at intervals greater than 4 days. The cli-ent should be monitored carefully for adverse toxic effects.
3. The chance of toxic effects in-creases if the trough plasma levels exceed 1 mcg/mL.
4. If client is being transferred to fle-cainide from another antiarrhythmic, at least two to four plasma half-lives should elapse for the drug being dis-continued before initiating flecainide therapy.

5. An occasional client may benefit from dosing at 8-hr intervals.
6. To minimize toxicity, the dose may be reduced once the arrhythmia is controlled.

Assessment
1. Document baseline physical as-sessment findings.
2. Obtain baseline ECG, CXR, electro-lytes, and liver and renal function studies prior to initiating therapy.
3. Review client history, echocardio-grams, and ECGs for evidence of CHF, ventricular arrhythmias, sinus node dysfunction, or abnormal ejec-tion fractions.

Interventions
1. Monitor ECG for increased ar-rhythmias or AV block and report if evident.
2. Check serum potassium levels. Preexisting hypokalemia or hyper-kalemia may alter the effects of the drug and should be corrected before starting therapy with flecainide.
3. Monitor for labile BP.
4. Note adverse CNS effects, such as client complaints of dizziness, visual disturbances, headaches, nausea, or depression and report.
5. Obtain urinary pH to detect alka-linity or acidity. Alkalinity of the urine decreases renal excretion and acidity increases renal excretion, which in turn affects the rate of drug elimination.
6. Observe for any S&S of CHF or pulmonary toxicity.
7. Concomitant administration of flecainide with disopyramide, pro-pranolol, or verapamil will promote additive negative inotropic effects.
8. Clients with pacemakers should have the pacing thresholds checked and adjusted before and 1 week fol-lowing drug therapy.

Evaluate
- Termination of lethal ventricular arrhythmias
- Maintenance of stable cardiac rhythm
- Therapeutic serum (trough) drug levels (0.2–1.0 mcg/mL)

Flucytosine
(flew-SYE-toe-seen)
Pregnancy Category: C
Ancobon, Ancotil ✹ **(Rx)**
Classification: Antibiotic, antifungal

Action/Kinetics: Flucytosine is indicated only for serious systemic fungal infections. The drug is less toxic than amphotericin B. Liver, renal system, and hematopoietic system must be monitored closely.

Flucytosine appears to penetrate the fungal cell membrane and then, after metabolism, to act as an antimetabolite interfering with nucleic acid and protein synthesis. It is well absorbed from the GI tract and is distributed to the joints, aqueous humor, peritoneal and other body fluids and tissues. **Peak plasma concentration:** 2–6 hr. **Therapeutic serum concentration:** 20–25 mcg/mL. t½: 2–5 hr, higher in presence of impaired renal function. Eighty percent to 90% of the drug is excreted unchanged in urine.

Uses: Serious systemic infections by susceptible strains of *Candida* (e.g., endocarditis, septicemia, UTIs) or *Cryptococcus* (pulmonary or UTIs, meningitis, septicemia).

Contraindications: Hypersensitivity to drug. Lactation.

Special Concerns: Safety and effectiveness have not been determined in children. Use with extreme caution in clients with kidney disease or history of bone marrow depression. The bone marrow depressant effects may cause an increased incidence of microbial infection, gingival bleeding, and delayed healing.

Side Effects: *GI:* N&V, diarrhea, abdominal pain, dry mouth, anorexia, duodenal ulcer, GI hemorrhage, ulcerative colitis. *Hematologic:* Anemia, leukopenia, thrombocytopenia, *aplastic anemia, agranulocytosis,* pancytopenia, eosinophilia. *CNS:* Headache, vertigo, confusion, sedation, hallucinations, paresthesia, parkinsonism, psychosis, pyrexia. *Hepatic:* Hepatic dysfunction, jaundice, ele-

vation of hepatic enzymes, increase in bilirubin. *GU:* Increase in BUN and creatinine, azotemia, crystalluria, renal failure. *Respiratory:* Chest pain, dyspnea, ***respiratory arrest.*** *Dermatologic:* Pruritus, rash, urticaria, photosensitivity. *Other:* Ataxia, hearing loss, peripheral neuropathy, weakness, hypoglycemia, fatigue, ***cardiac arrest,*** hypokalemia.

OD **Overdose Management:** *Symptoms (serum levels > 100 mcg/mL):* N&V, diarrhea, leukopenia, thrombocytopenia, hepatitis. *Treatment:* Prompt induction of vomiting or gastric lavage. Adequate fluid intake (by IV if necessary). Monitor blood, liver, and kidney parameters frequently. Hemodialysis will quickly decrease serum levels.

Drug Interactions
Amphotericin B / ↑ Effect and toxicity of flucytosine due to kidney impairment
Cytosine / Inactivates antifungal effect of flucytosine

Dosage ——————————
• **Capsules**
Adult and children: 50–150 mg/kg/day in four divided doses. Clients with renal impairment receive lower dosages.

RESPIRATORY CARE CONSIDERATIONS

See also *General Respiratory Care Considerations for All Anti-Infectives.*

Administration/Storage: Reduce or avoid nausea by administering capsules a few at a time over a 15-min period.

Assessment
1. Obtain baseline CBC and liver and renal function studies and monitor throughout therapy.
2. Before administering first dose, check that cultures have been taken.
3. Anticipate reduced dose with impaired renal function.

Evaluate: Resolution of fungal infection

✹ = Available in Canada   ***bold italic*** = life threatening side effect

Flumazenil

(floo-**MAZ**-eh-nill)
Pregnancy Category: C
Anexate ✦, Romazicon **(Rx)**
Classification: Benzodiazepine
receptor antagonist

Action/Kinetics: Flumazenil antagonizes the effects of benzodiazepines on the CNS by competitively inhibiting their action at the benzodiazepine recognition site on the GABA/benzodiazepine receptor complex. The drug does not antagonize the CNS effects of ethanol, general anesthetics, barbiturates, or opiates. Depending on the dose of flumazenil, there will be partial or complete antagonism of sedation, impaired recall, and psychomotor impairment. **Onset of reversal:** 1–2 min. **Peak effect:** 6–10 min. The duration of reversal is related to the plasma levels of the benzodiazepine and the dose of flumazenil. **Distribution t½, initial:** 7–15 min; **terminal t½:** 41–79 min. The drug is metabolized in the liver with 90%–95% excreted through the urine and 5%–10% excreted in the feces. Hepatic impairment prolongs the half-life of the drug. Ingestion of food results in a 50% increase in clearance of flumazenil.

Uses: Complete or partial reversal of benzodiazepine-induced depression of the ventilatory responses to hypercapnia and hypoxia. Situations include cases where general anesthesia has been induced or maintained by benzodiazepines, where sedation has been produced by benzodiazepines for diagnostic and therapeutic procedures, and for the management of benzodiazepine overdosage.

Contraindications: Use in clients given a benzodiazepine for control of intracranial pressure or status epilepticus. In clients manifesting signs of serious cyclic antidepressant overdose. Use during labor and delivery or in children as the risks and benefits are not known. To treat benzodiazepine dependence or for the management of protracted benzodiazepine

abstinence syndrome. Use until the effects of neuromuscular blockade have been fully reversed.

Special Concerns: The reversal of benzodiazepine effects may be associated with the onset of seizures in certain high-risk clients (e.g., concurrent major sedative-hypnotic drug withdrawal, recent therapy with repeated doses of parenteral benzodiazepines, myoclonic jerking or seizure activity prior to administration of flumazenil in cases of overdose, and concurrent cyclic antidepressant overdosage). Use with caution in clients with head injury as the drug may precipitate seizures or alter cerebral blood flow in clients receiving benzodiazepines. Use with caution in clients with alcoholism and other drug dependencies due to the increased frequency of benzodiazepine tolerance and dependence. Use with caution during lactation.

Flumazenil may precipitate a withdrawal syndrome if the client is dependent on benzodiazepines. Flumazenil may cause panic attacks in clients with a history of panic disorder.

Use with caution in mixed-drug overdosage as toxic effects (e.g., cardiac dysrhythmias, convulsions) may occur (especially with cyclic antidepressants).

Side Effects: *Deaths* have occurred in clients receiving flumazenil, especially in those with serious underlying disease or in those who have ingested large amounts of nonbenzodiazepine drugs (usually cyclic antidepressants) as part of an overdose. *Seizures are the most common serious side effect noted.*

CNS: Dizziness, vertigo, ataxia, anxiety, nervousness, tremor, palpitations, insomnia, dyspnea, hyperventilation, abnormal crying, depersonalization, euphoria, increased tears, depression, dysphoria, paranoia, delirium, difficulty concentrating, *seizures,* somnolence, stupor, speech disorder. *GI:* N&V, hiccoughs, dry mouth. *CV:* Sweating, flushing, hot flushes, *arrhythmias (atrial, nodal, ventricular extrasystoles),* bradycardia, tachycardia, hypertension, chest pain. *At injection site:* Pain, thrombophlebitis, rash, skin abnormality. *Body as a whole:* Headache, increased sweating, asthenia, malaise, rigors, shivering, paresthesia. *Ophthalmologic:* Abnormal vision including visual field defect and diplopia; blurred vision. *Otic:* Transient hearing impairment, tinnitus, hyperacusis.

Dosage
• **IV Only**

To reverse conscious sedation or in general anesthesia.

Adults, initial: 0.2 mg (2 mL) given IV over 15 sec. If the desired level of consciousness is not reached after waiting an additional 45 sec, a second dose of 0.2 mg (2 mL) can be given and repeated at 60-sec intervals, up to a maximum total dose of 1 mg (10 mL). Most clients will respond to doses of 0.6–1 mg. To treat resedation, give no more than 1 mg (given as 0.2 mg/min) at any one time and give no more than 3 mg in any 1 hr.

Management of suspected benzodiazepine overdose.

Adults, initial: 0.2 mg (2 mL) given IV over 30 sec; a second dose of 0.3 mg (3 mL) can be given over another 30 sec. Further doses of 0.5 mg (5 mL) can be given over 30 sec at 1-min intervals up to a total dose of 3 mg (although some clients may require up to 5 mg given slowly as described). If the client has not responded 5 min after receiving a cumulative dose of 5 mg, the major cause of sedation is probably not due to benzodiazepines and additional doses of flumazenil are likely to have no effect. For resedation, repeated doses may be given at 20-min intervals; no more than 1 mg (given as 0.5 mg/min) at any one time and no more than 3 mg in any 1 hr should be administered.

RESPIRATORY CARE CONSIDERATIONS
Administration/Storage
1. The dosage must be individualized. It is important to give only the smallest amount of flumazenil that is effective. The 1-min wait between individual doses in the dose-titration recommended for general uses may be too short for high-risk clients as it takes 6–10 min for any single dose of flumazenil to reach full effects. Thus, the rate of administration should be slowed in high-risk clients.

2. A major risk is resedation because the duration of effect of a long-acting or a large dose of a short-acting benzodiazepine may exceed that of flumazenil. If there is resedation, repeated doses may be given at 20-min intervals as needed.

3. Flumazenil is best given as a series of small injections to allow the physician to control the reversal of sedation to the end point desired and to decrease the possibility of side effects.

4. The dose of flumazenil should be reduced to 40%–60% of normal in clients with severe hepatic dysfunction.

5. Flumazenil should be given through a freely running IV infusion into a large vein to minimize pain at the injection site.

6. Doses larger than a total of 3 mg do not reliably produce additional effects.

7. Flumazenil is compatible with 5% dextrose in water, lactated Ringer's, and NSS solutions. If flumazenil is drawn into a syringe or mixed with any of these solutions, it should be discarded after 24 hr.

8. For optimum sterility, flumazenil should remain in the vial until just before use.

9. Before administering flumazenil, clients should have a secure airway and IV access; also, they should be awakened gradually.

Assessment
1. Review client history, noting any evidence of seizure disorder or panic attacks.

2. Determine type and amount of drug ingested and when; especially

note any overdose of tricyclic antidepressants or mixed-drug overdose.

3. Document any liver dysfunction as subsequent doses require adjustment.

4. Assess for any evidence of head injury or increased ICP.

5. Note any evidence of sedative or benzodiazepine dependence, alcohol abuse, or recent use of either as drug may precipitate withdrawal symptoms.

Interventions

1. The effects of flumazenil usually wear off before the effects of many benzodiazepines. Observe client closely for resedation, depressed respirations, or other residual benzodiazepine effects for up to 120 min after flumazenil administration. The availability of flumazenil does not decrease the need for prompt detection of hypoventilation and the need to establish an airway and assist with ventilation.

2. Flumazenil is intended as an adjunct to, not a substitute for, proper management of the airway, assisted breathing, circulatory access and support, use of lavage and charcoal, and adequate clinical evaluation. Prior to giving flumazenil, proper measures should be undertaken to secure an airway for ventilation and IV access. Be prepared for clients attempting to withdraw ET tubes or IV lines due to confusion and agitation following awakening; awakening should be gradual.

3. The drug should be used with caution in the intensive care unit (ICU) due to the increased risk of unrecognized benzodiazepine dependence in such settings. Drug may produce convulsions in benzodiazepine-dependent clients.

4. Flumazenil is not intended to be used to diagnose benzodiazepine-induced sedation in the ICU. Failure to respond may be masked by metabolic disorders, traumatic injury, or other drugs.

5. Incorporate seizure precautions. There is an increased risk for seizures with large overdoses of cyclic antidepressants and in clients on long-term sedation with benzodiazepines.

6. Convulsions associated with administration of flumazenil may be treated with benzodiazepines, phenytoin, or barbiturates. Higher than usual doses of benzodiazepines may be needed.

7. Flumazenil should not be used until the effects of neuromuscular blockade have been fully reversed.

8. Flumazenil does not consistently reverse amnesia. Therefore, clients cannot be expected to remember what is told to them in the postprocedure period. Instructions should be given in writing to the client or family member.

Evaluate: Reversal of benzodiazepine sedative and psychomotor effects

---

Flunisolide

(flew-**NISS**-oh-lyd)
Pregnancy Category: C
Inhalation: AeroBid, Bronalide Aerosol ✤, Rhinaris F ✤, Syn-Flunisolide ✤
(Rx), Intranasal: Nasalide, Nasarel, Rhinalar ✤ **(Rx)**
Classification: Corticosteroid

See also *Corticosteroids.*

Action/Kinetics: Produces anti-inflammatory effects intranasally with minimal systemic effects. Several days may be required for full beneficial effects. After inhalation, there is a significant first-pass effect through the liver and the drug is rapidly metabolized. **t½:** 1.8 hr.

Uses: Inhalation: Prophylaxis and treatment of bronchial asthma in combination with other therapy. Not used when asthma can be relieved by other drugs, in clients where systemic corticosteroid treatment is infrequent, and in nonasthmatic bronchitis. **Intranasal:** Seasonal or perennial rhinitis, especially if other treatment has proven unsatisfactory.

Contraindications: Active or quiescent tuberculosis, especially of the respiratory tract. Untreated fungal, bacterial, systemic viral infections. Ocular herpes simplex. Do not use until healing occurs following recent ulceration of nasal septum, nasal surgery, or trauma. Lactation.

Special Concerns: Safety and effectiveness in children less than 6 years of age have not been determined.

Additional Side Effects: *Respiratory:* Hoarseness, coughing, throat irritation; *Candida* infections of nose, larynx, and pharynx. *After intranasal use:* Nasopharyngeal irritation, stinging, burning, dryness, headache. *GI:* Dry mouth. Systemic corticosteroid effects, especially if recommended dose is exceeded.

Dosage ⎯⎯⎯⎯⎯⎯

• **Inhalation**

Bronchial asthma.

Adults: 2 inhalations (total of 500 mcg flunisolide) in a.m. and p.m., not to exceed 4 inhalations b.i.d. (i.e., total daily dose of 2 mg). **Pediatric, 6–15 years:** 2 inhalations in the morning and evening, with total daily dose not to exceed 1 mg.

• **Intranasal**

Rhinitis.

Adults, initial: 50 mcg (2 sprays) in each nostril b.i.d.; may be increased to 2 sprays t.i.d. up to maximum daily dose of 400 mcg (i.e., 8 sprays in each nostril). **Pediatric, 6–14 years, initial:** 25 mcg (1 spray) in each nostril t.i.d. or 50 mcg (2 sprays) in each nostril b.i.d., up to maximum daily dose of 200 mcg (i.e., 4 sprays in each nostril). **Maintenance, adults, children:** Smallest dose necessary to control symptoms. Some clients (approximately 15%) are controlled on 1 spray in each nostril daily.

RESPIRATORY CARE CONSIDERATIONS

See also *Respiratory Care Considerations* for *Corticosteroids.*

Administration/Storage

1. When initiating the inhalant in clients receiving corticosteroids systemically, the aerosol should be used concomitantly with the systemic steroid for 1 week. Then, slowly withdraw the systemic corticosteroid over several weeks.

2. If nasal congestion is present, use a decongestant before administration to ensure the drug reaches the site of action.

3. If beneficial effects do not occur within 3 weeks, discontinue therapy. Improvement of symptoms usually is seen within a few days, however.

Client/Family Teaching

1. Use a demonstrator and instruct client and family how to administer nasal spray or inhalant.

2. Remind clients to gargle and rinse their mouth with water after inhalation to prevent alterations in taste and to maintain adequate oral hygiene. Report any symptoms of fungal infections.

3. Advise that mild nasal bleeding may occur; this is usually transient.

4. Provide a printed list of drug side effects. Identify those that require immediate reporting.

Evaluate

• Improved airway exchange
• ↓ Allergic manifestations

Fluticasone propionate

(flu-**TIH**-kah-sohn)

Pregnancy Category: C

Flonase, Flovent **(Rx)**

Classification: Corticosteroid

See also *Corticosteroids.*

Action/Kinetics: Following intranasal use, a small amount is absorbed into the general circulation. **Onset:** Approximately 12 hr. **Maximum effect:** May take several days. Absorbed drug is metabolized in the liver and excreted in the urine.

Uses: Maintenance treatment of asthma in adults and children over 12 years of age. To manage seasonal and perennial allergic rhinitis in adults and children over 12 years of age.

Contraindications: Use for nonallergic rhinitis. Use following nasal septal ulcers, nasal surgery, or nasal trauma until healing has occurred.

Special Concerns: Safety and efficacy in children less than 12 years of age have not been determined. Clients on immunosuppressant drugs, such as corticosteroids, are more susceptible to infections. Use with caution, if at all, in active or quiescent tuberculosis infections; untreated fungal, bacterial, or systemic viral infections; or ocular herpes simplex. Use with caution during lactation.

Side Effects: *Allergic:* Rarely, immediate hypersensitivity reactions or contact dermatitis. *Respiratory:* Epistaxis, nasal burning, blood in nasal mucus, pharyngitis, irritation of nasal mucous membranes, sneezing, runny nose, nasal dryness, sinusitis, nasal congestion, bronchitis, nasal ulcer, nasal septum excoriation. *CNS:* Headache, dizziness. *Ophthalmologic:* Eye disorder, cataracts, glaucoma, increased intraocular pressure. *GI:* N&V, xerostomia. *Miscellaneous:* Unpleasant taste, urticaria. High doses have resulted in hypercorticism and adrenal suppression.

Dosage —————————————
• **Metered Dose Inhaler**
  Treatment of asthma.
Adults and children over 12 years of age, initial: 88 mcg b.i.d. for patients previously using only bronchodilators, and 88-220 mcg b.i.d. for those already using inhaled corticosteroids. For oral steroid sparing, the recommended dose is 880 mcg b.i.d.
• **Nasal Spray**
  Allergic rhinitis.
Adults and children over 12 years of age, initial: Two 50-mcg sprays in each nostril once a day, for a total daily dose of 200 mcg/day. Alternatively, one 50-mcg spray in each nostril twice a day (e.g., 8 a.m. and 8 p.m.), for a total dose of 200 mcg/day. Adolescents (i.e., those over 12 years) should be started on 50 mcg in each nostril once daily. **Maintenance, after 4–7 days:** 50 mcg in each nostril once daily, for a total dose of 100 mcg/day.
• **Ointment, Cream**

Apply sparingly to affected area 2–4 times daily.

RESPIRATORY CARE CONSIDERATIONS

See also *Respiratory Care Considerations* for *Corticosteroids.*
Administration/Storage
1. Effectiveness depends on regular use.
2. The spray should be stored at 4°C–30°C (39°F–86°F).
Assessment
1. Document indications for therapy, noting onset and duration of symptoms and other agents trialed.
2. Examine nostrils for any evidence of nasal septal ulcers and note turbinate findings.
3. Determine if client is immunocompromised or actively infected.
Client/Family Teaching
1. Review the technique for administration and observe client self-administer.
2. Advise to take at regular intervals to ensure effectiveness and not to exceed prescribed dose as it may take several days to achieve full benefits.
3. Remind not to interrupt therapy if side effects evident but to notify provider as drug may require slow withdrawal. The dosage should also be slowly reduced if symptoms of hypercorticism or adrenal suppression occur.
4. Review the S&S of adrenal insufficiency (depression, lassitude, joint and muscle pain) and advise to report if evident, especially when replacing systemic corticosteroids with topical.
5. Use adequate humidity, especially during winter months when dry heat may aggravate mucosa.
6. Avoid persons with active infections. Report exposure to chicken pox or measles. (If not immunized or previously infected with the disease, VZIG or IG prophylaxis may be administered to high risk-clients on long-term therapy).
7. Explain that height and weight will be monitored periodically in ad-

olescents to detect any evidence of growth suppression.

8. Review triggers that aggravate asthma (dust, pollen, smoke, chemicals, pets) and teach client how to use peak flow meter. Identify zones to assist client to better manage their asthma.

Evaluate

• Control of asthma
• Relief from symptoms of allergic rhinitis

Fosinopril sodium
(foh-**SIN**-oh-prill)
Pregnancy Category: D
Monopril **(Rx)**
Classification: Angiotensin-converting enzyme inhibitor

See also *Angiotensin-Converting Enzyme Inhibitors.*

Action/Kinetics: Onset: 1 hr. **Time to peak serum levels:** About 3 hr. Metabolized in the liver to the active fosinoprilat. Fosinoprilat is significantly bound to plasma proteins. **t½:** 12 hr for fosinoprilat (prolonged in impaired renal function) following IV administration. **Duration:** 24 hr. Approximately 50% excreted through the urine and 50% in the feces. Food decreases the rate, but not the extent, of absorption of fosinopril.

Uses: Alone or in combination with other antihypertensive agents (especially thiazide diuretics) for the treatment of hypertension. Adjunct in treating CHF in clients not responding adequately to diuretics and digitalis.

Contraindications: Use during lactation.

Side Effects: *CV:* Orthostatic hypotension, chest pain, hypotension, palpitations, angina pectoris, ***CVA, MI,*** rhythm disturbances, hypertensive crisis, claudication. *CNS:* Headache, dizziness, fatigue, confusion, memory disturbance, tremors, drowsiness, mood change, insomnia, vertigo, sleep disturbances. *GI:* N&V, diarrhea, abdominal pain, constipation, dry mouth, dysphagia, taste disturbance, abdominal distention, flatu-

lence, heartburn, appetite changes, weight changes. *Respiratory:* Cough, sinusitis, ***bronchospasm,*** asthma, pharyngitis, laryngitis. *Hematologic:* Leukopenia, eosinophilia, decreases in hemoglobin (mean of 0.1 g/dL) or hematocrit, neutropenia. *Dermatologic:* Diaphoresis, photosensitivity, flushing, pruritus, rash, urticaria. *Body as a whole:* Angioedema, muscle cramps, syncope, myalgia, arthralgia, edema, weakness, musculoskeletal pain. *GU:* Decreased libido, sexual dysfunction, renal insufficiency, urinary frequency. *Miscellaneous:* Paresthesias, hepatitis, pancreatitis, syncope, tinnitus, gout, lymphadenopathy, rhinitis, epistaxis, vision disturbances, eye irritation, laryngitis.

Laboratory Test Interferences: Transient ↓ H&H. False low measurement of serum digoxin levels with DigiTab RIA Kit for Digoxin.

Dosage

• **Tablets**

Hypertension.

Initial: 10 mg once daily; **then,** adjust dose depending on BP response at peak (2–6 hr after dosing) and trough (24 hr after dosing) blood levels. **Maintenance:** Usually 20–40 mg/day, although some clients manifest beneficial effects at doses up to 80 mg.

In clients taking diuretics.

Discontinue diuretic 2–3 days before starting fosinopril. If diuretic cannot be discontinued, use an initial dose of 10 mg fosinopril.

Congestive heart failure.

Initial: 10 mg once daily; **then,** following initial dose, observe the client for at least 2 hr for the presence of hypotension or orthostasis (if either is present, monitor until BP stabilizes). An initial dose of 5 mg is recommended in heart failure with moderate to severe renal failure or in those who have had significant diuresis. The dose is increased over several weeks, not to exceed a maximum of

40 mg daily (usual effective range is 20–40 mg once daily).

RESPIRATORY CARE CONSIDERATIONS

See also *Respiratory Care Considerations* for *Angiotensin-Converting Enzyme Inhibitors* and *Antihypertensive Agents.*

Administration/Storage

1. If the antihypertensive effect decreases at the end of the dosing interval in clients taking the medication once daily, b.i.d. administration should be considered.

2. If the client is taking a diuretic, the diuretic should be discontinued 2–3 days prior to beginning fosinopril therapy. If the BP is not controlled, the diuretic should be reinstituted. If the diuretic cannot be discontinued, an initial dose of fosinopril should be 10 mg.

3. The dose of fosinopril does not have to be adjusted in clients with renal insufficiency except as noted in Dosage.

Evaluate

- Control of hypertension
- Control of symptoms of CHF

Furosemide
(fur-**OH**-seh-myd)
Pregnancy Category: C
Apo-Furosemide ✚, Furoside ✚, Lasix, Myrosemide, Novo-Semide ✚, Uritol ✚ **(Rx)**
Classification: Loop diuretic

See also *Diuretics, Loop.*

Action/Kinetics: Furosemide inhibits the reabsorption of sodium and chloride in the proximal and distal tubules as well as the ascending loop of Henle; this results in the excretion of sodium, chloride, and, to a lesser degree, potassium and bicarbonate ions. The resulting urine is more acid. Diuretic action is independent of changes in clients' acid-base balance. Furosemide has a slight antihypertensive effect. **Onset: PO, IM:** 30–60 min; **IV:** 5 min. **Peak: PO, IM:** 1–2 hr; **IV:** 20–60 min. **t½:** About 2 hr after PO use.

Duration: PO, IM: 6–8 hr; **IV:** 2 hr. Metabolized in the liver and excreted through the urine. The drug may be effective for clients resistant to thiazides and for those with reduced GFRs.

Uses: Edema associated with CHF, nephrotic syndrome, hepatic cirrhosis, and ascites. IV for acute pulmonary edema. Furosemide can be used orally to treat hypertension in conjunction with spironolactone, triamterene, and other diuretics *except* ethacrynic acid. *Investigational:* Hypercalcemia.

Contraindications: Never use with ethacrynic acid. Anuria, hypersensitivity to drug, severe renal disease associated with azotemia and oliguria, hepatic coma associated with electrolyte depletion. Lactation.

Special Concerns: Use with caution in premature infants and neonates due to prolonged half-life in these clients (dosing interval must be extended). Geriatric clients may be more sensitive to the usual adult dose. Allergic reactions may be seen in clients who show hypersensitivity to sulfonamides.

Side Effects: *Electrolyte and fluid effects:* Fluid and electrolyte depletion leading to dehydration, hypovolemia, thromboembolism. Hypokalemia and hypochloremia may cause metabolic alkalosis. Hyperuricemia, azotemia, hyponatremia. *GI:* Nausea, oral and gastric irritation, vomiting, anorexia, diarrhea (especially in children) or constipation, cramps, pancreatitis, jaundice, ischemic hepatitis. *Otic:* Tinnitus, hearing impairment (may be reversible or permanent), reversible deafness. Usually following rapid IV or IM administration of high doses. *CNS:* Vertigo, headache, dizziness, blurred vision, restlessness, paresthesias, xanthopsia. *CV:* Orthostatic hypotension, thrombophlebitis, chronic aortitis. *Hematologic:* Anemia, thrombocytopenia, neutropenia, leukopenia, *agranulocytosis,* purpura. *Rarely, aplastic anemia. Allergic:* Rashes, pruritus, urticaria, photosensitivity, exfoliative dermatitis, vasculitis, erythema multiforme. *Miscellaneous:* Interstitial nephritis, fever, weakness, hyperglycemia, glycosuria, exacerbation of, aggravation of or worsening of SLE, increased perspiration, muscle spasms, urinary bladder spasm, urinary frequency.

Following IV use: Thrombophlebitis, ***cardiac arrest.*** *Following IM use:* Pain and irritation at injection site, ***cardiac arrest.***

Because this drug is resistant to the effects of pressor amines and potentiates the effects of muscle relaxants, it is recommended that the PO drug be discontinued 1 week before surgery and the IV drug 2 days before surgery.

OD **Overdose Management:** *Symptoms:* Profound water loss, electrolyte depletion (manifested by weakness, anorexia, vomiting, lethargy, cramps, mental confusion, dizziness), decreased blood volume, ***circulatory collapse (possibly vascular thrombosis and embolism).*** *Treatment:* Replace fluid and electrolytes. Monitor urine electrolyte output and serum electrolytes. Induce emesis or perform gastric lavage. Oxygen or assisted ventilation may be needed. Treat symptoms.

Additional Drug Interactions
Charcoal / ↓ Absorption of furosemide from the GI tract
Clofibrate / Enhanced diuretic effect
Hydantoins / Hydantoins ↓ the diuretic effect of furosemide
Propranolol / Furosemide may cause ↑ plasma levels of propranolol

Dosage ─────────────
• **Oral Solution, Tablets**
Edema.
Adults, initial: 20–80 mg/day as a single dose. For resistant cases, dosage can be increased by 20–40 mg q 6–8 hr until desired diuretic response is attained. Maximum daily dose should not exceed 600 mg. **Pediatric, initial:** 2 mg/kg as a single dose; **then,** dose can be increased by 1–2 mg/kg q 6–8 hr until desired re-

sponse is attained (up to 5 mg/kg may be required in children with nephrotic syndrome; maximum dose should not exceed 6 mg/kg). A dose range of 0.5–2 mg/kg b.i.d. has also been recommended.

Hypertension.
Adults, initial: 40 mg b.i.d. Adjust dosage depending on response.
CHF and chronic renal failure.
Adults: 2–2.5 g/day.
Antihypercalcemic.
Adults: 120 mg/day in one to three doses.

• **IV, IM**
Edema.
Adults, initial: 20–40 mg; if response inadequate after 2 hr, increase dose in 20-mg increments.
Pediatric, initial: 1 mg/kg given slowly; if response inadequate after 2 hr, increase dose by 1 mg/kg. Doses greater than 6 mg/kg should not be given.
Antihypercalcemic.
Adults: 80–100 mg for severe cases; dose may be repeated q 1–2 hr if needed.

• **IV**
Acute pulmonary edema.
Adults: 40 mg slowly over 1–2 min; if response inadequate after 1 hr, give 80 mg slowly over 1–2 min. Concomitant oxygen and digitalis may be used.
CHF, chronic renal failure.
Adults: 2–2.5 g/day. For IV bolus injections, the maximum should not exceed 1 g/day given over 30 min.
Hypertensive crisis, normal renal function.
Adults: 40–80 mg.
Hypertensive crisis with pulmonary edema or acute renal failure.
Adults: 100–200 mg.

RESPIRATORY CARE CONSIDERATIONS

See also *Respiratory Care Considerations* for *Diuretics, Loop.*
Administration/Storage
1. The drug should be given 2–4 days/week.

─────────────
bold italic = life threatening side effect

2. IV injections are given slowly over 1–2 min.

3. If used IV, furosemide should not be mixed with solutions with a pH below 5.5. After pH adjustment, furosemide can be mixed with sodium chloride injection, lactated Ringer's injection, and 5% dextrose injection and infused at a rate not to exceed 4 mg/min to prevent ototoxicity.

4. A precipitate may form if furosemide is mixed with gentamicin, netilmicin, or milrinone in either 5% dextrose or 0.9% sodium chloride.

5. Food decreases the bioavailability of furosemide and ultimately the degree of diuresis.

6. Slight discoloration resulting from light does not affect potency. However, discolored tablets or injection should not be dispensed.

7. If used with other antihypertensives, the dose of other agents reduced by at least 50% when furosemide is added in order to prevent an excessive drop in BP.

8. Store in light-resistant containers at room temperature (15°C–30°C, or 59°F–86°F).

9. In CHF or chronic renal failure oral and parenteral doses as high as 2–2.5 g/day (or higher) are well tolerated.

Interventions
1. Monitor serum electrolytes and observe for S&S of hypokalemia.

2. In clients with rapid diuresis, observe for dehydration and circulatory collapse. Monitor BP and pulse and document.

3. When more than 40 mg a day are required, give in divided doses, i.e., 40 mg PO b.i.d.

4. When the client has renal impairment or is receiving other ototoxic drugs, observe for ototoxicity.

5. Assess closely for signs of vascular thrombosis and embolism, particularly in the elderly.

6. With chronic use, assess for thiamine deficiency.

Evaluate
• Enhanced diuresis
• Resolution of pulmonary edema
• ↓ Dependent edema
• ↓ BP
• ↓ Serum calcium levels

G

Gentamicin sulfate
(jen-tah-**MY**-sin)
Pregnancy Category: C
Alcomicin ✷, Cidomycin ✷, Diogent ✷, Garamycin, Garamycin Cream or Ointment, Garamycin Intrathecal, Garamycin IV Piggyback, Garamycin Ophthalmic Ointment, Garamycin Ophthalmic Solution, Garamycin Pediatric, Garatec ✷, Genoptic Ophthalmic Liquifilm, Genoptic S.O.P. Ophthalmic, Gentacidin Ophthalmic, Gentafair, Gentak Ophthalmic, Gentamicin, Gentamicin Ophthalmic, Gentamicin Sulfate IV Piggyback, Gentrasul Ophthalmic, G-myticin Cream or Ointment, Jenamicin, Minims Gentamcin ✷, Ocugram ✷, Pediatric Gentamicin Sulfate, PMS-Gentamicin Sulfate ✷, R.O.-Gentycin ✷ **(Rx)**
Classification: Antibiotic, aminoglycoside

See also *Aminoglycosides*.
Action/Kinetics: Therapeutic serum levels: IM, 4–8 mcg/mL. **Toxic serum levels: >12 mcg/mL (peak) and >2 mcg/mL (trough). Prolonged serum levels above 12 mcg/mL should be avoided.** t½: 2 hr. The drug can be used concurrently with carbenicillin for the treatment of serious *Pseudomonas* infections. However, the drugs should not be mixed in the same flask because carbenicillin will inactivate gentamicin.
Uses: Systemic: Serious infections caused by *Pseudomonas aeruginosa, Proteus, Klebsiella, Enterobacter, Serratia, Citrobacter,* and *Staphylococcus.* Infections include bacterial neonatal sepsis, bacterial septicemia, and serious infections of the skin,

bone, soft tissue (including burns), urinary tract, GI tract (including peritonitis), and CNS (including meningitis). Should be considered as initial therapy in suspected or confirmed gram-negative infections. In combination with carbenicillin for treating life-threatening infections due to *P. aeruginosa*. In combination with penicillin for treating endocarditis caused by group D streptococci. In combination with penicillin for treating suspected bacterial sepsis or staphylococcal pneumonia in the neonate. Intrathecal administration is used in combination with systemic gentamicin for treating meningitis, ventriculitis, or other serious CNS infections due to *Pseudomonas. Investigational:* Pelvic inflammatory disease.

Ophthalmic: Ophthalmic infections due to *Staphylococcus, S. aureus, Streptococcus pneumoniae,* beta-hemolytic streptococci, *Corynebacterium* species, *Streptococcus pyogenes, Escherichia coli, Haemophilus influenzae, H. aegyptius, H. ducreyi, Klebsiella pneumoniae, Neisseria gonorrhoeae, Proteus* species, *Acinetobacter calcoaceticus, Enterobacter aerogenes, P. aeruginosa, Serratia marcescens, Moraxella lacunata.*

Topical: Prevention of infections following minor cuts, wounds, burns, and skin abrasions. Treatment of primary or secondary skin infections. Treatment of infected skin cysts and other skin abscesses when preceded by incision and drainage to permit adequate contact between the drug and the infecting bacteria, infected stasis and other skin ulcers, infected superficial burns, paronychia, infected insect bites and stings, infected lacerations and abrasions and wounds from minor surgery.

Contraindications: Ophthalmic use to treat dendritic keratitis, vaccinia, varicella, mycobacterial infections of the eye, fungal diseases of the eye, use with steroids after uncomplicated removal of a corneal foreign body.

Special Concerns: Use with caution in premature infants and neonates. Ophthalmic ointments may retard corneal epithelial healing.

Additional Side Effects: Muscle twitching, numbness, *seizures,* increased BP, alopecia, purpura, pseudotumor cerebri. Photosensitivity when used topically. *After ophthalmic use:* Transient irritation, burning, stinging, itching, inflammation, angioneurotic edema, urticaria, vesicular and maculopapular dermatitis, mydriasis, conjunctival paresthesia, conjunctival hyperemia, nonspecific conjunctivitis, conjunctival epithelial defects, lid itching and swelling, bacterial/fungal corneal ulcers.

Additional Drug Interactions: With carbenicillin or ticarcillin, gentamicin may result in increased effect when used for *Pseudomonas* infections.

Dosage
• **IM (usual), IV**
Adults with normal renal function.
Infections.
1 mg/kg q 8 hr, up to 5 mg/kg/day in life-threatening infections; **children:** 2–2.5 mg/kg q 8 hr; **infants and neonates:** 2.5 mg/kg q 8 hr; **premature infants or neonates less than 1 week of age:** 2.5 mg/kg q 12 hr. Therapy may be required for 7–10 days.
Prevention of bacterial endocarditis, dental or respiratory tract procedures.
Adults: 1.5 mg/kg gentamicin (not to exceed 80 mg) plus 1 g ampicillin, each IM or IV, 30–60 min before the procedure; one additional dose of each can be given 8 hr later (alternative: penicillin V, 1 g PO, 6 hr after initial dose).
Prophylaxis of bacterial endocarditis in GI or GU tract procedures or surgery.
Adults: 1.5 mg/kg gentamicin (not to exceed 80 mg) plus 2 g ampicillin, each IM or IV, 30–60 min before procedure; dose should be repeated

8 hr later. **Children:** 2 mg/kg gentamicin plus penicillin G, 30,000 units/kg, or ampicillin, 50 mg/kg in same dosage interval as for adults. Pediatric dosage should not exceed single or 24-hr adult doses.

NOTE: In clients allergic to penicillin, vancomycin, 1 g IV given slowly over 1 hr, may be substituted; the dose of vancomycin should be repeated 8–12 hr later. **Adults with impaired renal function:** To calculate interval (hr) between doses, multiply serum creatinine level (mg/100 mL) by 8.

• **IV**
  Septicemia.
Initially: 1–2 mg/kg infused over 30–60 min; **then,** maintenance doses may be administered.

• **Intrathecal**
  Meningitis.
Use only the intrathecal preparation. Adults, usual: 4–8 mg/day; **children and infants 3 months and older:** 1–2 mg/day
  Pelvic inflammatory disease.
Initial: 2 mg/kg IV; **then,** 1.5 mg/kg t.i.d. plus clindamycin, 500 mg IV q.i.d. Continue for at least 4 days and at least 48 hr after client improves. Continue clindamycin, 450 mg PO q.i.d. for 10–14 days.

• **Ophthalmic Solution (0.3%)**
  Acute infections.
Initially: 1–2 gtt in conjunctival sac q 15–30 min; **then,** as infection improves, reduce frequency.
  Moderate infections.
1–2 gtt in conjunctival sac 4–6 times/day.
  Trachoma.
2 gtt in each eye b.i.d.–q.i.d.; treatment should be continued for up to 1–2 months.

• **Ophthalmic Ointment (0.3%)**
Depending on the severity of infection, ½-in. ribbon from q 3–4 hr to 2–3 times/day.

• **Topical   Cream/Ointment (0.1%)**
Apply 3–4 times/day to affected area. The area may be covered with a sterile bandage.

RESPIRATORY CARE CONSIDERATIONS

See also Respiratory Care Considerations for Aminoglycosides.
Administration/Storage
1. For intermittent IV administration, the adult dose should be diluted in 50–200 mL of sterile 5% dextrose in water or isotonic saline and administered over a 30–120-min period. The volume should be less for infants and children.
2. Gentamicin should not be mixed with other drugs for parenteral use.
3. For parenteral use, the duration of treatment is 7–10 days, although a longer course of therapy may be required for severe or complicated infections.
4. When used intrathecally, the usual site is the lumbar area.
5. With topical administration:
• Remove the crusts of impetigo contagiosa before applying the cream or ointment to permit maximum contact between antibiotic and infection.
• Apply cream or ointment gently and cover with gauze dressing if desirable or as ordered.
• Avoid direct exposure to sunlight as photosensitivity reaction may occur.
• Avoid further contamination of infected skin.

Assessment
1. Document indications for therapy and type, duration, and onset of symptoms.
2. Obtain renal function studies and appropriate specimen for lab C&S.
3. With eye disorders, determine that ophthalmologic assessments and cultures have been performed before administering solution.
4. Assess for tinnitus, vertigo, or hearing losses during therapy. Persistently increased gentamycin levels have been associated with 8th CN dysfunction.

Evaluate
• Resolution of infection
• During systemic administration, therapeutic peak serum drug levels (4–8 mcg/mL); (peak 5–10 mcg/mL trough 1–2 mcg/mL)

Glycopyrrolate

(glye-koe-PYE-roe-late)
Pregnancy Category: B
Robinul, Robinul Forte

Action/Kinetics: Glycopyrrolate is related to atropine and ipratropium bromide and antagonizes the action of acetylcholine. The highly polar quarternary ammonium group of glycopyrrolate interferes with its passage across lipid barriers and therefore, it does not pass through the blood-brain barrier as readily as the non-polar tertiary amines, atropine sulfate and scopolamine hydrobromide. When given by IM, peak effects occur approximately 30-45 min. By IV onset of action is within one minute.

Uses: Tablets and parenteral: adjunctive therapy in treatment of peptic ulcers; parenteral (anesthesia): to reduce salivary, tracheobronchial, and pharyngeal secretions; to reduce volume and free acidity of gastric secretions; and to block cardiac vagal inhibitory reflexes during intubation and induction of anesthesia. Inhalation: has been given by aerosol for bronchodilation.

Contraindications: Known hypersensitivity to glycopyrrolate. Glaucoma; obstructive uropathy; obstructive disease of GI tract; paralytic ileus; intestinal atony of elderly or debilitated patient; unstable cardiovascular status in acute hemorrhage; severe ulcerative colitis; toxic megacolon complicating ulcerative colitis; myasthenia gravis.

Special Concerns: Use with caution in patients with glaucoma or asthma. Glycopyrrolate may cause drowsiness or blurred vision. Therefore, patient should be forewarned regarding activities requiring mental alertness, such as operating a motor vehicle or operating heavy machinery.

Side Effects: Xerostomia; decreased sweating; urinary hesitancy and retention; blurred vision; tachycardia; palpitations; dilation of pupil; cyclopegia; increased ocular tension; loss of taste; headaches; nervousness; mental confusion; drowsiness; weakness; dizziness; insomnia; nausea; vomiting; constipation; bloated feeling; impotence; suppression of lactation; severe allergic reaction or drug idiosyncrasies including anaphylaxis and urticaria.

OD **Overdose Management:** (1) gastric lavage (for oral route), cathartics, and/or enemas; (2) administer anticholinesterase, e.g., neostigmine methylsulfate; (3) for hypotension: use pressor amines, e.g., norepinephrine, metaraminol IV and supportive care; (4) for respiratory depression: use oxygen and assisted ventilation, give respiratory stimulant, e.g. doxapram hydrochloride; (5) treat fever symptomatically.

Dosage **For adults Robinul (1 mg) tablets: initial dose one tablet t.i.d.; some patients may require two tablets at bedtime; may be reduced to one tablet b.i.d. Robinul Forte (2 mg) tablets: one tablet b.i.d. or t.i.d. Injectable: (preanesthetic) 0.002 mg (0.01 ml) per pound of body weight by IM, 30 to 60 minutes prior to time of induction of anesthesia; (intraoperative for arrhythmias) 0.1 mg (0.5 ml) at 2-3 min. intervals; (reversal of neuromuscular blockade) 0.2 mg IV (1.0 ml) for each 1.0 mg of neostigmine or 5.0 mg of pyridostigmine. Robinul tablets are not recommended for use in children less than 12 years of age. Robinul injectable for children one month to 12 years: (preanesthetic) 0.002 mg (0.01) per pound of body weight except children 1 month to 2 years may require up to 0.004 mg (0.02 ml) per pound of body weight; (intraoperative) 0.002 mg (0.01 ml) per pound of body weight IV, not to exceed 0.1 mg (0.5 ml) in a single dose which may be repeated PRN every 2-3 min.; (reversal of neuromuscular blockade) same as**

adults. **Adults (peptic ulcer):** 0.1 mg (0.5 ml) q4h, t.i.d. or q.i.d. IV or IM, **max. dose 0.2 mg (1.0 ml).**

RESPIRATORY CARE CONSIDERATIONS

Administration/Storage: Store at controlled room temperature, 20-25°C.

Guaifenesin (Glyceryl guaiacolate)

(gwye-**FEN**-eh-sin)

Pregnancy Category: C

Anti-Tuss, Balminil Expectorant ✤, Benylin-E ✤, Breonesin, Calmylin Expectorant ✤, Fenesin, Gee-Gee, Genatuss, GG-Cen, Glyate, Glycotuss, Glytuss, Guiatuss, Halotussin, Humibid L.A., Humibid Sprinkle, Hytuss, Hytuss-2X, Mytussin, Naldecon Senior EX, Robitussin, Scot-tussin, Sinumist-SR Capsulets, Uni-tussin **(OTC)**

Classification: Expectorant

Action/Kinetics: Guaifenesin is said to increase the output of fluid of the respiratory tract by reducing the viscosity and surface tension of respiratory secretions, thereby facilitating their expectoration. Data on efficacy are lacking; however, guaifenesin is an ingredient of many nonprescription cough preparations.

Uses: Dry, nonproductive cough due to colds and minor upper respiratory tract infections when there is mucus in the respiratory tract.

Contraindications: Chronic cough (e.g., due to smoking, asthma, or emphysema), cough accompanied by excess secretions. Use in children under age 12 for persistent or chronic cough due to asthma or cough accompanied by excessive mucus (unless prescribed by a provider).

Special Concerns: Persistent cough may indicate a serious infection; thus, the provider should be consulted if cough lasts for more than 1 week, is recurring, or is accompanied by high fever, rash, or persistent headache.

Side Effects: *GI:* N&V, GI upset. *CNS:* Dizziness, headache. *Dermatologic:* Rash, urticaria.

OD **Overdose Management:** *Symptoms:* N&V. *Treatment:* Treat symptomatically.

Drug Interactions: Inhibition of platelet adhesiveness by guaifenesin may result in bleeding tendencies.

Laboratory Test Interferences: False + urinary 5-hydroxyindoleacetic acid. Color interference with determination of urinary vanillylmandelic acid.

Dosage

• **Capsules, Tablets, Oral Liquid, Syrup**

Expectorant.

Adults and children over 12 years: 100–400 mg q 4 hr, not to exceed 2.4 g/day; **pediatric, 6–12 years:** 100–200 mg q 4 hr, not to exceed 1.2 g/day; **pediatric, 2–6 years:** 50–100 mg q 4 hr, not to exceed 600 mg/day. If less than 2 years of age, the dosage must be individualized by the physician.

• **Sustained-Release Capsules, Sustained-Release Tablets**

Expectorant.

Adults and children over 12 years: 600–1,200 mg q 12 hr, not to exceed 2.4 g/day; **pediatric, 6–12 years:** 600 mg q 12 hr, not to exceed 1.2 g/day; **pediatric, 2–6 years:** 300 mg q 12 hr, not to exceed 600 mg/day. *NOTE:* The liquid dosage forms may be more suitable for children less than 6 years of age.

RESPIRATORY CARE CONSIDERATIONS

Assessment

1. Document pulmonary assessment findings.

2. Note type, frequency, duration, and characteristics of cough and sputum production.

Client/Family Teaching

1. Take only as directed and do not exceed prescribed dosing guidelines.

2. If symptoms persist more than 1 week, recur, or are accompanied by a persistent headache, fever, or rash, medical intervention should be sought as cough may indicate a more serious condition.

3. Any evidence of increased bleeding tendencies or increased bruising should be reported.

4. Do not perform activities that require mental alertness because drug may cause drowsiness.

5. Advise to increase fluid intake to 2.5 L/day to decrease viscosity of secretions.

6. Instruct to avoid triggers: dust, chemicals, cigarette smoke, pollutants, and perfumes.

Evaluate

• Control of coughing episodes

• Mobilization and expectoration of pulmonary mucus

Guanabenz acetate

(**GWON**-ah-benz)
Pregnancy Category: C
Wytensin **(Rx)**
Classification: Antihypertensive, centrally acting antiadrenergic

See also *Antihypertensive Agents.*

Action/Kinetics: Guanabenz stimulates alpha-adrenergic receptors in the CNS, resulting in a decrease in sympathetic impulses and in sympathetic tone. It also decreases the pulse rate, but postural hypotension has not been manifested. **Onset:** 60 min. **Peak effect:** 2–4 hr. **Peak plasma levels:** 2–5 hr. **t½:** 6 hr. **Duration:** 8–12 hr.

Uses: Hypertension, alone or as adjunct with thiazide diuretics.

Contraindications: Lactation, children under 12 years of age.

Special Concerns: Use with caution in severe coronary insufficiency, cerebrovascular disease, recent MI, hepatic or renal disease. Geriatric clients may be more sensitive to the hypotensive and sedative effects of guanabenz; also, it may be necessary to decrease the dose in these clients due to age-related decreases in renal function.

Side Effects: *CNS:* Drowsiness and sedation (common), dizziness, weakness, headache, ataxia, depression, disturbances in sleep, excitement. *GI:* Dry mouth (common), N&V, diarrhea, constipation, abdominal pain or discomfort. *CV:* Palpitations, chest pain, arrhythmias. *Miscellaneous:* Edema, blurred vision, muscle aches, dyspnea, rash, pruritus, nasal congestion, urinary frequency, gynecomastia, alterations in taste, disturbances of sexual function, taste disorders, aches in extremities.

OD   **Overdose Management:** *Symptoms:* Hypotension, sleepiness, irritability, miosis, lethargy, bradycardia. *Treatment:* Supportive treatment. VS and fluid balance should be monitored. Syrup of ipecac or gastric lavage followed by activated charcoal; administration of fluids, pressor agents, and atropine. Adequate airway should be maintained; assisted ventilation may be required.

Drug Interactions: Use with CNS depressants may result in significant sedation.

Dosage

• **Tablets**

Hypertension.

Adults, initial: 4 mg b.i.d. alone or with a diuretic; **then,** increase by 4–8 mg q 1–2 weeks until control achieved. Maximum recommended dose: 32 mg b.i.d.

RESPIRATORY CARE CONSIDERATIONS

See also *Respiratory Care Considerations* for *Antihypertensive Agents.*

Administration/Storage: The drug should be kept tightly closed and protected from light.

Evaluate: ↓ BP with control of hypertension

Guanadrel sulfate

(**GWON**-ah-drell)
Pregnancy Category: B
Hylorel **(Rx)**
Classification: Antihypertensive, peripherally acting antiadrenergic

See also *Antihypertensive Agents.*

Action/Kinetics: Similar to that of guanethidine. Inhibits vasoconstriction by blocking efferent, peripheral sympathetic pathways by depleting norepinephrine reserves and inhibiting norepinephrine release. Causes increased sensitivity to norepinephrine. **Onset:** 2 hr. **Peak plasma levels:** 1.5–2 hr. **Peak effect:** 4–6 hr. **t½:** Approximately 10 hr. **Duration:** 4–14 hr. Excreted through the urine as unchanged drug (40%) and metabolites.

Uses: Hypertension (usually step 2 therapy) in those not responding to a thiazide diuretic.

Contraindications: Pheochromocytoma, CHF, within 1 week of MAO drug use, within 2–3 days of elective surgery, lactation.

Special Concerns: Use with caution in bronchial asthma and peptic ulcer. Safety and efficacy not established in children. Geriatric clients may be more sensitive to the hypotensive effects.

Side Effects: *CNS:* Fainting, fatigue, headache, drowsiness, paresthesias, confusion, psychological problems, depression, syncope, sleep disorders, visual disturbances. *CV:* Chest pain, orthostatic hypotension, palpitations, peripheral edema. *Respiratory:* Exertional or resting SOB, coughing. *GI:* Increase in number of bowel movements, constipation, anorexia, indigestion, flatus, glossitis, N&V, dry mouth and throat, abdominal distress or pain. *GU:* Difficulty in ejaculation, impotence, nocturia, hematuria, urinary urgency or frequency. *Miscellaneous:* Leg cramps during both the day and night, excessive weight gain or loss, backache, neckache, joint pain or inflammation, aching limbs.

OD **Overdose Management:** *Symptoms:* Postural hypotension, syncope, dizziness, blurred vision. *Treatment:* Administration of a vasoconstrictor (e.g., phenylephrine) if hypotension persists. If used, monitor carefully as client may be hypersensitive.

Drug Interactions
Beta-adrenergic blocking agents / Excessive hypotension, bradycardia
Phenothiazines / Reverses effect of guanadrel

Phenylpropanolamine / ↓ Effect of guanadrel
Reserpine / Excessive hypotension, bradycardia
Sympathomimetics / Hypotensive effect of guanadrel may be reversed; also, guanadrel may ↑ the effects of directly acting sympathomimetics
Tricyclic antidepressants / Reverses effect of guanadrel
Vasodilators / ↑ Risk of orthostatic hypotension

Dosage —————————
• **Tablets**
Hypertension.
Individualized. Initial: 5 mg b.i.d.; **then,** increase dosage to maintenance level of 20–75 mg/day in two to four divided doses. For clients with a creatinine clearance of 30–60 mL/min, the initial dose should be 5 mg q 24 hr. If the creatinine clearance is less than 30 mL/min, the dosing interval should be increased to q 48 hr. Dose changes should be made carefully q 7 or more days for moderate renal insufficiency and q 14 or more days for severe insufficiency.

RESPIRATORY CARE CONSIDERATIONS

See also *Respiratory Care Considerations* for *Antihypertensive Agents.*
Administration/Storage
1. Tolerance may occur with long-term therapy, necessitating a dosage increase.
2. While adjusting dosage, both supine and standing BP should be monitored.
Evaluate: Control of hypertension

Guanethidine sulfate
(gwon-**ETH**-ih-deen)
Pregnancy Category: C
Apo-Guanethidine ✦, Ismelin Sulfate **(Rx)**
Classification: Antihypertensive, peripherally acting antiadrenergic

See also *Antihypertensive Agents.*
Action/Kinetics: Guanethidine produces selective adrenergic blockade of efferent, peripheral sympa-

thetic pathways by depleting norepinephrine reserve and inhibiting norepinephrine release. It induces a gradual, prolonged drop in both SBP and DBP, usually associated with bradycardia, decreased pulse pressure, a decrease in peripheral resistance, and small changes in CO. The drug is not a ganglionic blocking agent and does not produce central or parasympathetic blockade. In clients with depleted catecholamines, guanethidine can directly depress the myocardium and can cause an increase in the sensitivity of tissues to catecholamines. Incompletely and variably absorbed from the GI tract (3%–30%) but is relatively constant for any given client. **Peak effect:** 6–8 hr. **Duration:** 24–48 hr. **Maximum effect:** 1–3 weeks. **Duration:** 7–10 days after discontinuation. **t½:** 4–8 days. From 25% to 50% excreted through the kidneys unchanged. The drug is slowly excreted due to extensive tissue binding.

Uses: Moderate to severe hypertension—used alone or in combination. *NOTE:* The use of a thiazide diuretic may increase the effectiveness of guanethidine and reduce the incidence of edema. Also used for renal hypertension, including that secondary to pyelonephritis, renal artery stenosis, and renal amyloidosis.

Contraindications: Mild, labile hypertension; pheochromocytoma, CHF not due to hypertension, use of MAO inhibitors, lactation.

Special Concerns: Administer with caution and at a reduced rate to clients with impaired renal function, coronary disease, CV disease especially when associated with encephalopathy, or severe cardiac failure or to those who have suffered a recent MI. Use with caution in hypertensive clients with renal disease and nitrogen retention or increasing BUN levels. Fever decreases dosage requirements. During prolonged therapy, cardiac, renal, and blood tests should be performed. Used with caution in peptic ulcer. Geriatric cli-

ents may be more sensitive to the hypotensive effects of guanethidine; also, it may be necessary to decrease the dose in these clients due to age-related decreases in renal function. Safety and efficacy have not been determined in children.

Side Effects: *CNS:* Dizziness, weakness, lassitude. Rarely, fatigue, psychic depression. *CV:* Syncope due to exertional or postural hypotension, bradycardia, fluid retention and edema with possible CHF. Less commonly, angina. *Respiratory:* Dyspnea, nasal congestion, asthma in susceptible individuals. *GI:* Persistent diarrhea (may be severe enough to cause discontinuation of use), increased frequency of bowel movements. N&V, dry mouth, and parotid tenderness are less common. *GU:* Inhibition of ejaculation, nocturia, urinary incontinence, priapism, impotence. *Hematologic:* Anemia, thrombocytopenia, leukopenia (rare). *Miscellaneous:* Dermatitis, scalp hair loss, blurred vision, myalgia, muscle tremors, chest paresthesia, weight gain, ptosis of the lids.

OD Overdose Management: *Symptoms:* Bradycardia, postural hypotension, diarrhea (may be severe). *Treatment:* If the client was previously normotensive, keep in a supine position (symptoms usually subside within 72 hr). If the client was previously hypertensive (especially with impaired cardiac reserve or other CV problems or renal disease), intensive treatment may be needed. Vasopressors may be required. Severe diarrhea should be treated.

Drug Interactions
Alcohol, ethyl / Additive orthostatic hypotension
Amphetamines / ↓ Effect of guanethidine by ↓ uptake of the drug to its site of action
Anesthetics, general / Additive hypotension
Antidepressants, tricyclic / ↓ Effect of guanethidine by ↓ uptake of the drug to its site of action

Antidiabetic drugs / Additive effect ↓ in blood glucose

Cocaine / ↓ Effect of guanethidine by ↓ uptake of the drug at its site of action

Digitalis / Additive slowing of HR

Ephedrine / ↓ Effect of guanethidine by ↓ uptake of the drug at its site of action

Epinephrine / Guanethidine ↑ effect of epinephrine

Haloperidol / ↓ Effect of guanethidine by ↓ uptake of the drug at its site of action

Levarterenol / See *Norepinephrine*

MAO inhibitors / Reverse effect of guanethidine

Metaraminol / Guanethidine ↑ effect of metaraminol

Methotrimeprazine / Additive hypotensive effect

Methoxamine / Guanethidine ↑ effect of methoxamine

Methylphenidate / ↓ Effect of guanethidine

Minoxidil / Profound drop in BP

Norepinephrine / ↑ Effect of norepinephrine probably due to ↑ sensitivity of norepinephrine receptor and ↓ uptake of norepinephrine by the neuron

Oral contraceptives / ↓ Effect of guanethidine by ↓ uptake of the drug to its site of action

Phenothiazines / ↓ Effect of guanethidine by ↓ uptake of the drug to its site of action

Phenylephrine / ↑ Response to phenylephrine in guanethidine-treated clients

Phenylpropanolamine / ↓ Effect of guanethidine by ↓ uptake of the drug to its site of action

Procainamide / Additive hypotensive effect

Procarbazine / Additive hypotensive effect

Propranolol / Additive hypotensive effect

Pseudoephedrine / ↓ Effect of guanethidine by ↓ uptake of the drug at its site of action

Quinidine / Additive hypotensive effect

Reserpine / Excessive bradycardia, postural hypotension, and mental depression

Sympathomimetics / ↓ Effect of guanethidine; also, guanethidine potentiates the effects of directly acting sympathomimetics

Thiazide diuretics / Additive hypotensive effect

Thioxanthenes / ↓ Effect of guanethidine by ↓ uptake of the drug at its site of action

Tricyclic antidepressants / Inhibition of the effects of guanethidine

Vasodilator drugs, peripheral / Additive hypotensive effect

Vasopressor drugs / ↑ Effect of vasopressor agents probably due to ↑ sensitivity of norepinephrine receptor and ↓ uptake of vasopressor agent by the neuron

Laboratory Test Interferences: ↑ BUN, AST, and ALT. ↓ PT, serum glucose, and urine catecholamines. Alteration of electrolyte balance.

Dosage ————————
- **Tablets**
  Ambulatory clients.

Initial: 10–12.5 mg/day; increase in 10–12.5-mg increments q 5–7 days; **maintenance:** 25–50 mg/day.
  Hospitalized clients.

Initial: 25–50 mg; increase by 25 or 50 mg/day or every other day; **maintenance:** estimated to be approximately one-seventh of loading dose. **Pediatric, initial:** 0.2 mg/kg/day (6 mg/m²) given in one dose; **then,** dose may be increased by 0.2 mg/kg/day q 7–10 days to maximum of 3 mg/kg/day.

RESPIRATORY CARE CONSIDERATIONS

See also *Respiratory Care Considerations* for *Antihypertensive Agents*.

Administration/Storage

1. The loading dose for severe hypertension is given t.i.d. at 6-hr intervals with no nighttime dose.

2. The effects of guanethidine are cumulative; thus, initial doses should be small and increased gradually in small increments.

3. Often used concomitantly with thiazide diuretics to reduce severity of

sodium and water retention caused by guanethidine. When used together, the dose of guanethidine should be reduced.

4. When control is achieved, dosage should be reduced to the minimal dose required to maintain lowest possible BP.

5. Guanethidine sulfate should be discontinued or dosage decreased at least 2 weeks before surgery and MAO inhibitors should be discontinued at least 1 week before starting guanethidine.

Assessment

1. Ascertain that baseline hepatic and renal function studies are completed.

2. List drugs currently prescribed to ensure none interact unfavorably.

3. Perform baseline VS and report the presence of bradycardia. An anticholinergic drug, such as atropine, may be indicated for severe bradycardia.

4. Assess client for any undue stress, which could precipitate CV collapse. Assist to identify and reduce such stress whenever possible.

Evaluate: ↓ BP with control of hypertension

Guanfacine hydrochloride

(**GWON**-fah-seen)

Pregnancy Category: B

Tenex **(Rx)**

Classification: Antihypertensive, centrally acting

See also *Antihypertensive Agents.*

Action/Kinetics: Guanfacine is thought to act by central stimulation of alpha-2 receptors resulting in a decrease in peripheral sympathetic output and HR resulting in a decrease in BP. The drug may also manifest a direct peripheral alpha-2 receptor stimulant action. **Onset:** 2 hr. **Peak plasma levels:** 1–4 hr. **Peak effect:** 6–12 hr. **t½:** 12–23 hr. **Duration:** 24 hr. Approximately 50% is excreted through the kidneys unchanged.

Uses: Hypertension alone or with a thiazide diuretic. *Investigational:* Withdrawal from heroin use, to reduce the frequency of migraine headaches.

Contraindications: Hypersensitivity to guanfacine. Acute hypertension associated with toxemia. Children less than 12 years of age.

Special Concerns: Use with caution during lactation. Use with caution in clients with recent MI, cerebrovascular disease, chronic renal or hepatic failure, or severe coronary insufficiency. Geriatric clients may be more sensitive to the hypotensive and sedative effects. Safety and efficacy in children less than 12 years of age have not been determined.

Side Effects: *GI:* Dry mouth, constipation, nausea, abdominal pain, diarrhea, dyspepsia, dysphagia, taste perversion or alterations in taste. *CNS:* Sedation, weakness, dizziness, headache, fatigue, insomnia, amnesia, confusion, depression, vertigo, agitation, anxiety, malaise, nervousness, tremor. *CV:* Bradycardia, substernal pain, palpitations, syncope, chest pain, tachycarida, cardiac fibrillation, CHF, heart block, MI (rare), cardiovascular accident (rare). *Ophthalmic:* Visual disturbances, conjunctivitis, iritis, blurred vision. *Dermatologic:* Pruritus, dermatitis, purpura, sweating, skin rash with exfoliation, alopecia, rash. *GU:* Decreased libido, impotence, urinary incontinence or frequency, testicular disorder, nocturia, acute renal failure. *Musculoskeletal:* Leg cramps, hypokinesia, arthralgia, leg pain, myalgia. *Other:* Rhinitis, tinnitus, dyspnea, paresthesias, paresis, asthenia, edema, abnormal liver function tests.

OD **Overdose Management:** *Symptoms:* Drowsiness, bradycardia, lethargy, hypotension. *Treatment:* Gastric lavage. Supportive therapy, as needed. The drug is not dialyzable.

Drug Interactions: Additive sedative effects when used concomitantly with CNS depressants.

Dosage ————————
- **Tablets**

    Hypertension.

Initial: 1 mg/day alone or with other antihypertensives; if satisfactory results are not obtained in 3–4 weeks, dosage may be increased by 1 mg at 1–2-week intervals up to a maximum of 3 mg/day in one to two divided doses.

    Heroin withdrawal.

0.03–1.5 mg/day.

    Reduce frequency of migraine headaches.

1 mg/day for 12 weeks.

RESPIRATORY CARE CONSIDERATIONS

See also *Respiratory Care Considerations* for *Antihypertensive Agents.*

Administration/Storage

1. To minimize drowsiness, the daily dose should be given at bedtime.

2. If a decrease in BP is not maintained for over 24 hr, the daily dose may be more effective if divided, although the incidence of side effects increases.

3. Adverse effects increase significantly when the daily dose exceeds 3 mg.

4. Therapy for hypertension should be initiated in clients already taking a thiazide diuretic.

5. Abrupt cessation of therapy may result in increases in plasma and urinary catecholamines, symptoms of nervousness and anxiety, and increases in BP greater than those prior to therapy.

Assessment

1. Document indications for therapy, onset of symptoms, and any previous agents used and the outcome.

2. Determine the extent of CAD, and note any evidence of renal or liver dysfunction.

Evaluate

- ↓ BP to within desired range
- Control of S&S of heroin withdrawal
- ↓ Frequency of migraine headaches

Hydralazine hydrochloride

(hy-**DRAL**-ah-zeen)

Pregnancy Category: C

Apo-Hydralazine ✶, Apresoline, Novo-Hylazin ✶, Nu-Hydral ✶ **(Rx)**

Classification: Antihypertensive, direct action on vascular smooth muscle

See also *Antihypertensive Agents.*

Action/Kinetics: Exerts a direct vasodilating effect on vascular smooth muscle. The drug also alters cellular calcium metabolism that interferes with calcium movement within the vascular smooth muscle responsible for initiating or maintaining contraction. Hydralazine preferentially dilates arterioles compared with veins; this minimizes postural hypotension and increases CO. The drug increases renin activity in the kidney leading to an increase in angiotensin II, which then causes stimulation of aldosterone and thus sodium reabsorption. Because there is a reflex increase in cardiac function, hydralazine is commonly used with drugs that inhibit sympathetic activity (e.g., beta blockers, clonidine, methyldopa). The drug is rapidly absorbed after PO use. Food increases bioavailability of the drug. **PO: Onset:** 45 min; **peak plasma level:** 1–2 hr; **duration:** 3–8 hr. t½: 3–7 hr. **IM: Onset:** 10–30 min; **peak plasma level:** 1 hr; **duration:** 2–4 hr. **IV: Onset:** 10–20 min; **maximum effect:** 10–80 min; **duration:** 2–4 hr. Metabolized in the liver and excreted through the kidney (2%–5% unchanged after PO use and 11%–14% unchanged after IV administration).

Uses: *PO:* In combination with other drugs for essential hypertension. *Parenteral:* Severe essential hypertension when PO use is not possible or when there is an urgent need to lower BP. Hydralazine is the drug of choice for eclampsia. *Investigational:* To reduce afterload in CHF, severe aortic insufficiency, and after valve replacement.

Contraindications: Coronary artery disease, angina pectoris, advanced renal disease (as in chronic renal hypertension), rheumatic heart disease (e.g., mitral valvular) and chronic glomerulonephritis.

Special Concerns: Use with caution in stroke clients and in those with pulmonary hypertension. Use with caution during lactation, in clients with advanced renal disease, and in clients with tartrazine sensitivity. Safety and efficacy have not been established in children. Geriatric clients may be more sensitive to the hypotensive and hypothermic effects of hydralazine; also, a decrease in dose may be necessary in these clients due to age-related decreases in renal function.

Side Effects: *CV:* Orthostatic hypotension, hypotension, *MI,* angina pectoris, palpitations, paradoxical pressor reaction, tachycardia. *CNS:* Headache, dizziness, psychoses, tremors, depression, anxiety, disorientation. *GI:* N&V, diarrhea, anorexia, constipation, paralytic ileus. *Allergic:* Rash, urticaria, fever, chills, arthralgia, pruritus, eosinophilia. Rarely, hepatitis, obstructive jaundice. *Hematologic:* Decrease in hemoglobin and RBCs, purpura, agranulocytosis, leukopenia. *Other:* Peripheral neuritis (paresthesias, numbness, tingling), dyspnea, impotence, nasal congestion, edema, muscle cramps, lacrimation, flushing, conjunctivitis, difficulty in urination, lupus-like syndrome, lymphadenopathy, splenomegaly. Side effects are less severe when dosage is increased slowly. *NOTE:* Hydrala-

zine may cause symptoms resembling system lupus erythematosus (e.g., arthralgia, dermatoses, fever, splenomegaly, glomerulonephritis). Residual effects may persist for several years and long-term treatment with steroids may be necessary.

OD **Overdose** **Management:** *Symptoms:* Hypotension, tachycardia, skin flushing, headache. Also, myocardial ischemia, *cardiac arrhythmias, MI, and severe shock.* *Treatment:* If the CV status is stable, induce vomiting or perform gastric lavage followed by activated charcoal. Treat shock with volume expanders, without vasopressors; if a vasopressor is necessary, one should be used that is least likely to cause or aggravate tachycardia and cardiac arrhythmias. Renal function should be monitored.

Drug Interactions
Beta-adrenergic blocking agents / ↑ Effect of both drugs
Indomethacin / ↓ Effect of hydralazine
Methotrimeprazine / Additive hypotensive effect
Procainamide / Additive hypotensive effect
Quinidine / Additive hypotensive effect
Sympathomimetics / ↑ Risk of tachycardia and angina

Dosage ————
• **Tablets**
Hypertension.
Adult, initial: 10 mg q.i.d for 2–4 days; **then,** increase to 25 mg q.i.d. for rest of first week. For second and following weeks, increase to 50 mg q.i.d. **Maintenance:** individualized to lowest effective dose; maximum daily dose should not exceed 300 mg. **Pediatric, initial:** 0.75 mg/kg/day (25 mg/m²/day) in two to four divided doses; dosage may be increased gradually up to 7.5 mg/kg/day (or 300 mg/day). Food increases the bioavailability of the drug.
• **IV, IM**

Hypertensive crisis.
Adults, usual: 20–40 mg, repeated as necessary. BP may fall within 5–10 min, with maximum response in 10–80 min. Usually switch to PO medication in 1–2 days. Dosage should be decreased in clients with renal damage. **Pediatric:** 0.1–0.2 mg/kg q 4–6 hr as needed.

Eclampsia.
5–10 mg q 20 min as an IV bolus. If no effect after 20 mg, another drug should be tried.

RESPIRATORY CARE CONSIDERATIONS

See also *Respiratory Care Considerations* for *Antihypertensive Agents.*
Administration/Storage
1. Parenteral injections should be made as quickly as possible after being drawn into the syringe. Administer undiluted at a rate of 10 mg over at least 1 min.
2. The presence of a metal filter will cause a change in color of hydralazine.
3. The liquid formulation for parenteral use has been withdrawn from the market, although limited supplies may be available for emergency situations. A lyophilized formulation of the drug is being developed.
4. To enhance bioavailability, the tablets should be taken with food.
Assessment
1. Document indications for therapy, onset of symptoms, other agents trialed, and the outcome.
2. Assess VS, especially BP (lying, sitting, and standing).
3. Note any client history of hypersensitivity to the drug.
4. List any other drugs prescribed that may interact unfavorably with hydralazine.
5. Note any history of coronary or renal disease.
6. Document pulmonary assessment noting lung sounds, and the presence of rales, dyspnea, JVD, or edema.
7. Explore life-style and dietary and exercise habits and identify areas that need changes.

Interventions
1. During parenteral administration, take the BP every 5 min until stable, then every 15 min during hypertensive crisis.
2. Monitor electrolytes and I&O; report any reduction in urine output or electrolyte abnormality.
3. The BP should be taken several times a day under standardized conditions, lying, sitting, and/or standing.
4. Clients with cardiac conditions may require closer monitoring during drug therapy.
5. Observe for the development of arthralgia, dermatoses, fever, anemia, or splenomegaly since these may require discontinuation of drug therapy.
Evaluate
• ↓ BP with control of hypertension
• Improvement in S&S of CHF (↓ afterload, ↑ CO)

Hydrochlorothiazide
(**hy**-droh-klor-oh-**THIGH**-ah-zyd)
Pregnancy Category: B
Apo-Hydro ✸, Diuchlor H ✸, Esidrex, Ezide, Hydro-DIURIL, Hydro-Par, Neo-Codema ✸, Novo-Hydrazide ✸, Oretic, Urozide ✸ **(Rx)**
Classification: Diuretic, thiazide type

See also *Diuretics, Thiazide.*
Action/Kinetics: Onset: 2 hr. **Peak effect:** 4–6 hr. **Duration:** 6–12 hr. **t½:** 5.6–14.8 hr. Hydrochlorothiazide is also found in Aldactazide, Aldoril, Apresazide, Dyazide, Hydropres, and Ser-Ap-Es.
Special Concerns: Geriatric clients may be more sensitive to the usual adult dose.
Additional Side Effects: *CV:* Allergic myocarditis, hypotension. *Dermatologic:* Alopecia, exfoliative dermatitis, *toxic epidermal necrolysis,* erythema multiforme, ***Stevens-Johnson syndrome.*** *Miscellaneous:* ***Anaphylactic reactions, respiratory distress including pneumonitis and pulmonary edema.***

Dosage
• **Oral Solution, Tablets**
Diuretic.

Adults, initial: 25–200 mg/day for several days until dry weight is reached; **then,** 25–100 mg/day or intermittently. Some clients may require up to 200 mg/day.

Antihypertensive.
Adults, initial: 25 mg/day as a single dose. The dose may be increased to 50 mg/day in one to two doses. Doses greater than 50 mg are associated with significant reductions in serum potassium. **Pediatric, under 6 months:** 3.3 mg/kg/day in two doses; **up to 2 years of age:** 12.5–37.5 mg/day in two doses; **2–12 years of age:** 37.5–100 mg/day in two doses.

RESPIRATORY CARE CONSIDERATIONS

See also *Respiratory Care Considerations* for *Diuretics, Thiazide.*
Administration/Storage
1. Divide daily doses in excess of 100 mg.
2. Give b.i.d. at 6–12-hr intervals.
3. When used with other antihypertensives, clients usually do not require the dose of hydrochlorothiazide to be greater than 50 mg.
Evaluate
• ↓ BP
• ↑ Urine output with a reduction in refractory edema

————*COMBINATION DRUG*————

Hydrocodone bitartrate and Acetaminophen

(**high**-droh-**KOH**-dohn, ah-**seat**-ah-**MIN**-oh-fen)
Pregnancy Category: C
Anexia 5/500, Anexia 7.5/650, Anexsia 10 mg Hydrocodone bitartrate, Anexsia 660 mg Acetaminophen, Lorcet 10/650, Lorcet Plus, Lortab 10/500 10 mg Hydrocodone bitartrate, Lortab 500 mg Acetaminophen **(Rx) (C-III)**
Classification: Analgesic

See also *Narcotic Analgesics* and *Acetaminophen.*
Content: Anexia 5/500: *Narcotic analgesic:* Hydrocodone bitartrate, 5

mg, and *Nonnarcotic analgesic:* Acetaminophen, 500 mg.
Anexia 10/650 and Lorcet 10/650: *Narcotic analgesic:* Hydrocodone bitartrate, 10 mg, and *Nonnarcotic analgesic:* Acetaminophen, 650 mg. Anexia 7.5/650 and Lorcet Plus: *Narcotic analgesic:* Hydrocodone bitartrate, 7.5 mg, and *Nonnarcotic analgesic:* Acetaminophen, 650 mg. Lortab 10/500: *Narcotic analgesic:* Hydrocodone bitartrate, 10 mg, and *Nonnarcotic analgesic:* Acetaminophen, 500 mg.
Action/Kinetics: Hydrocodone produces its analgesic activity by an action on the CNS via opiate receptors. The analgesic action of acetaminophen is produced by both peripheral and central mechanisms.
Uses: Relief of moderate to moderately severe pain.
Contraindications: Hypersensitivity to acetaminophen or hydrocodone. Lactation.
Special Concerns: Use with caution, if at all, in clients with head injuries as the CSF pressure may be increased further. Use with caution in geriatric or debilitated clients; in those with impaired hepatic or renal function; in hypothyroidism, Addison's disease, prostatic hypertrophy, or urethral stricture; and in clients with pulmonary disease. Use shortly before delivery may cause respiratory depression in the newborn. Safety and efficacy have not been determined in children.
Side Effects: *CNS:* Lightheadedness, dizziness, sedation, drowsiness, mental clouding, lethargy, impaired mental and physical performance, anxiety, fear, dysphoria, psychologic dependence, mood changes. *GI:* N&V. *Respiratory:* Respiratory depression (dose-related), irregular and periodic breathing. *GU:* Ureteral spasm, spasm of vesical sphincters, urinary retention.
OD **Overdose Management:** *Symptoms:* **Acetaminophen overdose may result in potentially fatal hepatic necrosis.** Also, renal tubular necrosis,

hypoglycemic coma, and thrombocytopenia. Symptoms of hepatotoxic overdose include N&V, diaphoresis, and malaise. Symptoms of hydrocodone overdose include respiratory depression, somnolence progressing to stupor or **coma,** skeletal muscle flaccidity, cold and clammy skin, bradycardia, and hypotension. **Severe overdose may cause apnea, circulatory collapse, cardiac arrest, and death.** *Treatment (Acetaminophen):*

• Empty stomach promptly by lavage or induction of emesis with syrup of ipecac.

• Serum acetaminophen levels should be determined as early as possible but no sooner than 4 hr after ingestion.

• Determine liver function initially and at 24-hr intervals.

• The antidote, *N*-acetylcysteine, should be given within 16 hr of overdose for optimal results.

Treatment (Hydrocodone):

• Establish a patent airway and assisted or controlled ventilation as indicated.

• Respiratory depression can be reversed by giving naloxone IV.

• Oxygen, IV fluids, vasopressors, and other supportive measures may be instituted as required.

Drug Interactions
Anticholinergics / ↑ Risk of paralytic ileus
CNS depressants, including other narcotic analgesics, antianxiety agents, antipsychotics, alcohol / Additive CNS depression
MAO inhibitors / ↑ Effect of either the narcotic or the antidepressant
Tricyclic antidepressants / ↑ Effect of either the narcotic or the antidepressant

Dosage ————
• **Tablets**
Analgesia.
1 tablet of Anexsia 7.5/650, Lorcet 10/650, or Lorcet Plus q 4–6 hr as needed for pain. The total 24-hr dose should not exceed 6 tablets. 1–2 tablets of Anexsia 5/500 q 4–6 hr as needed for pain. The total 24-hr dose should not exceed 8 tablets.

RESPIRATORY CARE CONSIDERATIONS

See also *Respiratory Care Considerations* for *Narcotic Analgesics* and *Acetaminophen.*

Assessment
1. Document indications for therapy, noting onset, location, and duration of symptoms, any other agents prescribed, and the outcome. Determine if pain is acute or chronic in nature and rate pain level.
2. Note any history of hypothyroidism, prostatic hypertrophy or urethral stricture, Addison's disease, or pulmonary disease.
3. Obtain baseline liver and renal function studies.
4. Coadministration of an NSAID may reduce the dosage required for pain relief.

Evaluate: Desired level of pain control

Hydrocortisone (Cortisol)
(hy-droh-**KOR**-tih-zohn)

Pregnancy Category: C (topical and dental products)
Parenteral: Sterile Hydrocortisone Suspension. **Rectal:** Dermolate Anal-Itch, Cortenema ✶, Proctocort, Proc-toCream.HC 2.5%, Rectocort ✶. **Retention Enema:** Cortenema, Hycort ✶, Rectocort ✶. **Roll-on Applicator:** Cortaid FastStick, **Tablets:** Cortef, Hydrocortone. **Topical Aerosol Solution:** Aeroseb-HC, CaldeCORT Anti-Itch. **Topical Cream:** Ala-Cort, Allercort, Alphaderm, Bactine, Cortate ✶, Cort-Dome, Cortifair, Dermacort, DermiCort, Dermolate Anti-Itch, Dermtex HC, Emo-Cort ✶, H$_2$Cort, Hi-Cor 1.0 and 2.5, Hydro-Tex, Hytone, Nutracort, Penecort, Prevex HC ✶, Synacort. **Topical Lotion:** Acticort 100, Ala-Cort, Ala-Scalp HP, Allercort, Cetacort, Cortate ✶, Cort-Dome, Delacort, Dermacort, Dermolate Scalp-Itch, Emo-Cort ✶, Gly-Cort, Hytone, LactiCare-HC, Lemoderm, Lexocort Forte, My Cort, Nutracort, Pentacort, Rederm, S-T Cort. **Suppository:** Cortiment ✶. **Topical Ointment:** Allercort, Cortril, Hytone, Lemoderm, Penecort. **Topical Solution:** Penecort, Emo-Cort Scalp Solution, Texacort

Scalp Solution. **Topical Spray:** Cortaid, Dermolate Anti-Itch **(OTC) (Rx)**

Hydrocortisone acetate

(hy-droh-**KOR**-tih-zohn)
Pregnancy Category: C (topical and dental products)
Dental Paste: Orabase-HCA. **Intrarectal Foam:** Cortifoam. **Ophthalmic/Otic:** Cortamed ✿. **Parenteral:** Hydrocortone Acetate. **Rectal:** Cort-Dome High Potency, Cortenema, Corticaine, Cortifoam. **Suppository:** Cortiment ✿. **Topical Aerosol Foam:** Epifoam. **Topical Cream:** Allocort ✿, CaldeCORT Anti-Itch, CaldeCORT Light, Carmol-HC, Cortacet ✿, Cortaid, Cortef Feminine Itch, Corticaine, Corticreme ✿, FoilleCort, Gynecort, Hyderm ✿, Lanacort, Pharma-Cort, Rhulicort. **Topical Lotion:** Cortaid, Rhulicort. **Topical Ointment:** Cortaid, Cortef Acetate, Cortoderm ✿, Dermaflex HC 1% ✿, Lanacort, Nov-Hydrocort. **(OTC) (Rx)**

Hydrocortisone butyrate

(hy-droh-**KOR**-tih-zohn)
Pregnancy Category: C (topical products)
Topical Cream: Locoid **(Rx)**

Hydrocortisone cypionate

(hy-droh-**KOR**-tih-zohn)
Oral Suspension: Cortef **(Rx)**

Hydrocortisone sodium phosphate

(hy-droh-**KOR**-tih-zohn)
Parenteral: Hydrocortone Phosphate **(Rx)**

Hydrocortisone sodium succinate

(hy-droh-**KOR**-tih-zohn)
Parenteral: A-hydroCort, Solu-Cortef **(Rx)**

Hydrocortisone valerate

(hy-droh-**KOR**-tih-zohn)
Pregnancy Category: C (topical products)
Topical Cream/Ointment: Westcort **(Rx)**

Classification: Corticosteroid, naturally occurring; glucocorticoid-type

See also *Corticosteroids*.
Action/Kinetics: Short-acting. **t½:** 80–118 min. Topical products are available without a prescription in strengths of 0.5% and 1%.

Dosage
HYDROCORTISONE
• **Tablets**
20–240 mg/day, depending on disease.
• **IM Only**
One-third to one-half the PO dose q 12 hr.
• **Rectal**
100 mg in retention enema nightly for 21 days (up to 2 months of therapy may be needed; discontinue gradually if therapy exceeds 3 weeks).
• **Topical Ointment, Cream, Gel, Lotion, Solution, Spray**
Apply sparingly to affected area and rub in lightly t.i.d.–q.i.d.
HYDROCORTISONE ACETATE
• **Intralesional, Intra-articular, Soft Tissue**
5–50 mg, depending on condition.
• **Intrarectal Foam**
1 applicatorful (90 mg) 1–2 times/day for 2–3 weeks; **then** every second day.
• **Topical**
See *Hydrocortisone*.
HYDROCORTISONE BUTYRATE
• **Topical**
See *Hydrocortisone*.
HYDROCORTISONE CYPIONATE
• **Suspension**
20–240 mg/day, depending on the severity of the disease.
HYDROCORTISONE SODIUM PHOSPHATE
• **IV, IM, SC**
General uses.
Initial: 15–240 mg/day depending on use and on severity of the disease. Usually, one-half to one-third of the PO dose is given q 12 hr.
Adrenal insufficiency, acute.
Adults, initial: 100 mg IV; **then,** 100 mg q 8 hr in an IV fluid; **older children, initial:** 1–2 mg/kg by IV

✿ = Available in Canada **bold italic** = life threatening side effect bolus; **then,** 150–250 mg/kg/day **IV** in divided doses; **infants, initial:** 1–2 mg/kg by IV bolus; **then,** 25–150 mg/kg/day in divided doses.

HYDROCORTISONE SODIUM SUCCINATE

• **IM, IV**

Initial: 100–500 mg; **then,** may be repeated at 2-, 4-, and 6-hr intervals depending on response and severity of condition.

HYDROCORTISONE VALERATE

• **Topical Cream**

See *Hydrocortisone.*

RESPIRATORY CARE CONSIDERATIONS

See also *Respiratory Care Considerations* for *Corticosteroids.*

Administration/Storage

1. Check label of parenteral hydrocortisone to verify route that can be used for a particular preparation, because IM and IV preparations are not necessarily interchangeable.

2. Reconstituted direct IV solution may be administered at a rate of 100 mg over 30 sec. Doses larger than 500 mg should be infused over 10 min. Drug may be further diluted in 50–100 mL of dextrose or saline solutions and administered as ordered within 24 hr.

3. No part of the hydrocortisone acetate intrarectal foam aerosol container should be inserted into the anus.

4. When using topical products, washing the area prior to application may increase the penetration of the drug.

5. Topical products should not come in contact with the eyes.

6. Prolonged use of topical products should be avoided near the genital/rectal areas and eyes, on the face, and in creases of the skin.

Assessment

1. Document indications for therapy and type, location, onset, and duration of symptoms.

2. List other agents previously prescribed and the outcome.

3. Obtain baseline CBC, chemistry profile, and liver and renal function studies.

Evaluate

• Replacement therapy with adrenocortical deficiency
• Restoration of skin integrity
• Relief of allergic manifestations

Hydromorphone hydrochloride

(hy-droh-**MOR**-fohn)
Pregnancy Category: C
Dilaudid, Dilaudid-HP, PMS-Hydromorphone ✦ **(C-II) (Rx)**
Classification: Narcotic analgesic, morphine type

See also *Narcotic Analgesics.*

Action/Kinetics: Hydromorphone is 7–10 times more analgesic than morphine, with a shorter duration of action. It manifests less sedation, less vomiting, and less nausea than morphine, although it induces pronounced respiratory depression. **Onset:** 15–30 min. **Peak effect:** 30–60 min. **Duration:** 4–5 hr. **t½:** 2–3 hr. The drug can be given rectally for prolonged activity.

Uses: Analgesia for moderate to severe pain (e.g., surgery, cancer, biliary colic, burns, renal colic, MI, bone trauma). Dilaudid-HP is a concentrated solution intended for clients who are tolerant to narcotics.

Additional Contraindications: Migraine headaches. Use in children. Status asthmaticus, obstetrics, respiratory depression in absence of resuscitative equipment. Lactation.

Special Concerns: Do not confuse Dilaudid-HP with standard parenteral solutions of Dilaudid or with other narcotics as overdose and death can result. Use Dilaudid-HP with caution in clients with circulatory shock.

Additional Side Effects: Nystagmus.

Dosage

• **Tablets, Liquid**
Analgesia.

Adults: 2 mg q 4–6 hr as necessary. For severe pain, 4 or more mg q 4–6 hr.

• **Suppositories**

Analgesia.
Adults: 3 mg q 6–8 hr.
• **SC, IM, IV**
Analgesia.
Adults: 1–2 mg q 4–6 hr. For severe pain, 3–4 mg q 4–6 hr.

RESPIRATORY CARE CONSIDERATIONS

See also *Respiratory Care Considerations* for *Narcotic Analgesics.*
Administration/Storage
1. May be administered by slow IV injection. When using this route, administer the drug slowly to minimize hypotensive effects and respiratory depression. Dilute with 5 mL of sterile water or NSS and administer at a rate of 2 mg over 5 min.
2. Suppositories should be refrigerated.
3. Drug may be administered as Dilaudid brand cough syrup. Be alert to the possibility of an allergic response in people sensitive to yellow dye number 5.
4. Have naloxone available in the event of overdosage.
Assessment: Document indications for therapy and type, location, onset, and duration of symptoms. Use a pain rating scale to rate baseline pain.
Interventions
1. Observe closely for respiratory depression, as it is more profound with hydromorphone than with other narcotic analgesics. Encourage client to turn, cough, and deep breathe or use incentive spirometry every 2 hr to prevent atelectasis.
2. Assess abdomen carefully as drug may mask symptoms of acute pathology.
Evaluate: Relief of pain

Ibutilide fumarate
(ih-**BYOU**-tih-lyd)
Pregnancy Category: C
Corvert **(Rx)**
Classification: Antiarrhythmic agent

Action/Kinetics: Ibutilide is an antiarrhythmic agent with mostly class III properties. The drug delays repolarization by activation of a slow, inward current (mostly sodium), rather than by blocking outward potassium currents (the way other class III antiarrhythmics act). This results in prolongation in the duration of the atrial and ventricular action potential and refractoriness. There is also a dose-related prolongation of the QT interval. Ibutilide has a high systemic plasma clearance that approximates liver blood flow; protein binding is less than 40%. **t½, terminal:** 6 hr. Over 80% is excreted in the urine (with 7% excreted unchanged) and approximately 20% is excreted through the feces.

Uses: For rapid conversion of atrial fibrillation or atrial flutter of recent onset to sinus rhythm. Determination of clients to receive ibutilide should be based on expected benefits of maintaining sinus rhythm and whether this outweighs both the risks of the drug and of maintenance therapy.
Contraindications: Use of certain class Ia antiarrhythmic drugs (e.g., disopyramide, quinidine, procainamide) and certain class III drugs (e.g., amiodarone and sotalol) concomitantly with ibutilide or within 4 hr of postinfusion.
Special Concerns: Ibutilide may cause potentially fatal arrhythmias, especially sustained polymorphic ventricular tachycardia, usually in association with QT prolongation (torsades de pointes). Effectiveness has not been determined in clients with arrhythmias of more than 90 days in duration. Breast feeding

should be discouraged during therapy. Safety and efficacy have not been determined in children less than 18 years of age.

Side Effects: *CV: Life-threatening arrhythmias, either sustained or nonsustained polymorphic ventricular tachycardia (torsades de pointes).* Induction or worsening of ventricular arrhythmias. Nonsustained monomorphic ventricular extrasystoles, nonsustained monomorphic ventricular tachycardia, tachycardia, sinus tachycardia, SVT, hypotension, postural hypotension, bundle branch block, AV block, bradycardia, sinus bradycardia, QT-segment prolongation, hypertension, palpitation, supraventricular extrasystoles, nodal arrhythmia, CHF, idioventricular rhythm, sustained monomorphic ventricular tachycardia. *Miscellaneous:* Headache, nausea, syncope, renal failure.

OD **Overdose Management:** *Symptoms:* Increased ventricular ectopy, monomorphic ventricular tachycardia, AV block, nonsustained polymorphic ventricular tachycardia. *Treatment:* Use measures appropriate for the particular event.

Drug Interactions

Amiodarone / ↑ Risk of prolonged refractoriness

Antidepressants, tricyclic and tetracyclic / ↑ Risk of proarrhythmias

Digoxin / Supraventricular arrhythmias, due to ibutilide, may mask the cardiotoxicity due to high digoxin levels

Disopyramide / ↑ Risk of prolonged refractoriness

Histamne H₁ receptor antagonists / ↑ Risk of proarrhythmias

Quinidine / ↑ Risk of prolonged refractoriness

Phenothiazines / ↑ Risk of proarrhythmias

Procainamide / ↑ Risk of prolonged refractoriness

Sotalol / ↑ Risk of prolonged refractoriness

Dosage ———————————

• **IV Infusion**

Atrial fibrillation or atrial flutter of recent onset.

Clients weighing 60 kg or more, initial: 1 mg (one vial) infused over 10 min. **Clients weighing less than 60 kg, initial:** 0.01 mg/kg infused over 10 min. If the arrhythmia does not terminate within 10 min after the end of the initial infusion (regardless of the body weight), a second 10-min infusion of equal strength may be given 10 min after completion of the first infusion.

RESPIRATORY CARE CONSIDERATIONS
Administration/Storage

1. Clients with atrial fibrillation longer than 2–3 days duration must be anticoagulated adequately (usually for at least 2 weeks).

2. Ibutilide may be given undiluted or diluted in 50 mL of 0.9% sodium chloride injection or 5% dextrose injection before infusion. The contents of one vial (1 mg) mixed with 50 mL of diluent forms an admixture of approximately 0.017 mg/mL of ibutilide. Administer infusion over 10 min.

3. Either PVC plastic bags or polyolefin bags are compatible with admixtures of ibutilide.

4. Admixtures of ibutilide with approved diluents are chemically and physically stable for 24 hr at room temperature and for 48 hr if refrigerated.

Assessment

1. Document indications for therapy, onset of arrhythmia, and any associated symptoms.

2. List drugs currently prescribed to ensure none interact unfavorably.

3. Document baseline VS, ECG, and current arrhythmia on rhythm strip.

4. Anticipate that with more than 2–3 days duration of atrial fibrillation, client must be adequately anticoagulated for at least 2 weeks.

Interventions

1. Monitor VS, I&O, and cardiac rhythm.

2. Ibutilide must be given in a setting with continuous ECG monitoring and by those trained in the identification and treatment of acute ventricu-

lar arrhythmias, especially polymorphic ventricular tachycardia.

3. Document conversion to NSR (usually within 30–90 min). Infusion of the drug should cease as soon as the presenting arrhythmia is terminated or in the event of sustained or nonsustained ventricular tachycardia or marked prolongation of QT interval.

4. Observe clients carefully for at least 4 hr following infusion or until QT interval has returned to baseline. Longer monitoring is necessary if any arrhythmic activity is observed.

5. Have emergency equipment readily available.

Evaluate: Conversion of atrial fibrillation to stable sinus rhythm

---COMBINATION DRUG---

Imipenem-Cilastatin sodium

(em-ee-**PEN**-em, sigh-lah-**STAT**-in)
Pregnancy Category: C
Primaxin I.M., Primaxin I.V. **(Rx)**
Classification: Antibiotic combined with inhibitor of dehydropeptidase I

See also *Anti-Infectives*.

Content: The Powder for IV injection and the Powder for IM injection contain: imipenem, 500 mg, and cilastatin sodium, 500 mg, or imipenem, 750 mg, and cilastatin sodium, 750 mg.

Action/Kinetics: Imipenem, an antibiotic, inhibits cell wall synthesis and is thus bactericidal against a wide range of gram-positive and gram-negative organisms. It is stable in the presence of beta-lactamases. Addition of cilastatin prevents the metabolism of imipenem in the kidneys by dehydropeptidase I, thus ensuring high levels of the imipenem in the urinary tract. **t½, after IV:** 1 hr for each component. **Peak plasma levels of imipenem, after 20 min IV infusion:** 14–24 mcg/mL for the 250-mg dose, 21–58 mcg/mL for the 500-mg dose, and 41–83 mcg/mL for the 1-g dose. **Peak plasma levels, after IM:** 10–12 mcg/mL within 2 hr. Compared with IV administration, impenem is approximately 75% bioavailable after IM use with cilastatin being 95% bioavailable. **t½, imipenem:** 2–3 hr. About 70% of imipenem and cilastin is recovered in the urine within 10 hr of administration.

Uses: IV. To treat the following serious infections: lower respiratory tract, urinary tract, gynecologic, skin and skin structures, bone and joint, endocarditis, intra-abdominal, bacterial septicemia, and infections caused by more than one agent. Infections resistant to aminoglycosides, cephalosporins, or penicillins have responded to imipenem. Bacterial eradication may not be achieved in clients with cystic fibrosis, chronic pulmonary disease, and lower respiratory tract infections caused by *Pseudomonas aeruginosa*.

IM. This route of administration is not intended for severe or life-threatening infections (including endocarditis, or bacterial sepsis). Used for lower respiratory tract infections, intra-abdominal infections, skin and skin structure infections, gynecologic infections.

Contraindications: IM use in clients allergic to local anesthetics of the amide type and use in clients with heart block (due to the use of lidocaine HCl diluent) or severe shock. Use in clients with a creatinine clearance of less than or equal to 5 mL/min/1.73 m², unless hemodialysis is begun within 48 hr.

Special Concerns: Use with caution in pregnancy and lactation. Due to cross sensitivity, use with caution in clients with penicillin allergy. Safety and effectiveness have not been determined in children less than 12 years of age.

Side Effects: *GI: Pseudomembranous colitis,* nausea, diarrhea, vomiting, abdominal pain, heartburn, increased salivation, *hemorrhagic colitis,* gastroenteritis, glossitis, pharyngeal pain, tongue papillar hypertrophy, hepatitis, jaundice, staining of

---

the teeth. *CNS:* Fever, confusion, *seizures,* dizziness, sleepiness, myoclonus, headache, vertigo, paresthesia, encephalopathy, tremor, psychic disturbances (including hallucinations). *CV:* Hypotension, tachycardia, palpitations. *Dermatologic:* Rash, urticaria, pruritus, flushing, cyanosis, facial edema, erythema multiforme, skin texture changes, hyperhidrosis, *toxic epidermal necrolysis, Stevens-Johnson syndrome. CV:* Hypotension, palpitations, tachycardia. *Respiratory:* Chest discomfort, dyspnea, hyperventilation. *GU:* Pruritus vulvae, anuria/oliguria, acute renal failure, polyuria, urine discoloration. *Hematologic:* Pancytopenia, bone marrow depression, thrombocytopenia, neutropenia, leukopenia, hemolytic anemia. *Miscellaneous:* Candidiasis, superinfection, tinnitus, polyarthralgia, asthenia, muscle weakness, transient hearing loss in clients with existing hearing impairment, taste perversion, thoracic spine pain.

The following side effects may occur at the injection site: Thrombophlebitis, phlebitis, pain, erythema, vein induration, infused vein infection.
Drug Interactions: Use of ganciclovir with imipenem-cilastatin may result in generalized seizures.
Laboratory Test Interferences: ↑ AST, ALT, alkaline phosphatase, LDH, bilirubin, potassium, chloride, BUN, creatinine. Also, ↑ eosinophils, monocytes, lymphocytes, basophils. ↓ Serum sodium, neutrophils, hemoglobin, hematocrit. ↑ or ↓ WBCs, platelets. Positive Coombs' test and abnormal PT. Presence of protein, RBCs, WBCs, casts, bilirubin, or urobilinogen in the urine.

Dosage ————————
• **IV**
Fully susceptible gram-positive organisms, gram-negative organisms, anaerobes.
Mild: 250 mg q 6 hr; *moderate:* 500 mg q 6 hr or q 8 hr; *severe/life-threatening:* 500 mg q 6 hr.
Urinary tract infections due to fully susceptible organisms.

Uncomplicated: 250 mg q 6 hr; *complicated:* 500 mg q 6 hr.
Moderately susceptible organisms (especially some strains of P. aeruginosa).
Mild: 500 mg q 6 hr; *moderate,* 500 mg q 6 hr–1 g q 6 hr; *severe/life-threatening,* 1 g q 6 or 8 hr.
Urinary tract infections due to moderately susceptible organisms.
Uncomplicated: 250 mg q 6 hr; *complicated:* 500 mg q 6 hr.
The total daily dose should not exceed 50 mg/kg or 4 g, whichever is lower.
• **IM**
Lower respiratory tract, skin and skin structure, or gynecologic infections: mild to moderate.
500 or 750 mg q 12 hr depending on severity.
Intra-abdominal infections: mild to moderate.
750 mg q 12 hr. The total daily dose should not exceed 1.5 g.
Pediatric, 3 months to 3 years, all uses: 25 mg/kg q 6 hr, to a maximum of 2 g/day. **Pediatric, over 3 years, all uses:** 15 mg/kg q 6 hr.

RESPIRATORY CARE CONSIDERATIONS

See also *General Respiratory Care Considerations for All Anti-Infectives.*
Administration/Storage
1. Reconstitute for IV use by mixing with 100 mL of diluent. For IM use, prepare with 1% lidocaine HCl solution without epinephrine. The 500-mg vial is prepared with 2 mL while the 750-mg vial is prepared with 3 mL of lidocaine HCl.
2. The initial dose should be based on the type and severity of infection. Doses between 250 and 500 mg should be given by IV infusion over 20–30 min; doses of 1 g should be given by IV infusion over 40–60 min. If nausea develops, the infusion rate should be decreased.
3. The following solutions can be used as diluents: 0.9% sodium chloride injection, 5% or 10% dextrose injection, 5% dextrose and 0.9% sodi-

um chloride injection, 5% dextrose injection with either 0.225% or 0.45% saline solution, 5% dextrose with 0.15% potassium chloride solution, mannitol (2.5%, 5%, or 10%).

4. Reconstituted IV solutions vary from colorless to yellow while reconstituted IM solutions vary from white to light tan in color. Variations in color do not affect the potency.

5. Imipenem-cilastatin should not be physically mixed with other antibiotics; however, the drug may be administered with other antibiotics, if necessary.

6. Most reconstituted IV solutions can be stored at room temperature for 4 hr and, if refrigerated, for 24 hr. The exception is imipenem-cilastatin reconstituted with 0.9% sodium chloride solution, which is stable at room temperature for 10 hr and, if refrigerated, for 48 hr. Reconstituted IM solutions should be used within 1 hr of preparation.

7. When used IM, the dose should be given in a large muscle mass with a 21-gauge 2-in. needle.

8. IM use should be continued for at least 2 days after S&S of infection are absent. Safety and effectiveness have not been established for use for more than 14 days.

9. Dosage should be reduced in clients with a creatinine clearance of 70 mL/min/1.73 m² or less. Check package insert for specific dosage information.

Evaluate

- Resolution of infection
- Reports of symptomatic improvement

Indapamide

(in-**DAP**-ah-myd)
Pregnancy Category: B
Lozide ✦, Lozol **(Rx)**
Classification: Diuretic, thiazide type

See also *Diuretics, Thiazide.*
Action/Kinetics: Onset: 1–2 weeks after multiple doses. **Peak levels:** 2 hr. **Duration:** Up to 8 weeks with multiple doses. **t½:** 14 hr. Nearly 100% is absorbed from the GI tract. Excreted through the kidneys (70% with 7% unchanged) and the GI tract (23%).

Uses: Alone or in combination with other drugs for treatment of hypertension. Edema in CHF.

Special Concerns: Dosage has not been established in children. Geriatric clients may be more sensitive to the hypotensive and electrolyte effects.

Dosage
- **Tablets**
  Edema of CHF.
  Adults: 2.5 mg as a single dose in the morning. If necessary, may be increased to 5 mg/day after 1 week.
  Hypertension.
  Adults: 1.25 mg as a single dose in the morning. If the response is not satisfactory after 4 weeks, the dose may be increased to 2.5 mg taken once daily. If the response to 2.5 mg is not satisfactory after 4 weeks, the dose may be increased to 5 mg taken once daily (however, consideration should be given to adding another antihypertensive).

RESPIRATORY CARE CONSIDERATIONS

See also *Respiratory Care Considerations* for *Diuretics, Thiazide,* and *Antihypertensive Agents.*

Administration/Storage

1. May be combined with other antihypertensive agents if the response is inadequate. Initially, the dose of other agents should be reduced by 50%.

2. Doses greater than 5 mg/day do not increase effectiveness but may increase hypokalemia.

Assessment

1. Document indications for therapy and type, onset, and duration of symptoms.

2. List other drugs prescribed for these symptoms and the outcome.

Evaluate

- ↓ BP
- ↑ Urinary output with ↓ edema
- Improvement in S&S of CHF

Indomethacin

(in-doh-**METH**-ah-sin)

Apo-Indomethacin ✿, Indochron E-R, Indocid ✿, Indocid Ophthalmic Suspension ✿, Indocid SR ✿, Indocin, Indocin SR, Indotec ✿, Novo–Methacin ✿, Nu-Indo ✿, Pro-Indo ✿ **(Rx)**

Indomethacin sodium trihydrate

(in-doh-**METH**-ah-sin)

Indocin I.V. **(Rx)**

Classification: Nonsteroidal anti-inflammatory drug, analgesic, antipyretic

See also *Nonsteroidal Anti-Inflammatory Drugs.*

Action/Kinetics: Indomethacin is not considered to be a simple analgesic and should only be used for the conditions listed. **PO. Onset:** 30 min for analgesia and up to 1 week for anti-inflammatory effect. **Peak plasma levels:** 1–2 hr (2–4 hr for sustained-release). **Duration:** 4–6 hr for analgesia and 1–2 weeks for anti-inflammatory effect. **Therapeutic plasma levels:** 10–18 mcg/mL. **t½:** Approximately 5 hr (up to 6 hr for sustained-release). **Plasma t½ following IV in infants:** 12–20 hr, depending on age and dose. Approximately 90% plasma protein bound. The drug is metabolized in the liver and excreted in both the urine and feces.

Uses: Moderate to severe rheumatoid arthritis, osteoarthritis, and ankylosing spondylitis (drug of choice). Acute gouty arthritis and acute painful shoulder (tendinitis, bursitis). *IV:* Pharmacologic closure of persistent patent ductus arteriosus in premature infants. *Investigational:* Topically to treat cystoid macular edema (0.5% and 1% drops), sunburn, primary dysmenorrhea, prophylaxis of migraine, cluster headache, polyhydramnios.

Additional   Contraindications: Pregnancy and lactation. PO indomethacin in children under 14 years of age. GI lesions or history of recurrent GI lesions. *IV use:* GI or intracranial bleeding, thrombocytopenia, renal disease, defects of coagulation,

necrotizing enterocolitis. *Suppositories:* Recent rectal bleeding, history of proctitis.

Special Concerns: Use in children should be restricted to those unresponsive to or intolerant of other anti-inflammatory agents; efficacy has not been determined in children less than 14 years of age. Geriatric clients are at greater risk of developing CNS side effects, especially confusion. To be used with caution in clients with history of epilepsy, psychiatric illness, or parkinsonism and in the elderly. Indomethacin should be used with extreme caution in the presence of existing, controlled infections.

Additional Side Effects: Reactivation of latent infections may mask signs of infection. More marked CNS manifestations than for other drugs of this group. Aggravation of depression or other psychiatric problems, epilepsy, and parkinsonism.

Additional Drug Interactions

Captopril / Indomethacin ↓ effect of captopril, probably due to inhibition of prostaglandin synthesis

Diflunisal / ↑ Plasma levels of indomethacin; also, possible fatal GI hemorrhage

Diuretics (loop, potassium-sparing, thiazide) / Indomethacin may reduce the antihypertensive and natriuretic action of diuretics

Lisinopril / Possible ↓ effect of lisinopril

Prazosin / Indomethacin ↓ antihypertensive effects of prazosin

Dosage

- **Capsules, Oral Suspension**

  Moderate to severe arthritis, osteoarthritis, ankylosing spondylitis.

Adults, initial: 25 mg b.i.d.–t.i.d.; may be increased by 25–50 mg at weekly intervals, according to condition and, if tolerated, until satisfactory response is obtained. In those with persistent night pain or morning stiffness, a maximum of 100 mg of the total daily dose can be given at bedtime. **Maximum daily dosage:** 150–200 mg. In acute flares of chronic rheumatoid arthritis, the dose may need to be increased by

25–50 mg/day until the acute phase is under control.

Acute gouty arthritis.

Adults, initial: 50 mg t.i.d. until pain is tolerable; **then,** reduce dosage rapidly until drug is withdrawn. Pain relief usually occurs within 2–4 hr, tenderness and heat subside in 24–36 hr, and swelling disappears in 3–4 days.

Acute painful shoulder (bursitis/tendinitis).

75–150 mg/day in three to four divided doses for 1–2 weeks.

• **Sustained-Release Capsules**

Antirheumatic, anti-inflammatory.

Adults: 75 mg, of which 25 mg is released immediately, 1–2 times/day.

• **Suppositories**

Anti-inflammatory, antirheumatic, antigout.

Adults: 50 mg up to q.i.d. **Pediatric:** 1.5–2.5 mg/kg/day in three to four divided doses (up to a maximum of 4 mg/kg or 250–300 mg/day, whichever is less).

• **IV Only**

Patent ductus arteriosus.

3 IV doses, depending on age of the infant, are given at 12–24-hr intervals. **Infants less than 2 days:** first dose, 0.2 mg/kg, followed by two doses of 0.1 mg/kg each; **infants 2–7 days:** three doses of 0.2 mg/kg each; **infants more than 7 days:** first dose, 0.2 mg/kg, followed by two doses of 0.25 mg/kg each. If patent ductus arteriosus reopens, a second course of one to three doses may be given. Surgery may be required if there is no response after two courses of therapy.

RESPIRATORY CARE CONSIDERATIONS

See also *Respiratory Care Considerations* for *Nonsteroidal Anti-Inflammatory Drugs.*

Administration/Storage

1. Store in amber-colored containers.

2. The IV solution should be prepared with 1–2 mL of preservative-free sodium chloride injection or sterile water for injection.

3. IV solutions should be freshly prepared prior to use.

4. Reconstitute to 0.1 mg/mL or 0.05 mg/mL immediately before use and infuse over 5–10 sec.

5. Up to 100 mg of the total daily dose can be given at bedtime for clients with night pain or morning stiffness.

6. The sustained-release form should not be crushed and should not be used in clients with acute gouty arthritis.

7. If the client has difficulty swallowing capsules, the contents may be emptied into applesauce, food, or liquid to ensure that the client receives the prescribed dose.

8. Suppositories (50 mg) may be used in clients unable to take PO medication. They should be stored below 30°C (86°F).

9. Anticipate a peak action of drug to occur in 24–36 hr in clients taking the medication for gout. Swelling gradually disappears in 3–5 days. The sustained-release form should not be used to treat gout.

10. Peak drug activity in clients taking the medication for antirheumatic effect will occur in about 4 weeks.

11. The smallest effective dose of the drug should be administered, based on individual need. Adverse reactions are dose related.

Assessment

1. Document indications for therapy and type and onset of symptoms.

2. Determine any agents used for this condition and the outcome.

3. List other drugs prescribed to ensure none interact unfavorably.

4. Assess and document characteristics of involved joint(s), including goniometric measurements and ROM.

Evaluate

• Control of pain and inflammation with improved joint mobility

• Successful closure of patent ductus arteriosus with IV therapy

• Therapeutic serum drug levels (10–18 mcg/mL)

Ipratropium bromide
(eye-prah-**TROH**-pee-um)
Pregnancy Category: B
Atrovent **(Rx)**
Classification: Anticholinergic, quaternary ammonium compound

See also *Cholinergic Blocking Agents.*

Action/Kinetics: Ipratropium is chemically related to atropine; thus, it antagonizes the action of acetylcholine. The drug prevents the increase in intracellular levels of cyclic guanosine monophosphate, which is caused by the interaction of acetylcholine with muscarinic receptors in bronchial smooth muscle; this leads to bronchodilation which is primarily a local, site-specific effect. Ipratropium is not easily absorbed into the systemic circulation and is excreted through the feces. **t½, elimination:** 2 hr after inhalation.

Uses: Aerosol or solution: Bronchodilation in COPD, including chronic bronchitis and emphysema. **Nasal spray:** Symptomatic relief (using 0.06%) of rhinorrhea associated with allergic and nonallergic perennial rhinitis in clients over 12 years of age. Symptomatic relief (using 0.06%) of rhinorrhea associated with the common cold in those over 12 years of age. *NOTE:* The use of ipratropium with sympathomimetic bronchodilators, methylxanthines, steroids, or cromolyn sodium (all of which are used in treating COPD) are without side effects.

Contraindications: Hypersensitivity to atropine, ipratropium, or derivatives. Hypersensitivity to soya lecithin or related food products, including soy bean or peanut (inhalation aerosol).

Special Concerns: Use with caution in clients with narrow-angle glaucoma, prostatic hypertrophy, or bladder neck obstruction and during lactation. Safety and efficacy have not been determined in children.

Use of ipratropium as a single agent for the relief of bronchospasm in acute COPD has not been studied adequately.

Side Effects: *Inhalation aerosol. CNS:* Cough, nervousness, dizziness, headache, fatigue, insomnia, drowsiness, difficulty in coordination, tremor. *GI:* Dryness of oropharynx, GI distress, dry mouth, nausea, constipation. *CV:* Palpitations, tachycardia, flushing. *Dermatologic:* Itching, hives, alopecia. *Miscellaneous:* Irritation from aerosol, worsening of symptoms, rash, hoarseness, blurred vision, difficulty in accommodation, drying of secretions, urinary difficulty, paresthesias, mucosal ulcers.

Inhalation solution. CNS: Dizziness, insomnia, nervousness, tremor, headache. *GI:* Dry mouth, nausea, constipation. *CV:* Hypertension, aggravation of hypertension, tachycardia, palpitations. *Respiratory:* Worsening of COPD symptoms, coughing, dyspnea, bronchitis, bronchospasm, increased sputum, URI, pharyngitis, rhinitis, sinusitis. *Miscellaneous:* Urinary retention, UTIs, urticaria, pain, flu-like symptoms, back or chest pain, arthritis.

Nasal spray. CNS: Headache, dizziness. *GI:* Nausea, dry mouth, taste perversion. *CV:* Palpitation, tachycardia. *Respiratory:* URI, epistaxis, pharyngitis, nasal dryness, miscellaneous nasal symptoms, nasal irritation, blood-tinged mucus, dry throat, cough, nasal congestion, nasal burning, coughing. *Ophthalmic:* Ocular irritation, blurred vision, conjunctivitis. *Miscellaneous:* Hoarseness, thirst, tinnitis, urinary retention.

All products. Allergic: Skin rash; angioedema of the tongue, throat, lips, and face; urticaria, laryngospasm, **anaphylaxis.** *Anticholinergic reactions:* Precipitation or worsening of narrow angle glaucoma, prostatic disorders, tachycardia, urinary retention, constipation, and bowel obstruction.

Dosage
• **Respiratory Aerosol**
Treat bronchospasms.

Adults: 2 inhalations (36 mcg) q.i.d. Additional inhalations may be required but should not exceed 12 inhalations/day.

- **Solution for Inhalation**
  Treat bronchospasms.

Adults: 500 mcg (1-unit-dose vial) administered t.i.d.–q.i.d. by oral nebulization with doses 6–8 hr apart.

- **Nasal Spray, 0.03%**
  Perennial rhinitis.

2 sprays (42 mcg) per nostril b.i.d.–t.i.d. for a total daily dose of 168–252 mcg/day.

- **Nasal Spray, 0.06%**
  Rhinitis due to the common cold.

2 sprays (84 mcg) per nostril t.i.d.–q.i.d. for a total daily dose of 504–672 mcg/day. The safety and efficacy for use for the common cold for more than 4 days have not been determined.

RESPIRATORY CARE CONSIDERATIONS

See also *Respiratory Care Considerations* for *Cholinergic Blocking Agents.*

Administration/Storage

1. If clients are also taking albuterol, ipratropium may be mixed in the nebulizer with albuterol if used within 1 hr.

2. The aerosol should be stored below 30°C (86°F) and excessive humidity avoided.

3. The solution should be stored between 15°C and 30°C (59°F and 86°F) and protected from light. Unused vials should be stored in the foil pouch.

4. The nasal spray should be stored tightly closed between 15C and 30C (59F and 86F). Freezing should be avoided.

Assessment

1. Document indications for therapy, type, onset, and duration of symptoms, and any other agents used.

2. Perform full pulmonary assessment and review pulmonary function tests and X-ray reports.

3. Note any evidence of prostate enlargement or reports of difficulty urinating.

Client/Family Teaching

1. Take exactly as directed and shake well before using. Use a demonstrator to show client proper administration and observe client technique.

2. If directed to use more than one inhalation per dose, wait 3 min before administering the second inhalation.

3. Stress that drug is not for use in terminating an acute asthma attack as effects take up to 15 min. Have another prescribed agent readily available in this event.

4. Avoid contact with the eyes. A spacer may be useful with the inhaler and a mouthpiece with the nebulizer to help prevent solution (mist) contact with the eyes.

5. May experience a bitter taste and a dry mouth; frequent rinses and hard candy may relieve these symptoms.

6. Caution that transient dizziness, insomnia, blurred vision, or excessive weakness may occur.

7. Advise to stop smoking now to preserve current level of lung function and to prevent further damage. Refer to a formal smoking cessation group.

Evaluate

- Improved pulmonary function and breathing patterns with chronic airway conditions
- ↓ Wheezing, ↓ dyspnea
- Symptomatic relief of rhinorrhea

Ipratropium bromide and Albuterol sulfate

((eye-prah-**TROH**-pee-um, al-**BYOU**-ter-ohl))

Pregnancy Category: C

Combivent (R$_x$),

Classification: Anticholinergic and direct-acting adrenergic (sympathomimetic) agents

See also *Cholinergic Blocking Agents* and *Sympathomimetic Drugs.*

Action/Kinetics: Ipratropium antagonizes the action of acetylcholine. It prevents an increase in intracellular levels of cyclic guanosine monophosphate, which normally results from the interaction of acetylcholine with muscarinic receptors in bronchial smooth muscles; this leads to bronchodilation which is primarily a local, site-specific effect. Ipratropium is not readily absorbed into the systemic circulation and is excreted through the feces. t½, **elimination: 2 hr.** Albuterol stimulates beta-2 receptors of the bronchi, leading to bronchodilation. It causes less tachycardia and is longer-acting them isoproterenol. Beta-1 activity is minimal. **t½ elimination: 3.9 hr.** The combination product, Combivent (R_x), is expected to maximize the response to treatment in COPD patients by treating bronchospasm through two different mechanisms. The two agents apparently act to produce an overall bronchodilator effect that is greater than when either drug is administered alone at recommended dosages.

Uses: Treat bronchospasm in COPD patients who continue to have bronchospasm while on a regular inhaled bronchodilator and the addition of a second bronchodilator is indicated.

Contraindications: Hypersensitivity to atropine, ipratropium, or related anticholinergics. Hypersensitivity to soya lecithin or related food products (e.g. soybeans and peanuts) or hypersensitivity to any other component.

Special Concerns: Use with caution in clients with narrow-angle glaucoma, prostatic hypertrophy, or bladder neck obstruction. Safety and efficacy have not been determined in children. Teratogenic effects of albuterol have been demonstrated in animal studies, but there have been no adequate studies in humans. Therefore, its use in pregnant women should weigh potential benefits to risk to the fetus. Combivent (R_x) use has not been studied in clients with hepatic or renal insufficiency and,

therefore, it should be used with caution in such cases.

Side Effects: See Sympathomimetic Drugs, Albuterol and Ipratropium bromide.

OD Overdose Management: The effects of overdosage are expected to be primarily due to albuterol which may include anginal pain, hypertension, hypokalemia, tachycardia, and exageration of side effects. Dialysis is *not* appropriate treatment, but the judicious use of a beta-1 selective blocker, such as metoprolol, may be indicated.

Dosage ──────────────
• **Metered Dose Inhaler**
Two inhalation (42 mcg of ipratropium and 240 mcg of albuterol) QID. Clients may take additional inhalations PRN, but total number of inhalations should not exceed 12 in 24 hours.

RESPIRATORY CARE CONSIDERATIONS

See *Sympathomimentic Drugs, Cholinergic Blocking Agents, Albuterol,* and *Ipratropium bromide.*

Administration/Storage
1. Do not exceed the recommended dosage.
2. If the dose of drug used previously does not provide relief, contact the provider immediately.
3. Do not use Combivent (R_x) with other inhalation medications unless specifically prescribed.
4. The contents of the container are under pressure. Therefore, do not store near heat or open flames and do not puncture the container.
5. The inhaler should be stored between 15°C and 30°C and excess humidity should be avoided.
6. The MDI may be administered to a client on mechanical ventilation with an adapter. Actuation should be timed to be delivered just prior to or with inspiration.

Client/Family Teaching
1. Take exactly as directed and shake well before using. Use a demonstrator to show client proper admin-

istration and observe client technique.

2. Wait at least 3 minutes between inhalations.

3. Avoid contact with the eyes. A spacer may be useful to improve deposition in the airways, as well as, preventing contact of mist with eyes.

4. Advise of possibility of paradoxical bronchospasm which may occur with any inhaled formulation. It frequently occurs with the first use of a new cannister. Use of drug should be terminated immediately followed by contact with provider and use of alternate therapy.

5. Review side effects associated with both ipratropium and albuterol.

Evaluate
• Improved gas exchange and breathing patterns
• ↓ wheezing, ↓ dyspnea
• Heart rate and other signs of side effects

Isoetharine hydrochloride
(eye-so-**ETH**-ah-reen)
Pregnancy Category: C
Arm-a-Med Isoetharine HCl, Beta-2, Bronkosol **(Rx)**

Isoetharine mesylate
(eye-so-**ETH**-ah-reen)
Pregnancy Category: C
Bronkometer **(Rx)**
Classification: Adrenergic agent, bronchodilator

See also *Sympathomimetic Drugs.*

Action/Kinetics: Isoetharine has a greater stimulating activity on beta-2 receptors of the bronchi than on beta-1 receptors of the heart. Causes relief of bronchospasms. **Inhalation: Onset,** 1–6 min; **peak effect:** 15–60 min; **duration:** 1–3 hr. Partially metabolized; excreted in urine.

Uses: Bronchial asthma, bronchospasms due to chronic bronchitis or emphysema, bronchiectasis, pulmonary obstructive disease.

Special Concerns: Dosage has not been established in children less than 12 years of age.

Dosage ———
• **Inhalation Solution**
Hand nebulizer.
Adults: 3–7 inhalations (use undiluted) of the 0.5% or 1% solution.
Aerosolization or IPPB.
Adults: Dose depends on strength of solution used (range: 0.062%–1%) and whether the solution is used undiluted or diluted according to the following: **1%:** 0.25–1 mL by IPPB or 0.25–0.5 mL by aerosolization diluted 1:3 with saline or other diluent. **0.2–0.5%:** 2 mL used undiluted; **0.2%:** 1.25–2.5 mL used undiluted; **0.167 or 0.17%:** 3 mL used undiluted; **0.125%:** 2–4 mL used undiluted; **0.1%:** 2.5-5 mL used undiluted; **0.08%:** 3 mL used undiluted; **0.062%:** 4 mL used undiluted.

• **Mesylate Metered Dose Inhaler**
Adults: 0.34 mg (1 inhalation) repeated after 1–2 min if needed; **then,** dose may be repeated q 4 hr.

RESPIRATORY CARE CONSIDERATIONS

See *Special Respiratory Care Considerations for Adrenergic Bronchodilators* under *Sympathomimetic Drugs.*

Administration/Storage
1. One or 2 inhalations are usually sufficient. Wait 1 min after giving initial dose to ensure necessity of another dose.

2. Treatment usually does not need to be repeated more than q 4 hr.

3. Do not use if solution contains a precipitate or is brown.

Assessment
1. Note any allergy to sulfites.

2. Document indications for therapy and note pulmonary function and assessments.

Client/Family Teaching
1. Review proper technique for administration and observe client in self-administration.

2. Instruct client to stop smoking and refer to a formal smoking cessation program.

Evaluate: Evidence of improved pulmonary funcion with ↓ airway resistance

---

Isoniazid (INH, Isonicotinic acid hydrazide)

(eye-so-**NYE**-ah-zid)
Pregnancy Category: C
Isotamine ✥, Laniazid, Laniazid C.T., Nydrazid Injection, PMS-Isoniazid ✥
(Rx)
Classification: Primary antitubercular agent

General Statement: Isoniazid is the most effective tuberculostatic agent. The metabolism of isoniazid is genetically determined and involves the level of a hepatic enzyme. Clients on isoniazid fall into two groups, depending on the manner in which they metabolize isoniazid. As a rule, 50% of whites and blacks inactivate the drug slowly, whereas the majority of American Indians, Eskimos, Japanese, and Chinese are rapid acetylators (inactivators).

1. **Slow acetylators:** These clients show earlier, favorable response but have more toxic reactions (e.g., neuropathies because of higher blood levels of drug).

2. **Rapid acetylators:** These clients have possible poor clinical response due to rapid inactivation, which is 5–6 times faster than slow acetylators. This group requires an increased daily dose of the drug. They are more likely to develop hepatitis.

Action/Kinetics: Isoniazid probably interferes with lipid and nucleic acid metabolism of growing bacteria, resulting in alteration of the bacterial wall. The drug is tuberculostatic. It is readily absorbed after PO and parenteral (IM) administration and is widely distributed in body tissues, including cerebrospinal, pleural, and ascitic fluids. **Peak plasma concentration: PO,** 1–2 hr. **t½, fast acetylators:** 0.5–6 hr; **t½, slow acetylators:** 2–5 hr. These values are increased in association with liver and kidney impairment. Drug is metabolized in liver and excreted primarily in urine.

Uses: Tuberculosis caused by human, bovine, and BCG strains of My-cobacterium tuberculosis. The drug should not be used as the sole tuberculostatic agent. Prophylaxis of tuberculosis. *Investigational:* To improve severe tremor in clients with multiple sclerosis.

Contraindications: Severe hypersensitivity to isoniazid or in clients with previous isoniazid-associated hepatic injury or side effects.

Special Concerns: Severe, and sometimes fatal, hepatitis may occur even after several months of therapy; incidence is age-related and current alcohol use increases the risk. Extreme caution should be exercised in clients with convulsive disorders, in whom the drug should be administered only when the client is adequately controlled by anticonvulsant medication. Also, use with caution for the treatment of renal tuberculosis and, in the lowest dose possible, in clients with impaired renal function and in alcoholics.

Side Effects: *Neurologic:* Peripheral neuropathy characterized by symmetrical numbness and tingling of extremities (dose-related). Rarely, toxic encephalopathy, optic neuritis, optic atrophy, **seizures,** impaired memory, toxic psychosis. *GI:* N&V, epigastric distress, xerostomia. *Hypersensitivity:* Fever, skin rashes and eruptions, vasculitis, lymphadenopathy. *Hepatic:* Liver dysfunction, jaundice, bilirubinemia, bilirubinuria, *serious and sometimes fatal hepatitis (especially in clients over 50 years of age).* Increases in serum AST and ALT. *Hematologic: Agranulocytosis,* eosinophilia, thrombocytopenia, *hemolytic, sideroblastic, or aplastic anemia. Metabolic/Endocrine:* Metabolic acidosis, pyridoxine deficiency, pellagra, hyperglycemia, gynecomastia. *Miscellaneous:* Tinnitus, urinary retention, rheumatic syndrome, lupus-like syndrome, arthralgia.

NOTE: Pyridoxine, 10–50 mg/day, may be given concomitantly with isoniazid to decrease CNS side effects. Ophthalmologic and liver function tests are recommended periodically.

OD Overdose Management:
Symptoms: N&V, dizziness, blurred vision, slurred speech, visual hallucinations within 30–180 min. Severe overdosage may cause respiratory distress, *CNS depression (coma can occur), severe seizures,* metabolic acidosis, acetonuria, hyperglycemia. *Treatment:* Maintain respiration and undertake gastric lavage (within first 2–3 hr providing seizures are not present). To control seizures, give diazepam or a short-acting IV barbiturate followed by pyridoxine (1 mg IV/1 mg isoniazid ingested). Sodium bicarbonate, IV, to correct metabolic acidosis. Forced osmotic diuresis; monitor fluid I&O. For severe cases, hemodialysis or peritoneal dialysis should be considered.

Drug Interactions
Aluminum salts / ↓ Effect of isoniazid due to ↓ absorption from GI tract
Anticoagulants, oral / ↓ Anticoagulant effect
Atropine / ↑ Side effects of isoniazid
Benzodiazepines / ↑ Effect of benzodiazepines that undergo oxidative metabolism (e.g., diazepam, triazolam)
Carbamazepine / ↑ Risk of both carbamazepine and isoniazid toxicity
Cycloserine / ↑ Risk of cycloserine CNS side effects
Disulfiram / ↑ Risk of acute behavioral and coordination changes
Enflurane / Isoniazid may produce high levels of hydrazine, which increases defluorination of enflurane
Ethanol / ↑ Chance of isoniazid-induced hepatitis
Halothane / ↑ Risk of hepatotoxicity and hepatic encephalopathy
Hydantoins (phenytoin) / ↑ Effect of hydantoins due to ↓ breakdown in liver
Ketoconazole / ↓ Serum levels of ketoconazole → ↓ effect
Meperidine / ↑ Risk of hypotension or CNS depression

PAS / ↑ Effect of isoniazid by ↑ blood levels
Rifampin / Additive liver toxicity
Laboratory Test Interferences: Altered liver function tests. False + or ↑ potassium, AST, ALT, urine glucose (Benedict's test, Clinitest).

Dosage
• **Syrup, Tablets**
  Active tuberculosis.
Adults: 5 mg/kg/day (up to 300 mg/day) as a single dose; **children and infants:** 10–20 mg/kg/day (up to 300 mg total) in a single dose.
  Prophylaxis.
Adults: 300 mg/day in a single dose; **children and infants:** 10 mg/kg/day (up to 300 mg total) in a single dose.
• **IM**
  Active tuberculosis.
Adults: 5 mg/kg (up to 300 mg) once daily. **Pediatric:** 10–20 mg/kg (up to 300 mg) once daily.
  Prophylaxis.
Adults/adolescents: 300 mg/day. **Pediatric:** 10 mg/kg/day.
  NOTE: Pyridoxine, 6–50 mg/day, is recommended in the malnourished and those prone to neuropathy (e.g., alcoholics, diabetics).

RESPIRATORY CARE CONSIDERATIONS

See also *General Respiratory Care Considerations for All Anti-Infectives.*
Administration/Storage
1. Store in dark, tightly closed containers.
2. Solutions for IM injection may crystallize at low temperature and should be allowed to warm to room temperature if precipitation is evident.
3. Anticipate a slight local irritation at the site of injection. Rotate and document injection sites.
4. Isoniazid should be administered with pyridoxine, 10–50 mg/day, in malnourished, alcoholic, or diabetic clients to prevent symptoms of peripheral neuropathy.

Assessment

1. Document indications for therapy and type and onset of symptoms.
2. Determine any other agents used previously for these symptoms and the outcome.
3. Obtaine baseline lab studies, CXR, and sputum cultures. Note date of PPD conversion. Monitor liver and renal function studies and anticipate reduced dose with renal dysfunction.
4. Perform a thorough pulmonary assessment and describe the characteristics of any sputum produced.

Interventions

1. If CNS stimulation is marked, withhold drug and report.
2. Assess clients with diabetes closely because it is more difficult to control when isoniazid is administered.
3. Monitor I&O to ascertain that renal output is adequate to prevent systemic accumulation of the drug.
4. Provide client with only a 1-month supply of the drug because client should be examined and evaluated monthly while on isoniazid.

Client/Family Teaching

1. Take drug on an empty stomach 1 hr before or 2 hr after meals.
2. Consume 2–3 L/day of fluids to ensure adequate hydration.
3. Explain that pyridoxine is given to prevent neurotoxic effects (peripheral neuritis) of isoniazid.
4. Avoid alcohol while on drug therapy to prevent hepatic toxicity.
5. Withhold drug and report fatigue, weakness, malaise, and anorexia immediately because these may be S&S of hepatitis.
6. Report any visual disturbances as these may precede optic neuritis.
7. Stress the importance of taking drugs as ordered and of reporting for monthly follow-up and periodic lab and ophthalmic assessments.

Evaluate

• Negative sputum cultures for acid-fast bacilli
• Prevention of neurotoxic drug side effects
• Reports of symptomatic improvement (↓ fever, ↓ pulmonary secretions, ↑ appetite)

Isoproterenol
(eye-so-proh-**TER**-ih-nohl)
Pregnancy Category: C
Isuprel Glossets **(Rx)**

Isoproterenol hydrochloride
(eye-so-proh-**TER**-ih-nohl)
Pregnancy Category: C
Dispos-a-Med Isoproterenol HCl, Isuprel, Isuprel Mistometer, Norisodrine Aerotrol **(Rx)**

Isoproterenol sulfate
(eye-so-proh-**TER**-ih-nohl)
Pregnancy Category: C
Medihaler-Iso **(Rx)**
Classification: Sympathomimetic, direct-acting

See also *Sympathomimetic Drugs.*

Action/Kinetics: Isoproterenol produces pronounced stimulation of both beta-1 and beta-2 receptors of the heart, bronchi, skeletal muscle vasculature, and the GI tract. The drug has both positive inotropic and chronotropic activity; systolic BP may increase while diastolic BP may decrease. Thus, mean arterial BP may not change or may be decreased. It also causes less hyperglycemia than epinephrine, but produces bronchodilation and the same degree of CNS excitation. **Inhalation: Onset,** 2–5 min; **peak effect:** 3–5 min; **duration:** 30–120 min. **IV: Onset,** immediate; **duration:** less than 1 hr. **Sublingual: Onset,** 15–30 min; **duration:** 1–2 hr. Partially metabolized; excreted in urine.

Uses: Bronchodilator in asthma, chronic pulmonary emphysema, bronchiectasis, bronchitis, and other conditions involving bronchospasms (e.g., during surgery). Treat bronchospasms during anesthesia. Cardiac arrest, heart block, syncope due to complete heart block, Adams-Stokes syndrome. Certain cardiac arrhythmias including ventricular tachycardia, ventricular arrhythmias; syncope due to carotid sinus hypersensitivity. Hypoperfusion shock syndrome. Hypovolemic and septic shock as an adjunct to fluid and electrolyte replacement. Use in cardiac arrest until electric shock or pacemaker therapy are available.

Contraindications: Tachyarrhythmias, tachycardia, or heart block caused by digitalis intoxication, ventricular arrhythmias that require inotropic therapy, and angina pectoris.

Special Concerns: Use with caution in the presence of tuberculosis. Safety and effectiveness have not been determined in children less than 12 years of age. Use with caution during lactation.

Additional Side Effects: *CV: Cardiac arrest,* Adams-Stokes attack, hypotension, precordial pain or distress. *CNS:* Hyperactivity, hyperkinesia. *Respiratory:* Wheezing, bronchitis, increase in sputum, *bronchial edema and inflammation, pulmonary edema, paradoxical airway resistance.* Excessive inhalation causes refractory bronchial obstruction. *Miscellaneous:* Flushing, sweating, swelling of the parotid gland. Sublingual administration may cause buccal ulceration. Side effects of drug are less severe after inhalation.

Drug Interactions

Bretylium / Possibility of arrhythmias

Guanethidine / ↑ Pressor response of isoproterenol

Halogenated hydrocarbon anesthetics / Sensitization of the heart to catecholamines which may cause serious arrhythmias

Oxytocic drugs / Possibility of severe, persistent hypertension

Tricyclic antidepressants / Potentiation of pressor effect

Dosage ————————
Isoproterenol hydrochloride
• **IV Infusion**
 Shock.
5 mcg/min (1.25 mL/min of solution prepared by diluting 10 mL of 1:5,000 solution in 500 mL of D5W or 5 mL of 1:5,000 solution in 250 mL of D5W).
 Cardiac standstill and cardiac arrhythmias.

Adults: 5 mcg/min (1.25 mL of either 1.25 mL/min of solution prepared by diluting 10 mL of 1:5,000 solution in 500 mL of D5W or 5 mL of 1:5,000 solution in 250 mL of D5W).
• **IV**
 Cardiac standstill and cardiac arrhythmias.
1–3 mL (0.02–0.06 mg) of solution prepared by diluting 1 mL of 1:5,000 solution to 10 mL with sodium chloride or 5% dextrose solution. Dosage range: 0.01–0.2 mg.
 Bronchospasm during anesthesia.
Adults: Dilute 1 mL of the 1:5,000 solution to 10 mL with sodium chloride injection or 5% dextrose solution and given an initial dose of 0.01–0.02 mg IV; repeat when necessary.
• **IM, SC**
 Cardiac standstill and cardiac arrhythmias.
Adults: 1 mL (0.2 mg) of 1:5,000 solution (range: 0.02–1 mg).
 Intracardiac (in extreme emergencies): 0.1 mL (0.02 mg) of 1:5,000 solution.
• **Hand Bulb Nebulizer**
 Acute bronchial asthma.
Adults and children: 5–15 deep inhalations of the 1:200 solution. In adults 3–7 inhalations of the 1:100 solution may be useful. If there is no relief after 5–10 min, the doses may be repeated one more time. Repeat treatment up to 5 times/day may be necessary if there are repeat attacks.
 Bronchospasm in chronic obstructive lung disease.
Adults and children: 5–15 deep inhalations of the 1:200 solution (in clients with severe attacks, 3–7 inhalations of the 1:100 solution may be useful). An interval of 3–4 hr should elapse between uses.
• **Metered-Dose Inhalation**
 Acute bronchial asthma.
Adults, usual: 1–2 inhalations beginning with 1 inhalation, and if no relief occurs within 2–5 min, a second inhalation may be used. **Maintenance:** 1–2 inhalations 4–6 times/day. No more than 2 inhala-

tions at any one time or more than 6 inhalations in 1 hr should be taken.

Bronchospasm in chronic obstructive lung disease.

Adults and children: 1–2 inhalations repeated at no less than 3–4 hr intervals (i.e., 4–6 times/day).

• **Nebulization by Compressed Air or Oxygen**

Bronchospasms in chronic obstructive lung disease.

Adults and children: 0.5 mL of the 1:200 solution is diluted to 2–2.5 mL (for a concentration of 1:800–1:1,000). The solution is delivered over 15–20 min and may be repeated up to 5 times/day.

• **IPPB**

Bronchospasms in chronic obstructive lung disease.

Adults and children: 0.5 mL of a 1:200 solution diluted to 2–2.5 mL with water or isotonic saline. The solution is delivered over 10–20 min and may be repeated up to 5 times/day.

Isoproterenol sulfate
Dispensed from metered aerosol inhaler for bronchospasms. See preceding dosage for *Hydrochloride.*

RESPIRATORY CARE CONSIDERATIONS

See also *Special Respiratory Care Considerations for Adrenergic Bronchodilators* under *Sympathomimetic Drugs.*

Administration/Storage

1. Administration to children, except where noted, is the same as that for adults, because a child's smaller ventilatory exchange capacity will permit a proportionally smaller aerosol intake. For acute bronchospasms in children, use 1:200 solution.

2. In children, no more than 0.25 mL of the 1:200 solution should be used for each 10–15 min of programmed treatment.

3. Elderly clients usually receive a lower dose.

4. The sublingual tablets should not be crushed or chewed; rather, they should be placed under the tongue

and allowed to disintegrate. Clients should not swallow saliva until absorption has taken place.

5. The injection should not be used if it is pinkish to brownish in color. It should be protected from light and stored at 15°C–30°C (59°F–86°F).

Assessment

1. Document indications for therapy, any causative factors, and type and onset of symptoms.

2. Perform a thorough pulmonary assessment. Note pulmonary function tests and CXR reports. Report respiratory problems that seem to worsen after the administration of isoproterenol. Refractory reactions may necessitate withdrawal of the drug.

3. List drugs currently prescribed.

4. Identify arrhythmias (especially ventricular) and note any evidence of angina as these may preclude drug therapy.

Client/Family Teaching

1. Review and demonstrate the appropriate method for using the inhaler and provide a spacer to enhance instillation. Observe client in self-administration to ensure proper technique.

2. Rinse mouth and equipment with water to remove any drug residue and to minimize dryness, after inhalation therapy.

3. Maintain an adequate fluid intake of 2-3 L/day to help liquefy secretions.

4. The sputum and saliva may appear pink after inhalation therapy. This is due to the drug and the client should not become alarmed.

5. When also taking inhalant glucocorticoids advise to take isoproterenol first and to wait 15 min before using the second inhaler.

6. Do not use inhaler therapy more frequently than prescribed. Excessive use can cause severe cardiac and respiratory problems.

7. Avoid all OTC agents without provider approval.

8. Identify the parotid gland. Instruct client to withhold the drug and report immediately if it becomes enlarged.

Evaluate
- Improved pulmonary function
- ↓ Bronchoconstriction and bronchospasms
- Restoration of stable cardiac rhythm with ↑ HR and ↑ CO

Isosorbide dinitrate chewable tablets
(eye-so-**SOR**-byd)
Pregnancy Category: C
Sorbitrate **(Rx)**

Isosorbide dinitrate extended-release capsules
(eye-so-**SOR**-byd)
Pregnancy Category: C
Dilatrate-SR, Isordil Tembids **(Rx)**

Isosorbide dinitrate extended-release tablets
(eye-so-**SOR**-byd)
Pregnancy Category: C
Cedocard-SR ✿, Coradur ✿, Isordil Tembids **(Rx)**

Isosorbide dinitrate sublingual tablets
(eye-so-**SOR**-byd)
Pregnancy Category: C
Apo-ISDN ✿, Coronex ✿, Isordil, Sorbitrate **(Rx)**

Isosorbide dinitrate tablets
(eye-so-**SOR**-byd)
Pregnancy Category: C
Apo-ISDN ✿, Coronex ✿, Isordil Titradose, Sorbitrate **(Rx)**
Classification: Coronary vasodilator, antianginal drug

See also *Antianginal Drugs, Nitrates/Nitrites.*
Action/Kinetics: **Sublingual, chewable. Onset:** 2–5 min; **duration:** 1–3 hr. **Oral Capsules/Tablets. Onset:** 20–40 min; **duration:** 4–6 hr. **Extended-release. Onset:** up to 4 hr; **duration:** 6–8 hr.

Additional Use: Diffuse esophageal spasm. Oral tablets are only for prophylaxis while sublingual and chewable forms may be used to terminate acute attacks of angina.
Special Concerns: Use with caution during lactation. Safety and efficacy have not been established in children.
Additional Side Effects: Vascular headaches occur especially frequently.
Additional Drug Interactions
Acetylcholine / Isosorbide antagonizes the effect of acetylcholine
Norepinephrine / Isosorbide antagonizes the effect of norepinephrine

Dosage ————————
- **Tablets**
  Antianginal.
Initial: 5–20 mg q 6 hr; **maintenance:** 10–40 mg q 6 hr (usual: 20–40 mg q.i.d.
- **Chewable Tablets**
  Antianginal, acute attack.
Initial: 5 mg q 2–3 hr. The dose can be titrated upward until angina is relieved or side effects occur.
  Prophylaxis.
5–10 mg q 2–3 hr.
- **Extended-Release Capsules**
  Antianginal.
Initial: 40 mg; **maintenance:** 40–80 mg q 8–12 hr.
- **Extended-Release Tablets**
  Antianginal.
Initial: 40 mg; **maintenance:** 40–80 mg q 8–12 hr.
- **Sublingual**
  Acute attack.
2.5–5 mg q 2–3 hr as required. The dose can be titrated upward until angina is relieved or side effects occur.
  Prophylaxis.
5–10 mg q 2–3 hr.

RESPIRATORY CARE CONSIDERATIONS

See also *Respiratory Care Considerations* for *Antianginal Drugs, Nitrates/Nitrites.*

Evaluate
- ↓ Frequency and severity of anginal attacks
- ↑ Exercise tolerance
- Resolution of esophageal spasm

Isosorbide mononitrate, oral

(eye-so-**SOR**-byd)
Pregnancy Category: C
Imdur, ISMO, Monoket **(Rx)**
Classification: Coronary vasodilator, antianginal drug

See also *Antianginal Drugs, Nitrates/Nitrites,* and *Isosorbide Dinitrate.*

Action/Kinetics: Isosorbide mononitrate is the major metabolite of isosorbide dinitrate. The mononitrate is not subject to first-pass metabolism. Bioavailability is nearly 100%. **Onset:** 30–60 min. **t½:** About 5 hr.

Uses: Prophylaxis of angina pectoris.

Contraindications: To abort acute anginal attacks. Use in acute MI or CHF.

Special Concerns: Use with caution in clients who may be volume depleted or who are already hypotensive. Use with caution during lactation. Safety and effectiveness have not been determined in children. The benefits have not been established in acute MI or CHF.

Side Effects: *CV:* Hypotension (may be accompanied by paradoxical bradycardia and increased angina pectoris). *CNS:* Headache, lightheadedness, dizziness. *GI:* N&V. *Miscellaneous:* Possibility of methemoglobinemia.

OD **Overdose Management:** *Symptoms:* Increased intracranial pressure manifested by throbbing headache, confusion, moderate fever. Also, vertigo, palpitations, visual disturbances, N&V, syncope, air hunger, dyspnea (followed by reduced ventilatory effort), diaphoresis, skin either flushed or cold and clammy, heart block, bradycardia, paralysis, ***coma, seizures, death.*** *Treatment:* Therapy should be directed toward an increase in central fluid volume. Vasoconstrictors should *not* be used.

Drug Interactions
Ethanol / Additive vasodilation
Calcium channel blockers / Severe orthostatic hypotension
Organic nitrates / Severe orthostatic hypotension

Dosage
IMDUR TABLETS
  Prophylaxis of angina.
Initial: 30 mg (given as one-half of the 60-mg tablet) or 60 mg once daily; **then,** dosage may be increased to 120 mg given as 2–60-mg tablets once daily. Rarely, 240 mg daily may be needed.
ISMO, MONOKET TABLETS
  Prevention and treatment of angina.
Adults: 20 mg b.i.d. with the doses 7 hr apart (it is preferable that first dose be given on awakening). An initial dose of 5 mg may be best for clients of small stature; the dose should then be increased to at least 10 mg by the second or third day of therapy.

RESPIRATORY CARE CONSIDERATIONS

See also *Respiratory Care Considerations* for *Antianginal Drugs, Nitrates/Nitrites,* and *Isosorbide Dinitrate.*

Administration/Storage
1. The treatment regimen provided minimizes the development of refractory tolerance.
2. The extended release tablet should be given in the morning on arising. These tablets should not be crushed or chewed. They should be taken with a half glass of water.

Interventions
1. Determine that the client is adequately hydrated.
2. Ensure that SBP > 100 mm Hg as drug may cause marked hypotension.

Evaluate: Desired prophylaxis of angina pectoris

Isradipine

(iss-**RAD**-ih-peen)
Pregnancy Category: C
DynaCirc **(Rx)**
Classification: Calcium channel blocking agent

See also *Calcium Channel Blocking Agents.*

Action/Kinetics: Isradipine binds to calcium channels resulting in the inhibition of calcium influx into cardiac and smooth muscle and subsequent arteriolar vasodilation. The reduced systemic resistance leads to a decrease in BP with a small increase in resting HR. In clients with normal ventricular function, the drug reduces afterload leading to some increase in CO. Isradipine is well absorbed from the GI tract although it undergoes significant first-pass metabolism. **Peak plasma levels:** 1 ng/mL after 1.5 hr. **Onset:** 2–3 hr. When taken with food, the time to peak effect is increased by approximately 1 hr, although the total bioavailability does not change. **t½, initial:** 1.5–2 hr; **terminal,** 8 hr. The drug is completely metabolized in the liver with 60%–65% excreted through the kidneys and 25%–30% through the feces. The maximum effect may not be observed for 2–4 wk.

Uses: Alone or with thiazide diuretics in the management of essential hypertension. *Investigational:* Chronic stable angina.

Contraindications: Lactation.

Special Concerns: Safety and effectiveness have not been determined in children. Use with caution in clients with CHF, especially those taking a beta-adrenergic blocking agent. The bioavailability of isradipine increases in geriatric clients over 65 years of age, clients with impaired hepatic function, and those with mild renal impairment.

Side Effects: *CV:* Palpitations, edema, flushing, tachycardia, SOB, hypotension, transient ischemic attack, **stroke,** atrial fibrillation, **ventricular fibrillation, MI,** CHF, angina. *CNS:* Headache, dizziness, fatigue, drowsiness, insomnia, lethargy, nervousness, depression, syncope, amnesia, psychosis, hallucinations, weakness, jitteriness, paresthesia. *GI:* Nausea, abdominal discomfort, diarrhea, vomiting, constipation, dry mouth. *Respiratory:* Dyspnea, cough. *Dermatologic:* Pruritus, urticaria. *Miscellaneous:* Chest pain, rash, pollakiuria, cramps of the legs and feet, nocturia, polyuria, hyperhidrosis, visual disturbances, numbness, throat discomfort, leukopenia, sexual difficulties.

Drug Interactions: Severe hypotension has been observed during fentanyl anesthesia with concomitant use of a beta-blocker and a calcium channel blocking agent.

Laboratory Test Interferences: ↑ Liver function tests.

Dosage ─────────
• **Capsules**
  Hypertension.
Adults, initial: 2.5 mg b.i.d. alone or in combination with a thiazide diuretic. If BP is not decreased satisfactorily after 2–4 weeks, the dose may be increased in increments of 5 mg/day at 2 *to* 4-week intervals up to a maximum of 20 mg/day. Adverse effects increase, however, at doses above 10 mg/day.

RESPIRATORY CARE CONSIDERATIONS

See *Respiratory Care Considerations* for *Calcium Channel Blocking Agents.*

Administration/Storage: The drug should be stored in a tight container protected from light.

Evaluate: ↓ BP with control of hypertension

Itraconazole

(**ih**-trah-**KON**-ah-zohl)
Pregnancy Category: C
Sporanox **(Rx)**
Classification: Antifungal

Action/Kinetics: The drug is believed to inhibit cytochrome P-450-dependent synthesis of ergosterol, which is a necessary component of fungal cell membranes. The absorption appears to increase when taken with a cola beverage. The drug concentrates in fatty tissues, omentum, liver, kidney, and skin. **t½, at steady-state:** 64 hr. Extensively metabolized by the liver; the major metabolite is hydroxyitraconazole, which also has antifungal activity. The drug and major metabolite are extensively bound (over 99%) to plasma proteins. Metabolites are excreted in both the urine and feces.

Uses: Treatment of blastomycosis (pulmonary and extrapulmonary) and histoplasmosis (including chronic cavitary pulmonary disease and disseminated, nonmeningeal histoplasmosis) in both immunocompromised and nonimmunocompromised clients. To treat aspergillus infections (pulmonary and extrapulmonary) in clients intolerant or refractory to amphotericin B. Onychomycosis due to tinea unguium of the toenail with or without fingernail involvement. The drug is effective against *Blastomyces dermatitidis, Histoplasma capsulatum* and *H. duboisii, Aspergillus flavus* and *A. fumigatis,* and *Cryptococcus neoformans.* In vitro activity has also been found for a number of other organisms, including *Sporothirx scheneckii, Trochophyton* species, *Candida albicans,* and *Candida species. Investigational:* (1) Superficial mycoses including dermatophytoses (tinea capitis, tinea corporis, tinea cruris, tinea pedis, and tinea manuum), pityriasis versicolor, candidiasis (vaginal, oral, chronic mucocutaneous), and sebopsoriasis. (2) Systemic mycoses including dimorphic infections (paracoccidioidomycosis, coccidioidomycosis), cryptococcal infections (meningitis, disseminated), and candidiasis. (3) Miscellaneous mycoses including fungal keratitis, alternariosis, leishmaniasis (cutaneous), subcutaneous mycoses (chromomycosis, sporotrichosis), and zygomycosis.

Contraindications: Concomitant use of astemizole, cisapride, triazolam, oral midazolam, or terfenadine. Hypersensitivity to the drug or its excipients. Lactation. Use for the treatment of onychomycosis in pregnant women or in women wishing to become pregnant.

Special Concerns: Safety and efficacy have not been determined in children although pediatric clients have been treated for systemic fungal infections.

Side Effects: *GI:* N&V, diarrhea, abdominal pain, anorexia, general GI disorders, flatulence, constipation, gastritis. *CNS:* Headache, dizziness, vertigo, insomnia, decreased libido, somnolence, depression. *CV:* Hypertension, orthostatic hypotension, vasculitis. *Dermatologic:* Rash (occurs more frequently in immunocompromised clients also taking immunosuppressant drugs), pruritus. *Allergic:* Rash, pruritus, urticaria, angioedema, and rarely, ***anaphylaxis and Stevens-Johnson syndrome.*** *Miscellaneous:* Edema, fatigue, fever, malaise, abnormal hepatic function, hypokalemia, albuminuria, tinnitus, impotence, adrenal insufficiency, gynecomastia, breast pain in males, menstrual disorder, hepatitis (rare), neuropathy (rare).

OD **Overdose Management:** *Symptoms:* Extension of side effects. *Treatment:* Use supportive measures, including gastric lavage and sodium bicarbonate. Dialysis will not remove itraconazole.

Drug Interactions

Astemizole / ↑ Astemizole levels → serious CV toxicity including ventricular tachycardia, torsades de pointes, and death.

Calcium blockers (especially amlodipine and nifedipine) / Development of edema

Cisapride / Cisapride levels serious CV toxicity including ventricular tachycardia, torsades de pointes, and death.

Cyclosporine and HMG-CoA reductase inhibitors / Possible development of rhabdomyolysis. ↑ Cyclosporine levels (dose of cyclosporine should be ↓ by 50% if itraconazole doses are much greater than 100 mg/day)

Digoxin / ↑ Digoxin levels

H₂ Antagonists / ↓ Plasma levels of itraconazole

Midazolam, oral / ↑ Levels of oral midazolam → potentiation of sedative and hypnotic effects

Isoniazid / ↓ Plasma levels of itraconazole

Phenytoin / ↓ Plasma levels of itraconazole; also, metabolism of phenytoin may be altered

Rifampin / ↓ Plasma levels of itraconazole

Quinidine / Tinnitus and decreased hearing

Sulfonylureas / ↑ Risk of hypoglycemia

Tacrolimus / ↑ Levels of tacrolimus

Terfenadine / ↑ Terfenadine levels → serious CV toxicity including ventricular tachycardia, torsades de pointes, and death

Triazolam / Levels of triazolam potentiation of sedative and hypnotic effects

Warfarin / ↑ Anticoagulant effect of warfarin

Laboratory Test Interferences: Liver enzymes

Dosage ———————
- **Capsules**

   Blastomycosis or histoplasmosis.
Adults: 200 mg once daily. If there is no improvement or the disease is progressive, the dose may be increased in 100-mg increments to a maximum of 400 mg/day. **Children, 3–16 years of age:** 100 mg/day (for systemic fungal infections).

   Aspergillosis.
200–400 mg daily.

   Life-threatening infections.
Adults: A loading dose of 200 mg t.i.d. for the first 3 days should be given.

   Onychomycosis.
200 mg once a day for 12 consecutive weeks.

   Unlabeled uses.
Adults: 50–400 mg/day for 1 day to more than 6 months, depending on the condition and the response.

RESPIRATORY CARE CONSIDERATIONS
Administration/Storage
1. The drug should be taken with food to ensure maximal absorption.
2. Daily doses greater than 200 mg should be given in two divided doses.
3. Treatment should be continued for a minimum of 3 months and until symptoms and lab tests indicate the active fungal infection has subsided. Recurrence of active infection may occur if there is an inadequate period of treatment.

Assessment
1. Document indications for therapy, onset and duration of symptoms, and other agents prescribed, noting compliance and outcome. Drug is extremely expensive and should not generally be considered first-line therapy with typical fungal infections.
2. List drugs currently prescribed to prevent any unfavorable interactions.
3. Obtain baseline CBC, electrolytes, fungal cultures/scrapings, and liver and renal function studies.
4. Drug is not intended for pregnant or nursing mothers.

Interventions
1. Monitor hepatic enzyme test values in clients with preexisting abnormal liver function.
2. The response rate of histoplasmosis in HIV-infected clients is similar to non-HIV-infected clients, although the clinical course of histoplasmosis in HIV-infected clients is more severe and usually requires maintenance therapy to prevent relapse.
3. Absorption may be decreased in HIV-infected clients with hypochlorhydria.

Evaluate: Eradication of infecting organisms and reports of symptomatic relief

K

Kanamycin sulfate
(kan-ah-**MY**-sin)
Pregnancy Category: D
Kantrex, Klebcil **(Rx)**
Classification: Aminoglycoside antibiotic and antitubercular agent (tertiary)

See also *Anti-Infectives* and *Aminoglycosides*.

Action/Kinetics: The activity of kanamycin resembles that of neomycin and streptomycin. **Peak therapeutic serum levels: IM,** 15–40 mcg/mL. **t½:** 2–3 hr. Toxic serum levels: >35 mcg/mL (peak) and >10 mcg/mL (trough).

Uses: Parenteral: As initial therapy for infections due to *Escherichia coli, Proteus, Enterobacter aerogenes, Klebsiella pneumoniae, Serratia marcescens,* and *Acinetobacter.* May be combined with a penicillin or cephalosporin before knowing results of susceptibility tests. *Investigational:* As part of a multiple-drug regimen for *Mycobacterium avium* complex in AIDS clients.

PO: As an adjunct to mechanical cleansing of large bowel for suppression of intestinal bacteria; hepatic coma.

Special Concerns: Use with caution in premature infants and neonates.

Additional Side Effects: Sprue-like syndrome with steatorrhea, malabsorption, and electrolyte imbalance.

Additional Drug Interactions: Procainamide ↑ muscle relaxation.

Dosage ⎯⎯⎯⎯⎯⎯

• **Capsules**

Intestinal bacteria suppression.
1 g every hour for 4 hr; **then,** 1 g q 6 hr for 36–72 hr.
Hepatic coma.
8–12 g/day in divided doses.

• **IM, IV**
Adults and children: 15 mg/kg/day in two to three equal doses. Maximum daily dose should not exceed 1.5 g regardless of route of administration.

For calculating dosage interval (in hr) in clients with impaired renal function, multiply serum creatinine (mg/100 mL) by 9.

• **IM**
Tuberculosis.
Adults: 15 mg/kg/day. Not recommended for use in children.

• **Intraperitoneal**
500 mg diluted in 20 mL sterile distilled water.

• **Inhalation**
250 mg in saline—nebulize b.i.d.–q.i.d.
Irrigation of abscess cavities, pleural space, ventricular cavities.
0.25% solution.

RESPIRATORY CARE CONSIDERATIONS

See also *General Respiratory Care Considerations for All Anti-Infectives* and *Aminoglycosides.*

Assessment
1. Document indications for therapy, and onset, duration, and characteristics of symptoms.
2. Anticipate reduced dosage with renal dysfunction

Evaluate
• Negative followup culture reports
• Desired bowel cleansing

L

Labetalol hydrochloride
(lah-**BET**-ah-lohl)
Pregnancy Category: C
Normodyne, Trandate **(Rx)**
Classification: Alpha- and beta-adrenergic blocking agent

See also *Beta-Adrenergic Blocking Agents* and *Antihypertensive Agents.*
Action/Kinetics: Labetalol decreases BP by blocking both alpha- and beta-adrenergic receptors. Significant reflex tachycardia and bradycardia do not occur although AV conduction may be prolonged. **Onset: PO,** 2–4 hr; **IV,** 5 min. **Peak plasma levels, PO:** 1–2 hr. **Duration: PO,** 8–12 hr. **t½: PO,** 6–8 hr; **IV,** 5.5 hr. Significant first-pass effect; metabolized in liver. Food increases bioavailability of the drug.
Uses: PO: Alone or in combination with other drugs for hypertension. **IV:** Hypertensive emergencies. *Investigational:* Pheochromocytoma, clonidine withdrawal hypertension.
Contraindications: Cardiogenic shock, cardiac failure, bronchial asthma, bradycardia, greater than first-degree heart block.
Special Concerns: Use with caution during lactation, in impaired renal and hepatic function, and diabetes (may prevent premonitory signs of acute hypoglycemia). Safety and efficacy in children have not been established.
Side Effects: *CV:* Postural hypotension, edema, flushing, ***ventricular arrhythmias, intensification of AV block.*** *GI:* N&V, diarrhea, altered taste, dyspepsia. *CNS:* Headache, drowsiness, fatigue, sleepiness, dizziness, vertigo, paresthesias, numbness. *GU:* Impotence, urinary bladder retention, difficulty in urination, failure to ejaculate, priapism, Peyronie's disease. *Dermatologic:* Rashes, facial erythema, alopecia, urticaria, pruritus, psoriasis-like syn-

drome, bullous lichen planus. *Respiratory:* **Bronchospasm,** dyspnea, wheezing. *Musculoskeletal:* Muscle cramps, asthenia, toxic myopathy. *Other:* SLE, jaundice, cholestasis, difficulties with vision, dry eyes, nasal stuffiness, tingling of skin or scalp, sweating, fever. Possible changes in laboratory values include increased serum transaminase, positive antinuclear factor, antimitochondrial antibodies, and increases in blood urea and creatine.

OD **Overdose Management:**
Symptoms: Excessive hypotension and bradycardia. *Treatment:* Induce vomiting or perform gastric lavage. Clients should be placed in a supine position with legs elevated. If required, the following treatment can be used:
• Epinephrine or a beta-2 agonist (aerosol) to treat bronchospasm.
• Atropine or epinephrine to treat bradycardia.
• Digitalis glycoside and a diuretic for cardiac failure; dopamine or dobutamine may also be used.
• Diazepam to treat seizures.
• Norepinephrine (or another vasopressor) to treat hypotension.
• Administration of glucagon (5–10 mg rapidly over 30 sec), followed by continuous infusion of 5 mg/hr, may be effective in treating severe hypotension and bradycardia.
Drug Interactions
Beta-adrenergic bronchodilators / Labetalol ↓ bronchodilator effect of these drugs
Cimetidine / ↑ Bioavailability of oral labetalol
Glutethimide / ↓ Effects of labetalol due to ↑ breakdown by liver
Halothane / ↑ Risk of severe myocardial depression → hypotension
Nitroglycerin / Additive hypotension
Tricyclic antidepressants / ↑ Risk of tremors

Laboratory Test Interferences: False + increase in urinary catecholamines.

Dosage

- **Tablets**

Hypertension.
Initial: 100 mg b.i.d. alone or with a diuretic; **maintenance:** 200–400 mg b.i.d. up to 1,200–2,400 mg/day for severe cases.

- **IV**

Hypertension.
Individualize. Initial: 20 mg slowly over 2 min; **then,** 40–80 mg q 10 min until desired effect occurs or a total of 300 mg has been given.

- **IV Infusion**

Hypertension.
Initial: 2 mg/min; **then,** adjust rate according to response. **Usual dose range:** 50–300 mg.

Transfer from IV to PO therapy.
Initial: 200 mg; **then,** 200–400 mg 6–12 hr later, depending on response. Thereafter, dosage based on response.

RESPIRATORY CARE CONSIDERATIONS

See also *Respiratory Care Considerations* for *Beta-Adrenergic Blocking Agents* and *Antihypertensive Agents.*

Administration/Storage

1. When transferring to oral labetalol from other antihypertensive therapy, slowly reduce dosage of current therapy.
2. To transfer from IV to PO therapy in hospitalized clients, begin when supine BP begins to increase.
3. Labetalol is not compatible with 5% sodium bicarbonate injection.
4. The full antihypertensive effect of labetalol is usually seen within the first 1–3 hr after the initial dose or dose increment.
5. May give IV undiluted (20 mg over 2 min) or reconstituted with dextrose or saline solutions (infuse at a rate of 2 mg/min). When given by IV infusion, labetalol should be administered using an infusion pump, a micro-drip regulator, or similar type device that allows precise control of flow rate.

Interventions

1. The effect of labetalol tablets on standing BP should be assessed before the client is discharged from the hospital. Perform measurements with the client standing at several different times during the day to determine full effects of the drug.
2. To reduce the chance of orthostatic hypotension, clients should remain supine for 3 hr after receiving parenteral labetalol.

Evaluate: ↓ BP and control of hypertension

Levarterenol bitartrate (Norepinephrine bitartrate)
(lee-var-**TER**-ih-nohl)
Levophed **(Rx)**
Classification: Adrenergic agent, direct-acting

See also *Sympathomimetic Drugs.*
Action/Kinetics: Levarterenol produces vasoconstriction (increase in BP) by stimulating alpha-adrenergic receptors. Also causes a moderate increase in contraction of heart by stimulating beta-1 receptors. Minimal hyperglycemic effect. **Onset:** immediate; **duration:** 1–2 min. Metabolized in liver and other tissues by the enzymes MAO and catechol-O-methyltransferase; however, the pharmacologic activity is terminated by uptake and metabolism in sympathetic nerve endings. Metabolites excreted in urine.

Uses: Hypotensive states caused by trauma, septicemia, blood transfusions, drug reactions, spinal anesthesia, poliomyelitis, central vasomotor depression, and MIs. Adjunct to treatment of cardiac arrest and profound hypotension.

Additional Contraindications: Hypotension due to blood volume deficiency (except in emergencies), mesenteric or peripheral vascular thrombosis, in halothane or cyclopropane anesthesia (due to possibilities of fatal arrhythmias). Pregnancy (may cause fetal anoxia or hypoxia).

Special Concerns: Use with caution in clients taking MAO inhibitors or tricyclic antidepressants.
Additional Side Effects: Drug may cause bradycardia that can be abolished by atropine.

Dosage ————————
• **IV Infusion Only**
Effect on BP determines dosage, initial: 8–12 mcg/min or 2–3 mL of a 4-mcg/mL solution/min; **maintenance,** 2–4 mcg/min with the dose determined by client response.

RESPIRATORY CARE CONSIDERATIONS

See also *Respiratory Care Considerations* for *Sympathomimetic Drugs.*
Administration/Storage
1. Discard solutions that are brown or that have a precipitate.
2. Do not administer through the same tube as blood products.
3. The infusion should be continued until BP is maintained without therapy. Abrupt withdrawal of levarterenol should be avoided.
4. Levarterenol should be diluted in either D5W or 5% dextrose in saline.
5. For IV administration, a large vein should be used, preferably the antecubital or subclavian. Veins with poor circulation should be avoided.
6. Administer IV solutions with an electronic infusion device. Monitor the rate of flow constantly.
7. Have phentolamine available for use at the site of extravasation to dilate local blood vessels and to minimize local necrosis.
Assessment
1. Document indications for therapy, onset of symptoms, and causative factors.
2. Determine that client is adequately hydrated.
Interventions
1. During administration of levarterenol, the client should be in a closely monitored environment.
2. Monitor BP frequently. An arterial line or *Dinemapp* for continuous BP determinations should be used. ECG

tracings, CVP, and PA wedge pressure readings are useful.
3. Monitor the pulse frequently, noting any signs of bradycardia. Have atropine readily available.
4. Monitor I&O. Report if urine output is less than 30 cc/hr.
5. Observe infusion site frequently for evidence of extravasation because ischemia and sloughing may occur. Check the area for blanching along the course of the vein. This could indicate permeability of the vein wall, which could allow leakage to occur. As a result, the IV site would need to be changed and phentolamine administered to the site of the extravasation.
6. The drug should be gradually withdrawn. Avoid an abrupt withdrawal. Clients may experience an initial rebound drop in BP.
7. Extra fluids parenterally may diminish rebound hypotension and help stabilize BP during withdrawal of the drug.
Evaluate
• ↑ BP
• Evidence of improved tissue perfusion
• Adequate urinary output (>30 mL/hr)

Levofloxacin
(lee-voh-**FLOX**-a-sin)
Pregnancy Category:
Levaquin **(Rx)**
Classification: Fluoroquinolone antibiotic

See also Fluoroquinolones.
Uses: Acute maxillary sinusitis due to *Streptococcus pneumoniae, Haemophilus influenzae,* or *Moraxella catarrhalis.* Acute bacterial exacerbation of chronic bronchitis due to *Staphylococcus aureus, S. pneumoniae, H. influenzae, Haemophilus parainfluenzae,* or *M. catarrhalis.* Community acquired pneumonia due to *S. aureus, S. pneumoniae, H. influenzae, H. parainfluenzae, Klebsiella pneumoniae, M. catarrhalis, Chlamydia*

pneumoniae, Legionella pneumonophila, or *Mycoplasma pneumoniae.* Uncomplicated mild to moderate infections of the skin and skin structures, including abscesses, cellulitis, furuncles, impetigo, pyoderma, and wound infections due to *S. aureus* or *Streptococcus pyogenes.* Mild to moderate complicated urinary tract infections due to *Enterococcus faecalis, Enterobacter cloacae, Escherichia coli, Klebsiella pneumoniae, Proteus mirabilis,* or *Pseudomonas aeruginosa.* Acute mild to moderate pyelonephritis due to E. coli.

Special Concerns: The dose must be reduced in clients with impaired renal function (See Administration/Storage).

Dosage ───────────────
• **Injection, Tablets**
  Acute maxillary sinusitis.
500 mg once daily for 10–14 days.
  Acute bacterial exacerbation of chronic bronchitis.
500 mg once daily for 7 days.
  Community acquired pneumonia.
500 mg once daily for 7–14 days.
  Uncomplicated skin and skin structure infections.
500 mg once daily for 7–10 days.
  Complicated urinary tract infections.
250 mg once daily for 10 days.
  Acute pyelonephritis.
250 mg once daily for 10 days.

RESPIRATORY CARE CONSIDERATIONS

See also *Respiratory Care Considerations* for Fluoroquinolones, .

Administration/Storage

1. The dose must be reduced as indicated in clients with impaired renal function when used for acute maxillary sinusitis, acute bacterial exacerbation of chronic bronchitis, community acquired pneumonia, and uncomplicated skin and skin structure infections. If creatinine clearance is between 20 and 49 mL/min, the initial dose is 500 mg and subsequent doses are 250 mg q 24 hr. If creatinine clearance is between 10 and 19 mL/min, the initial dose is 500 mg and subsequent doses are 250 mg q 48 hr. If the client is on hemodialysis or chronic ambulatory peritoneal dialysis, the initial dose is 500 mg and subsequent doses are 250 mg q 48 hr.

2. Oral doses are given at least 2 hr before or 2 hr after antacids containing magnesium or aluminum, as well as sucralfate, iron products, and multivitamin preparations containing zinc.

3. The injectable form may be mixed with 0.9% sodium chloride injection, 5% dextrose injection, 5% dextrose and 0.9% sodium chloride injection, 5% dextrose in lactated Ringers, Plasma-Lyte 56/5% dextrose injection, 5% dextrose and 0.45% sodium chloride injection, 0.15% potassium chloride injection, or M/6 sodium lactate injection.

4. Diluted solutions for IV use are stable for 72 hr up to a concentration of 5 mg/mL when stored in IV containers at 25°C or less (77°F or less). Such solutions are stable for 14 days when stored under refrigeration at 5°C (41°F). Diluted solutions that are frozen in glass bottles or plastic IV containers are stable for 6 months when stored at –20°C (–4°F).

5. Frozen solutions should be thawed at room temperature or in a refrigerator. They should not be thawed in a microwave or by bath immersion. After initial thawing, these solutions should not be refrozen.

6. Levofloxacin tablets should be stored in a tight container at 15°C–30°C (59°F–85°F).

Assessment

1. Document indications for therapy and type, onset, location, and duration of symptoms.

2 Obtain baseline CBC, cultures, and renal function studies.

Evaluate

• Reports of symptomatic improvement
• Resolution of infective organism

Levomethadyl acetate hydrochloride
(lee-voh-**METH**-ah-dill)
ORLAAM **(Rx)**
Classification: Narcotic analgesic only for use in opiate dependence

See also *Narcotic Analgesics.*
Uses: Treatment of opiate dependence. *NOTE:* This drug can be dispensed only by treatment programs approved by the FDA, DEA, and the designated state authority. The drug can be dispensed only in the oral form and according to treatment requirements stated in federal regulations. The drug has no approved uses outside of the treatment of opiate dependence.
Special Concerns: Usual dose must not be given on consecutive days due to the risk of fatal overdosage.
Side Effects: See *Narcotic Analgesics.* Induction with levomethadyl that is too rapid for the level of tolerance of the client may result in overdosage, including symptoms of both *respiratory and CV depression.*

Dosage ────────────
• **Oral Solution**
Induction.
Initial: 20–40 mg administered at 48–72-hr intervals; **then,** dose may be increased in increments of 5–10 mg until steady state is reached (usually within 1–2 weeks). Clients dependent on methadone may require higher initial doses of levomethadyl; the suggested initial 3-times/week dose for such clients is 1.2–1.3 times the daily methadone maintenance dose being replaced. This initial dose should not exceed 120 mg with subsequent doses given at 48- or 72-hr intervals, depending on the response. If additional opioids are required, supplemental amounts of methadone should be given rather than giving levomethadyl on 2 consecutive days.
Maintenance.
Most clients are stabilized on doses of 60–90 mg 3 times/week although

the dose may range from 10 to 140 mg 3 times/week. The maximum *total* amount of levomethadyl recommended for any client is either 140, 140, 140 mg or 130, 130, 180 mg on a thrice-weekly schedule.
Reinduction after an unplanned lapse in dosing: following a lapse of one levomethadyl dose.
If the client comes to the clinic the day following a missed scheduled dose (e.g., misses Monday and arrives at clinic on Tuesday), the regular Monday dose is given, with the scheduled Wednesday dose given on Thursday and the Friday dose given on Saturday. The client's regular schedule can be resumed the following Monday. If the client misses one dose and comes to the clinic the day of the next scheduled dose (i.e., misses Monday, comes to clinic on Wednesday), the usual dose will be well tolerated in most cases although some clients will need a reduced dose.
Reintroduction after a lapse of more than one levomethadyl dose.
Restart the client at an initial dose of 50%–75% of the previous dose, followed by increases of 5–10 mg every dosing day (i.e., intervals of 48–72 hr) until the previous maintenance dose is reached.
Transfer from levomethadyl to methadone.
Transfer can be done directly, although the dose of methadone should be 80% of the levomethadyl dose being replaced. The first methadone dose should not be given sooner than 48 hr after the last levomethadyl dose. Increases or decreases of 5–10 mg may be made in the daily methadone dose to control symptoms of withdrawal or symptoms of excessive sedation.
Detoxification from levomethadyl.
Both gradual reduction (i.e., 5%–10% a week) and abrupt withdrawal have been used successfully.

L

RESPIRATORY CARE CONSIDERATIONS
Administration/Storage
1. The drug is usually given 3 times/week—either on Monday, Wednesday, and Friday or on Tuesday, Thursday, and Saturday. If withdrawal is a problem with this interval, the preceding dose may be increased.

2. If the degree of tolerance is not known, clients can be started on methadone to facilitate more rapid titration to an effective dose. They can then be converted to levomethadyl after a few weeks. The cross-over from methadone to levomethadyl should be accomplished in a single dose.

3. If clients on maintenance therapy complain of withdrawal symptoms (e.g., those on a Monday, Wednesday, and Friday schedule) on Sunday, the Friday dose may be increased in 5- to 10-mg increments up to 40% over the Monday/Wednesday dose up to a maximum of 140 mg.

4. Levomethadyl take-home doses are not permitted. If a situation arises where the client cannot come to the clinic for a regular dose of levomethadyl, that client may be switched to receive one or more doses of methadone. Methadone doses should be 80% of the client's Monday/Wednesday levomethadyl dose; the first dose of methadone should be taken no sooner than 48 hr after the last dose of levomethadyl. The number of take-home doses of methadone should be two less than the number of days expected absence and should not exceed the number of take-home doses allowed in the methadone regulations. Upon return to the clinic, the client should resume levomethadyl maintenance following the same dosage schedule prior to the temporary interruption. If more than 48 hr has elapsed since the last methadone dose, the client should be reintroduced on levomethadyl at a dose determined by the clinical evaluation.

Assessment
1. Document that client is opiate dependent, length of dependence, and specific drugs used.

2. Determine methadone usage as drug requirements may be higher.

3. Identify that client has been accepted/approved for drug through a federally approved treatment protocol.

4. In clients who have missed scheduled doses, follow administration guidelines carefully.

Evaluate: Freedom from drug (opiate) dependence

Lidocaine hydrochloride
(**LYE**-doh-kayn)
Pregnancy Category: B
IM: LidoPen Auto-Injector, **(Rx)**. Direct **IV or IV Admixtures:** Lidocaine HCl for Cardiac Arrhythmias, Xylocaine HCl IV for Cardiac Arrhythmias, Xylocard ✤ **(Rx)**. **IV Infusion:** Lidocaine HCl in 5% Dextrose **(Rx)**
Classification: Antiarrhythmic, class IB

See also *Antiarrhythmic Agents*.

Action/Kinetics: Lidocaine shortens the refractory period and suppresses the automaticity of ectopic foci without affecting conduction of impulses through cardiac tissue. The drug increases the electrical stimulation threshold of the ventricle during diastole. It does not affect BP, CO, or myocardial contractility. **IV: Onset,** 45–90 sec; **duration:** 10–20 min. **IM, Onset,** 5–15 min; **duration,** 60–90 min. **t½:** 1–2 hr. **Therapeutic serum levels:** 1.5–6 mcg/mL. **Time to steady-state plasma levels:** 3–4 hr (8–10 hr in clients with AMI). **Protein-binding:** 40%–80%. Ninety percent of lidocaine is rapidly metabolized in the liver to active metabolites. Since lidocaine has little effect on conduction at normal antiarrhythmic doses, it should be used in acute situations (instead of procainamide) in instances in which heart block might occur.

Uses: IV: Treatment of acute ventricular arrhythmias such as those following MIs or occurring during surgery. The drug is ineffective against atrial arrhythmias. **IM:** Certain emergency situations (e.g., ECG equipment not available; mobile coronary care unit, under advice of a physician).

Investigational: IV in children who develop ventricular couplets or frequent premature ventricular beats.

Contraindications: Hypersensitivity to amide-type local anesthetics, Stokes-Adams syndrome, Wolff-Parkinson-White syndrome, severe SA, AV, or intraventricular block (when no pacemaker is present).

Special Concerns: Use with caution during labor and delivery, during lactation, and in the presence of liver or severe kidney disease, CHF, marked hypoxia, digitalis toxicity with AV block, severe respiratory depression, or shock. In geriatric clients, the rate and dose for IV infusion should be decreased by one-half and slowly adjusted. Safety and efficacy have not been determined in children; the IM autoinjector product should not be used for children.

Side Effects: *Body as a whole:* Malignant hyperthermia characterized by tachycardia, tachypnea, labile BP, metabolic acidosis, temperature elevation. *CV: **Precipitation or aggravation of arrhythmias (following IV use),** hypotension, **bradycardia (with possible cardiac arrest), CV collapse.** CNS:* Dizziness, apprehension, euphoria, lightheadedness, nervousness, drowsiness, confusion, changes in mood, hallucinations, twitching, "doom anxiety," **convulsions,** unconsciousness. *Respiratory:* Difficulties in breathing or swallowing, **respiratory depression or arrest.** *Allergic:* Rash, cutaneous lesions, urticaria, edema, **anaphylaxis.** *Other:* Tinnitus, blurred or double vision, vomiting, numbness, sensation of heat or cold, twitching, tremors, soreness at IM injection site, fever, **venous thrombosis or phlebitis (extending from site of injection),** extravasation. During anesthesia, CV depression may be the first sign of lidocaine toxicity. During other usage, convulsions are the first sign of lidocaine toxicity.

OD   **Overdose   Management:**

Symptoms: Symptoms are dependent on plasma levels. If plasma levels range from 4 to 6 mcg/mL, mild CNS effects are observed. Levels of 6 to 8 mcg/mL may result in significant CNS and CV depression while levels greater than 8 mcg/mL cause hypotension, decreased CO, respiratory depression, obtundation, **seizures, and coma.** *Treatment:* Discontinue the drug and begin emergency resuscitative procedures. Seizures can be treated with diazepam, thiopental, or thiamylal. Succinylcholine, IV, may be used if the client is anesthetized. IV fluids, vasopressors, and CPR are used to correct circulatory depression.

Drug Interactions

Aminoglycosides / ↑ Neuromuscular blockade

Beta-adrenergic blockers / ↑ Lidocaine levels with possible toxicity

Cimetidine / ↓ Clearance of lidocaine → possible toxicity

Phenytoin / IV phenytoin → excessive cardiac depression

Procainamide / Additive cardiodepressant effects

Succinylcholine / ↑ Action of succinylcholine by ↓ plasma protein binding

Tocainide / ↑ Risk of side effects

Tubocurarine / ↑ Neuromuscular blockade

Laboratory Test Interferences: ↑ CPK following IM use.

Dosage ─────────────
• **IV Bolus**
   Antiarrhythmic.
Adults: 50–100 mg at rate of 25–50 mg/min. Bolus is used to establish rapid therapeutic plasma levels. Repeat if necessary after 5-min interval. Onset of action is 10 sec. **Maximum dose/hr:** 200–300 mg.
• **Infusion**
   Antiarrhythmic.
20–50 mcg/kg at a rate of 1–4 mg/min. No more than 200–300 mg/hr should be given. **Pediatric, loading dose:** 1 mg/kg IV or intratracheally q 5–10 min until desired ef-

fect reached (maximum total dose: 5 mg/kg).

- **IV Continuous Infusion**

Maintain therapeutic plasma levels following loading doses.

Adults: Give at a rate of 1–4 mg/min (20–50 mcg/kg/min). Dose should be reduced in clients with heart failure, with liver disease, or who are taking drugs that interact with lidocaine. **Pediatric:** 20–50 mcg/kg/min (usual is 30 mcg/kg/min).

- **IM**

Antiarrhythmic.

Adults: 4.5 mg/kg (approximately 300 mg for a 70-kg adult). Switch to IV lidocaine or oral antiarrhythmics as soon as possible although an additional IM dose may be given after 60–90 min.

RESPIRATORY CARE CONSIDERATIONS

See also *Respiratory Care Considerations* for *Antiarrhythmic Agents.*

Administration/Storage

1. *Do not add lidocaine to blood transfusion assembly.*

2. Lidocaine solutions that contain epinephrine should not be used to treat arrhythmias. Make certain that vial states, "For Cardiac Arrhythmias." Check prefilled syringes closely to ensure the appropriate dose has been obtained. (Lidocaine prefilled syringes come in both milligrams and grams).

3. Use D5W to prepare solution; this is stable for 24 hr.

4. IV infusions should be administered with an electronic infusion device.

5. IV bolus dosage should be reduced in clients over 70 years of age, in those with CHF or liver disease, and in clients taking cimetidine or propranolol (i.e., where metabolism of lidocaine is reduced).

Assessment

1. Document indications for therapy and onset of symptoms.

2. Note any client history of hypersensitivity to amide-type local anesthetics.

3. Note client age. Elderly clients

who have hepatic or renal disease or who weigh less than 45.5 kg will need to be watched especially closely for adverse side effects; adjust dosage as directed.

4. Document CNS status and pulmonary findings; obtain baseline liver and renal function studies, electrolytes, and ECG.

Interventions

1. Monitor VS frequently during IV therapy. Clients on antiarrhythmic drug therapy are particularly susceptible to hypotension and cardiac collapse.

2. Observe for myocardial depression, variations of rhythm, or aggravation of the arrhythmia and report as drug administration may need to be altered.

3. Note evidence of dizziness or visual disturbances, and report any CNS effects such as twitching and tremors. These symptoms may precede convulsions.

4. Assess for any respiratory depression, characterized by slow, shallow respirations.

5. Note any sudden changes in mental status and report immediately because the dose of drug may need to be decreased.

6. The administration of the drug should be titrated to the client's response and within established written guidelines.

Evaluate

- Restoration of stable cardiac rhythm with control of ventricular arrhythmias
- Therapeutic serum drug levels (1.5–6 mcg/mL)

Lincomycin hydrochloride

(link-oh-**MY**-sin)
Lincocin **(Rx)**
Classification: Anti-infective

See also *Anti-Infectives.*

Action/Kinetics: Lincomycin is isolated from *Streptomyces lincolnensis.* Its spectrum resembles that of the erythromycins and includes a variety of gram-positive organisms, in particular staphylococci, streptococci, and pneumococci, and some gram-negative organisms. Lincomycin suppresses protein synthesis by microorganisms by binding to ribosomes (50S subunit), which is essential for transmittal of genetic information. It is both bacteriostatic and bactericidal. Lincomycin is absorbed rapidly from the GI tract and is widely distributed. **Peak serum levels: PO,** 2.6 mcg/mL after 500 mg; **IM,** 9.5 mcg/mL after 600 mg; **IV,** 19 mcg/mL after 600 mg. **t½:** 4.4–6.4 hr. This drug should not be used for trivial infections.

Uses: Not a first-choice drug but useful for clients allergic to penicillin. Used for serious respiratory tract, skin, and soft tissue infections due to staphylococci, streptococci, or pneumococci. Septicemia. In conjunction with diphtheria antitoxin in the treatment of diphtheria.

Contraindications: Hypersensitivity to drugs. Use in infants up to 1 month of age.

Special Concerns: Safe use during pregnancy has not been established. Use with caution in clients with GI disease, liver or renal disease, or a history of allergy or asthma. Not for use in treating viral and minor bacterial infections.

Side Effects: *GI:* N&V, diarrhea, abdominal pain, tenesmus, flatulence, bloating, anorexia, weight loss, esophagitis. Nonspecific colitis, pseudomembranous colitis (may be severe). *Allergic:* Morbilliform rash (most common). Also, maculopapular rash, urticaria, pruritus, fever, hypotension. Rarely, polyarteritis, ***anaphylaxis,*** erythema multiforme. *Hematologic:* Leukopenia, neutropenia, eosinophilia, thrombocytopenia, ***agranulocytosis.*** *Miscellaneous:* Superinfection.

Following IV use: Thrombophlebitis, erythema, pain, swelling. IV lincomycin may cause hypotension, syncope, and ***cardiac arrest*** (rare). *Following IM use:* Pain, induration, sterile abscesses. *Following topical use:* Erythema, irritation,

dryness, peeling, itching, burning, oiliness. Also, sore throat, fatigue, urinary frequency, headache.

NOTE: The injection contains benzyl alcohol, which has been associated with a fatal gasping syndrome in infants.

Drug Interactions
Antiperistaltic antidiarrheals (opiates, Lomotil) / ↑ Diarrhea due to ↓ removal of toxins from colon
Erythromycin / Cross-interference → ↓ effect of both drugs
Kaolin (e.g., Kaopectate) / ↓ Effect due to ↓ absorption from GI tract
Neuromuscular blocking agents / ↑ Effect of blocking agents
Laboratory Test Interferences: ↓ Levels of AST, ALT, NPN, alkaline phosphatase, bilirubin, BSP retention, and ↓ platelet count.

Dosage ⸺
• **Capsules**
  Infections.
  Adults: 500 mg t.i.d.–q.i.d.; **children over 1 month of age:** 30–60 mg/kg/day in three to four divided doses, depending on severity of infection.
• **IM**
  Infections.
  Adults: 600 mg q 12–24 hr; **children over 1 month of age:** 10 mg/kg q 12–24 hr, depending on severity of infection.
• **IV**
  Infections.
  Adults: 0.6–1.0 g q 8–12 hr up to 8 g/day, depending on severity of infection; **children over 1 month of age:** 10–20 mg/kg/day, depending on severity of infection.
  NOTE: In impaired renal function, reduce dosage by 70%–75%.
• **Subconjunctival Injection**
  0.75 mg/0.25 mL.

RESPIRATORY CARE CONSIDERATIONS

See also *General Respiratory Care Considerations for All Anti-Infectives.*

Administration/Storage

1. Prepare drug for administration as directed on package insert.

2. Administer slowly IM to minimize pain.

3. For IV use, carefully follow concentration and recommended rate for administration to prevent severe cardiopulmonary reactions.

4. Injection contains benzyl alcohol.

Interventions

1. Be prepared to manage colitis, which can occur 2–9 days to several weeks after initiation of therapy, by providing fluids, electrolytes, protein supplements, systemic corticosteroids, and vancomycin.

2. Do not administer, and caution client against using, antiperistaltic agents if diarrhea occurs, because these agents can prolong or aggravate condition.

3. Do not use any acne or topical mercury preparations containing a peeling agent in an area affected by medication because severe irritation can occur.

4. Do not administer kaolin concomitantly because it will reduce absorption of lincomycin. If kaolin is required, administer 3 hr before antibiotic.

5. Observe for adverse drug interactions caused by concurrent administration of neuromuscular blocking agents. Be alert to hypotension, bronchospasms, cardiac disturbances, hyperthermia, and respiratory depression.

6. Assess for transient flushing and sensations of warmth and cardiac disturbances, which may accompany IV infusions. Monitor pulse rate before, during, and after infusion until rate is stable at levels normal for client.

7. CBC and liver function tests should be done periodically during long-term therapy.

Evaluate

- Negative lab culture reports
- Resolution of infection

Lisinopril

(lie-**SIN**-oh-prill)

Pregnancy Category: C

Prinivil, Zestril **(Rx)**

Classification: Antihypertensive, ACE inhibitor

See also *Angiotensin-Converting Enzyme Inhibitors.*

Action/Kinetics: Both supine and standing BPs are reduced, although the drug is less effective in blacks than in Caucasians. Although food does not alter the bioavailability of lisinopril, only 25% of a PO dose is absorbed. **Onset:** 1 hr. **Peak serum levels:** 7 hr. **Duration:** 24 hr. t½: 12 hr. 100% of the drug is excreted unchanged in the urine.

Uses: Alone or in combination with a diuretic (usually a thiazide) to treat hypertension (step I therapy). In combination with digitalis and a diuretic for treating CHF not responding to other therapy. Use within 24 hr of acute MI to improve survival in hemodynamically stable clients (clients should receive the standard treatment, including thrombolytics, aspirin, and beta blockers).

Special Concerns: Use with caution during lactation. Safety and efficacy have not been established in children. Geriatric clients may manifest higher blood levels. Dosage should be reduced in clients with impaired renal function.

Side Effects: *CNS:* Dizziness, headache, fatigue, vertigo, insomnia, depression, sleepiness, paresthesias, malaise, nervousness, confusion. *GI:* Diarrhea, N&V, dyspepsia, anorexia, constipation, dysgeusia, dry mouth, abdominal pain, flatulence. *Respiratory:* Cough, dyspnea, bronchitis, upper respiratory symptoms, nasal congestion, sinusitis, pharyngeal pain, **bronchospasm, asthma.** *CV:* Hypotension, orthostatic hypotension, angina, tachycardia, palpitations, rhythm disturbances, **stroke,** chest pain, orthostatic effects, peripheral edema, **MI, CVA.** *Musculoskeletal:* Asthenia, muscle cramps, joint pain, shoulder and back pain, myalgia, arthralgia, arthritis. *Hepatic:* Hepatitis, cholestatic jaundice, pancreatitis. *Dermatologic:* Rash, pruritus, flushing, increased sweating, urticaria. *GU:* Impotence, oliguria, progressive azotemia, acute renal failure, UTI. *Miscellaneous: Angioedema (may be fatal if laryngeal edema occurs),* hyperkalemia, neutropenia, anemia, **bone marrow depression,** decreased libido, chest pain, fever, blurred vision, syncope, vasculitis of the legs, gout.

OD **Overdose Management:** *Symptoms:* Hypotension. *Treatment:* Supportive. To correct hypotension, IV normal saline is treatment of choice. Lisinopril may be removed by hemodialysis.

Drug Interactions
Diuretics / Excess ↓ BP
Indomethacin / Possible ↓ effect of lisinopril
Potassium-sparing diuretics / Significant ↑ serum potassium
Laboratory Test Interferences: ↑ Serum potassium, BUN, serum creatinine. ↓ H&H.

Dosage
• **Tablets**
Essential hypertension, used alone.
10 mg once daily. Adjust dosage depending on response (range: 20–40 mg/day given as a single dose). Doses greater than 80 mg/day do not give a greater effect.
Essential hypertension in combination with a diuretic.
Initial: 5 mg. The BP-lowering effects of the combination are additive. Dosage should be reduced in clients with renal impairment.
CHF.
Initial: 5 mg once daily (2.5 mg/day in clients with hyponatremia) in combination with diuretics and digitalis. **Dosage range:** 5–20 mg/day as a single dose.
Acute MI.
First dose: 5 mg; **then,** 5 mg after 24 hr, 10 mg after 48 hr, and then 10 mg daily. Continue dosing for 6 weeks. In clients with a systolic pressure less than 120 mm Hg when treatment is started or within 3 days after the infarct should be given 2.5 mg. If hypo-

tension occurs (systolic BP less than 100 mm Hg), the dose may be temporarily reduced to 2.5 mg. If prolonged hypotension occurs, the drug should be withdrawn.

RESPIRATORY CARE CONSIDERATIONS

See also *Respiratory Care Considerations* for *Angiotensin-Converting Enzyme Inhibitors* and *Antihypertensive Agents.*
Administration/Storage
1. When considering use of lisinopril in a client taking diuretics, discontinue the diuretic, if possible, 2–3 days before beginning lisinopril therapy. If the diuretic cannot be discontinued, the initial dose of lisinopril should be 5 mg and the client should be closely observed for at least 2 hr.
2. In some clients, maximum antihypertensive effects may not be observed for 2–4 weeks.
3. When starting treatment for CHF, give under medical supervision, especially in clients with a systolic blood pressure less than 100 mm Hg.
4. With clients whose BP is controlled with lisinopril, 20 mg plus hydrochlorothiazide, 25 mg given separately should be given a trial of Prinzide 12.5 mg or Zestoretic 20–12.5 mg before Prinzide 25 mg or Zestoretic 20–25 mg is used.
5. The maximum recommended daily dose of lisinopril is 80 mg in a single daily dose. However, clients usually do not require hydrochlorothiazide in doses exceeding 50 mg/day, especially if combined with other antihypertensives.
6. Use of potassium supplements, potassium-sparing diuretics, or potassium salt substitutes with Prinzide or Zestoretic may lead to increases in serum potassium.
7. Prinzide or Zestoretic is recommended for those clients with a creatinine clearance greater than 30 mL/min.
8. Anticipate reduced dosage if the client has renal insufficiency—initial

dose of 10 mg/day if creatinine clearance is greater than 30 mL/min, 5 mg/day if creatinine clearance is between 10 and 30 mL/min, and 2.5 mg/day in dialysis clients (i.e., less than 10 mL/min).

Evaluate
- ↓ BP to within desired range
- Resolution of S&S of CHF
- Improved survival with acute MI

Lomefloxacin hydrochloride

(**loh**-meh-**FLOX**-ah-sin)
Pregnancy Category:C
Maxaquin **(Rx)**
Classification: Antibacterial, fluoroquinolone derivative

See also *Fluoroquinolones.*
Action/Kinetics: Mean peak plasma levels: 4.2 mcg/mL after a 400-mg dose. The rate and extent of absorption is decreased if taken with food. **t½:** 8 hr. The drug is metabolized in the liver with 65% excreted unchanged through the urine and 10% excreted unchanged in the feces.
Uses: Acute bacterial exacerbation of chronic bronchitis caused by *Haemophilus influenzae* or *Morazella catarrhalis.* Uncomplicated UTIs due to *Escherichia coli, Klebsiella pneumoniae, Proteus mirabilis,* or *Staphylococcus saprophyticus.* Complicated UTIs due to *E. coli, K. pneumoniae, P. mirabilis, Pseudomonas aeruginosa, Citrobacter diversus,* or *Enterobacter cloacae.* Preoperatively to decrease the incidence of UTIs 3–5 days after surgery in clients undergoing transurethral procedures. *NOTE:* Not to be used for the empiric treatment of acute bacterial exacerbation of chronic bronchitis if the probable cause is Streptococcus pneumoniae.
Contraindications: Use in minor urologic procedures for which prophylaxis is not indicated (e.g., simply cystoscopy, retrograde pyelography). Use for the empiric treatment of acute bacterial exacerbation of chronic bronchitis due to *S. pneumoniae.* Lactation.

Special Concerns: Plasma clearance is reduced in the elderly. Safety and efficacy have not been determined in children less than 18 years of age. Serious hypersensitivity reactions that are occasionally fatal have occurred, even with the first dose. No dosage adjustment is needed for elderly clients with normal renal function. Lomefloxacin is not efficiently removed from the body by hemodialysis or peritoneal dialysis.
Additional Side Effects: *CNS:* Confusion, tremor, vertigo, nervousness, anxiety, hyperkinesia, anorexia, agitation, increased appetite, depersonalization, paranoia, **coma.** *GI:* GI inflammation or bleeding, dysphagia, tongue discoloration, bad taste in mouth. *GU:* Dysuria, hematuria, micturition disorder, anuria, strangury, leukorrhea, intermenstrual bleeding perineal pain, vaginal moniliasis, orchitis, epididymitis, proteinuria, albuminuria. *Hypersensitivity Reactions:* Urticaria, itching, pharyngeal or facial edema, *CV collapse,* tingling, loss of consciousness, dyspnea. *CV:* Hypotension, tachycardia, bradycardia, extrasystoles, cyanosis, *arrhythmia, cardiac failure,* angina pectoris, *MI, pulmonary embolism, cardiomyopathy,* phlebitis, cerebrovascular disorder. *Respiratory:* Dyspnea, respiratory infection, epistaxis, *bronchospasm,* cough, increased sputum, respiratory disorder, stridor. *Hematologic:* Eosinophilia, leukopenia, increase or decrease in platelets, increase in ESR, lymphocytopenia, decreased hemoglobin, anemia, bleeding, increased PT, increase in monocytes. *Dermatologic:* Urticaria, eczema, skin exfoliation, skin disorder. *Ophthalmologic:* Conjunctivitis, eye pain. *Otic:* Earache, tinnitus. *Musculoskeletal:* Back or chest pain, asthenia, leg cramps, arthralgia, myalgia. *Miscellaneous:* Increase or decrease in blood glucose, flushing, increased sweating, facial edema, influenza-like symptoms, decreased heat tolerance, purpura, lymphadenopathy, increased fibrinolysis, thirst, gout, hypoglycemia, phototoxicity.

Laboratory Test Interferences: ↑ ALT, AST, alkaline phosphatase, bilirubin, BUN, gamma-glutamyltransferase. ↑ or ↓ Potassium. Abnormalities of urine specific gravity or serum electrolytes.

Dosage —————————————
• **Tablets**

Acute bacterial exacerbation of chronic bronchitis. Cystitis. Complicated UTIs.

Adults: 400 mg once daily for 10 days.

Prophylaxis of infection before surgery for transurethral procedures. Single 400-mg dose 2–6 hr before surgery.

Uncomplicated gonococcal infections.

400 mg as a single dose (as an alternative to ciprofloxacin or ofloxacin).

RESPIRATORY CARE CONSIDERATIONS

See also *General Respiratory Care Considerations for All Anti-Infectives* and *Fluoroquinolones.*

Administration/Storage

1. Can be taken without regard for meals.

2. Dosage modification is required for clients with creatinine clearance less than 40 mL/min/1.73 m² and more than 10 mL/min/1.73 m². Following an initial loading dose of 40 mg, daily maintenance doses of 200 mg should be given for the duration of treatment. Lomefloxacin levels should be performed to determine any necessary alteration in the next dosing interval. This same regimen should be followed for clients on hemodialysis.

Assessment

1. Document indications for therapy and type and onset of symptoms.

2. Obtain baseline cultures and renal function studies. Modify dosage in clients with renal dysfunction.

Evaluate

• UTI prophylaxis during transurethral procedures

• Reports of symptomatic relief (↓ frequency and burning) with UTIs
• Improved breathing patterns with lower respiratory tract infections
• Negative follow-up culture reports

Loracarbef
(**lor**-ah-**KAR**-bef)
Pregnancy Category: B
Lorabid **(Rx)**
Classification: Beta-lactam antibiotic

See also *Anti-Infectives.*

Action/Kinetics: Loracarbef is related chemically to the cephalosporin antibiotics. The drug acts by inhibiting cell wall synthesis; it is stable in the presence of certain bacterial beta-lactamases. **Average peak plasma levels:** 8 mcg/mL following a single 200-mg dose in a fasting subject after 90 min and 14 mcg/mL following a single 400-mg dose in a fasting subject after 90 min. Following doses of 7.5 mg/kg and 15 mg/kg of the oral suspension to children, average peak plasma levels were 13 and 19 mcg/mL, respectively, within 40–60 min. **Elimination t½:** 1 hr (increased to 5.6 hr in clients with a creatinine clearance from 10 to 50 mL/min/1.73 m² and to 32 hr in clients with a creatinine clearance of less than 10 mL/min/1.73 m²). The drug is not metabolized in humans.

Uses: Secondary bacterial infections of acute bronchitis caused by *Streptococcus pneumoniae, Haemophilus influenzae,* or *Morazella catarrhalis* (including beta-lactamase-producing strains of both organisms). Acute bacterial exacerbations of chronic bronchitis caused by *S. pneumoniae, H. influenzae,* or *M. catarrhalis* (including beta-lactamase-producing strains of both organisms). Pneumonia caused by *S. pneumoniae* or *H. influenzae* (only non-beta-lactamase-producing strains). Otitis media caused by *S. pneumoniae, Streptococcus pyogenes, H. influenzae,* or *M. catarrhalis* (including beta-lactamase-producing strains of both organisms). Acute maxillary sinusitis caused by *S. pneumoniae, H. influenzae* (only non-beta-lactamase-producing strains), or *M. catarrhalis* (including beta-lactamase-producing strains). Pharyngitis and tonsillitis caused by *S. pyogenes.* Uncomplicated skin and skin structure infections caused by *Staphylococcus aureus* (including penicillinase-producing strains) or *S. pyogenes.* Uncomplicated UTIs caused by *Escherichia coli* or *Staphylococcus saprophyticus.* Uncomplicated pyelonephritis caused by E. coli.

Contraindications: Hypersensitivity to loracarbef or cephalosporin-class antibiotics.

Special Concerns: Use during labor and delivery only if clearly needed. Pseudomembranous colitis is possible with most antibacterial agents. Use with caution and at reduced dosage in clients with impaired renal function, in those with a history of colitis, in clients receiving concurrent treatment with potent diuretics, during lactation, and in clients with known penicillin allergies. Safety and efficacy in children less than 6 months of age have not been determined.

Side Effects: The incidence of certain side effects is different in the pediatric population compared with the adult population. *GI:* Diarrhea, N&V, abdominal pain, anorexia, pseudomembranous colitis. *Hypersensitivity:* Skin rashes, urticaria, pruritus, erythema multiforme. *CNS:* Headache, somnolence, nervousness, insomnia, dizziness. *Hematologic:* Transient thrombocytopenia, leukopenia, eosinophilia. *Miscellaneous:* Vasodilation, vaginitis, vaginal moniliasis, rhinitis.

OD **Overdose Management:** *Symptoms:* N&V, epigastric distress, diarrhea. *Treatment:* Hemodialysis may be effective in increasing the elimination of loracarbef from plasma from clients with chronic renal failure.

Drug Interactions
Diuretics, potent / ↑ Risk of renal dysfunction

Probenecid / ↓ Renal excretion resulting in ↑ plasma levels of loracarbef

Dosage
• **Capsules, Oral Suspension**
Secondary bacterial infection of acute bronchitis.
Adults 13 years of age and older: 200–400 mg q 12 hr for 7 days.
Acute bacterial exacerbation of chronic bronchitis.
Adults 13 years of age and older: 400 mg q 12 hr for 7 days.
Pneumonia.
Adults 13 years of age and older: 400 q 12 hr for 14 days.
Pharyngitis, tonsillitis.
Adults 13 years of age and older: 200 mg q 12 hr for 10 days. **Infants and children, 6 months–12 years:** 15 mg/kg/day in divided doses q 12 hr for 10 days.
Sinusitis.
Adults 13 years of age and older: 400 mg q 12 hr for 10 days.
Acute otitis media.
Infants and children, 6 months–12 years: 30 mg/kg/day in divided doses q 12 hr for 10 days. The suspension should be used as it is more rapidly absorbed than the capsules, resulting in higher peak plasma levels when given at the same dose.
Skin and skin structure infections (impetigo).
Infants and children, 6 months–12 years: 15 mg/kg/day in divided doses q 12 hr for 7 days.

RESPIRATORY CARE CONSIDERATIONS

See also *General Respiratory Care Considerations for All Anti-Infectives.*

Administration/Storage

1. Should be taken at least 1 hr before or at least 2 hr after meals.
2. The manufacturer provides a chart to assist with establishing the dosage regimen for pediatric clients.
3. Clients with creatinine clearance levels of 10–49 mL/min may be given one-half the recommended dose at the usual dosage interval. Clients with creatinine clearance less than

10 mL/min may be treated with the recommended dose given every 3–5 days. Clients on hemodialysis should receive another dose following dialysis.

4. The oral suspension is reconstituted by adding 30 mL water to the 50-mL bottle or 60 mL water to the 100-mL bottle. After mixing, the suspension may be kept at room temperature for 14 days without significant loss of potency. The bottle should be kept tightly closed. After 14 days any unused portion should be discarded.

Assessment

1. Note any history or evidence of sensitivity to cephalosporins and penicillin derivatives.

2. Obtain baseline cultures and renal function studies.

3. List drugs currently prescribed to ensure that none interact unfavorably.

Evaluate

• Negative lab C&S reports with resolution of infection

• Relief of ear pain and/or sore throat

• Improved breathing patterns

• Evidence of wound healing

Loratidine

(loh-**RAH**-tih-deen)
Pregnancy Category: B
Claritin **(Rx)**
Classification: Antihistamine

See also Antihistamines

Action/Kinetics: Loratidine is metabolized in the liver to an active metabolite (descarboethoxyloratidine). The drug has low to no sedative and anticholinergic effects. It has not been shown to alter cardiac repolarization and has not been linked to development of torsades de pointes as seen with astemizole and terfenadine. **Onset:** 1–3 hr. **Maximum effect:** 8–12 hr. **t½, loratidine:** 8.4 hr; **t½, descarboethoxyloratidine:** 28 hr. **Duration:** 24 hr. Excreted through both the urine and feces.

Uses: Relief of nasal and nonnasal symptoms of seasonal allergic rhinitis, including runny nose, itchy and watery eyes, itchy palate, and sneezing. Treatment of chronic idiopathic urticaria.

Special Concerns: Use with caution, if at all, during lactation. Clients with liver impairment should be given a lower initial dose. Safety and efficacy have not been determined in children less than 2 years of age.

Side Effects: Most commonly, headache, somnolence, fatigue, and dry mouth. *GI:* Altered salivation, gastritis, dyspepsia, stomatitis, tooth ache, thirst, altered taste, flatulence. *CNS:* Hypoesthesia, hyperkinesia, migraine, anxiety, depression, agitation, paroniria, amnesia, impaired concentration. *Ophthalmologic:* Altered lacrimation, conjunctivitis, blurred vision, eye pain, blepharospasm. *Respiratory:* Upper respiratory infection, epistaxis, pharyngitis, dyspnea, coughing, rhinitis, sinusitis, sneezing, bronchitis, ***bronchospasm,*** hemoptysis, laryngitis. *Body as a whole:* Asthenia, increased sweating, flushing, malaise, rigors, fever, dry skin, aggravated allergy, pruritus, purpura. *Musculoskeletal:* Back/chest pain, leg cramps, arthralgia, myalgia. *GU:* Breast pain, menorrhagia, dysmenorrhea, vaginitis. *Miscellaneous:* Earache, dysphonia, dry hair, urinary discoloration.

Dosage

• **Syrup, Tablets**

  Allergic rhinitis, chronic idiopathic urticaria.

  Adults and children 6 years and older: 10 mg once daily on an empty stomach. **Children, 2 to 6 years (less than 30 kg):** 5 mg daily. *In clients with impaired liver function (GFR less than 30 mL/min):* 10 mg every other day.

RESPIRATORY CARE CONSIDERATIONS

See also *Respiratory Care Considerations* for *Antihistamines.*

Assessment

1. Document indications for therapy and type, onset, and duration of symptoms. List other agents trialed and the outcome.

2. Note any evidence or history of liver dysfunction. Obtain baseline liver function studies and anticipate reduced dosage with dysfunction.

3. Document pulmonary findings; assess throat and turbinates.

4. Perform a drug profile. Cautiously coadminister with drugs that inhibit hepatic metabolism (i.e., macrolide antibiotics, cimetidine, ranitidine, ketoconazole, or theophylline).

Interventions: The elderly and clients with hepatic and renal impairment warrant close observation for increasing somnolence.

Evaluate

• Subjective reports of relief of nasal congestion and seasonal allergic manifestations

• Control of eruption R/T antigenic offender

Losartan potassium

(loh-**SAR**-tan)
Pregnancy Category: C (first trimester), D (second and third trimesters)
Cozaar **(Rx)**
Classification: Antihypertensive

See also *Antihypertensive Agents*.

Action/Kinetics: Angiotensin II is a potent vasoconstrictor, is the primary vasoactive hormone of the renin-angiotensin system, and is involved in the pathophysiology of hypertension. Angiotensin II increases systemic vascular resistance, causes sodium and water retention, and leads to increased heart rate and vasoconstriction. Losartan competitively blocks the angiotensin AT_1 receptor located in vascular smooth muscle and the adrenal glands, which is involved in mediating the effects of angiotensin II. Thus, BP is reduced. The drug does not have significant effects on heart rate, has minimal orthostatic effects, and does not affect potassium levels significantly. Also, losartan does not have effects on the AT_2 receptor. Losartan undergoes significant first-pass metabolism in the liver, where it is converted to an active carboxylic acid metabolite that is responsible for most of the angiotensin receptor blockade. The drug is rapidly absorbed after PO administration, although food slows absorption. **Peak plasma levels of losartan and metabolite:** 1 hr and 3–4 hr, respectively. **t½, losartan:** 2 hr; **t½, metabolite:** 6–9 hr. The drug and metabolite are highly bound to plasma proteins. Maximum effects are usually seen within 1 week, although from 3 to 6 weeks may be required in some clients. The drug and metabolites are excreted through both the urine (35%) and feces (60%).

Uses: Treatment of hypertension, alone or in combination with other antihypertensive agents.

Contraindications: Lactation. Use after pregnancy is discouraged.

Special Concerns: When used alone, the effect to decease BP in blacks was less than in non-blacks. Dosage adjustments are not required in clients with renal impairment, unless they are volume depleted. In clients with severe CHF, there is a risk of oliguria and/or progressive azotemia with acute renal failure and/or death (which are rare). In those with unilateral or bilateral renal artery stenosis, there is a risk of increased serum creatinine or BUN. Lower doses are recommended in those with hepatic insufficiency. Safety and efficacy have not been determined in children less than 18 years of age.

Side Effects: *GI:* Diarrhea, dyspepsia, anorexia, constipation, dental pain, dry mouth, flatulence, gastritis, vomiting, taste perversion. *CV:* Angina pectoris, second-degree AV block, **CVA, MI, ventricular tachycardia, ventricular fibrillation,** hypotension, palpitation, sinus bradycardia, tachycardia, orthostatic effects. *CNS:* Dizziness, insomnia, anxiety, anxiety disorder, ataxia, confusion, depression, abnormal dreams, hypesthesia, decreased libido, impaired memory, migraine, nervousness, paresthesia, peripheral neuropathy, panic disorder, sleep disorder, somnolence, tremor, vertigo. *Respiratory:* Upper respiratory infection, cough, nasal congestion, sinus disorder, sinusitis, dyspnea, bronchitis, pharyngeal discomfort, epistaxis, rhinitis, respiratory congestion. *Musculoskeletal:* Muscle cramps, myalgia, joint swelling, musculoskeletal pain, stiffness, arthralgia, arthritis, fibromyalgia, muscle weakness; pain in the back, legs, arms, hips, knees, shoulders. *Dermatologic:* Alopecia, dermatitis, dry skin, ecchymosis, erythema, flushing, photosensitivity, pruritus, rash, sweating, urticaria. *GU:* Impotence, nocturia, urinary frequency, UTI. *Ophthalmologic:* Blurred vision, burning/stinging in the eye, conjunctivitis, decrease in visual acuity. *Miscellaneous:* Gout, anemia, tinnitus, facial edema, fever, syncope.

OD **Overdose Management:** *Symptoms:* Hypotension, tachycardia, bradycardia (due to vagal stimulation). *Treatment:* Supportive treatment. Hemodialysis is not indicated.

Drug Interactions: Administration of losartan and phenobarbital resulted in a decreased plasma level (20%) of losartan.

Laboratory Test Interferences: Minor ↑ BUN, serum creatinine. Occasional ↑ liver enzymes and/or serum bilirubin. Small ↓ hemoglobin, hematocrit.

Dosage ─────────────
• **Tablets**

Hypertension.
Adults: 50 mg once daily. In those with possible depletion of intravascular volume (e.g., clients treated with a diuretic), use 25 mg once daily. If the antihypertensive effect (measured at trough) is inadequate, a twice-a-day regimen, using the same dose, may be tried; or an increase in dose may give a more satisfactory result. If BP is not controlled by losartan alone, a diuretic (e.g., hydrochlorothiazide) may be added.

RESPIRATORY CARE CONSIDERATIONS

See also *Respiratory Care Considerations* for *Antihypertensive Agents.*
Administration/Storage
1. Losartan may be given with other antihypertensive drugs.
2. The drug may be taken with or without food.
Assessment
1. Document indications for therapy, onset and duration of disease, and previous agents used and the outcome.
2. Obtain baseline CBC and liver and renal function studies. Anticipate reduced starting dose in clients with volume depletion or hepatic impairment.
Interventions
1. Correct any volume depletion prior to using losartan in order to prevent sympathomimetic hypotension.
2. Observe closely for any S&S of fluid or electrolyte imbalance.
Evaluate: Desired level of BP control

Mannitol
(**MAN**-nih-tol)
Pregnancy Category: C
Osmitrol **(Rx)**
Classification: Diuretic, osmotic

Action/Kinetics: Mannitol increases

the osmolarity of the glomerular filtrate, which decreases the reabsorption of water while increasing excretion of sodium and chloride. It also increases the osmolarity of the plasma, which causes enhanced flow of water from tissues into the interstitial fluid and plasma. Thus, cerebral edema, increased ICP, and CSF volume and pressure are decreased. **Onset, IV:** 30–60 min for diuresis and within 15 min for reduction of cerebrospinal and intraocular pressures. **Peak:** 30–60 min. **Duration:** 6–8 hr diuresis and 4–8 hr for reduction of intraocular pressure. **t½:** 15–100 min. Over 90% excreted through the urine unchanged. A test dose is given in clients with impaired renal function or oliguria.

Uses: Diuretic to prevent or treat the oliguric phase of acute renal failure before irreversible renal failure occurs. Decrease ICP and cerebral edema by decreasing brain mass. Decrease elevated intraocular pressure when the pressure cannot be lowered by other means. To promote urinary excretion of toxic substances. As a urinary irrigant to prevent hemolysis and hemoglobin buildup during transurethral prostatic resection or other transurethral surgical procedures. *Investigational:* Prevent hemolysis during cardiopulmonary bypass surgery.

Contraindications: Anuria, pulmonary edema, severe dehydration, active intracranial bleeding except during craniotomy, progressive heart failure or pulmonary congestion after mannitol therapy, progressive renal damage following mannitol therapy.

Special Concerns: Use with caution during lactation. If blood is given simultaneously with mannitol, add at least 20 mEq of sodium chloride to each liter of mannitol solution to avoid pseudoagglutination. Sudden expansion of the extracellular volume that occurs after rapid IV mannitol may lead to fulminating CHF. Mannitol may obscure and intensify inadequate hydration or hypovolemia.

Side Effects: *Electrolyte:* Fluid and electrolyte imbalance, acidosis, loss of electrolytes, dehydration. *GI:* Nausea, vomiting, dry mouth, thirst, diarrhea. *CV:* Edema, hypotension or hypertension, increase in heart rate, angina-like chest pain, CHF, thrombophlebitis. *CNS:* Dizziness, head-

aches, blurred vision, **seizures.** *Miscellaneous:* Pulmonary congestion, marked diuresis, rhinitis, chills, fever, urticaria, pain in arms, skin necrosis.

OD **Overdose Management:** *Symptoms:* Increased electrolyte excretion, especially sodium, chloride, and potassium. Sodium depletion results in orthostatic tachycardia or hypotension and decreased CVP. Potassium loss can impair neuromuscular function and cause intestinal dilation and ileus. If urine flow is inadequate, pulmonary edema or water intoxication may occur. Other symptoms include hypotension, polyuria that rapidly becomes oliguria, stupor, **seizures,** hyperosmolality, and hyponatremia. *Treatment:* Discontinue the infusion immediately and begin supportive measures to correct fluid and electrolyte imbalances. Hemodialysis is effective.

Drug Interactions: May cause deafness when used in combination with kanamycin.

Laboratory Test Interferences: ↑ or ↓ Inorganic phosphorus. ↑ Ethylene glycol values because mannitol also is oxidized to an aldehyde during test.

Dosage ——————————
• **IV Infusion Only**
  Test dose (oliguria or reduced renal function).
Either 50 mL of a 25% solution, 75 mL of a 20% solution, or 100 mL of a 15% solution infused over 3–5 min. If urine flow is 30–50 mL/hr, therapeutic dose can be given. If urine flow does not increase, give a second test dose; if still no response, client must be reevaluated.
  Prevention of acute renal failure (oliguria).
Adults: 50–100 g, as a 5%–25% solution, given at a rate to maintain urine flow of at least 30–50 mL/hr.
  Treatment of oliguria.
Adults: 50–100 g of a 15%–25% solution.
  Reduction of intracranial pressure and brain mass.

Adults: 1.5–2 g/kg as a 15%–25% solution, infused over 30–60 min.

Reduction of intraocular pressure.
Adults: 1.5–2 g/kg as a 20% solution (7.5–10 mL/kg) or as a 15% solution (10–13 mL/kg) given over 30–60 min. When used preoperatively, the dose should be given 1–1.5 hr before surgery to maintain the maximum effect.

Antidote to remove toxic substances.
Adults: Dose depends on the fluid requirement and urinary output. IV fluids and electrolytes are given to replace losses. If a beneficial effect is not seen after 200 g mannitol, the infusion should be discontinued.

• **Irrigation Solution**
Urologic irrigation.
Adults: Use as a 2.5% irrigating solution for the bladder (this concentration minimizes the hemolytic effect of water alone).

RESPIRATORY CARE CONSIDERATIONS
Administration/Storage
1. If concentrated mannitol is used (15%, 20%, and 25%), a filter should be used.
2. If the concentration of mannitol is greater than 15%, it may crystallize. To redissolve, warm the bottle in a hot water bath or autoclave. Then cool to body temperature before administering to the client.
3. IV administration can reduce cerebrospinal and intraocular pressures within 15 min. Onset of diuresis occurs in about 1–3 hr.
4. Mannitol should not be added to other IV solutions nor should it be mixed with other medications.
5. If blood is to be administered at the same time, add 20 mEq of sodium chloride to each liter of mannitol to prevent pseudoagglutination.
Assessment
1. Document indications for therapy and type and onset of symptoms.
2. List other medications prescribed that can be affected by mannitol. Lithium, for example, can be excret-ed more rapidly than normal, thereby impairing the therapeutic effects of the drug.
3. Carefully assess and document neurologic findings.
4. When used to reduce ICP and brain mass, evaluate the circulatory and renal reserve, fluid and electrolyte balance, body weight, and total I&O before and after mannitol infusion.
5. Ensure that appropriate baseline lab data have been performed. Note any evidence of renal failure.
6. Determine that client is not dehydrated as drug may mask this clinical presentation.
Interventions
1. Monitor carefully and record VS and I&O.
2. If renal failure or oliguria is present, ensure that test dose is performed.
3. Observe the client for S&S of electrolyte imbalances and dehydration and replace as needed.
4. Monitor serum electrolytes and renal function throughout the drug therapy.
5. Observe for S&S of pulmonary edema manifested by dyspnea, cyanosis, rales, and/or frothy sputum. Slow the rate of infusion, and notify the provider immediately.
Evaluate
• Desired diuresis with ↓ edema
• ↓ ICP
• ↓ Intraocular pressures

Mecamylamine hydrochloride
(mek-ah-**MILL**-ah-meen)
Pregnancy Category: C
Inversine **(Rx)**
Classification: Antihypertensive

Action/Kinetics: The drug is less apt than other ganglionic blocking agents to induce tolerance. Withdraw or substitute mecamylamine slowly because sudden withdrawal or switching to other antihypertensive agents may result in severe hypertensive rebound. Since mecamylamine reduces peristalsis, it is a useful addition to a thiazide-guanethidine regimen in clients who experience persistent diarrhea with guanethidine. **Onset (gradual):** –2 hr. **Duration:** 6–12 hr. May take 2–3 days to achieve full therapeutic potential. Mecamylamine is excreted unchanged by the kidneys. The rate of excretion is influenced by urinary pH in that alkalinization of the urine decreases, and acidification increases, renal excretion.

Uses: Moderate to severe hypertension including uncomplicated malignant hypertension.

Contraindications: Mild, moderate, labile hypertension; coronary insufficiency, clients with recent MI, uremia, clients being treated with antibiotics and sulfonamides, glaucoma, organic pyloric stenosis, uncooperative clients. Lactation.

Special Concerns: Dosage has not been established in children. Geriatric clients may be more sensitive to the hypotensive effects of mecamylamine; also, a decrease in dose may be required in these clients due to age-related decreases in renal function. Use with caution in marked cerebral and coronary arteriosclerosis, after recent CVA, prostatic hypertrophy, urethral stricture, bladder neck obstruction. Abdominal distention, decreased bowel signs, and other symptoms of adynamic ileus are reasons for discontinuing the drug.

Side Effects: *GI:* N&V, constipation (may be preceded by small, frequent, liquid stools), dry mouth, glossitis, anorexia, ileus. *CNS:* Sedation, weakness, fatigue. Rarely, choreiform movements, mental aberrations, tremors, **seizures.** *Respiratory:* Fibrosis, interstitial pulmonary edema. *CV:* Postural hypotension, orthostatic dizziness, syncope. *GU:* Urinary retention, decreased libido, impotence. *Miscellaneous:* Paresthesia, blurred vision, dilated pupils.

OD **Overdose Management:** *Symptoms:* Hypotension, *peripheral vascular collapse,* orthostatic hypotension, N&V, diarrhea, constipation, paralytic ileus, dizziness, anxiety, dry mouth, mydriasis, blurred vision, palpitations, increased intraocular pressure, urinary retention. *Treatment:* Vasopressors to treat hypotension.

Dosage
- **Tablets**
  Hypertension.
  Adults, initial: 2.5 mg b.i.d. Increase by increments of 2.5 mg q 2 or more days; **maintenance:** 25 mg/day in three divided doses.

RESPIRATORY CARE CONSIDERATIONS

See also *Respiratory Care Considerations* for *Antihypertensive Agents.*

Administration/Storage
1. For better control of hypertension, administer after meals.
2. The morning dose may be small or omitted; larger doses are given at noon and in the evening.

Evaluate: ↓ BP with control of hypertension

Meperidine hydrochloride (Pethidine hydrochloride)

(meh-**PER**-ih-deen)

Pregnancy Category: C
Demerol Hydrochloride **(C-II) (Rx)**
Classification: Narcotic analgesic, synthetic

See also *Narcotic Analgesics.*

Action/Kinetics: The pharmacologic activity of meperidine is similar to that of the opiates; however, meperidine is only one-tenth as potent an analgesic as morphine. Its analgesic effect is only one-half when given PO rather than parenterally. Meperidine has no antitussive effects and does not produce miosis. The drug does produce moderate spasmogenic effects on smooth muscle. The duration of action of meperidine is less than that of most opiates, and this must be kept in mind when a dosing schedule is being established. Meperidine will produce both psychologic and physical dependence; overdosage is manifested by severe respiratory depression (see *Narcotic Overdose*). **Onset:** 10–45 min. **Peak effect:** 30–60 min. **Duration:** 2–4 hr. **t½:** 3–4 hr.

Uses: Any situation that requires a narcotic analgesic: severe pain, hepatic and renal colic, obstetrics, preanesthetic medication, adjunct to anesthesia. These drugs are particularly useful for minor surgery, as in orthopedics, ophthalmology, rhinology, laryngology, and dentistry, and for diagnostic procedures such as cystoscopy, retrograde pyelography, and gastroscopy. Spasms of GI tract, uterus, urinary bladder. Anginal syndrome and distress of CHF.

Additional   Contraindications: Hypersensitivity to drug, convulsive states as in epilepsy, tetanus and strychnine poisoning, children under 6 months, diabetic acidosis, head injuries, shock, liver disease, respiratory depression, increased cranial pressure, and before labor during pregnancy.

Special Concerns: To be used with caution in lactating mothers and in older or debilitated clients. Use with extreme caution in clients with asthma. Meperidine has atropine-like effects that may aggravate glaucoma, especially when given with other drugs, which should be used with caution in glaucoma.

Additional Side Effects: Transient hallucinations, transient hypotension (high doses), visual disturbances. Meperidine may accumulate in clients with renal dysfunction, leading to an increased risk of CNS toxicity.

OD Overdose Management: *Treatment:* Naloxone 0.4 mg IV is effective in the treatment of acute overdosage. In PO overdose, gastric lavage and induced emesis are indicated. Treatment, however, is aimed at combating the progressive respiratory depression usually through assisted ventilation.

Additional Drug Interactions
Antidepressants, tricyclic / Additive anticholinergic side effects
Hydantoins / ↓ Effect of meperidine due to ↑ breakdown by liver
MAO inhibitors / ↑ Risk of severe symptoms including hyperpyrexia, restlessness, hyper- or hypotension, convulsions, or coma

Dosage ——————————
• **Tablets, Syrup, IM, SC**
Analgesic.
Adults: 50–100 mg q 3–4 hr as needed; **pediatric:** 1.1–1.8 mg/kg, up to adult dosage, q 3–4 hr as needed.
Preoperatively.
Adults, IM, SC: 50–100 mg 30–90 min before anesthesia; **pediatric, IM, SC:** 1–2 mg/kg 30–90 min before anesthesia.
Obstetrics.
Adults, IM, SC: 50–100 mg q 1–3 hr.
• **IV**
Support of anesthesia.
IV infusion: 1 mg/mL or **slow IV injection:** 10 mg/mL until client needs met.

RESPIRATORY CARE CONSIDERATIONS

See also *Respiratory Care Considerations* for *Narcotic Analgesics.*

Administration/Storage
1. For repeated doses, IM administration is preferred over SC use.
2. Meperidine is more effective when given parenterally than when given PO.
3. The syrup should be taken with ½ glass of water to minimize anesthetic effect on mucous membranes.
4. If used concomitantly with phenothiazines or antianxiety agents, the dose of meperidine should be reduced by 25%–50%.
5. Meperidine for IV use is incompatible with the following drugs: aminophylline, barbiturates, heparin, iodide, methicillin, morphine sulfate, phenytoin, sodium bicarbonate, sulfadiazine, and sulfisoxazole.

Assessment
1. Document intensity, location, onset, duration, and level of pain (use a rating scale).

2. Note any evidence of head injury or history of seizure disorder.

3. Record any history of asthma or other conditions that tend to compromise respirations.

4. Obtain baseline renal function studies and note any history of glaucoma.

5. Determine if client is a candidate for PCA via pump.

Evaluate: Desired level of analgesia without compromise in level of consciousness or respirations

---

Mephentermine sulfate
(meh-**FEN**-ter-meen)
Pregnancy Category: C
Wyamine Sulfate **(Rx)**
Classification: Adrenergic agent, indirectly acting; vasopressor

---

See also *Sympathomimetic Drugs*.

Action/Kinetics: Mephentermine acts both indirectly by releasing norepinephrine from its storage sites and directly by exerting a slight effect on alpha and beta-1 receptors and a moderate effect on beta-2 receptors mediating vasodilation. The drug causes increased CO; also elicits slight CNS effects. **IV: Onset,** immediate; **duration:** 15–30 min. **IM: Onset,** 5–15 min; **duration:** 1–2 hr. Metabolized in liver. Excreted in urine within 24 hr (rate increased in acidic urine).

Uses: Hypotension due to anesthesia, ganglionic blockade, or hemorrhage (only as emergency treatment until blood or blood substitutes can be given).

Contraindications: To treat hypotension caused by chlorpromazine. In combination with MAO inhibitors.

Special Concerns: Use with caution in CV disease and in chronically ill clients. Use with caution in treating shock secondary to hemorrhage. Safety and efficacy have not been demonstrated in children.

Side Effects: Anxiety, cardiac arrhythmias, increased BP (especially in those with heart disease).

Additional Drug Interactions: Me-

phentermine will potentiate hypotensive effects of phenothiazines.

Dosage ——————————
• **IV, IM**
   Hypotension during spinal anesthesia.
IV, Adults: 30–45 mg; 30-mg doses may be repeated as required; or, **IV infusion, Adults and children:** 0.1% (1 mg/mL) mephentermine in D5W with the rate of infusion and duration dependent on client response.
IV, Pediatric: 0.4 mg/kg (12 mg/m²) as a single dose.
   Prophylaxis of hypotension in spinal anesthesia.
IM, Adults: 30–45 mg 10–20 min before anesthesia. **IM, Pediatric:** 0.4 mg/kg (12 mg/m²) as a single dose.
   Shock following hemorrhage.
Not recommended, but IV infusion of 0.1% in D5W may maintain BP until blood volume is replaced.

RESPIRATORY CARE CONSIDERATIONS

See also *Respiratory Care Considerations* for *Sympathomimetic Drugs*.
Administration/Storage
1. The preferable method of administration for shock is either injection of the undiluted parenteral solution containing 30 mg/mL or a continuous infusion of a 1-mg/mL solution in D5W directly into the vein.
2. The 0.1% solution can be prepared by adding 10 or 20 mL of mephentermine (the 30-mg/mL strength) to either 250 or 500 mL of D5W, respectively.
Assessment
1. Determine cause of hypotensive episode; rule out chlorpromazine induced.
2. Note any history or evidence of CV disease, hemorrhage, or chronic illness.
Interventions: Record BP every 5 min until stable. Once BP has stabilized, take a reading every 15–30 min beyond the duration of the drug's action (IM 1–4 hr; IV 5–15 min).
Evaluate: Stabilization of BP

Metaproterenol sulfate (Orciprenaline sulfate)

(met-ah-proh-**TER**-ih-nohl)

Pregnancy Category: C

Alupent, Arm-A-Med Metaproterenol Sulfate, Metaprel **(Rx)**

Classification: Adrenergic agent, direct-acting; bronchodilator

See also *Sympathomimetic Drugs.*

Action/Kinetics: Metaproterenol markedly stimulates beta-2 receptors, resulting in relaxation of smooth muscles of the bronchial tree, as well as peripheral vasodilation. It has minimal effects on beta-1 receptors. It is similar to isoproterenol, but it has a longer duration of action and fewer side effects. Has minimal beta-1 activity. **Onset: Inhalation aerosol,** within 1 min; **peak effect:** 1 hr; **duration:** 1–5 hr. **Onset, hand bulb nebulizer or IPPB:** 5–30 min; **duration:** 4–6 hr after repeated doses. **PO: Onset,** 15–30 min; **peak effect:** 1 hr. **Duration:** 4 hr. PO administration produces a marked first-pass effect. Metabolized in the liver and excreted through the kidney.

Uses: Bronchodilator in asthma, bronchitis, emphysema, and other conditions associated with reversible bronchospasms. Treatment of acute asthmatic attacks in children over 6 years of age.

Special Concerns: Dosage of syrup or tablets not determined in children less than 6 years of age.

Additional Side Effects: *GI:* Diarrhea, bad taste or taste changes. *Respiratory:* Worsening of asthma, nasal congestion, hoarseness. *Miscellaneous:* Hypersensitivity reactions, rash, fatigue, backache, skin reactions.

Drug Interactions: Possible potentiation of adrenergic effects if used before or after other sympathomimetic bronchodilators.

Dosage

- **Syrup, Tablets**
  Bronchodilation.

Adults and children over 27.2 kg or 9 years: 20 mg t.i.d.–q.i.d.; **children under 27.2 kg or 6–9 years of age:** 10 mg t.i.d.–q.i.d.; **children less than 6 years of age:** 1.3–2.6 mg/kg/day of the syrup has been studied.

- **Inhalation. Hand Nebulizer**
  Bronchodilation.

Usual dose is 10 inhalations (range: 5–15 inhalations) of undiluted 5% solution.

- **IPPB**
  Bronchodilation.

0.3 mL (range: 0.2–0.3 mL) of 5% solution diluted to 2.5 mL saline or other diluent.

- **MDI**
  Bronchodilation.

2–3 inhalations (1.30–2.25 mg) q 3–4 hr. Total daily dose should not exceed 12 inhalations (9 mg).

RESPIRATORY CARE CONSIDERATIONS

See also *Special Respiratory Care Considerations for Adrenergic Bronchodilators* under *Sympathomimetic Drugs.*

Administration/Storage

1. Instruct client to shake the container.

2. Unit dose vials should be refrigerated at 2°C–8°C (35°F–46°F).

3. The inhalant solution can be stored at room temperature, but excessive heat and light should be avoided.

4. The solution should not be used if it is brown or shows a precipitate.

5. The inhalant solutions should not be used more often than q 4 hr to relieve acute bronchospasms. In chronic bronchospastic disease, the dose can be given t.i.d.–q.i.d. A single dose of the nebulized drug may not completely abort an attack of acute asthma.

Client/Family Teaching

1. Review appropriate method for administration; use a demonstrator if possible. Observe client self-administer to ensure proper technique.

2. Report any loss of effectiveness with prescribed dosage and frequency.

M

3. Review drug side effects that should be reported if evident.

Evaluate

• Reports of symptomatic relief and improved pulmonary function
• Improved oxygen saturation levels

Metaraminol bitartrate

(met-ah-**RAM**-ih-nohl)
Pregnancy Category: C
Aramine **(Rx)**
Classification: Adrenergic agent, direct-acting; vasopressor

See also *Sympathomimetic Drugs.*

Action/Kinetics: Metaraminol indirectly releases norepinephrine from storage sites and directly stimulates primarily alpha receptors and, to a slight extent, beta-1 receptors. The drug causes marked increases in BP due primarily to vasoconstriction and to a slight increase in CO. Reflex bradycardia is also manifested. Metaraminol increases venous tone, causes pulmonary vasoconstriction, and increases pulmonary pressure, even if CO is decreased. CNS stimulation usually does not occur. **Onset: IV:** 1–2 min; **IM:** 10 min; **SC:** 5–20 min. **Duration, IV:** 20 min; **IM, SC:** About 60 min. Metabolized in the liver and excreted through the urine and feces. Urinary excretion of unchanged drug can be enhanced by acidifying the urine.

Uses: Hypotension associated with surgery, spinal anesthesia, hemorrhage, trauma, infections, tumors, and adverse drug reactions. Adjunct to the treatment of either septicemia or cardiogenic shock. *Investigational:* Injected intracavernosally to treat priapism due to phentolamine, papaverine, or other causes.

Contraindications: Use with cyclopropane or halothane anesthesia (unless clinical conditions mandate such use). As a substitute for blood or fluid replacement.

Special Concerns: Use with caution in cirrhosis, malaria, heart or thyroid disease, hypertension, or diabetes. Hypertension and ischemic ECG changes may occur when used to treat priapism. Use with caution during lactation. Use is not a substitute for the replacement of blood, plasma, fluids, and electrolytes.

Additional Side Effects: Rapidly induced hypertension may cause acute pulmonary edema, arrhythmias, and *cardiac arrest.* Due to its long duration of action, cumulative effects are possible with prolonged increases in BP.

Drug Interactions

Digitalis glycosides / ↑ Risk of ectopic arrhythmias
Furazolidone / Possible hypertensive crisis and intracranial hemorrhage
Guanethidine / Antihypertensive effects of guanethidine may be partially or totally reversed
Halogenated hydrocarbons / Sensitization of the heart to catecholamines; use of metaraminol may cause serious arrhythmias
MAO Inhibitors / Possible hypertensive crisis and intracranial hemorrhage
Oxytocic drugs / Possiblity of severe, persistent hypertension
Tricyclic antidepressants / ↓ Pressor effect of metaraminol

Dosage

• **IM, SC**

Prophylaxis of hypotension.

Adults: 2–10 mg given IM or SC; **pediatric:** 0.01 mg/kg (3 mg/m^2) IM or SC.

• **IV Infusion**

Hypotension.

Adults: 15–100 mg in 250–500 mL of 0.9% sodium chloride injection or 5% dextrose injection by IV infusion at a rate to maintain desired BP (up to 500 mg/500 mL has been used). **Pediatric:** 0.4 mg/kg (12 mg/m^2) by IV infusion in a solution containing 1 mg/25 mL 0.9% sodium chloride injection or 5% dextrose injection.

• **Direct IV**

Severe shock.

Adults: 0.5–5.0 mg by direct IV followed by IV infusion of 15–100 mg in 250–500 mL fluid. **Pediatric:** 0.01 mg/kg (0.3 mg/m^2) by direct IV.

• **Endotracheal Tube**
If IV access is not possible, meta-raminol may be given by an ET tube. Perform five quick insufflations; forcefully expel 5 mg diluted to 10 mL into the ET tube and follow with five quick insufflations.

RESPIRATORY CARE CONSIDERATIONS

See also *Respiratory Care Considerations* for *Sympathomimetic Drugs*.
Administration/Storage
1. Do not inject IM in areas that seem to have poor circulation because sloughing has occurred with extravasation.
2. Use an electronic infusion device when administering IV drug therapy for more adequate control and titration of drug.
3. The following solutions may be used to dilute metaraminol: sodium chloride injection, 5% dextrose injection, Ringer's injection, lactated Ringer's injection, 5% dextran in saline, Normosol-R pH 7.4, and Normosol-M in 5% dextrose injection.
4. Storage at temperatures below –20 ° C (–4 ° F) should be avoided.
5. Infusion solutions should be used within 24 hr.
Assessment
1. Document indications for therapy and type and onset of symptoms as well as any precipitating factors.
2. Ensure that client is adequately hydrated.
Interventions
1. Take BP every 15 min. Obtain written parameters for maintaining the SBP. Monitor ECG, I&O, and VS.
2. Frequently assess administration site because extravasation may result in tissue necrosis.
Evaluate: Effective management of hypotension with desired ↑ in SBP

Methadone hydrochloride
(**METH**-ah-dohn)
Pregnancy Category: C
Dolophine, Methadose **(C-II) (Rx)**
Classification: Narcotic analgesic, morphine type

See also *Narcotic Analgesics*.
Action/Kinetics: Methadone produces only mild euphoria, which is the reason it is used as a heroin withdrawal substitute and for maintenance programs. Methadone produces physical dependence, but the abstinence syndrome develops more slowly upon termination of therapy; also, withdrawal symptoms are less intense but more prolonged than those associated with morphine. Methadone does not produce sedation or narcosis. Methadone is not effective for preoperative or obstetric anesthesia. When administered PO, it is only one-half as potent as when given parenterally. **Onset:** 30–60 min. **Peak effects:** 30–60 min. **Duration:** 4–6 hr. **t½:** 15–30 hr. Both the duration and half-life increase with repeated use due to cumulative effects.

Uses: Severe pain. Drug withdrawal and maintenance of narcotic dependence.

Additional Contraindications: Intravenous use, liver disease; give rarely, if at all, during pregnancy. Use in children. Use in obstetrics (due to long duration of action and chance of respiratory depression in the neonate).

Special Concerns: Use with caution during lactation.

Additional Side Effects: Marked constipation, excessive sweating, pulmonary edema, choreic movements.

Drug Interactions: Rifampin and phenytoin ↓ plasma methadone levels by ↑ breakdown by liver; thus, possible symptoms of narcotic withdrawal may develop.

Laboratory Test Interferences: ↑ Immunoglobulin G.

Dosage ─────────
• **Tablets, Oral Solution, Oral Concentrate**
  Analgesia.

M

Adults, individualized: 2.5–10 mg q 3–4 hr, although higher doses may be necessary for severe pain or due to development of tolerance.

Narcotic withdrawal.

Initial: 15–20 mg/day PO (some may require 40 mg/day); **then,** depending on need of the client, slowly decrease dosage.

Maintenance following narcotic withdrawal.

Adults, individualized, initial: 20–40 mg PO 4–8 hr after heroin is stopped; **then,** adjust dosage as required up to 120 mg/day.

RESPIRATORY CARE CONSIDERATIONS

See also *Respiratory Care Considerations* for *Narcotic Analgesics.*

Administration/Storage

1. PO concentrations of solution should be diluted in at least 90 mL of water prior to administration.

2. If the client is taking dispersible tablets, the tablets should be diluted in 120 mL of water, orange juice, citrus-flavored drink, or other acidic fruit drink. Allow at least 1 min for complete dispersion of the drug.

3. For repeated analgesic doses, IM administration is preferred over SC administration. Inspect injection sites for signs of irritation.

4. Clients receiving methadone for detoxification purposes should be on the drug no longer than 21 days. The treatment should not be repeated until 4 weeks have elapsed.

Evaluate

• Control of severe pain
• Successful detoxification and maintenance in narcotic-dependent individual

Methicillin sodium

(meth-ih-**SILL**-in)
Staphcillin **(Rx)**
Classification: Antibiotic, penicillin

See also *Anti-Infectives* and *Penicillins.*

Action/Kinetics: This drug is a semisynthetic, penicillinase-resistant salt suitable for soft tissue, penicillin G-resistant, and resistant staphylococcal infections. **Peak plasma levels: IM,** 10–20 mcg/mL after 30–60 min; **IV,** 15 min. **t½:** 30 min. Excreted chiefly in the urine.

Additional Use: Infections by penicillinase-producing staphylococci, osteomyelitis, septicemia, enterocolitis, bacterial endocarditis.

Special Concerns: Use with caution in clients with renal failure. Safe use in neonates has not been established. Periodic renal function tests are indicated for long-term therapy.

Dosage ───────────

• **IM, Continuous IV Infusion**
General infections.

Adults: 4–12 g/day, depending on the infection, in divided doses q 4–6 hr. (*NOTE:* If creatinine clearance is less than 10 mL/min, the dose should not exceed 2 g q 12 hr.) **Pediatric:** 100–300 mg/kg/day in divided doses q 4–6 hr. **Infants over 7 days of age and weighing more than 2 kg:** 100 mg/kg/day in divided doses q 6 hr. **Infants more than 7 days of age and weighing less than 2 kg or less than 7 days of age and weighing more than 2 kg:** 75 mg/kg/day in divided doses q 8 hr. **Infants under 7 days of age and weighing less than 2 kg:** 50 mg/kg/day in divided doses q 12 hr.

Meningitis.

Infants over 7 days of age and weighing more than 2 kg: 150–200 mg/kg/day. **Infants more than 7 days of age and weighing less than 2 kg or less than 7 days and weighing more than 2 kg:** 150 mg/kg/day. **Infants under 7 days of age and weighing less than 2 kg:** 100 mg/kg/day.

RESPIRATORY CARE CONSIDERATIONS

See also *General Respiratory Care Considerations for All Anti-Infectives* and for *Penicillins.*

Administration/Storage

1. Do not use dextrose solutions for diluting methicillin because their low acidity may destroy the antibiotic.

2. Inject medication slowly. Methicillin injections are particularly painful.

3. Inject deeply into gluteal muscle. Use caution to avoid sciatic nerve injury.

4. To prevent sterile abscesses at injection site, include 0.2–0.3 mL of air in syringe before starting injection so that when the needle is withdrawn the irritating solution will not leak into tissue.

5. If used IV, care should be taken as thrombophlebitis can occur, especially in geriatric clients.

6. Check for redness or edema at site of injection and for pain along the course of the vein into which the drug is administered. Methicillin is a vesicant.

7. Methicillin is sensitive to heat when dissolved. Therefore, solutions for IM administration must be used within 24 hr if standing at room temperature or within 4 days if refrigerated. Solutions for IV use must be used within 8 hr.

8. For IV administration, dilute 1 mL (500 mg) with 20–25 mL of sterile water for injection or sodium chloride injection USP and administer at a rate of 10 mL/min. May further dilute and administer IVPB over 30 min.

9. Do not mix methicillin with any other drug in the same syringe or IV solution.

Assessment

1. Document indications for therapy and type and onset of symptoms.

2. Ensure that blood cultures and CBC are taken prior to start of therapy and weekly during therapy. Many strains of methicillin-resistant staphylococci have been identified. It has been recommended that these clients be isolated until appropriate antibiotic therapy can be instituted to prevent major institutional outbreaks.

3. Obtain CBC, electrolytes, and liver and renal function studies.

Interventions

1. Monitor I&O. Note any evidence of hematuria or casts in the urine.

2. Observe for any evidence of pallor, ecchymosis, or bleeding tendencies (drug enhances anticoagulants); monitor CBC.

3. Observe for fever, nausea, and other signs of hepatotoxicity, especially with prolonged therapy; monitor liver function.

4. Drug contains sodium; calculate accordingly for clients on strict sodium restrictions; monitor electrolytes.

Evaluate

• Negative lab C&S reports and no evidence of organism resistance

• Eradication of infection and evidence of ↓ fever, ↓ WBC, and ↓ symptoms

Methyldopa
(meth-ill-**DOH**-pah)
Pregnancy Category: B
Aldomet, Apo-Methyldopa ♣, Dopamet ♣, Medimet ♣, Novo–Medopa ♣, Nu-Medopa ♣ **(Rx)**

Methyldopate hydrochloride
(meth-ill-**DOH**-payt)
Pregnancy Category: B
Aldomet Hydrochloride **(Rx)**
Classification: Antihypertensive, centrally acting antiadrenergic

See also *Antihypertensive Agents*.

Action/Kinetics: Primary mechanism thought to be that the active metabolite, alpha-methylnorepinephrine, lowers BP by stimulating central inhibitory alpha-adrenergic receptors, false neurotransmission, and/or reduction of plasma renin. It causes little change in CO. **PO: Onset:** 7–12 hr. **Duration:** 12–24 hr. All effects terminated within 48 hr. Absorption is variable. **IV: Onset:** 4–6 hr. **Duration:** 10–16 hr. Seventy percent of drug excreted in urine. **Full therapeutic effect:** 1–4 days. t½: 1.7 hr. *NOTE:* Methyldopa is a component of Aldoril.

Uses: Moderate to severe hypertension. Particularly useful for clients with impaired renal function, renal hypertension, resistant cases of hypertension complicated by stroke, CAD, or nitrogen retention, and for hypertensive crisis (parenterally).

Contraindications: Sensitivity to drug, labile and mild hypertension, pregnancy, active hepatic disease, or pheochromocytoma.

Special Concerns: Use with caution in clients with a history of liver or kidney disease. Geriatric clients may be more sensitive to the hypotensive and sedative effects of guanabenz; also, it may be necessary to decrease the dose in these clients due to age-related decreases in renal function.

Side Effects: *CNS:* Sedation (disappears with use), weakness, headache, asthenia, dizziness, paresthesias, Parkinson-like symptoms, psychic disturbances, choreoathetotic movements, Bell's palsy, decreased mental acuity, verbal memory impairment. *CV:* Bradycardia, orthostatic hypotension, hypersensitivity of carotid sinus, worsening of angina, hypertensive response (paradoxical), myocarditis. *GI:* N&V, abdominal distention, diarrhea or constipation, flatus, colitis, dry mouth, "black tongue," pancreatitis, sialoadenitis. *Hematologic:* **Hemolytic anemia,** leukopenia, granulocytopenia, thrombocytopenia, **bone marrow depression.** *Endocrine:* Gynecomastia, amenorrhea, galactorrhea, lactation, hyperprolactinemia. *Miscellaneous:* Edema, jaundice, hepatitis, liver disorders, abnormal liver function tests, rash (eczema, lichenoid eruption), **toxic epidermal necrolysis,** fever, lupus-like symptoms, impotence, failure to ejaculate, decreased libido, nasal stuffiness, joint pain, myalgia, **septic shock-like syndrome.**

OD **Overdose Management:** *Symptoms:* CNS, GI, and CV effects including sedation, weakness, lightheadedness, dizziness, coma, bradycardia, acute hypotension, impairment of AV conduction, constipation, diarrhea, distention, flatus, N&V. *Treatment:* Induction of vomiting or gastric lavage if detected early. General supportive treatment with special attention to HR, CO, blood volume, urinary function, electrolyte imbalance, paralytic ileus, and CNS activity. In severe cases, hemodialysis is effective.

Drug Interactions
Anesthetics, general / Additive hypotension
Antidepressants, tricyclic / Tricyclic antidepressants may block hypotensive effect of methyldopa
Ephedrine / ↓ Action of ephedrine in methyldopa-treated clients
Fenfluramine / ↑ Effect of methyldopa
Haloperidol / Methyldopa ↑ toxic effects of haloperidol
Levodopa / ↑ Effect of both drugs
Lithium / ↑ Possibility of lithium toxicity
MAO inhibitors / May reverse hypotensive effect of methyldopa and cause headache and hallucinations
Methotrimeprazine / Additive hypotensive effect
Norepinephrine / ↑ Pressor response to norepinephrine
Phenoxybenzamine / Urinary incontinence
Phenylpropanolamine / ↑ Pressor response to phenylpropanolamine
Propranolol / Paradoxical hypertension
Sympathomimetics / Potentiation of hypertensive effect of sympathomimetics
Thiazide diuretics / Additive hypotensive effect
Thioxanthenes / Additive hypotensive effect
Tolbutamide / ↑ Hypoglycemia due to ↓ breakdown by liver
Tricyclic antidepressants / ↓ Effect of methyldopa
Vasodilator drugs / Additive hypotensive effect
Verapamil / ↑ Effect of methyldopa

Laboratory Test Interferences: False + or ↑ : Alkaline phosphatase, bilirubin, BUN, BSP, cephalin flocculation, creatinine, AST, ALT, uric acid, Coombs' test, PT. Positive lupus erythematosus cell preparation and antinuclear antibodies.

Dosage

• **Methyldopa. Oral Suspension, Tablets**

Hypertension.

Initial: 250 mg b.i.d.–t.i.d. for 2 days. Adjust dose q 2 days. If increased, start with evening dose. **Usual maintenance:** 0.5–3.0 g/day in two to four divided doses; **maximum:** 3 g/day. Transfer to and from other antihypertensive agents should occur gradually, with initial dose of methyldopa not exceeding 500 mg. *NOTE:* Do not use combination medication to initiate therapy. **Pediatric, initial:** 10 mg/kg/day in two to four divided doses, adjusting maintenance to a maximum of 65 mg/kg/day (or 3 g/day, whichever is less).

• **Methyldopate HCl. IV Infusion**

Hypertension.

Adults: 250–500 mg q 6 hr; **maximum:** 1 g q 6 hr for hypertensive crisis.

Switch to PO methyldopa, at same dosage level, when BP is brought under control. **Pediatric:** 20–40 mg/kg/day in divided doses q 6 hr; **maximum:** 65 mg/kg/day (or 3 g/day, whichever is less).

RESPIRATORY CARE CONSIDERATIONS

See also *Respiratory Care Considerations* for *Antihypertensive Agents.*
Administration/Storage
1. If the drug is to be administered by IV, methyldopate HCl should be mixed with 100 mL of 5% dextrose or administered in D5W at a concentration of 10 mg/mL.
2. The IV should be diluted in 100 mL of D5W and infused over 30–60 min.
3. Tolerance may occur following 2–3 months of therapy.
4. Increasing the dose or adding a diuretic often restores effect on BP.
Assessment
1. Document indications for therapy, onset of symptoms, and other agents prescribed and the outcome.
2. Ascertain that hematologic studies, liver function tests, and a

Coombs' test are done before and during drug therapy.
3. If the client requires a blood transfusion, ascertain that both direct and indirect Coombs' tests are done. If the indirect and direct Coombs' tests are positive, anticipate consultation with a hematologist.
4. Assess for signs of drug tolerance. These may occur during the second or third month of drug therapy.
5. Note any evidence of jaundice. The drug is contraindicated when the client has active hepatic disease.
Evaluate: ↓ BP with control of hypertension

Methylprednisolone

(meth-ill-pred-**NISS**-oh-lohn)
Tablets: Medrol, Meprolone **(Rx)**

Methylprednisolone acetate

(meth-ill-pred-**NISS**-oh-lohn)
Cream: Medrol Veriderm Cream ✦.
Enema: Medrol Enpak **(Rx)**. **Parenteral:** depMedalone-40 and -80, Depoject 40 and 80, Depo-Medrol, D-Med 80, Duralone-40 and -80, Medralone-40 and -80, M-Prednisol-40 and -80 **(Rx)**

M

Methylprednisolone sodium succinate

(meth-ill-pred-**NISS**-oh-lohn)
Parenteral: A-methaPred, Solu-Medrol **(Rx)**
Classification: Glucocorticoid

See also *Corticosteroids.*
Action/Kinetics: Low incidence of increased appetite, peptic ulcer, and psychic stimulation. Also, low degree of sodium and water retention. May mask negative nitrogen balance. **Onset:** Slow, 12–24 hr. **t½, plasma:** 78–188 min. **Duration:** Long, up to 1 week. The sodium succinate product has a rapid onset by both the IM and IV routes. Methylprednisolone acetate has a long duration of action.

Additional Use: Severe hepatitis due to alcoholism. Within 8 hr of severe spinal cord injury (to improve neurologic function). Septic shock (controversial).

Special Concerns: Use during pregnancy only if benefits outweigh risks.

Additional Drug Interactions

Erythromycin / ↑ Effect of methylprednisolone due to ↓ breakdown by liver

Troleandomycin / ↑ Effect of methylprednisolone due to ↓ breakdown by liver

Laboratory Test Interferences: ↓ Immunoglobulins A, G, M.

Dosage ———————————

METHYLPREDNISOLONE

• **Tablets**

Rheumatoid arthritis.

Adults: 6–16 mg/day. Decrease gradually when condition is under control. **Pediatric:** 6–10 mg/day.

SLE.

Adults, acute: 20–96 mg/day; **maintenance:** 8–20 mg/day.

Acute rheumatic fever.

1 mg/kg body weight daily. Drug is always given in four equally divided doses after meals and at bedtime.

METHYLPREDNISOLONE ACETATE

• **IM**

Adrenogenital syndrome.

40 mg q 2 weeks.

Rheumatoid arthritis.

40–120 mg/week.

Dermatologic lesions, dermatitis.

40–120 mg/week for 1–4 weeks; for severe cases, a single dose of 80–120 mg should provide relief.

Seborrheic dermatitis.

80 mg/week.

Asthma, rhinitis.

80–120 mg.

• **Intra-articular, Soft Tissue and Intralesional Injection**

4–80 mg, depending on site.

• **Retention Enema**

40 mg 3–7 times/week for 2 or more weeks.

METHYLPREDNISOLONE SODIUM SUCCINATE

• **IM, IV**

Most conditions.

Adults, initial: 10–40 mg, depending on the disease; **then,** adjust dose depending on response, with subsequent doses given either **IM, IV.**

Severe conditions.

Adults: 30 mg/kg infused IV over 10–20 min; may be repeated q 4–6 hr for 2–3 days only. **Pediatric:** not less than 0.5 mg/kg/day.

RESPIRATORY CARE CONSIDERATIONS

See also *Respiratory Care Considerations* for *Corticosteroids.*

Administration/Storage

1. Dosage must be highly individualized.

2. Methylprednisolone acetate is not for IV use.

3. Solutions of methylprednisolone sodium succinate should be used within 48 hr after preparation.

4. For alternate day therapy using methylprednisolone, twice the usual PO dose is given every other morning (the client receives the beneficial effect while minimizing side effects).

Assessment

1. Document indications for treatment and describe clinical presentation.

2. Obtain baseline CBC, HbA1-C, glucose, and electrolytes and monitor with long-term therapy.

Evaluate

• Relief of allergic manifestations

• Control of pain and inflammation with improved mobility

• ↓ Destruction of nerve fibers in spinal cord injury

Metolazone

(meh-**TOH**-lah-zohn)

Pregnancy Category: B

Mykrox, Zaroxolyn **(Rx)**

Classification: Diuretic, thiazide

See also Diuretics, Thiazide.

Action/Kinetics: Onset: 1 hr. **Peak blood levels, rapid availability tablets:** 2–4 hr; **t½, elimination:** About 14 hr. **Peak blood levels, slow availability tablets:** 8 hr. **Duration, rapid or slow availablity tablets:** 24 hr or more. Most of the drug is excreted unchanged through the urine.

Uses: *Slow availability tablets:* Edema accompanying CHF; edema accompanying renal diseases, including nephrotic syndrome and conditions of reduced renal function. Alone or in combination with other drugs for the treatment of hypertension.

Rapid availability tablets: Treatment of newly diagnosed mild to moderate hypertension alone or in combination with other drugs. The rapid availability tablets are not to be used to produce diuresis.

Investigational: Alone or as an adjunct to treat calcium nephrolithiasis, premanagement of menstrual syndrome, and adjunct treatment of renal failure.

Contraindications: Anuria, prehepatic and hepatic coma, allergy or hypersensitivity to metolazone. Routine use during pregnancy. Lactation.

Special Concerns: Use with caution in those with severely impaired renal function. Safety and effectiveness have not been determined in children.

Side Effects: See *Diuretics, Thiazide.* The most commonly reported side effects are dizziness, headache, muscle cramps, malaise, lethargy, lassitude, joint pain/swelling, and chest pain.

Additional Drug Interactions

Alcohol / ↑ Hypotensive effect
Barbiturates / Hypotensive effect
Narcotics / Hypotensive effect
NSAIDs / ↓ Hypotensive effect of metolazone
Salicylates / Hypotensive effect of metolazone

Dosage ─────────────────

• **Slow Availability Tablets**

Edema due to cardiac failure or renal disease.

Adults: 5–20 mg once daily. For those who experience paroxysmal nocturnal dyspnea, a larger dose may be required to ensure pro-

longed diuresis and saluresis for a 24-hr period.

Mild to moderate essential hypertension.

Adults: 2.5–5 mg once daily.

• **Rapid Availability Tablets**

Mild to moderate essential hypertension.

Adults, initial: 0.5 mg once daily, usually in the morning. If inadequately controlled, the dose may be increased to 1 mg once a day. Increasing the dose higher than 1 mg does not increase the effect.

RESPIRATORY CARE CONSIDERATIONS

See also *Respiratory Care Considerations* for Diuretics, Thiazide, .

Administration/Storage

1. *Formulations of slow availability tablets should not be interchanged with formulations of rapid availability tablets as they are not therapeutically equivalent.*

2. The antihypertensive effect may be observed from three to four days to three to six weeks.

3. If BP is not controlled with 1 mg of the rapid availability tablets, another antihypertensive drug, with a different mechanism of action, should be added to the therapy.

4. Tablets should be stored at room temperature in a tight, light-resistant container.

Assessment

1. Document indications for therapy, noting onset, duration, and characteristics of symptoms.

2. Note any sulfonamide allergy.

3. List drugs prescribed to ensure none interact unfavorably, especially lithium, lasix, and antihypertensive agents.

4. Obtain baseline CBC, liver and renal function studies and monitor.

5. Obtain BP and ECG and assess for symptoms of electrolyte imbalance (i.e. ↓ Na, ↓ K, ↓ Mg and hypochloremic alkalosis).

Evaluate

• ↓ Edema
• ↓ BP

Metoprolol succinate

(me-toe-**PROH**-lohl)
Pregnancy Category: C
Toprol XL **(Rx)**

Metoprolol tartrate

(me-toe-**PROH**-lohl)
Pregnancy Category: B
Apo-Metoprolol ✿, Apo-Metoprolol
(Type L) ✿, Betaloc ✿, Betaloc Du-
rules ✿, Lopressor, Novo–Metoprol ✿,
Nu-Metop ✿ **(Rx)**
Classification: Beta-adrenergic
blocking agent

See also *Beta-Adrenergic Blocking Agents.*

Action/Kinetics: Exerts mainly beta-1-adrenergic blocking activity although beta-2 receptors are blocked at high doses. Has no membrane stabilizing or intrinsic sympathomimetic effects. Moderate lipid solubility. **Onset:** 15 min. **Peak plasma levels:** 90 min. **t½:** 3–7 hr. Effect of drug is cumulative. Food increases bioavailability. Exhibits significant first-pass effect. Metabolized in liver and excreted in urine.

Uses: Metoprolol Succinate: Alone or with other drugs to treat hypertension. Chronic management of angina pectoris.

Metoprolol Tartrate: Hypertension (either alone or with other antihypertensive agents, such as thiazide diuretics). Acute MI in hemodynamically stable clients. Angina pectoris. *Investigational:* IV to suppress atrial ectopy in COPD, aggressive behavior, prophylaxis of migraine, ventricular arrhythmias, enhancement of cognitive performance in geriatric clients, essential tremors.

Additional Contraindications: Myocardial infarction in clients with a HR of less than 45 beats/min, in second- or third-degree heart block, or if SBP is less than 100 mm Hg. Moderate to severe cardiac failure.

Special Concerns: Safety and effectiveness have not been established in children. Use with caution in impaired hepatic function and during lactation.

Additional Drug Interactions

Cimetidine / May ↑ plasma levels of metoprolol
Contraceptives, oral / May ↑ effects of metoprolol
Methimazole / May ↓ effects of metoprolol
Phenobarbital / ↓ Effect of metoprolol due to ↑ breakdown by liver
Propylthiouracil / May ↓ the effects of metoprolol
Quinidine / May ↑ effects of metoprolol
Rifampin / ↓ Effect of metoprolol due to ↑ breakdown by liver
Laboratory Test Interferences: ↑ Serum transaminase, LDH, alkaline phosphatase.

Dosage

- **Metoprolol Succinate Tablets**
  Angina pectoris.
Individualized. Initial: 100 mg/day in a single dose. Dose may be increased slowly, at weekly intervals, until optimum effect is reached or there is a pronounced slowing of HR. Doses above 400 mg/day have not been studied.
  Hypertension.
Initial: 50–100 mg/day in a single dose with or without a diuretic. Dosage may be increased in weekly intervals until maximum effect is reached. Doses above 400 mg/day have not been studied.

- **Metoprolol Tartrate Tablets**
  Hypertension.
Initial: 100 mg/day in single or divided doses; **then,** dose may be increased weekly to maintenance level of 100–450 mg/day. A diuretic may also be used.
  Aggressive behavior.
200–300 mg/day.
  Essential tremors.
50–300 mg/day.
  Prophylaxis of migraine.
50–100 mg b.i.d.
  Ventricular arrhythmias.
200 mg/day.

- **Metoprolol Tartrate Injection (IV) and Tablets**
  Early treatment of MI.
3 IV bolus injections of 5 mg each at approximately 2-min intervals. If cli-

ents tolerate the full IV dose, give 50 mg q 6 hr PO beginning 15 min after the last IV dose (or as soon as client's condition allows). This dose is continued for 48 hr followed by **late treatment:** 100 mg b.i.d. as soon as feasible; continue for 1–3 months (although data suggest treatment should be continued for 1–3 years). In clients who do not tolerate the full IV dose, begin with 25–50 mg q 6 hr PO beginning 15 min after the last IV dose or as soon as the condition allows.

RESPIRATORY CARE CONSIDERATIONS

See also *Respiratory Care Considerations* for *Beta-Adrenergic Blocking Agents* and *Antihypertensive Agents.*
Assessment
1. Document indications for therapy and type and onset of symptoms.
2. Document any history of cardiac disease.
3. Obtain baseline liver and renal function studies, ECG, and VS prior to initiating therapy and monitor during therapy.
Evaluate
- ↓ BP
- ↓ Frequency of anginal attacks
- Prevention of myocardial reinfarction and associated mortality

Mexiletine hydrochloride

(mex-**ILL**-eh-teen)
Pregnancy Category: C
Mexitil **(Rx)**
Classification: Antiarrhythmic, class IB

See also *Antiarrhythmic Drugs.*
Action/Kinetics: Mexiletine is similar to lidocaine but is effective PO. The drug inhibits the flow of sodium into the cell, thereby reducing the rate of rise of the action potential. The drug decreases the effective refractory period in Purkinje fibers. BP and pulse rate are not affected following use, but there may be a small decrease in CO and an increase in peripheral vascular resistance. The drug also has both local anesthetic and anticonvulsant effects. **Onset:** 30–120 min. **Peak blood levels:** 2–3 hr. **Therapeutic plasma levels:** 0.5–2 mcg/mL. **Plasma t½:** 10–12 hr. Approximately 10% excreted unchanged in the urine; acidification of the urine enhances excretion, whereas alkalinization decreases excretion.

Uses: Documented life-threatening ventricular arrhythmias (such as ventricular tachycardia). *Investigational:* Prophylactically to decrease the incidence of ventricular tachycardia and other ventricular arrhythmias in the acute phase of MI. To reduce pain, dysesthesia, and paresthesia associated with diabetic neuropathy.

Contraindications: Cardiogenic shock, preexisting second- or third-degree AV block (if no pacemaker is present). Use with lesser arrhythmias. Lactation.

Special Concerns: There is the possibility of increased risk of death when used in clients with non-life-threatening cardiac arrhythmias. Use with caution in hypotension, severe CHF, or known seizure disorders. Dosage has not been established in children.

Side Effects: *CV: Worsening of arrhythmias,* palpitations, chest pain, increased ventricular arrhythmias (PVCs), CHF, angina or angina-like pain, hypotension, bradycardia, syncope, *AV block or conduction disturbances,* atrial arrhythmias, hypertension, *cardiogenic shock,* hot flashes, edema. *GI:* High incidence of N&V, heartburn. Also, diarrhea or constipation, changes in appetite, dry mouth, abdominal cramps or pain, abdominal discomfort, salivary changes, dysphagia, altered taste, pharyngitis, changes in oral mucous membranes, upper GI bleeding, peptic ulcer, esophageal ulceration. *CNS:* High incidence of lightheadedness, dizziness, tremor, coordination difficulties, and nervousness. Also, changes in sleep habits, headache, fatigue, weakness, tinnitus, paresthesias, numbness, depression, confu-

M

sion, difficulty with speech, short-term memory loss, hallucinations, malaise, psychosis, *seizures,* loss of consciousness. *Hematologic:* Leukopenia, neutropenia, agranulocytosis, thrombocytopenia. *GU:* Decreased libido, impotence, urinary hesitancy or retention. *Dermatologic:* Rash, dry skin. Rarely, exfoliative dermatitis, and *Stevens-Johnson syndrome. Miscellaneous:* Blurred vision, visual disturbances, dyspnea, arthralgia, fever, diaphoresis, loss of hair, hiccoughs, laryngeal or pharyngeal changes, syndrome of SLE, myelofibrosis.

OD **Overdose Management:** *Symptoms:* CNS symptoms (dizziness, drowsiness, paresthesias, seizures) usually precede CV symptoms (hypotension, sinus bradycardia, intermittent left bundle branch block, *temporary asystole). Massive overdoses cause coma and respiratory arrest. Treatment:* General supportive treatment. Give atropine to treat hypotension or bradycardia. Acidification of the urine may increase rate of excretion.

Drug Interactions
Aluminum hydroxide / ↓ Absorption of mexiletine
Atropine / ↓ Absorption of mexiletine
Cimetidine / ↑ or ↓ Plasma levels of mexiletine
Magnesium hydroxide / ↓ Absorption of mexiletine
Metoclopramide / ↑ Absorption of mexiletine
Narcotics / ↓ Absorption of mexiletine
Phenobarbital / ↓ Plasma levels of mexiletine
Phenytoin / ↑ Clearance → ↓ plasma levels of mexiletine
Rifampin / ↑ Clearance → ↓ plasma levels of mexiletine
Theophylline / ↑ Effect of theophylline due to ↑ serum levels
Urinary acidifiers / ↑ Rate of excretion of mexiletine
Urinary alkalinizers / ↓ Rate of excretion of mexiletine
Laboratory Test Interferences: ↑ AST. Positive ANA.

Dosage ⎯⎯⎯⎯⎯⎯
• **Capsules**
  Antiarrhythmic.
Adults, individualized, initial: 200 mg q 8 hr if rapid control of arrhythmia not required; dosage adjustment may be made in 50- or 100-mg increments q 2–3 days, if required. **Maintenance:** 200–300 mg q 8 hr, depending on response and tolerance of client. If adequate response is not achieved with 300 mg or less q 8 hr, 400 mg q 8 hr may be tried although the incidence of CNS side effects increases. If the drug is effective at doses of 300 mg or less q 8 hr, the same total daily dose may be given in divided doses q 12 hr (e.g., 450 mg q 12 hr). Maximum total daily dose: 1,200 mg.
  Rapid control of arrhythmias.
Initial loading dose: 400 mg followed by a 200-mg dose in 8 hr.
  Diabetic neuropathy.
Initial: 150 mg/day for 3 days; **then,** 300 mg/day for 3 days. **Maintenance:** 10 mg/kg/day.

RESPIRATORY CARE CONSIDERATIONS

See also *Respiratory Care Considerations* for *Antiarrhythmic Drugs.*
Administration/Storage
1. The dose should be reduced in clients with severe liver disease and marked right-sided CHF.
2. If transferring to mexiletine from other class I antiarrhythmics, mexiletine may be initiated at a dose of 200 mg and then titrated according to the response at the following times: 6–12 hr after the last dose of quinidine sulfate, 3–6 hr after the last dose of procainamide, 6–12 hr after the last dose of disopyramide, or 8–12 hr after the last dose of tocainide.
3. When transferring to mexiletine, the client should be hospitalized if there is a chance that withdrawal of the previous antiarrhythmic may produce life-threatening arrhythmias.
Assessment
1. Document indications for therapy and type and onset of symptoms.

2. List any other agents trialed and the outcome.

3. Note any evidence of CHF and assess ECG for evidence of AV block.

4. Document pulmonary assessment findings; note arterial oxygen percent return(SaO$_2$) and/or partial pressure of oxygen (PO$_2$).

5. Obtain baseline ECG, CXR, CBC, electrolytes, and liver and renal function studies and monitor throughout therapy.

Interventions

1. Review ECG for increased arrhythmias and report.

2. Observe for adverse CNS effects such as dizziness, tremor, impaired coordination, and N&V and supervise activity.

3. Obtain urinary pH to determine alkalinity or acidity. Alkalinity decreases renal excretion and acidity increases renal excretion of the drug.

Evaluate

• Control of ventricular arrhythmias
• Restoration of stable cardiac rhythm
• Therapeutic serum drug levels (0.5–2 mcg/mL)
• Control of symptoms of diabetic neuropathy

Mezlocillin sodium
(mez-low-**SILL**-in)
Pregnancy Category: B
Mezlin **(Rx)**
Classification: Antibiotic, penicillin

See also *Anti-Infectives* and *Penicillins*.

Action/Kinetics: Mezlocillin is a broad-spectrum (gram-negative and gram-positive organisms, including aerobic and anaerobic strains) antibiotic used parenterally. **Therapeutic serum levels:** 35–45 mcg/mL. t½: **IV,** 55 min. Excreted mostly unchanged by the kidneys. Penetration to CSF is poor unless meninges are inflamed.

Uses: Septicemia and infections of the lower respiratory tract, urinary tract, abdomen, skin, and female genital tract caused by *Klebsiella, Proteus, Pseudomonas, Escherichia coli, Bacteroides, Peptococcus, Streptococcus faecalis* (enterococcus), *Peptostreptococcus,* and *Enterobacter.* Also, *Neisseria gonorrhoeae* infections of the urinary tract and female genital system. Infections caused by *Streptococcus pneumoniae* and group A beta-hemolytic streptococcus.

Additional Side Effects: Bleeding abnormalities. Decreased hemoglobin or hematocrit values.

Laboratory Test Interferences: ↑ AST, ALT, serum alkaline phosphatase, serum bilirubin, serum creatinine, and/or BUN. ↓ Serum potassium.

Dosage ─────────

• **IV, IM**
Serious infections.
Adults: 200–300 mg/kg/day in four to six divided doses; **usual:** 3 g q 4 hr or 4 g q 6 hr. **Infants and children, 1 month–12 years:** 50 mg/kg q 4 hr given IM or IV over 30 min; **infants more than 2 kg and less than 1 week of age or less than 2 kg and less than 1 week of age:** 75 mg/kg q 12 hr; **infants less than 2 kg and more than 1 week of age:** 75 mg/kg q 8 hr; **infants more than 2 kg and more than 1 week of age:** 75 mg/kg q 6 hr.
Life-threatening infections.
Adults: Up to 350 mg/kg/day, not to exceed 24 g/day.
Gonococcal urethritis.
Adults: Single dose of 1–2 g with probenecid, 1 g.
Prophylaxis of postoperative infection.
Adults: 4 g 30–90 min prior to start of surgery; **then,** 4 g, IV, 6 and 12 hr later.
Prophylaxis of infection in clients undergoing cesarean section.
First dose: 4 g IV when cord is clamped; **second and third doses:** 4 g IV 4 and 8 hr after the first dose.

RESPIRATORY CARE CONSIDERATIONS

See also *Respiratory Care Considerations* for *Penicillins*.

Administration/Storage

1. When given by IV infusion (including piggyback), administration of other drugs should be discontinued during administration of mezlocillin.
2. Drug is very irritating to veins. Direct IV administration should be slow to prevent phlebitis; 1 g over 3–5 min. May further dilute in 50–100 mL of dextrose or saline solution and administer over 30 min.
3. For pediatric IV administration, infuse over 30 min.
4. Vials and infusion bottles should be stored at temperatures below 30°C (86°F).
5. The powder and reconstituted solution may darken slightly, but potency is not affected.
6. IM doses should not exceed 2 g/injection. Mezlocillin should be continued for at least 2 days after symptoms of infection have disappeared.
7. For group A beta-hemolytic streptococcus, therapy should continue for at least 10 days.

Assessment

1. Note any sensitivity to penicillin or cephalosporins.
2. Obtain appropriate specimens for culture prior to initiating therapy.
3. Obtain baseline CBC, PT, PTT, electrolytes, and renal function studies and monitor during therapy.
4. Anticipate reduced dosage in clients with impaired renal function.

Evaluate

- Negative culture reports
- Reports of symptomatic improvement
- Serum drug levels within therapeutic range (35–45 mcg/mL)

Milrinone lactate

(**MILL**-rih-nohn)
Pregnancy Category: C
Primacor **(Rx)**
Classification: Inotropic/vasodilator

Action/Kinetics: Milrinone is a selective inhibitor of peak III cyclic AMP phosphodiesterase isozyme in cardiac and vascular muscle. This results in a direct inotropic effect and a direct arterial vasodilator activity. In addition to improving myocardial contractility, milrinone improves diastolic function as manifested by improvements in LV diastolic relaxation. In clients with depressed myocardial function, the drug produces a prompt increase in CO and a decrease in pulmonary wedge pressure and vascular resistance, without a significant increase in HR or myocardial oxygen consumption. Milrinone has an inotropic effect in clients who are fully digitalized without causing signs of glycoside toxicity. Also, LV function has improved in clients with ischemic heart disease. **Therapeutic plasma levels:** 150–250 ng/mL. **t½:** 2.3 hr following doses of 12.5–125 mcg/kg to clients with CHF. The drug is metabolized in the liver and excreted primarily through the urine.

Uses: Short-term treatment of CHF, usually in clients receiving digoxin and diuretics.

Contraindications: Hypersensitivity to the drug. Use in severe obstructive aortic or pulmonic valvular disease in lieu of surgical relief of the obstruction.

Special Concerns: Use with caution during lactation. Safety and efficacy have not been determined in children.

Side Effects: *CV: Ventricular and supraventricular arrhythmias, including ventricular ectopic activity, nonsustained ventricular tachycardia, sustained ventricular tachycardia, and ventricular fibrillation. Infrequently, life-threatening arrhythmias associated with preexisting arrhythmias,* metabolic abnormalities, abnormal digoxin levels, and catheter insertion. Also, hypotension, angina, chest pain. *Miscellaneous:* Mild to moderately severe headaches, hypokalemia, tremor, thrombocytopenia, bronchospasm (rare).

OD **Overdose Management:** *Symptoms:* Hypotension. *Treatment:* If hypotension occurs, reduce or temporarily discontinue administration of milrinone until the condition of the client stabilizes. General measures should be used for supporting circulation.

Dosage ⎯⎯⎯⎯⎯⎯⎯⎯⎯
• **IV Infusion**
Adults, loading dose: 50 mcg/kg administered slowly over 10 min. **Maintenance, minimum:** 0.59 mg/kg/24 hr (infused at a rate of 0.375 mcg/kg/min); **maintenance, standard:** 0.77 mg/kg/24 hr (infused at a rate of 0.5 mcg/kg/min); **maintenance, maximum:** 1.13 mg/kg/24 hr (infused at a rate of 0.75 mcg/kg/min).

RESPIRATORY CARE CONSIDERATIONS
Administration/Storage
1. IV infusions should be administered at rates described in the package insert.
2. The infusion rate should be adjusted depending on the hemodynamic and clinical response.
3. Dilutions of milrinone may be prepared using 0.45% or 0.9% sodium chloride injection or 5% dextrose injection.
4. Clients with renal impairment require a reduced infusion rate (see package insert for chart).
5. Furosemide should not be given in IV lines containing milrinone as a precipitate will form.
6. Store at room temperatures of 15°C–30 °C (59° F–86°F).
Assessment
1. Document indications for therapy and type and onset of symptoms.
2. Identify other medications used and the outcome.
3. Obtain baseline CBC, electrolytes, and liver and renal function studies.
4. Document baseline ECG, CO, CVP, and PCWP and ensure that acute MI has been ruled out.
Interventions
1. Monitor and record I&O, electrolyte

levels, and renal function. If diuresis is excessive, assess for hypokalemia.
2. Potassium loss due to excessive diuresis may result in arrhythmias in digitalized clients. Thus, hypokalemia must be corrected before or during milrinone use.
3. Monitor VS closely during milrinone infusion. Obtain written parameters for interruption of infusion (e.g., SBP < 80; HR < 50).
4. Observe cardiac rhythm for evidence of increased supraventricular and ventricular arrhythmias.
Evaluate
• ↑ CO and ↓ PCWP
• Resolution of S&S of CHF
• Therapeutic serum drug levels (150–250 ng/mL)

Minoxidil, oral
(mih-**NOX**-ih-dil)
Pregnancy Category: C
Loniten **(Rx)**
Classification: Antihypertensive, depresses sympathetic nervous system

See also *Antihypertensive Agents*.
Action/Kinetics: Decreases elevated BP by decreasing peripheral resistance by a direct effect. Drug causes increase in renin secretion, increase in cardiac rate and output, and salt/water retention. It does not cause orthostatic hypotension. **Onset:** 30 min. **Peak plasma levels:** reached within 60 min; **plasma t½:** 4.2 hr. **Duration:** 24–48 hr. Ninety percent absorbed from GI tract; excretion: renal (90% metabolites). The time needed to reach the maximum effect is inversely related to the dose.
Uses: Severe hypertension not controllable by the use of a diuretic plus two other antihypertensive drugs. Usually taken with at least two other antihypertensive drugs (a diuretic and a drug to minimize tachycardia such as a beta-adrenergic blocking agent). Minoxidil can produce severe side effects; it should be reserved for resistant cases of hypertension. Close medical supervision re-

quired, including possible hospitalization during initial administration. Topically to promote hair growth in balding men.

Contraindications: Pheochromocytoma. Within 1 month after a MI. Dissecting aortic aneurysm.

Special Concerns: Safe use during lactation not established. Use with caution and at reduced dosage in impaired renal function. Geriatric clients may be more sensitive to the hypotensive and hypothermic effects of minoxidil; also, it may be necessary to decrease the dose in these clients due to age-related decreases in renal function. BP controlled too rapidly may cause syncope, stroke, MI, and ischemia of affected organs. Experience with use in children is limited.

Side Effects: *CV:* Edema, *pericardial effusion that may progress to tamponade* (acute compression of heart caused by fluid or blood in pericardium), CHF, angina pectoris, changes in direction of T waves, increased HR. In children, rebound hypertension following slow withdrawal. *GI:* N&V. *CNS:* Headache, fatigue. *Hypersensitivity:* Rashes, including bullous eruptions and *Stevens-Johnson syndrome.* *Hematologic:* Initially, decrease in hematocrit, hemoglobin, and erythrocyte count but all return to normal. Rarely, thrombocytopenia and leukopenia. *Other:* Hypertrichosis (enhanced hair growth, pigmentation and thickening of fine body hair 3–6 weeks after initiation of therapy), breast tenderness, darkening of skin.

OD **Overdose Management:** *Symptoms:* Excessive hypotension. *Treatment:* Give NSS IV (to maintain BP and urine output). Vasopressors, such as phenylephrine and dopamine, can be used but only in underperfusion of a vital organ.

Drug Interactions: Concomitant use with guanethidine may result in severe hypotension.

Laboratory Test Interferences: Nonspecific changes in ECG. ↑ Alkaline phosphatase, serum creatinine, and BUN.

Dosage ———————————
- **Tablets**
  Hypertension.
Adults and children over 12 years, Initial: 5 mg/day. For optimum control, dose can be increased to 10, 20, and then 40 mg in single or divided doses/day. Daily dosage should not exceed 100 mg. **Children under 12 years: Initial,** 0.2 mg/kg/day. Effective dose range: 0.25–1.0 mg/kg/day. Dosage must be titrated to individual response. Daily dosage should not exceed 50 mg.

RESPIRATORY CARE CONSIDERATIONS

See also *Respiratory Care Considerations* for *Antihypertensive Agents.*

Administration/Storage
1. Can be taken with fluids and without regard to meals.
2. The drug should be given once daily if the supine diastolic pressure has been reduced less than 30 mm Hg and twice daily (in two equal doses) if it has been reduced more than 30 mm Hg.
3. The interval between dosage adjustments should be at least 3 days as the full response is not obtained until then. However, if more rapid control is required, adjustments can be made q 6 hr but with careful monitoring.

Assessment
1. Anticipate that minoxidil therapy will be initiated in the hospital. After medication administration, BP decreases within 30 min and the client reaches minimum BP within 2–3 hr.
2. List all agents prescribed for this condition, length of use, and the outcome.
3. Determine if concomitant diruetic is prescribed.
4. Note cardiopulmonary findings.
5. Clients receiving guanethidine concomitantly may experience severe hypotensive effects that may be precipitated by a drug interaction.
6. Obtain baseline CBC, glucose, electrolytes, and renal function studies.

Evaluate: ↓ BP with control of refractory hypertension

Mivacurium chloride
(**mih**-vah-**KYOUR**-ee-um)
Pregnancy Category: C
Mivacron **(Rx)**
Classification: Neuromuscular blocking agent

See also *Neuromuscular Blocking Agents.*

Action/Kinetics: Mivacurium competitively inhibits the action of acetylcholine on the motor end plate, resulting in a block of neuromuscular transmission. The time to maximum neuromuscular blockade is similar to atracurium (2.3–4.9 min in adults depending on the dose and 1.6–2.8 min in children depending on the dose). **Clinically effective neuromuscular block, adults:** 15–20 min after 0.15 mg/kg; **children:** 6–15 min after 0.2 mg/kg. Spontaneous recovery may be 95% complete in 25–30 min after an initial dose of 0.15 mg/kg in adults during opioid/nitrous oxide/oxygen anesthesia. Repeated administration or continuous infusion (for up to 2.5 hr) does not cause tachyphylaxis or cumulative neuromuscular blockade. Higher doses may cause transient decreases in mean arterial BP (especially seen in obese clients) and increases in HR in some clients within 1–3 min following the dose (can be minimized by giving the drug over 30–60 sec). The product is actually a mixture of isomers with varying elimination half-lives. The drug is inactivated by plasma cholinesterase with metabolites excreted in the urine and bile.

Uses: Adjunct to general anesthesia to facilitate tracheal intubation and to provide relaxation of skeletal muscle during surgery or mechanical ventilation.

Contraindications: Sensitivity to mivacurium or other similar agents. Use of multidose vials in clients with allergy to benzyl alcohol.

Special Concerns: Use with caution during lactation. Use with caution in clients with significant CV disease and in those with any history of a greater sensitivity to the release of histamine or related mediators such as asthma. Volatile anesthetics may decrease the dosing requirement and prolong the duration of action. The duration of action of mivacurium may be prolonged in clients with decreased plasma cholinesterase. Reduced clearance of one or more isomers is observed in clients with end-stage kidney or liver disease. Geriatric clients show a longer duration of neuromuscular blockade. Acid-base or serum electrolyte abnormalities may potentiate or antagonize the action of neuromuscular blocking agents. Antagonism of neuromuscular blockade may be delayed in the presence of debilitation, carcinomatosis, and concomitant use of certain broad-spectrum antibiotics, anesthetic agents, and other drugs that enhance neuromuscular blockade. In children 2–12 years of age, mivacurium has a faster onset, shorter duration, and a faster recovery following reversal than adults. The drug has not been studied in children less than 2 years of age.

Side Effects: *Neuromuscular:* Prolonged neuromuscular blockade, muscle spasms. *CV:* Flushing of face, neck, or chest; hypotension, tachycardia, bradycardia, cardiac arrhythmias, phlebitis. *Respiratory:* **Bronchospasm,** wheezing, hypoxemia. *Dermatologic:* Rash, urticaria, erythema, reaction at injection site. *CNS:* Dizziness.

OD **Overdose Management:** *Symptoms:* Neuromuscular blockade beyond the time needed for surgery and anesthesia. Increased risk of hemodynamic side effects such as hypotension. *Treatment:*

• Primary treatment is maintenance of a patent airway and controlled ventilation until there is recovery of normal neuromuscular function.

• Neostigmine (0.03–0.064 mg/kg) or edrophonium (0.5 mg/kg) can be given once there is evidence of recovery from neuromuscular blockade.

• A peripheral nerve stimulator can be used to assess recovery and antagonism of neuromuscular block.

Drug Interactions

See *Neuromuscular Blocking Agents.*

Also, there is enhanced neuromuscular blockade when magnesium is given to pregnant women for toxemia.

Dosage ————————————

• **IV Only**

Facilitation of tracheal intubation.

Adults: 0.15 mg/kg given over 5–15 sec. Maintenance doses of 0.1 mg/kg provide about 15 min of additional clinically effective blockade.

Children, 2–12 years: The dosage requirements on a mg/kg basis are higher in children and onset and recovery occur more rapidly. **Initial:** 0.2 mg/kg given over 5–15 sec.

Facilitation of tracheal intubation using continuous IV infusion.

Continuous IV infusion may be used to maintain neuromuscular block. **Adults:** On evidence of spontaneous recovery from an initial dose, an initial infusion rate of 9–10 mcg/kg/min is recommended. If continuous infusion is started at the same time as the administration of an initial dose, a lower initial infusion rate (such as 4 mcg/kg/min) should be used. In either case, the initial infusion rate should be adjusted according to the response to peripheral nerve stimulation and to clinical criteria. An average infusion rate of 6–7 mcg/kg/min will maintain neuromuscular block within the range of 89%–99% for extended periods of time in adults receiving opioid/nitrous oxide/oxygen anesthesia. **Children:** Require higher infusion rates. During opioid/nitrous oxide/oxygen anesthesia, the infusion rate needed to maintain 89%–99% blockade averages 14 mcg/kg/min (range: 5–31 mcg/kg/min).

Tracheal intubation in clients with renal or hepatic impairment.

0.15 mg/kg. Infusion rates should be decreased by as much as 50% in these clients depending on the degree of renal or hepatic impairment.

Use in clients with reduced cholinesterase activity.

Initial doses greater than 0.03 mg/kg are not recommended.

Use in clients who are cachectic, are debilitated, or have carcinomatosis or neuromuscular disease.

A test dose of 0.015–0.02 mg/kg is recommended.

Use with isoflurane or enflurane anesthesia.

An initial dose of 0.15 mg/kg may be used for intubation prior to administration of the isoflurane or enflurane. If mivacurium is given after establishment of anesthesia, the initial dose should be reduced by as much as 25% and the infusion rate should be decreased by as much as 35%–40%. When used with halothane, no adjustment of the initial dose is necessary but the infusion rate should be decreased by as much as 20%.

Use in burn clients.

A test dose of not more than 0.015–0.02 mg/kg is recommended, followed by additional dosing guided by the use of a neuromuscular block monitor.

Use in obese clients weighing equal to or greater than 30% more than their ideal body weight (IBW).

The initial dose is calculated using the IBW according to the following formulas:

Men: IBW in kg = (106 + [6 × height in inches above 5 ft])/2.2

Women: IBW in kg = (100 + [5 × height in inches above 5 ft])/2.2

Use in clients with clinically significant CV disease or in those with any history of a greater sensitivity to the release of histamine or related mediators (asthma).

An initial dose less than or equal to 0.15 mg/kg given over 60 sec.

RESPIRATORY CARE CONSIDERATIONS

See also *Respiratory Care Considera-*

tions for *Neuromuscular Blocking Agents.*

Administration/Storage
1. The drug should only be given in carefully adjusted dosage under the supervision of trained clinicians who know the action of the drug as well as possible complications from its use. The drug should only be given if personnel and facilities for resuscitation and life support are available immediately.
2. For adults and children, the amount of infusion solution required per hour depends on the clinical requirements, the concentration of mivacurium in the infusion solution, and the weight of the client. Tables provided by the manufacturer should be consulted to determine the infusion rates using either the premixed infusion of 0.5 mg/mL or the injection containing 2 mg/mL.
3. Dosage adjustment may be necessary in the presence of significant liver, kidney, or CV disease; in obese clients weighing more than 30% of their ideal body weight for height; asthma; those with reduced plasma cholinesterase activity; and the use of inhalation general anesthetics.
4. Additives should not be introduced into mivacurium premixed infusion in flexible plastic containers.
5. Mivacurium premixed infusion should be clear and the container undamaged. It is intended for use in a single client only and any unused portion should be discarded.
6. Mivacurium in vials (2 mg/mL) may be diluted to 0.5 mg/mL with 5% dextrose injection, 5% dextrose and 0.9% sodium chloride injection, 0.9% sodium chloride injection, lactated Ringer's injection, or 5% dextrose in lactated Ringer's injection and then given by Y-site injection and titrated to desired response. The dilution is stable when stored in polyvinyl chloride bags at 5°C–25°C (41°F–77°F). The dilution should be used within 24 hr and is intended

for use in a single client only with any unused portion discarded.
7. Mivacurium injection is compatible with sufentanil citrate injection, alfentanil hydrochloride injection, fentanyl citrate injection, midazolam hydrochloride injection, and droperidol injection. However, it may not be compatible with alkaline solutions having a pH greater than 8.5 (e.g., barbiturate solutions).
8. The injection and premixed infusion are stored at 15°C–25°C (59°F–77°F); exposure to direct ultraviolet light should be avoided and the products should not be frozen or exposed to excessive heat.

Assessment
1. Note indications for therapy. Review conditions and drugs that antagonize and enhance neuromuscular blockade and assess for their presence.
2. Note any history of CV disease or asthma.
3. Obtain baseline ABGs, electrolytes, and liver and renal function studies.
4. Multidose vials contain benzyl alcohol; assess for any client intolerance.
5. Clients homozygous for the atypical plasma cholinesterase gene are quite sensitive to mivacurium neuromuscular blocking effects.
6. Burn clients may show resistance depending on the time elapsed since the burn and the size of the burn; however, clients with burns may have decreased plasma cholinesterase, which offsets the resistance.

Interventions
1. Mivacurium should only be administered in a carefully monitored environment and by persons specially trained in the use of neuromuscular blocking agents.
2. Anticipate reduced dose with liver or renal dysfunction.
3. To avoid distress, ensure that client is unconscious or sedated before administering mivacurium.
4. Use a peripheral nerve stimulator to measure neuromuscular function

(assess response), adjust dosage, and confirm recovery (5-sec head lift and grip strength).

5. Geriatric clients show a longer duration of neuromuscular blockade.

6. Monitor VS. Mivacurium will not counteract the bradycardia produced by many anesthetic agents or by vagal stimulation.

7. Advise that transient flushing, wheezing, and tachycardia may be experienced.

Evaluate

• Desired skeletal muscle relaxation

• Successful tracheal intubation

• Adequate suppression of twitch response on peripheral nerve stimulation tests

Moexipril hydrochloride

(moh-**EX**-ih-prill)

Pregnancy Category: C (first trimester), D (second and third trimesters)

Univasc **(Rx)**

Classification: Angiotensin-converting enzyme inhibitor

See also *Angiotensin-Converting Enzyme Inhibitors.*

Action/Kinetics: Moexipril is converted in the liver to the active moexiprilat. **Onset:** 1 hr. **Duration:** 24 hr. Food decreases absorption of the drug. **t½, moexiprilat:** 2–9 hr. About 50% is bound to plasma protein. The active metabolite is excreted through both the urine and feces.

Uses: Treatment of hypertension alone or in combination with thiazide diuretics.

Contraindications: In those with a history of angioedema as a result of previous treatment with ACE inhibitors. Lactation.

Special Concerns: Use with caution in clients with impaired renal function or renal artery stenosis, hyperkalemia, CHF, severe hepatic impairment, and volume depletion. Those who are salt or volume depleted are at a greater risk of developing hypotension. Safety and efficacy have not been determined in children.

Side Effects: *GI:* Abdominal pain, N&V, diarrhea, dysgeusia, constipation, dry mouth, dyspepsia, pancreatitis, hepatitis, changes in appetite, weight changes. *CNS:* Insomnia, sleep disturbances, headache, dizziness, fatigue, drowsiness/sleepiness, malaise, nervousness, anxiety, mood changes. *CV:* Chest pain, hypotension, palpitations, angina pectoris, **CVA, MI,** orthostatic hypotension, rhythm disturbances, peripheral edema. *Respiratory:* Cough, bronchospasm, dyspnea, upper respiratory infection, sinusitis. *GU:* Oliguria, urinary frequency, renal insufficiency. *Dermatologic:* Flushing, rash, diaphoresis, photosensitivity, pruritus, urticaria, pemphigus. *Musculoskeletal:* Myalgia, arthralgia. *Miscellaneous:* Angioedema, neutropenia, syncope, anemia, tinnitus, flu syndrome, pharyngitis, pain, rhinitis.

Drug Interactions

Diuretics / Excessive hypotension

Lithium / Moexipril ↑ serum levels of lithium → lithium toxicity

Potassium-sparing diuretics / ↑ Hyperkalemic effect of moexipril

Potassium supplements / ↑ Hyperkalemic effect of moexipril

Dosage —————————

• **Tablets**

Hypertension.

Initial, adults not receiving diuretics: 7.5 mg 1 hr before meals once daily. Dose is adjusted depending on response. **Maintenance:** 7.5–30 mg daily in one or two divided doses 1 hr before meals.

Initial, adults receiving diuretics: Discontinue diuretic 2–3 days before beginning moexipril at a dose of 7.5 mg. If BP is not controlled, diuretic therapy can be resumed. If diuretic cannot be discontinued, give moexipril in an initial dose of 3.75 mg once daily 1 hr before meals. In those with impaired renal function, start with 3.75 mg once daily if creatinine clearance is less than 40 mL/min/1.73 m². The dose may be increased to a maximum of 15 mg/day.

RESPIRATORY CARE CONSIDERATIONS

See also *Respiratory Care Considerations* for *Angiotensin-Converting Enzyme Inhibitors*.

Administration/Storage: The drug should be taken on an empty stomach 1 hr before meals.

Assessment

1. Document indications for therapy, onset and duration of disease, and other agents trialed and the outcome.

2. Note any evidence of dehydration, CHF, or hyperkalemia.

3. Obtain baseline ECG, electrolytes, and liver and renal function studies and monitor periodically during therapy.

4. Anticipate reduced dosage with renal impairment.

Evaluate: ↓ BP with control of hypertension

Montelukast sodium

(MAHN-teh-loo-kast)
Pregnancy Category: B
Singulair

Action/Kinetics: Cysteinyl leukotrienes (LTC$_4$, LTD$_4$, LTE$_4$) are products of arachidonic acid metabolism. These eicosanoids are released from various cells, especially mast cells and eosinophils, and bind to cysteinyl leukotriene receptors (CysLT) in the human airways. This type of reaction is associated with the pathophysiology of asthma, contributing to airways edema, smooth muscle contraction, and inflammatory processes. Montelukast binds to the CysLT$_1$ receptor and thereby blocks the physiologic actions of LTD$_4$. Montelukast is rapidly absorbed via the oral route. Mean peak plasma concentration (C$_{max}$) is achieved in 3 to 4 hours with the 10 mg tablet with a mean bioavailability of 64%. C$_{max}$ and mean bioavailability with the 5 mg tablet is 2 to 2.5 hours and 73% with fasting and 63% with a standard meal in the morning. The bi-oavailability and C$_{max}$ are not influenced by a standard meal in the morning with the 10 mg tablet. The drug is readily metabolized and eliminated primarily via the bile. t½: 2.7 to 5.5 hours in healthy young adults.

Uses: Prophylaxis and chronic treatment of asthma in patients 6 years of age or older.

Contraindications: Hypersensitivity to any component of montelukast.

Special Concerns: Montelukast should not be used for the reversal of bronchospasm in acute asthmatic episodes. Though inhaled and oral corticosteroids may be tapered over time with the use of montelukast, montelukast should not be an abrupt substitute for corticosteroids. Montelukast should not be used as monotherapy for exercise-induced bronchospasm. Patients susceptible to exercise-induced asthma attacks should continue their usual regimen of β-agonists for prophylaxis and rescue therapy. Though montelukast has been demonstrated to reduce bronchoconstrictor response to aspirin in those asthmatics with known aspirin sensitivity, these patients should continue to adhere to a regimen of avoidance of aspirin and other non-steroidal anti-inflammatory agents while taking montelukast. Reduction in corticosteroid use with the use of another leukotriene antagonist has on rare occurrences been associated with the development of Churg-Strauss syndrome, a systemic eosinophilic vasculitis which is manifested as eosinophilia, vasculitic rash, worsening pulmonary symptoms, cardiac symptoms, and/or neuropathy. A causal relationship with leukotriene receptor antagonism has not been established and the phenomenon was not seen during clinical trials with montelukast.

Side Effects: The following experiences were noted in adult (15 years or older) clinical trials at greater than

M

1% of patients with an incidence greater than placebo: asthenia/fatigue, fever, abdominal pain, trauma, dyspepsia, infections gastroenteritis, dental pain, dizziness, headache, nasal congestion, cough, influenza, rash, and pyuria. In the pediatric patients, the following events were noted with a frequency of greater than 2% with incidence reater than placebo: diarrhea, laryngitis, pharyngitis, nausea, otitis, sinusitis, and vial finection. No causal relationships were established for the noted side effects and prolonged treatment did not significantly alter the adverse experience profiles.

OD **Overdose Management:** In chronic asthma studies, patients received up to 200 mg/day for 22 weeks and, in short-term studies, dosages up to 900 mg/day were administered without clinically important adverse effects. In the event of overdose, usual supportive measures should be considered, e.g., removal of unabsorbed material from the GI tract, clinical monitoring, and supportive therapy as indicated. The effectiveness of peritoneal dialysis or hemodialysis is unknown.

Laboratory Test Interferences: ↑ ALT and ↑ AST.

Dosage ————————————
• **Tablets**
Patients 15 years of age and older: one 10 mg tablet daily in the evening. Patients 6 to 14 years of age: one 5 mg chewable tablet daily in the evening. Safety and efficacy in children less than 6 years of age have not been established.

RESPIRATORY CARE CONSIDERATIONS
Administration/Storage: Tablets should be stored at room temperature (15-30°C) and protected from moisture and light.
Assessment
1. Note any hepatic impairment though no dosage adjustment has been necessary for mild-to-moderate hepatic impairment.
2. Note use of drugs such as pheno-

barbital and rifampin which induce hepatic metabolism and invoke appropriate clinical monitoring.
3. Institute monitoring of daytime asthma symptoms, use of PRN β-agonists, AM and PM peak flows, and nocturnal awakenings with use of montelukast.

Client/Family Teaching
1. Take montelukast daily as prescribed, even when symptomatic, as well as during asthma exacerbations. Contact physician if asthma is not well controlled.
2. Do not use montelukast tablets for the treatment of acute asthma attacks. Rather, short-acting β-agonists should be employed for acute exacerbations.
3. Medical attention should be sought while using montelukast if short-acting inhaled bronchodilators are employed more often than usual or if the maximum number of inhalations prescribed are exceeded during any 24-hour period.
4. Patients taking montelukast should not decrease or stop dosage of other antiasthmatic medications without instructions from a physician.
5. Patients susceptible to exercise-induced bronchospasm should continue to use inhaled β-agonists as prophylaxis unless otherwise instructed by a physician. Short-acting inhaled β-agonists for rescue treatment should always be available.
6. Aspirin and NSAID avoidance should be continued by those patients with known aspirin sensitivity.

Moricizine hydrochloride
(mor-**IS**-ih-zeen)
Pregnancy Category: B
Ethmozine **(Rx)**
Classification: Antiarrhythmic, class I

See also *Antiarrhythmic Agents*.
Action/Kinetics: Moricizine causes a stabilizing effect on the myocardial membranes as well as local anesthetic activity. The drug shortens phase II and III repolarization leading to a decreased duration of the action

potential and an effective refractory period. Also, there is a decrease in the maximum rate of phase O depolarization and a prolongation of AV conduction in clients with ventricular tachycardia. Whether the client is at rest or is exercising, moricizine has minimal effects on cardiac index, stroke index volume, systemic or pulmonary vascular resistance or ejection fraction, and pulmonary capillary wedge pressure. There is a small increase in resting BP and HR. The time, course, and intensity of antiarrhythmic and electrophysiologic effects are not related to plasma levels of the drug. **Onset:** 2 hr. **Peak plasma levels:** 30–120 min. **t½:** 1.5–3.5 hr (reduced after multiple dosing). **Duration:** 10–24 hr. 95% is protein bound. Significant first-pass effect. Metabolized almost completely by the liver with metabolites excreted through both the urine and feces; the drug induces its own metabolism. Food delays the rate of absorption resulting in lower peak plasma levels; however, the total amount absorbed is not changed.

Uses: Documented life-threatening ventricular arrhythmias (e.g., sustained ventricular tachycardia) where benefits of the drug are determined to outweigh the risks. *Investigational:* Ventricular premature contractions, couplets, and nonsustained ventricular tachycardia.

Contraindications: Preexisting second- or third-degree block, right bundle branch block when associated with bifascicular block (unless the client has a pacemaker), cardiogenic shock. Use during lactation.

Special Concerns: There is the possibility of increased risk of death when used in clients with non-life-threatening cardiac arrhythmias. Safety and effectiveness in children less than 18 years of age have not been determined. Geriatric clients have a higher rate of side effects. Increased survival rates following use of antiarrhythmic drugs have not been proven in clients with ventricular arrhythmias. Use with caution in clients with sick sinus syndrome due to the possibility of sinus bradycardia, sinus pause, or sinus arrest. Use with caution in clients with CHF.

Side Effects: *CV: **Proarrhythmias, including new rhythm disturbances or worsening of existing arrhythmias;** ECG abnormalities, including conduction defects, sinus pause, junctional rhythm, AV block; palpitations, **sustained ventricular tachycardia,** cardiac chest pain, CHF, **cardiac death,** hypotension, hypertension, atrial fibrillation, atrial flutter, syncope, bradycardia, **cardiac arrest, MI, pulmonary embolism,** vasodilation, thrombophlebitis, **cerebrovascular events.** CNS:* Dizziness (common), anxiety, headache, fatigue, nervousness, paresthesias, sleep disorders, tremor, anxiety, hypoesthesias, depression, euphoria, somnolence, agitation, confusion, *seizures,* hallucinations, loss of memory, vertigo, coma. *GI:* Nausea, dry mouth, abdominal pain, vomiting, diarrhea, dyspepsia, anorexia, ileus, flatulence, dysphagia, bitter taste. *Musculoskeletal:* Asthenia, abnormal gait, akathisia, ataxia, abnormal coordination, dyskinesia, pain. *GU:* Urinary retention, dysuria, urinary incontinence, urinary frequency, impotence, kidney pain, decreased libido. *Respiratory:* Dyspnea, apnea, asthma, hyperventilation, pharyngitis, cough, sinusitis. *Opthalmologic:* Nystagmus, diplopia, blurred vision, eye pain, periorbital edema. *Dermatologic:* Rash, pruritus, dry skin, urticaria. *Miscellaneous:* Sweating, drug fever, hypothermia, temperature intolerance, swelling of the lips and tongue, speech disorder, tinnitus, jaundice.

OD **Overdose Management:** *Symptoms:* Vomiting, hypotension, lethargy, worsening of CHF, **MI, conduction disturbances, arrhythmias (e.g., junctional bradycardia, ventricular tachycardia, ventricular fibrillation, asystole), sinus arrest, respiratory failure.** *Treatment:* In acute over-

M

dose, induce vomiting, taking care to prevent aspiration. Client should be hospitalized and closely monitored for cardiac, respiratory, and CNS changes. Provide life support, including an intracardiac pacing catheter, if necessary.

Drug Interactions
Cimetidine / ↑ Plasma levels of moricizine due to ↓ excretion
Digoxin / Additive prolongation of the PR interval (but no significant increase in the rate of second- or third-degree AV block)
Propranolol / Additive prolongation of the PR interval
Theophylline / ↓ Plasma levels of theophylline due to ↑ rate of clearance
Laboratory Test Interferences: ↑ Bilirubin and liver transaminases.

Dosage ———————
- **Tablets**
  Antiarrhythmic.
Adults: 600–900 mg/day in equally divided doses q 8 hr. If needed, the dose can be increased in increments of 150 mg/day at 3-day intervals until the desired effect is obtained. In clients with hepatic or renal impairment, the initial dose should be 600 mg or less with close monitoring and dosage adjustment.

RESPIRATORY CARE CONSIDERATIONS

See also *Respiratory Care Considerations* for *Antiarrhythmic Agents.*
Administration/Storage
1. When transferring clients from other antiarrhythmics to moricizine, the previous drug should be withdrawn for one to two plasma half-lives before starting moricizine. For example, when transferring from quinidine or disopyramide, moricizine can be started 6–12 hr after the last dose; when transferring from procainamide, moricizine can be initiated 3–6 hr after the last dose; when transferring from mexiletine, propafenone, or tocainide, moricizine can be started 8–12 hr after the last dose; and, when transferring from flecai-

nide, moricizine can be started 12–24 hr after the last dose.
2. If clients are well controlled on an 8-hr regimen, they might be given the same total daily dose q 12 hr to increase compliance.
Assessment
1. Document cardiac history and note any preexisting conditions and ECG abnormalities.
2. Obtain baseline ECG, electrolytes, CXR, pulmonary function tests, and liver and renal function studies.
3. List drugs client currently taking to determine any potential adverse interactions.
Interventions
1. Monitor cardiac rhythm closely to observe for drug-induced rhythm disturbances during therapy.
2. Anticipate lower initial doses in clients with impaired hepatic or renal function.
3. Clients should be hospitalized for initial dosing because they will be at high risk. Antiarrhythmic response may be determined by ECG, exercise testing, or programmed electrical stimulation testing.
4. Correct any electrolyte imbalance before initiating drug therapy.
5. Document and monitor pacing parameters in clients with pacemakers.
6. Monitor VS and report any persistent temperature elevations.
Evaluate: Termination of life-threatening ventricular arrhythmias

Morphine hydrochloride
(**MOR**-feen)
Pregnancy Category: C
Morphitec ✦, M.O.S. ✦, M.O.S.-S.R. ✦ **(Rx)**

Morphine sulfate
(**MOR**-feen **SUL**-fayt)
Pregnancy Category: C
Astramorph PF, Duramorph, Epimorph ✦, Infumorph, Kadian, M-Eslon ✦, Morphine HP ✦, MS Contin, MS-IR, MSIR Capsules, Oramorph SR, RMS, RMS Rectal Suppositories, Roxanol, Roxanol 100, Roxanol Rescudose, Roxanol UD, Statex ✦ **(C-II) (Rx)**

Classification: Narcotic analgesic, morphine type

See also *Narcotic Analgesics.*
Action/Kinetics: Morphine is the prototype for opiate analgesics. **Onset:** approximately 15–60 min, based on epidural or intrathecal use. **Peak effect:** 30–60 min. **Duration:** 3–6 hr. **t½:** 1.5–2 hr. Oral morphine is only one-third to one-sixth as effective as parenteral products.
Uses: Intrathecally, epidurally, PO (including sustained-release products), or by continuous IV infusion for acute or chronic pain. In low doses, morphine is more effective against dull, continuous pain than against intermittent, sharp pain. Large doses, however, will dull almost any kind of pain. Preoperative medication. To facilitate induction of anesthesia and reduce dose of anesthetic. *Investigational:* Acute LV failure (for dyspneic seizures) and pulmonary edema. Morphine should not be used with papaverine for analgesia in biliary spasms but may be used with papaverine in acute vascular occlusions.
Additional   Contraindications: Epidural or intrathecal morphine if infection is present at injection site, in clients on anticoagulant therapy, bleeding diathesis, if client has received parenteral corticosteroids within the past 2 weeks.
Special Concerns: Morphine may increase the length of labor. Clients with known seizure disorders may be at greater risk for morphine-induced seizure activity.

Dosage
• **Capsules, Tablets, Oral Solution, Soluble Tablets, Syrup**
Analgesia.
10–30 mg q 4 hr.
• **Sustained-Release Tablets**
Analgesia.
30 mg q 8–12 hr, depending on client needs and response. Kadian is indicated for once-daily dosing at doses of 20, 50, or 100 mg where analgesia is indicated for just a few days.

• **IM, SC**
Analgesia.
Adults: 5–20 mg/70 kg q 4 hr as needed; **pediatric:** 100–200 mcg/kg up to a maximum of 15 mg.
• **IV Infusion**
Analgesia.
Adults: 2.5–15 mg/70 kg in 4–5 mL of water for injection (should be administered slowly over 4–5 min).
• **IV Infusion, Continuous**
Analgesia.
Adults: 0.1–1 mg/mL in D5W by a controlled-infusion pump.
• **Rectal Suppositories**
Adults: 10–20 mg q 4 hr.
• **Intrathecal**
Adults: 0.2–1 mg as a single daily injection.
• **Epidural**
Initial: 5 mg/day in the lumbar region; if analgesia is not manifested in 1 hr, increasing doses of 1–2 mg can be given, not to exceed 10 mg/day. For continuous infusion, 2–4 mg/day with additional doses of 1–2 mg if analgesia is not satisfactory.

RESPIRATORY CARE CONSIDERATIONS

See also *Respiratory Care Considerations* for *Narcotic Analgesics.*
Administration/Storage
1. May be administered with food to diminish GI upset. Controlled-release tablets should not be crushed or chewed.
2. Immediate-release capsules may be swallowed intact or the contents of the capsule may be sprinkled on food or stirred in juice to avoid the bitter taste. The contents of the capsule may also be delivered through a nasogastric or a gastric tube.
3. For IV use, dilute 2–10 mg with at least 5 mL sterile water or NSS and administer over 4–5 min. For continous infusions, reconstitute to a concentration of 0.1–1 mg/mL and administer as prescribed to control symptoms.
4. Rapid IV administration increases the risk of adverse effects; a narcotic antagonist (e.g., naloxone) should

M

be available at all times if morphine is given IV.

5. For intrathecal use, no more than 2 mL of the 5-mg/10 mL preparation or 1 mL of the 10-mg/10 mL product should be given.

6. Intrathecal administration should be only in the lumbar region; repeated injections are not recommended.

7. To reduce the chance of side effects with intrathecal administration, a constant IV infusion of naloxone (0.6 mg/hr for 24 hr after intrathecal injection) is recommended.

8. In certain circumstances (e.g., tolerance, severe pain), the physician may prescribe doses higher than those listed under *Dosage*.

9. Use an electronic infusion device for IV solutions. May also be administered by PCA pump.

10. Obtain written parameters for BP and respirations during IV infusions.

11. Dose may be lower in geriatric clients or those with respiratory disease.

12. Have respiratory support and naloxone available in the event of overdose.

Assessment

1. Document indications for therapy and type, onset, location, and characteristics of pain. Rate pain utilizing a pain-rating scale.

2. List other agents prescribed and the outcome.

3. Note any history of seizure disorder.

4. Determine if client is a candidate for PCA via pump.

Evaluate

• Relief of pain

• Control of respirations during mechanical ventilation

N

Nadolol

(**NAY**-doh-lohl)
Pregnancy Category: C
Apo-Nadol ✦, Corgard, Syn-Nadolol ✦ **(Rx)**
Classification: Beta-adrenergic blocking agent

See also *Beta-Adrenergic Blocking Agents.*

Action/Kinetics: Manifests both beta-1- and beta-2-adrenergic blocking activity. Has no membrane stabilizing or intrinsic sympathomimetic activity. Low lipid solubility. **Peak serum concentration:** 3–4 hr. **t½:** 20–24 hr (permits once-daily dosage). **Duration:** 17–24 hr. Absorption variable, averaging 30%; steady plasma level achieved after 6–9 days of administration. Excreted unchanged by the kidney.

Uses: Hypertension, either alone or with other drugs (e.g., thiazide diuretic). Angina pectoris. *Investigational:* Prophylaxis of migraine, ventricular arrhythmias, aggressive behavior, essential tremor, tremors associated with lithium or parkinsonism, antipsychotic-induced akathisia, rebleeding of esophageal varices, situational anxiety, reduce intraocular pressure.

Contraindications: Bronchial asthma or bronchospasm, including severe COPD.

Special Concerns: Dosage has not been established in children.

Dosage

• **Tablets**

Hypertension.

Initial: 40 mg/day; **then,** may be increased in 40- to 80-mg increments until optimum response obtained. **Maintenance:** 40–80 mg/day although up to 240–320 mg/day may be needed.

Angina.

Initial: 40 mg/day; **then,** increase dose in 40- to 80-mg increments q 3–7 days until optimum response obtained. **Maintenance:** 40–80

mg/day, although up to 160–240 mg/day may be needed.
Aggressive behavior.
40–160 mg/day.
Antipsychotic-induced akathisia.
40–80 mg/day.
Essential tremor.
120–240 mg/day.
Lithium-induced tremors.
20–40 mg/day.
Tremors associated with parkinsonism.
80–320 mg/day.
Prophylaxis of migraine.
40–80 mg/day.
Rebleeding from esophageal varices.
40–160 mg/day.
Situational anxiety.
20 mg.
Ventricular arrhythmias.
10–640 mg/day.
Reduction of intraocular pressure.
10–20 mg b.i.d.
NOTE: Dosage for all uses should be decreased in clients with renal failure.

RESPIRATORY CARE CONSIDERATIONS

See also *Respiratory Care Considerations* for *Beta-Adrenergic Blocking Agents* and *Antihypertensive Agents.*
Evaluate
• ↓ BP, ↓ HR
• ↓ Frequency and intensity of angina attacks

Nafcillin sodium

(naf-**SILL**-in)
Nafcil, Nallpen, Unipen **(Rx)**
Classification: Antibiotic, penicillin

See also *Anti-Infectives* and *Penicillins.*
Action/Kinetics: Nafcillin is penicillinase-resistant and acid stable. Used for resistant staphylococcal infections. Parenteral therapy is recommended initially for severe infections. **Peak plasma levels: PO,** 7 mcg/mL after 30–60 min; **IM,** 14–20 mcg/mL after 30–60 min. **t½:** 60

min. Significantly bound to plasma proteins.
Uses: Infections by penicillinase-producing staphylococci; also certain pneumococci and streptococci. As initial therapy if staphylococcal infection is suspected (i.e., until results of culture have been obtained).
Additional Side Effects: Sterile abscesses and thrombophlebitis occur frequently, especially in the elderly.

Dosage ───────────
• **IV**
Adults: 0.5–1 g q 4 hr.
• **IM**
Adults: 0.5 g q 4–6 hr. **Children and infants:** 25 mg/kg b.i.d. **Neonates:** 10 mg/kg b.i.d. Or, for neonates weighing less than 2,000 g and less than 7 days of age, a dose of 25 mg/kg b.i.d. can be given; for neonates weighing more than 2,000 g but older than 7 days, a dose of 75 mg/kg/day divided q 6 hr.
• **Capsules**
Mild to moderate infections.
Adults: 250–500 mg q 4–6 hr.
Severe infections.
Adults: Up to 1 g q 4–6 hr.
Pneumonia/scarlet fever.
Children: 25 mg/kg/day in four divided doses.
Staphylococcal infections.
Children: 50 mg/kg/day in four divided doses. **Neonates:** 10 mg/kg t.i.d.–q.i.d.
Streptococcal pharyngitis.
Children: 250 mg t.i.d.
NOTE: IV administration is not recommended for neonates or infants.

RESPIRATORY CARE CONSIDERATIONS

See also *Respiratory Care Considerations* for *Penicillins.*
Administration/Storage
1. Reconstitute for PO use by adding powder to bottle of diluent. Replace cap tightly. Then shake thoroughly until all powder is in solution. Check carefully for undissolved powder at the bottom of bottle. Solution must be

N

stored in refrigerator and unused portion discarded after 1 week.

2. Reconstitute for parenteral use by adding required amount of sterile water. Shake vigorously. Date, time, and initial bottle. Refrigerate after reconstitution and discard unused portion after 48 hr.

3. For direct IV administration, dissolve powder in 15–30 mL of sterile water for injection or isotonic sodium chloride solution and inject over 5- to 10-min period into the tubing of flowing IV infusion. For IV drip, dissolve the required amount in 100–150 mL of isotonic sodium chloride injection and administer by IV drip over a period of 30–90 min.

4. IV use should be reserved for therapy of 24–48 hr duration due to the possibility of thrombophlebitis, especially in geriatric clients. Reduce rate of flow and report any pain, redness, or edema at site of IV administration.

5. Do not administer IV to newborn infants.

6. Administer IM by deep intragluteal injection.

7. Serum levels after PO administration are low and unpredictable.

Evaluate

• Laboratory evidence of negative C&S results

• ↓ WBC, ↓ temperature, and reports of symptomatic improvement

---

Nalbuphine hydrochloride
(**NAL**-byou-feen)
Nubain **(Rx)**
Classification: Narcotic agonist/antagonist

See also *Narcotic Analgesics*.

Action/Kinetics: Nalbuphine, a synthetic compound resembling oxymorphone and naloxone, is a potent analgesic with both narcotic agonist and antagonist actions. Its analgesic potency is approximately equal to that of morphine, while its antagonistic potency is approximately one-fourth that of nalorphine. **Onset: IV,** 2–3 min; **SC or IM,** <15 min. **Peak effect: 30–60 min. Duration: 3–6 hr; t½:** 5 hr.

Uses: Moderate to severe pain. Preoperative analgesia, anesthesia adjunct, obstetric analgesia.

Contraindications: Hypersensitivity to drug. Children under 18 years.

Special Concerns: Safe use during pregnancy (except for delivery) and lactation not established. Use with caution in presence of head injuries and asthma, MI (if client is nauseous or vomiting), biliary tract surgery (may induce spasms of sphincter of Oddi), renal insufficiency. Clients dependent on narcotics may experience withdrawal symptoms following use of nalbuphine.

Additional Side Effects: Even though nalbuphine is an agonist-antagonist, it may cause dependence and may precipitate withdrawal symptoms in an individual physically dependent on narcotics. *CNS:* Sedation is common. Crying, feelings of unreality, and other psychologic reactions. *GI:* Cramps, dry mouth, bitter taste, dyspepsia. *Skin:* Itching, burning, urticaria, sweaty, clammy skin. *Other:* Blurred vision, difficulty with speech, urinary frequency.

Drug Interactions: Concomitant use with CNS depressants, other narcotics, phenothiazines, may result in additive depressant effects.

Dosage ————
• **SC, IM, IV**
  Analgesia.
Adults: 10 mg/70 kg q 3–6 hr as needed (single dose should not exceed 20 mg q 3–6 hr; total daily dose should not exceed 160 mg).

RESPIRATORY CARE CONSIDERATIONS

See also *Respiratory Care Considerations* for *Narcotic Analgesics*.

Administration/Storage: Nalbuphine hydrochloride may be administered IV, undiluted. Administer each 10 mg or less over a 3- to 5-min period.

Assessment

1. Take a complete history, noting any evidence of dependence on nar-

cotics. Nalbuphine may precipitate withdrawal symptoms in clients with narcotic addiction.

2. Note any history of head injuries, asthma, or cardiac dysfunction because the drug may be contraindicated.

3. Document any sulfite sensitivity.

4. Determine onset, location, duration, and intensity of pain. Use a pain-rating scale to assess pain.

Evaluate: Desired level of pain control

Nalmefene hydrochloride
(**NAL**-meh-feen)
Pregnancy Category: B
Revex **(Rx)**
Classification: Narcotic antagonist

See also *Narcotic Antagonists.*

Action/Kinetics: Nalmefene prevents or reverses respiratory depression, sedation, and hypotension due to opioids, including propoxyphene, nalbuphine, pentazocine, and butorphanol. Nalmefene has a significantly longer duration of action than naloxone. The drug does not produce respiratory depression, psychotomimetic effects, or pupillary constriction (i.e., it has no intrinsic activity). Also, tolerance, physical dependence, or abuse potential have not been noted. **Onset, after IV:** 2 min. **Duration:** Up to 8 hr. **t½:** 10.8 hr. Nalmefene is metabolized by the liver and is excreted in the urine.

Uses: For complete or partial reversal of the effects of opioid drugs postoperatively. Management of known or suspected overdose of opiates.

Special Concerns: Nalmefene will precipitate acute withdrawal symptoms in those who have some degree of tolerance and dependence on opioids. Use with caution in high CV risk clients or in those who have received potentially cardiotoxic drugs. Reversal of buprenorphine-induced respiratory depression may be incomplete; therefore artificial respiration may be necessary. Use with caution during lactation. Safety

and effectiveness have not been determined in children.

Side Effects: *CV:* Tachycardia, hypertension, hypotension, vasodilation, bradycardia, arrhythmia. *GI:* N&V, diarrhea, dry mouth. *CNS:* Dizziness, somnolence, depression, agitation, nervousness, tremor, confusion, withdrawal syndrome, myoclonus. *Body as a whole:* Fever, headache, chills, postoperative pain. *Miscellaneous:* Pharyngitis, pruritus, urinary retention.

Laboratory Test Interferences: ↑ AST.

Dosage

• **IV**

Reversal of postoperative depression due to opiates.

Adults: Titrate in 0.25-mcg/kg incremental doses at 2–5-min intervals until the desired degree of reversal is achieved (i.e., adequate ventilation and alertness without significant pain or discomfort). In cases where the client is known to be at an increased CV risk, the incremental dose should be 0.1 mcg/kg (the drug may be diluted 1:1 with saline or sterile water). A total dose greater than 1 mcg/kg does not provide additional effects.

Management of known or suspected overdose of opiates.

Adults, initial: 0.5 mg/70 kg; **then,** 1 mg/70 kg 2–5 min later, if needed. Doses greater than 1.5 mg/70 kg do not increase the beneficial effect. If there is a reasonable suspicion of dependence on opiates, a challenge dose of nalmefene of 0.1 mg/70 kg should be given first; if there is no evidence of withdrawal in 2 min, the recommended dose can be given.

RESPIRATORY CARE CONSIDERATIONS

See also *Respiratory Care Considerations* for *Narcotic Antagonists.*
Administration/Storage
1. Treatment with nalmefene should follow, not precede, the establishment of a patent airway, ventilatory

bold italic = life threatening side effect

assistance, administration of oxygen, and establishment of circulatory access.

2. Nalmefene is supplied in two concentrations—ampules containing 1 mL (blue label) at a concentration suitable for postoperative use (100 mcg) and ampules containing 2 mL (green label) suitable for management of overdose (1 mg/mL), i.e., **10 times as concentrated.** Specific guidelines should be followed, depending on the use.

3. Should IV access be lost or not readily obtainable, nalmefene can be given by the SC or IM route at doses of 1 mg. This dose is effective in 5–15 min.

Assessment

1. Document type of agent used, when administered/ingested, and amount (dosage).

2. Note any history or evidence of opioid dependence as drug may induce acute withdrawal symptoms.

3. Identify clients at high CV risk or those who have received potentially cardiotoxic drugs as the risk for cardiac complications may be increased.

Interventions

1. Ensure that ventilatory assistance, patent airway, and circulatory access are established.

2. Observe client carefully to ensure there is no risk of recurrent respiratory depression.

3. Compared to naloxone (1.1 hr) the half-life of nalmefene is much longer (10.8 hr). Even though nalmefene has a long duration of action, overdose with long-acting opiates (e.g., methadone, LAAM) may cause recurrence of respiratory depression.

4. With renal failure, if more than one dose is required, administer incremental doses slowly (over 60 sec) to prevent the occurrence of dizziness and hypertension.

5. Advise client of side effects that may be experienced (N&V, fever, headaches, chills, pain, dizziness, and tachycardia) with this drug therapy.

Evaluate

• Reversal of opioid-induced drug effects
• ↓ Risk of renarcotization

Naloxone hydrochloride
(nal-**OX**-ohn)
Pregnancy Category: B
Narcan **(Rx)**
Classification: Narcotic antagonist

See also *Narcotic Antagonists.*

Action/Kinetics: Naloxone, administered by itself, does not produce significant pharmacologic activity. Since the duration of action of naloxone is shorter than that of the narcotic analgesics, the respiratory depression may return when the narcotic antagonist has worn off. **Onset: IV,** 2 min; **SC, IM: <5 min. Time to peak effect: 5–15 min. Duration: Dependent on dose and route of administration but may be as short as 45 min. t½:** 60–100 min. Metabolized in the liver to inactive products that are eliminated through the kidneys.

Uses: Respiratory depression induced by natural and synthetic narcotics, including butorphanol, methadone, nalbuphine, pentazocine, and propoxyphene. Drug of choice when nature of depressant drug is not known. Diagnosis of acute opiate overdosage. Not effective when respiratory depression is induced by hypnotics, sedatives, or anesthetics and other nonnarcotic CNS depressants. Adjunct to increase BP in septic shock. *Investigational:* Treatment of Alzheimer's dementia, alcoholic coma, and schizophrenia.

Contraindications: Sensitivity to drug. Narcotic addicts (drug may cause severe withdrawal symptoms). Not recommended for use in neonates.

Special Concerns: Safe use during lactation and in children is not established.

Side Effects: N&V, sweating, hypertension, tremors, sweating due to reversal of narcotic depression. If used postoperatively, excessive doses may cause ***ventricular tachycardia and fibrillation,*** hypo- or hypertension, pulmonary edema, and ***seizures (infrequent)***.

Dosage
- **IV, IM, SC**
  Narcotic overdose.
Initial: 0.4–2 mg IV; if necessary, additional IV doses may be repeated at 2- to 3-min intervals. If no response after 10 mg, reevaluate diagnosis. **Pediatric, initial:** 0.01 mg/kg IV; **then,** 0.1 mg/kg IV, if needed. The SC or IM route may be used if an IV route is not available.
  To reverse postoperative narcotic depression.
Adults: IV, initial, 0.1- to 0.2-mg increments at 2- to 3-min intervals; **then,** repeat at 1- to 2-hr intervals if necessary. Supplemental IM dosage increases the duration of reversal. **Children: Initial,** 0.005–0.01 mg IV at 2- to 3-min intervals until desired response is obtained.
  Reverse narcotic-induced depression in neonates.
Initial: 0.01 mg/kg IV, IM, or SC. May be repeated using adult administration guidelines.

RESPIRATORY CARE CONSIDERATIONS

See also *Respiratory Care Considerations* for *Narcotic Antagonists.*
Administration/Storage
1. May administer undiluted at a rate of 0.4 mg over 15 sec with narcotic overdosage. The drug may be reconstituted, 2 mg in 500 mL of NSS or 5% dextrose to provide a concentration of 4 mcg/mL or 0.004 mg/mL. The rate of administration varies with the response of the client.
2. Do not mix naloxone with preparations containing bisulfite, metabisulfite, long-chain or high molecular weight anions, or solutions with an alkaline pH.
3. When naloxone is mixed with other solutions, they should be used within 24 hr.

4. Naloxone is effective within 2 min after IV administration.
Assessment
1. Document indications for therapy and type, onset, and duration of symptoms.
2. Identify any evidence of narcotic addiction.
3. Note baseline cardiopulmonary and neurologic assessments.
Interventions
1. The duration of the effects of the narcotic may exceed the effects of naloxone (the antagonist). Therefore, more than one dose may be necessary to counteract the effects of the narcotic. Observe client closely and determine narcotic half-life.
2. Monitor VS at 5-min intervals, then every 30 min once stabilized.
3. For acutely ill clients or those who are in a coma, attach to a cardiac monitor and have a suction machine immediately available.
4. Titrate drug to avoid interfering with pain control or readminister narcotic at a lower dosage to maintain desired level of pain control.
Evaluate: Reversal of narcotic-induced respiratory depression

Naltrexone
(nal-**TREX**-ohn)
Pregnancy Category: C
ReVia **(Rx)**
Classification: Narcotic antagonist

See also *Narcotic Antagonists.*
Action/Kinetics: Naltrexone binds to opiate receptors, thereby reversing or preventing the effects of narcotics. This is an example of competitive inhibition. **Peak plasma levels:** 1 hr. **Duration:** 24–72 hr. Metabolized in the liver; a major metabolite—6-beta-naltrexol—is active. **Peak serum levels, after 50 mg: naltrexone,** 8.6 ng/mL; **6-beta-naltrexol,** 99.3 ng/mL. **t½: naltrexone,** approximately 4 hr; **6-beta-naltrexol,** 13 hr. Naltrexone and its metabolites are excreted in the urine.
Uses: To prevent narcotic use in former narcotic addicts. Adjunct to the

psychosocial treatment for alcoholism. *Investigational:* To treat eating disorders and postconcussional syndrome not responding to other approaches.

Contraindications: Clients taking narcotic analgesics, those dependent on narcotics, those in acute withdrawal from narcotics. Liver failure, acute hepatitis.

Special Concerns: Use with caution during lactation. Safety during lactation and in children under 18 years of age has not been established.

Side Effects: *CNS:* Headache, anxiety, nervousness, sleep disorders, dizziness, change in energy level, depression, confusion, restlessness, disorientation, hallucinations, nightmares, bad dreams, paranoia, fatigue, drowsiness. *GI:* N&V, diarrhea, constipation, anorexia, abdominal pain or cramps, flatulence, ulcers, increased appetite, weight gain or loss, increased thirst, xerostomia, hemorrhoids. *CV:* Phlebitis, edema, increased BP, changes in ECG, palpitations, epistaxis, tachycardia. *GU:* Delayed ejaculation, increased urinary frequency or urinary discomfort, increased or decreased interest in sex. *Respiratory:* Cough, sore throat, nasal congestion, rhinorrhea, sneezing, excess secretions, hoarseness, SOB, heaving breathing, sinus trouble. *Dermatologic:* Rash, oily skin, itching, pruritus, acne, cold sores, alopecia, athlete's foot. *Musculoskeletal:* Joint/muscle pain, muscle twitches, tremors, pain in legs, knees, or shoulders. *Ophthalmologic:* Blurred vision, aching or strained eyes, burning eyes, lightsensitive eyes, swollen eyes. *Other:* Hepatotoxicity, tinnitus, painful or clogged ears, chills, swollen glands, inguinal pain, cold feet, "hot" spells, "pounding" head, fever, yawning, side pains.

A severe narcotic withdrawal syndrome may be precipitated if naltrexone is administered to a dependent individual. The syndrome may begin within 5 min and may last for up to 2 days.

Dosage ⎯⎯⎯⎯⎯⎯⎯

• **Tablets**

To produce blockade of opiate actions.

Initial: 25 mg followed by an additional 25 mg in 1 hr if no withdrawal symptoms occur. **Maintenance:** 50 mg/day.

Alternate dosing schedule for blockade of opiate actions.

The weekly dose of 350 mg may be given as: (a) 50 mg/day on weekdays and 100 mg on Saturday; (b) 100 mg/48 hr; (c) 100 mg every Monday and Wednesday and 150 mg on Friday; or, (d) 150 mg q 72 hr.

Alcoholism.

50 mg once daily for up to 12 weeks. Treatment for longer than 12 weeks has not been studied.

RESPIRATORY CARE CONSIDERATIONS

See also *Respiratory Care Considerations* for *Narcotic Antagonists.*

Administration/Storage

1. Naltrexone therapy should **never** be initiated until it has been determined that the individual is not dependent on narcotics (i.e., a naloxone challenge test should be completed).

2. The client should be opiate free for at least 7–10 days before beginning naltrexone therapy.

3. When initiating naltrexone therapy, begin with 25 mg and observe for 1 hr for any signs of narcotic withdrawal.

4. The blockade produced by naltrexone may be overcome by taking large doses of narcotics. Such doses may be fatal.

5. Clients taking naltrexone may not respond to preparations containing narcotics for use in coughs, diarrhea, or pain.

Assessment

1. Determine if addicted to opiates and when the last dose was ingested as client must be opiate free for 7–10 days before initiating therapy.

2. Obtain VS and monitor daily. Report if the respirations are severely lowered or if the client complains of difficulty breathing.

3. Obtain baseline ECG prior to initiating therapy.
4. Perform baseline liver function studies and monitor monthly during the first 6 months of therapy.
5. Ensure that urinalysis confirms absence of opiates and that naloxone challenge test has been performed before initiating drug therapy.
Evaluate: Maintenance of narcotic-free state in detoxified addicts

Nedocromil sodium
(neh-**DAH**-kroh-mill)
Pregnancy Category: B
Tilade **(Rx)**
Classification: Antiasthmatic

Action/Kinetics: Nedocromil is an inhalation anti-inflammatory drug for the prophylaxis of asthma. It inhibits the release of various mediators, such as histamine, leukotriene C_4, and prostaglandin D_2, from a variety of cell types associated with asthma. The drug has no intrinsic bronchodilator, antihistamine, or glucocorticoid activity; also, systemic bioavailability is low. **t½:** 3.3 hr. Nedocromil is about 89% bound to plasma protein; it is excreted unchanged.
Uses: Maintenance therapy in clients with mild to moderate bronchial asthma.
Contraindications: Use for the reversal of acute bronchospasms, especially status asthmaticus.
Special Concerns: Use with caution during lactation. Safety and efficacy have not been established in children less than 12 years of age. Nedocromil has not been shown to be able to substitute for the total dose of corticosteroids.
Side Effects: *Respiratory:* Coughing, pharyngitis, rhinitis, upper respiratory tract infection, increased sputum, bronchitis, dyspnea, ***bronchospasm.*** *GI tract:* N&V, dyspepsia, abdominal pain, dry mouth, diarrhea. *CNS:* Dizziness, dysphonia. *Skin:* Rash, sensation of warmth. *Body as a whole:* Headache, chest pain, fatigue, arthritis. *Miscellaneous:* Viral infection, unpleasant taste.
Laboratory Test Interferences: ↑ ALT.

Dosage ————
• **Metered Dose Inhaler**
  Bronchial asthma.
Adults and children over 12 years of age: Two inhalations q.i.d. at regular intervals in order to provide 14 mg/day. If the client is under good control on q.i.d. dosing (i.e., requiring inhaled or oral beta agonist no more than twice a week or no worsening of symptoms occur with respiratory infections), a lower dose can be tried. In such instances, the dose should first be reduced to 10.5 mg/day (i.e., used t.i.d.); then, after several weeks with good control, the dose can be reduced to 7 mg/day (i.e., used b.i.d.).

RESPIRATORY CARE CONSIDERATIONS
Administration/Storage
1. Each actuation releases 1.75 mg.
2. Nedocromil must be used regularly, even during symptom-free period, in order to achieve beneficial effects.
3. Clients must be taught the proper method of use of the drug. An illustrated pamphlet is included in each pack of nedocromil.
4. Nedocromil should be added to the existing treatment (e.g., bronchodilators). When a clinical response is seen and if the asthma is under good control, a gradual decrease in the concomitant medication can be tried.
5. The drug should be stored between 2°C and 30°C (36°F and 86°F) and should not be frozen.
Assessment
1. Document symptoms, noting type, onset, and duration. List other agents trialed and the outcome.
2. Assess respiratory status thoroughly; drug is not for use with status asthmaticus or for reversal of

acute bronchospasm since drug is not a bronchodilator.

3. Note peak flow and vital capacity measurements and monitor.

4. Document systemic and inhaled steroid therapy accurately. When a reduction is in progress, remind provider that nedocromil cannot substitute for total steroid dose/requirements.

5. Review drug usage and time between prescriptions to ensure proper use by client.

Client/Family Teaching

1. Review correct procedure for administration and observe client technique. Instruct client to use the step-by-step instructions provided with the medication to ensure desired effects.

2. Stress that beneficial *preventative* effects will not be obtained if drug is not correctly administered by topical lung application.

3. Explain that drug is an inhaled anti-inflammatory that reduces lung inflammation.

4. Advise not to stop therapy during symptom-free periods. In order to achieve benefits, drug must be taken at regular intervals.

5. Instruct client to continue to use nedocromil inhaler along with other prescribed therapies unless otherwise specified.

6. Report any persistent headaches, unpleasant taste in mouth that interferes with nutrition, severe nausea, or chest pain.

7. Advise client to report any coughing or bronchospasm following use of nedocromil as drug should be discontinued, lungs assessed, and alternative therapy substituted.

Evaluate: ↓ Severity and frequency of asthmatic episodes

Neostigmine bromide

(nee-oh-**STIG**-meen)
Pregnancy Category: C
Prostigmin Bromide **(Rx)**

Neostigmine methylsulfate

(nee-oh-**STIG**-meen)
Pregnancy Category: C
Prostigmin Injection, PMS-Neostigmine Methylsulfate ✱ **(Rx)**
Classification: Indirectly acting cholinergic-acetylcholinesterase inhibitor

Action/Kinetics: By inhibiting the enzyme acetylcholinesterase, these drugs cause an increase in the concentration of acetylcholine at the myoneural junction, thus facilitating transmission of impulses across the myoneural junction. In myasthenia gravis, muscle strength is increased. The drug may also act on the autonomic ganglia of the CNS. Neostigmine also prevents or relieves postoperative distention by increasing gastric motility and tone and prevents or relieves urinary retention by increasing the tone of the detrusor muscle of the bladder. Shorter acting than ambenonium chloride and pyridostigmine. Atropine is often given concomitantly to control side effects. **Onset:** PO, 45–75 min; **IM,** 20–30 min; **IV,** 4–8 min. **Time to peak effect, parenteral:** 20–30 min. **Duration:** All routes, 2–4 hr. t½, PO: 42–60 min; **IM:** 51–90 min; **IV:** 47–60 min. Eliminated through the urine (about 40% unchanged).

Uses: Diagnosis and treatment of myasthenia gravis. Prophylaxis and treatment of postoperative GI ileus or urinary retention. Antidote for tubocurarine and other nondepolarizing drugs.

Contraindications: Hypersensitivity, mechanical obstruction of GI or urinary tract, peritonitis, history of bromide sensitivity. Vesical neck obstruction of urinary bladder.

Special Concerns: Safe use during lactation not established. Safety and effectiveness in children have not been established. Use with caution in clients with bronchial asthma, bradycardia, vagotonia, epilepsy, hyperthyroidism, peptic ulcer, cardiac arrhythmias, or recent coronary occlusion. May cause uterine irritability and premature labor if given IV to pregnant women near term. In geriatric clients, the duration of action may be increased.

Side Effects: *GI:* N&V, diarrhea, abdominal cramps, involuntary defecation, salivation, dysphagia, flatulence, increased gastric and intestinal secretions. *CV:* Bradycardia, tachycardia, hypotension, ECG changes, nodal rhythm, **cardiac arrest,** syncope, **AV block,** substernal pain, thrombophlebitis after IV use. *CNS:* Headache, **seizures,** malaise, weakness, dysarthria, dizziness, drowsiness, loss of consciousness. *Respiratory:* Increased oral, pharyngeal, and bronchial secretions; **bronchospasms, skeletal muscle paralysis, laryngospasm, central respiratory paralysis, respiratory depression or arrest,** dyspnea. *Ophthalmologic:* Miosis, double vision, lacrimation, accommodation difficulties, hyperemia of conjunctiva, visual changes. *Musculoskeletal:* Muscle fasciculations or weakness, muscle cramps or spasms, arthralgia. *Other:* Skin rashes, urinary frequency and incontinence, sweating, flushing, allergic reactions, anaphylaxis, urticaria. These effects can usually be reversed by parenteral administration of 0.6 mg of atropine sulfate, which should be readily available.

Cholinergic crisis, due to overdosage, must be distinguished from myasthenic crisis (worsening of the disease), since cholinergic crisis involves removal of drug therapy, while myasthenic crisis involves an increase in anticholinesterase therapy.

OD **Overdose Management:** *Symptoms:* Abdominal cramps, vomiting, diarrhea, epigastric distress, excessive salivation, cold sweating, pallor, blurred vision, urinary urgency, fasciculation and **paralysis of voluntary muscles (including the tongue),** miosis, increased BP (may be accompanied by bradycardia), sensation of internal trembling, panic, severe anxiety. *Treatment:* Discontinue medication temporarily. Give atropine, 0.5–1 mg IV (up to 5–10 or more mg may be needed to get the HR to 80 beats/min). Supportive treatment including artificial respiration and oxygen.

Drug Interactions
Aminoglycosides / ↑ Neuromuscular blockade
Atropine / Atropine suppresses symptoms of excess GI stimulation caused by cholinergic drugs
Corticosteroids / ↓ Effect of neostigmine
Magnesium salts / Antagonize the effects of anticholinesterases
Mecamylamine / Intense hypotensive response
Organophosphate-type insecticides/pesticides / Added systemic effects with cholinesterase inhibitors
Succinylcholine / ↑ Neuromuscular blocking effects

Dosage ⎯⎯⎯⎯⎯⎯
NEOSTIGMINE BROMIDE
• **Tablets**
Treat myasthenia gravis.
Adults: 15 mg q 3–4 hr; adjust dose and frequency as needed. **Usual maintenance:** 150 mg/day with dosing intervals determined by client response. **Pediatric,** 2 mg/kg (60 mg/m²) daily in six to eight divided doses.
NEOSTIGMINE METHYLSULFATE
• **IM, IV, SC**
Diagnosis of myasthenia gravis.
Adults, IM, SC: 1.5 mg given with 0.6 mg atropine; **pediatric, IM:** 0.04 mg/kg (1 mg/m²); or, **IV:** 0.02 mg/kg (0.5 mg/m²).
Treat myasthenia gravis.
Adults, IM, SC: 0.5 mg. **Pediatric, IM, SC:** 0.01–0.04 mg/kg q 2–3 hr.
Antidote for tubocurarine.
Adults, IV: 0.5–2 mg slowly with 0.6–1.2 mg atropine sulfate. Can repeat if necessary to total dose of 5 mg. **Pediatric, IV:** 0.04 mg/kg with 0.02 mg/kg atropine sulfate.
Prevention of postoperative GI distention or urinary retention.
Adults, IM, SC: 0.25 mg (1 mL of the 1:4,000 solution) immediately after

surgery repeated q 4–6 hr for 2–3 days.

Treatment of postoperative GI distention.

Adults, IM, SC: 0.5 mg (1 mL of the 1:2,000 solution) as required.

Treatment of urinary retention.

Adults, IM, SC: 0.5 mg (1 mL of the 1:2,000 solution). If urination does not occur within 1 hr after 0.5 mg, the client should be catheterized. After the bladder is emptied, 0.5 mg is given q 3 hr for at least five injections.

RESPIRATORY CARE CONSIDERATIONS
Administration/Storage
1. The interval between doses must be individually determined to achieve optimum effects.
2. If greater fatigue occurs at certain times of the day, a larger part of the daily dose can be administered at these times.
3. Neostigmine should not be given if high concentrations of halothane or cyclopropane are present.
4. May administer IV form undiluted at a rate of 0.5 mg/min.

Assessment
1. Note any history of hypersensitivity to drugs in this category.
2. Identify any drugs the client is taking to determine if they may interact unfavorably with neostigmine.
3. Note any history of bromide sensitivity as drug is contraindicated.

Interventions
1. Observe and report symptoms of generalized cholinergic stimulation; evidence of a toxic reaction.
2. Assess for stability and vision. If the client has difficulty with coordination or vision caution him to avoid use of heavy machinery until the effects of the medication wear off.
3. Monitor VS for the first hour after drug administration. Report if the pulse is less than 80 as the drug should be withheld. If hypotension occurs, have the client remain recumbent until BP stabilizes.
4. When the medication is used as an antidote for nondepolarizing drugs,

assist in the ventilation of the client and maintain a patent airway.
5. If the client is taking the medication for treatment of myasthenia gravis, any onset of weakness 1 hr after administration usually indicates overdosage of drug. The onset of weakness 3 hr or more after administration usually indicates underdosage and/or resistance and should also be documented as well as any associated difficulty with respirations or increase in muscle weakness.

Evaluate
• ↑ Muscle strength and function with myasthenia gravis
• Relief of postoperative ileus or urinary retention
• Reversal of respiratory depression R/T nondepolarizing drugs

Nicardipine hydrochloride
(nye-**KAR**-dih-peen)
Pregnancy Category: C
Cardene, Cardene IV, Cardene SR **(Rx)**
Classification: Calcium channel blocking agent (antianginal, antihypertensive)

See also *Calcium Channel Blocking Agents.*

Action/Kinetics: The drug moderately increases CO and significantly decreases peripheral vascular resistance. **Onset of action:** 20 min. **Maximum plasma levels:** 30–120 min. Significant first-pass metabolism by the liver. Food (especially fats) will decrease the amount of drug absorbed from the GI tract. Steady-state plasma levels are reached after 2–3 days of therapy. **Therapeutic serum levels:** 0.028–0.050 mcg/mL. **t½, at steady state:** 8.6 hr. **Duration:** 8 hr. The drug is highly bound to plasma protein (> 95%) and is metabolized by the liver with excretion through both the urine and feces.

Uses: *Immediate release:* Chronic stable angina (effort-associated angina) alone or in combination with beta-adrenergic blocking agents.

Immediate and sustained released: Hypertension alone or in combination with other antihypertensive drugs.

IV: Short-term treatment of hypertension when PO therapy is not desired or possible.

Investigational: CHF.

Contraindications: Clients with advanced aortic stenosis due to the effect on reducing afterload. During lactation.

Special Concerns: Safety and efficacy in children less than 18 years of age have not been established. Use with caution in clients with CHF, especially in combination with a beta blocker due to the possibility of a negative inotropic effect. Use with caution in clients with impaired liver function, reduced hepatic blood flow, or impaired renal function. Initial increase in frequency, duration, or severity of angina.

Side Effects: *CV:* Pedal edema, flushing, increased angina, palpitations, tachycardia, other edema, abnormal ECG, hypotension, postural hypotension, syncope, ***MI, AV block,*** ventricular extrasystoles, peripheral vascular disease. *CNS:* Dizziness, headache, somnolence, malaise, nervousness, insomnia, abnormal dreams, vertigo, depression, confusion, amnesia, anxiety, weakness, psychoses, hallucinations, paranoia. *GI:* N&V, dyspepsia, dry mouth, constipation, sore throat. *Neuromuscular:* Asthenia, myalgia, paresthesia, hyperkinesia, arthralgia. *Miscellaneous:* Rash, dyspnea, SOB, nocturia, polyuria, allergic reactions, abnormal liver chemistries, hot flashes, impotence, rhinitis, sinusitis, nasal congestion, chest congestion, tinnitus, equilibrium disturbances, abnormal or blurred vision, infection, atypical chest pain.

OD **Overdose Management:** *Symptoms:* Marked hypotension, bradycardia, palpitations, flushing, drowsiness, confusion, and slurred speech following PO overdose. Lethal overdose may cause systemic hypotension, bradycardia (following initial tachycardia), and progressive AV block. *Treatment:*
• Treatment is supportive. Monitor cardiac and respiratory function.
• If client is seen soon after ingestion, emetics or gastric lavage should be considered, followed by cathartics.
• *Hypotension:* IV calcium, dopamine, isoproterenol, metaraminol, or norepinephrine. Also, provide IV fluids. Place client in Trendelenburg position.
• *Ventricular tachycardia:* IV procainamide or lidocaine; also, cardioversion may be necessary. Also, provide slow-drip IV fluids.
• *Bradycardia, asystole, AV block:* IV atropine sulfate (0.6–1 mg), calcium gluconate (10% solution), isoproterenol, norepinephrine; also, cardiac pacing may be indicated. Provide slow-drip IV fluids.

Drug Interactions
Cimetidine / ↑ Bioavailability of nicardipine → ↑ plasma levels
Cyclosporine / ↑ Plasma levels of cyclosporine possibly leading to renal toxicity
Ranitidine / ↑ Bioavailability of nicardipine

Dosage ———————————
• **Capsules, Immediate Release**
Angina, hypertension.
Initial, usual: 20 mg t.i.d. (range: 20–40 mg t.i.d.). Wait 3 days before increasing dose to ensure steady-state plasma levels.
• **Capsules, Sustained Release**
Hypertension.
Initial: 30 mg b.i.d. (range: 30–60 mg b.i.d.).
NOTE: In renal impairment, the initial dose should be 20 mg t.i.d. In hepatic impairment, the initial dose should be 20 mg b.i.d.
• **IV**
Hypertension.
Individualize dose. Initial: 5 mg/hr; the infusion rate may be increased to a maximum of 15 mg/hr (by 2.5-mg/hr increments q 15 min). For a more rapid reduction in BP, in-

itiate at 5 mg/hr but increase the rate q 5 min in 2.5-mg/hr increments until a maximum of 15 mg/hr is reached. **Maintenance:** 3 mg/hr. The IV infusion rate to produce an average plasma level similar to a particular PO dose is as follows: 20 mg q 8 hr is equivalent to 0.5 mg/hr; 30 mg q 8 hr is equivalent to 1.2 mg/hr; and 40 mg q 8 hr is equivalent to 2.2 mg/hr.

RESPIRATORY CARE CONSIDERATIONS

See also *Respiratory Care Considerations* for *Calcium Channel Blocking Agents*.

Administration/Storage

1. The maximum BP-lowering effects for immediate release are seen 1–2 hr after dosing; the maximum BP-lowering effects for sustained release are seen in 2–6 hr.
2. When used for treating clients with angina, nicardipine may be administered safely along with sublingual nitroglycerin, prophylactic nitrates, or beta blockers.
3. When used to treat clients with hypertension, nicardipine may be administered safely along with diuretics or beta blockers.
4. During initial therapy and when dosage is increased, clients may experience an increase in the frequency, duration, or severity of angina.
5. If transfer to PO antihypertensives other than nicardipine is planned, therapy should be initiated after discontinuing the infusion. If PO nicardipine is to be used at a dosage regimen of three times daily, give the first dose 1 hr prior to discontinuing IV infusion.
6. Ampules must be diluted before infusion. Acceptable diluents are 5% dextrose, 5% dextrose and 0.45% sodium chloride, 5% dextrose with 40 mEq potassium, 0.45% sodium chloride, and 0.9% sodium chloride. Nicardipine is incompatible with 5% sodium bicarbonate and lactated Ringer's solution.
7. The infusion concentration should be 0.1 mg/mL. The diluted product is stable at room temperature for 24 hr.
8. Ampules should be stored at room temperature although freezing does not affect the product. Ampules should be protected from light and elevated temperatures.

Assessment

1. Document indications for therapy and type and onset of symptoms.
2. List other agents prescribed and the outcome.
3. Note any history of CHF and if beta blockers prescribed, as this warrants close monitoring.
4. Obtain baseline ECG and renal and liver function studies, noting any evidence of dysfunction.

Interventions

1. Monitor VS. When the immediate-release product is used for hypertension, the maximum lowering of BP occurs 1–2 hr after dosing. Thus, during initiation of therapy BP should be monitored at this interval. Also, BP should be evaluated at the trough (8 hr after dosing). When the sustained-release product is used, maximum lowering of BP occurs 2–6 hr after dosing.
2. Monitor BP frequently during and following IV infusion. Avoid too rapid or excessive decrease in BP and discontinue infusion if there is significant hypotension or tachycardia.

Evaluate

- Control of hypertension
- ↓ Frequency and intensity of anginal attacks
- Therapeutic serum drug levels (0.028–0.050 mcg/mL)

Nicotine polacrilex (Nicotine Resin Complex)

(**NIK**-oh-teen)
Pregnancy Category: X
Nicorette, Nicorette DS, Nicorette Plus ✦ **(OTC)**
Classification: Smoking deterrent

Action/Kinetics: Following chewing, nicotine is released from an ion exchange resin in the gum product, providing blood nicotine levels approximating those produced by smoking cigarettes. The amount of nicotine released depends on the rate and duration of chewing. Following repeated administration q 30 min, nicotine blood levels reach 25–50 ng/mL. If the gum is swallowed, only a minimum amount of nicotine is released. Nicotine is metabolized mainly by the liver, with about 10%–20% excreted unchanged in the urine.

Uses: Adjunct with behavioral modification in smokers wishing to give up the smoking habit. Is considered only as an initial aid, with the ultimate goal being abstention from all forms of nicotine. Most likely to benefit are individuals with the following characteristics:

a. smoke brands of cigarettes containing more than 0.9 mg nicotine;

b. smoke more than 15 cigarettes daily;

c. inhale cigarette smoke deeply and frequently;

d. smoke most frequently during the morning;

e. smoke the first cigarette of the day within 30 min of arising;

f. indicate cigarettes smoked in the morning are the most difficult to give up;

g. smoke even if the individual is ill and confined to bed;

h. find it necessary to smoke in places where smoking is not allowed. *NOTE:* Nicotine may be effective in improving the course of difficult-to-treat ulcerative colitis.

Contraindications: Pregnancy, lactation, nonsmokers, serious arrhythmias, angina, vasospastic disease, active temporomandibular joint disease. Use in individuals less than 18 years of age.

Special Concerns: Safety and effectiveness in children and adolescents who smoke have not been determined. Use with caution in hypertension, PUD, oral or pharyngeal inflammation, gastritis, stomatitis, hyperthyroidism, insulin-dependent diabetes, and pheochromocytoma.

Side Effects: *CNS:* Dizziness, irritability, headache. *GI:* N&V, indigestion, GI upset, salivation, eructation. *Other:* Sore mouth or throat, hiccoughs, sore jaw muscles.

OD   **Overdose Management:** *Symptoms: GI:* N&V, diarrhea, salivation, abdominal pain. *CNS:* Headache, dizziness, confusion, weakness, fainting, **seizures.** *Respiratory:* Labored breathing, ***respiratory paralysis (cause of death).*** *Other:* Cold sweat, disturbed hearing and vision, hypotension, and rapid, weak pulse. *Treatment:* Syrup of ipecac if vomiting has not occurred, saline laxative, gastric lavage followed by activated charcoal (if client is unconscious), support of ventilation, maintenance of CV function.

Drug Interactions
Caffeine / Possibly ↓ blood levels of caffeine due to ↑ rate of breakdown by liver
Catecholamines / ↑ Levels of catecholamines
Cortisol / ↑ Levels of cortisol
Furosemide / Possible ↓ diuretic effect of furosemide
Glutethimide / Possible ↓ absorption of glutethimide
Imipramine / Possibly ↓ blood levels of imipramine due to ↑ rate of breakdown by liver
Pentazocine / Possibly ↓ blood levels of pentazocine due to ↑ rate of breakdown by liver
Theophylline / Possibly ↓ blood levels of theophylline due to ↑ rate of breakdown by liver

Dosage
• **Gum**
Initial: One piece of gum chewed whenever the urge to smoke occurs; however, best results are obtained when the gum is chewed on a fixed schedule, at intervals of 1 to 2 hr, with at least 9 pieces chewed per day. **maintenance:** 9–12 pieces of gum daily during the first month, not to exceed 30 pieces daily of the 2-mg strength and 20 pieces daily of the 4-mg strength.

N

RESPIRATORY CARE CONSIDERATIONS

Administration/Storage

1. Nicotine polacrilex is available as a 2-mg (Nicorette) and 4-mg (Nicorette DS) gum. The 4-mg dosage form was introduced since those heavily addicted to smoking had adapted and their symptoms could not be managed by the 2-mg dosage form. Thus, those who smoke more than 25 cigarettes/day should be started on the 4-mg dose.

2. The individual must want to stop smoking and should do so immediately.

3. Each piece of gum should be chewed slowly for about 30 min.

4. Acidic beverages, such as coffee, juices, soft drinks, and wine, interfere with buccal absorption of nicotine from the gum; thus, eating and drinking 15 min before and during chewing of the nicotine gum should be avoided.

5. Clients should be evaluated monthly and if the individual has not smoked for 3 months, the gum should be slowly withdrawn. Nicotine should not be used for longer than 6 months.

6. Suggested procedures for gradual withdrawal of the gum include:

• decreasing the total number of pieces/day by one or more pieces q 4–7 days.

• decreasing the chewing time with each piece from the normal 30 min to 10–15 min for 4–7 days; then gradually decreasing the number of pieces used per day.

• increasing the chewing time for more than 30 min and reducing the number of pieces used per day.

• substituting one or more pieces of sugarless gum for an equal number of pieces of nicotine gum; then, increasing the number of pieces of sugarless gum substituted for nicotine gum q 4–7 days.

• replacing the 4-mg gum with the 2-mg gum and applying any of the first four procedures listed in the preceding.

Assessment

1. Document nicotine profile: type and brand (cigarettes, chewing tobacco, or cigars), amount used per day, when used, and what increases usage.

2. Note if any temporomandibular joint syndrome or cardiac arrhythmia, as either precludes gum therapy.

Client/Family Teaching

1. Use the gum only as directed. When client has the urge to smoke, chew one piece slowly. When a slight tingling becomes evident, stop chewing until sensation subsides.

2. Advise that too vigorous chewing can increase adverse effects. Provide a printed list of drug (gum) side effects and instruct to report any that are bothersome or of concern.

3. Do not ingest food or liquids 15 min before and during ingestion of the gum as effects may be diminished.

4. Advise that gum will not stick to dentures or appliances.

5. Provide the client with names of local support groups that can help with smoking cessation and provide emotional and psychologic support throughout the endeavor.

6. Advise and support participation and enrollment in a formal smoking cessation program.

Evaluate:
Evidence of control of nicotine withdrawal symptoms with ↓ number of cigarettes smoked per day or complete smoking cessation

Nicotine transdermal system
(**NIK**-oh-teen)
Pregnancy Category: D
Habitrol, Prostep **(Rx)**, Nicoderm QC, Nicotrol **(OTC)**
Classification: Smoking deterrent

Action/Kinetics: Nicotine transdermal system is a multilayered film that provides systemic delivery of varying amounts of nicotine over a 24-hr period after applying to the skin. Nicotine's reinforcing activity is due to two CNS effects. The first is stimulation of the cortex (via the locus ceruleus), producing increased alertness and cognitive performance. The second is a "reward" effect due to an action in the limbic system. At low doses the stimulatory effects predominate, whereas at high doses the reward effects predominate. The nicotine transdermal system produces an initial (first day of use) increase in BP, an increase in HR (3%–7%), and a decrease in SV after 10 days. Nicotine is metabolized in the liver to a large number of metabolites, all of which are less active than nicotine. **t½, following removal of the system from the skin:** 3–4 hr.

Uses: As an aid to stopping smoking for the relief of nicotine withdrawal symptoms. Should be used in conjunction with a comprehensive behavioral smoking cessation program.

Contraindications: Hypersensitivity or allergy to nicotine or any components of the therapeutic system. Use in children and during pregnancy, labor, and delivery. Lactation. Use in those with heart disease, hypertension, a recent MI, severe or worsening angina pectoris, and those taking certain antidepressants or antiasthmatic drugs. Use in severe renal impairment.

Special Concerns: Pregnant smokers should be encouraged to try to stop smoking using educational and behavioral interventions before using the nicotine transdermal system. The product should only be used during pregnancy if the potential benefit outweighs the potential risk of nicotine to the fetus. The use of nicotine transdermal systems for longer than 3 months has not been studied. Clients with coronary heart disease (history of MI and/or angina pectoris), serious cardiac arrhythmias, or vasospastic diseases (e.g., Buerger's disease, Prinzmetal's variant angina) should be screened carefully before using the transdermal system. Use with caution in clients with hyperthyroidism, pheochromocytoma, or insulin-dependent diabetes (nicotine causes the release of catecholamines). Use with caution in clients with active peptic ulcers, in accelerated hypertension, and during lactation.

Side Effects: *NOTE:* The incidence of side effects is complicated by the fact that clients manifest effects of nicotine withdrawal or by concurrent smoking.

Dermatologic: Erythema, pruritus, or burning at the site of application; cutaneous hypersensitivity, sweating, rash at application site. *Body as a whole:* Allergy, back pain. *GI:* Diarrhea, dyspepsia, dry mouth, abdominal pain, constipation, N&V. *Musculoskeletal:* Arthralgia, myalgia. *CNS:* Abnormal dreams, somnolence, dizziness, impaired concentration, headache, insomnia. *CV:* Tachycardia, hypertension. *Respiratory:* Increased cough, pharyngitis, sinusitis. *GU:* Dysmenorrhea.

OD **Overdose Management:** *Symptoms:* Pallor, cold sweat, N&V, abdominal pain, salivation, diarrhea, headache, dizziness, disturbed hearing and vision, mental confusion, weakness, tremor. Large overdoses may cause prostration, hypotension, ***respiratory failure, seizures, and death.*** *Treatment:* Remove the transdermal system immediately. The surface of the skin may be flushed with water and dried; soap should not be used as it may increase the absorption of nicotine. Diazepam or barbiturates may be used to treat seizures and atropine can be given for excessive bronchial secretions or diarrhea. Respiratory support for respiratory failure and fluid support for hypotension and CV collapse. If transdermal systems are ingested PO, activated charcoal should be given to prevent seizures. If the client is unconscious, the charcoal should be administered by an NGT. A saline cathartic or sorbitol added to the first dose of activated charcoal may hasten GI passage of the system. Doses of activated charcoal should be repeated as long as the system remains in the GI tract as nicotine will continue to be released for many hours.

N

Dosage
• Transdermal System
HABITROL OR NICODERM

Initial: 21 mg/day for the first 6 weeks, followed by 14 mg/day for the next 2 weeks and 7 mg/day for last 2 weeks.

Clients weighing less than 45.5 kg, those who smoke fewer than 10 cigarettes daily, or clients with CV disease.
Initial: 14 mg/day for the first 6 weeks, followed by 7 mg/day for the next 2 weeks. The entire course of therapy should be from 8 to 12 weeks.

NICOTROL

Adults: 15 mg/day for 6 weeks. The patch is to be worn for 16 hr and removed at bedtime.

PROSTEP

Initial: 22 mg/day for 4–8 weeks followed by 11 mg/day for 2–4 additional weeks. The entire course of therapy should be from 6 to 12 weeks.

RESPIRATORY CARE CONSIDERATIONS
Administration/Storage
1. There will be differences in the duration and length of therapy, depending on the product prescribed.
2. The transdermal system should be applied promptly after its removal from the protective pouch to prevent loss of nicotine due to evaporation. Systems should only be used when the pouch is intact.
3. The system should be applied once daily to a nonhairy, clean, and dry site on the trunk or upper, outer arm. After 24 hr, the system should be removed and a new system applied to an alternate skin site when using Habitrol, Nicoderm, or ProStep. Skin sites should not be reused for at least a week. For Nicotrol, a new system should be applied each day upon waking and removed at bedtime.
4. When a used system is removed, it should be folded over and placed in the protective pouch that contained the new system. The used system should be disposed of to ensure access is prevented by children or pets.
5. The goal of therapy with nicotine transdermal systems is complete abstinence. If the client has not stopped smoking by the fourth week of therapy, treatment should be discontinued.
6. The need for adjustment of the dose should be assessed during the first 2 weeks of therapy.
7. Nicotine will continue to be absorbed from the skin for several hours after removal of the system.
8. Use beyond 3 months for Habitrol, Nicoderm, and ProStep and use beyond 5 months for Nicotrol has not been studied.
9. Systems should not be stored above 30°C (86°F) because they are sensitive to heat.

Assessment:
1. Document nicotine profile: type and brand (cigarettes, chewing tobacco, or cigars), amount used per day, when used, and what increases usage.
2. Determine any evidence of renal or liver dysfunction.
3. Note any history of CAD.
4. List all medications client currently prescribed. Cessation of smoking, with or without nicotine replacement, may alter the response to certain drugs. For example, a decrease in the dosage of acetaminophen, caffeine, imipramine, insulin, oxazepam, pentazocine, propranolol, theophylline, and certain adrenergic blockers (e.g., prazosin, labetalol) may be required. An increase in the dose of adrenergic agonists (e.g., isoproterenol, phenylephrine) may be required.
5. Document any skin disorders as nicotine transdermal systems may be irritating for clients with skin disorders such as atopic or eczematous dermatitis.

Client/Family Teaching
1. Use extreme caution during application and advise all to avoid contact with active systems. If contact does occur, wash the area with water only. The eyes should not be touched.

2. These systems can be a dermal irritant and can cause contact dermatitis. Instruct clients on the proper use of the systems using a return demonstration technique.

3. Any persistent skin irritations such as erythema, edema, or pruritus at the application site as well as any generalized skin reactions such as hives, urticaria, or a generalized rash should be reported and the system should be removed.

4. Advise client to follow the manufacturer's guidelines for proper system application. Review the information sheet that comes with the product as it contains instructions on how to use and dispose of the transdermal systems properly.

5. Stop smoking completely when initiating the nicotine transdermal system. If smoking continues, advise clients that they may experience side effects due to higher nicotine levels in the body.

6. Encourage participation in a formal smoking cessation program. The success or failure of smoking cessation depends on the quality, intensity, and frequency of supportive care. Stress that clients are more likely to stop smoking if they are seen frequently and are active in a formal smoking cessation program.

7. Advise client that nicotine in any form can be toxic and addictive. Review the risks of therapy and stress that the use of nicotine transdermal systems may lead to dependence. To minimize this risk, clients should be encouraged to withdraw use of the transdermal system gradually after 4–8 weeks of use.

8. Review the symptoms of nicotine withdrawal, which include craving, nervousness, restlessness, irritability, mood lability, anxiety, drowsiness, sleep disturbances, impaired concentration, increased appetite, headache, myalgia, constipation, fatigue, and weight gain and advise client to report if evident as dosage may require adjustment.

9. Remind client to change sites of application daily and not to reuse this site for 1 week.

10. Client prescribed Nicotrol should remove patch at bedtime and apply upon arising.

11. Keep all products used and unused away from children and pets. Advise that sufficient nicotine is still present in used systems to cause toxicity.

12. If therapy is unsuccessful after 4 weeks, discontinue and identify reasons for failure so that a later attempt may be more successful.

Evaluate: Successful smoking cessation with control of symptoms of nicotine withdrawal

Nifedipine
(nye-**FED**-ih-peen)
Pregnancy Category: C
Adalat, Adalat CC, Adalat P.A. 10 and 20 ✤, Adalat XL ✤, Apo-Nifed ✤, Gen-Nifedipine ✤, Novo-Nifedin ✤, Nu-Nifed ✤, Procardia, Procardia XL, Taro-Nifedipine ✤ **(Rx)**
Classification: Calcium channel blocking agent (antianginal, antihypertensive)

See also *Calcium Channel Blocking Agents.*

Action/Kinetics: Variable effects on AV node effective and functional refractory periods. CO is moderately increased while peripheral vascular resistance is significantly decreased. **Onset:** 20 min. **Peak plasma levels:** 30 min (up to 4 hr for extended-release). **t½:** 2–5 hr. **Therapeutic serum levels:** 0.025–0.1 mcg/mL. **Duration:** 4–8 hr (12 hr for extended-release). Low-fat meals may slow the rate but not the extent of absorption. Metabolized in the liver to inactive metabolites.

Uses: Vasospastic (Prinzmetal's or variant) angina. Chronic stable angina without vasospasm, including angina due to increased effort (especially in clients who cannot take beta blockers or nitrates or who remain symptomatic following clinical doses of these drugs). Essential hypertension (sustained-release only). *Investigational:* PO, sublingually, or chewed in hypertensive emergencies. Also prophylaxis of migraine headaches, primary pulmonary hypertension, severe pregnancy-associated hypertension, esophageal diseases, Raynaud's phenomenon, CHF, asthma, premature labor, biliary and renal colic, and cardiomyopathy. To prevent strokes and to decrease the risk of CHF in geriatric hypertensives.

Contraindications: Hypersensitivity. Lactation.

Special Concerns: Use with caution in impaired hepatic or renal function and in elderly clients. Initial increase in frequency, duration, or severity of angina (may also be seen in clients being withdrawn from beta blockers and who begin taking nifedipine).

Side Effects: *CV:* Peripheral and pulmonary edema, MI, hypotension, palpitations, syncope, CHF (especially if used with a beta blocker), decreased platelet aggregation, arrhythmias, tachycardia. Increased frequency, length, and duration of angina when beginning nifedipine therapy. *GI:* Nausea, diarrhea, constipation, flatulence, abdominal cramps, dysgeusia, vomiting, dry mouth, eructation, gastroesophageal reflux, melena. *CNS:* Dizziness, lightheadedness, giddiness, nervousness, sleep disturbances, headache, weakness, depression, migraine, psychoses, hallucinations, disturbances in equilibrium, somnolence, insomnia, abnormal dreams, malaise, anxiety. *Dermatologic:* Rash, dermatitis, urticaria, pruritus, photosensitivity, erythema multiforme, ***Stevens-Johnson syndrome.*** *Respiratory:* Dyspnea, cough, wheezing, SOB, respiratory infection, throat, nasal, or chest congestion. *Musculoskeletal:* Muscle cramps or inflammation, joint pain or stiffness, arthritis, ataxia, myoclonic dystonia, hypertonia, asthenia. *Hematologic:* Thrombocytopenia, leukopenia, purpura, anemia. *Other:* Fever, chills, sweating, blurred vision, sexual difficulties, flushing, transient blindness, hyperglycemia, hypokalemia, gingival hyperplasia, allergic hepatitis, hepatitis, tinnitus, gynecomastia, polyuria, nocturia, erythromelalgia, weight gain, epistaxis, facial and periorbital edema, hypoesthesia, gout, abnormal lacrimation, breast pain, dysuria, hematuria.

Additional Drug Interactions
Anticoagulants, oral / Possibility of ↑ PT
Cimetidine / ↑ Bioavailability of nifedipine
Digoxin / ↑ Effect of digoxin by ↓ excretion by kidney
Magnesium sulfate / ↑ Neuromuscular blockade and hypotension
Quinidine / Possible ↓ effect of quinidine due to ↓ plasma levels; ↑ risk of hypotension, bradycardia, AV block, pulmonary edema, and ventricular tachycardia
Ranitidine / ↑ Bioavailability of nifedipine
Theophylline / Possible ↑ effect of theophylline

Laboratory Test Interferences: ↑ Alkaline phosphatase, CPK, LDH, AST, ALT. Positive Coombs' test.

Dosage ——————————

• **Capsules**
Individualized. Initial: 10 mg t.i.d. (range: 10–20 mg t.i.d.); **maintenance:** 10–30 mg t.i.d.–q.i.d. Clients with coronary artery spasm may respond better to 20–30 mg t.i.d.–q.i.d. Doses greater than 120 mg/day are rarely needed while doses greater than 180 mg/day are not recommended.

• **Sustained-Release Tablets**
Initial: 30 or 60 mg once daily for Procardia XL and 30 mg once daily for Adalat CC. Titrate over a 7- to 14-day period. Dosage can be increased as required and as tolerated, to a maximum of 120 mg/day for Procardia XL and 90 mg/day for Adalat CC.

Investigational, hypertensive emergencies.
10–20 mg given PO, sublingually (by puncturing capsule and squeezing contents under the tongue), or chewed (capsule is punctured several times and then chewed).

RESPIRATORY CARE CONSIDERATIONS

See also *Respiratory Care Considerations* for *Calcium Channel Blocking Agents*.

Administration/Storage

1. A single dose (other than sustained-released) should not exceed 30 mg.
2. Before increasing the dose of drug, BP should be carefully monitored.
3. Only the sustained-release tablets should be used to treat hypertension.
4. Sublingual nitroglycerin and long-acting nitrates may be used concomitantly with nifedipine.
5. Concomitant therapy with beta-adrenergic blocking agents may be used. In these cases, note any potential drug interactions.
6. Clients withdrawn from beta blockers may manifest symptoms of increased angina which cannot be prevented by nifedipine; in fact, nifedipine may increase the severity of angina in this situation.
7. Clients with angina may be switched to the sustained-release product at the nearest equivalent total daily dose. However, doses greater than 90 mg/day should be used with caution.
8. Protect capsules from light and moisture and store at room temperature in the original container.
9. During initial therapy and when dosage is increased, clients may experience an increase in the frequency, duration, or severity of angina.
10. Food may decrease the rate but not the extent of absorption. Thus, the drug can be taken without regard to meals.

Assessment

1. Document any history of hypersensitivity to other calcium channel blocking agents.
2. Note any evidence of pulmonary edema, ECG abnormalities, or palpitations.

3. Document cardiopulmonary assessment findings.
4. When working with women of childbearing age, determine if pregnant because drug is contraindicated.

Interventions

1. During the titration period, note evidence of hypotensive response and increased HR that result from peripheral vasodilation. These side effects may precipitate angina.
2. Although beta-blocking drugs may be used concomitantly in clients with chronic stable angina, the combined effects of the drugs cannot be predicted (especially in clients with compromised LV function or cardiac conduction abnormalities). Pronounced hypotension, heart block, and CHF may occur.
3. If therapy with a beta blocker is to be discontinued, gradually decrease dosage to prevent withdrawal syndrome.
4. Determine if client is able to swallow before administering sublingually.

Evaluate

- ↓ Frequency and intensity of anginal episodes
- ↓ BP
- Improved peripheral circulation
- Prevention of strokes and ↓ risk of CHF in geriatric hypertensives
- Therapeutic serum drug levels (0.025–0.1 mcg/mL)

Nisoldipine

(**NYE**-sohl-dih-peen)
Pregnancy Category: C
Sular **(Rx)**
Classification: Calcium channel blocking drug

Action/Kinetics: Nisoldipine inhibits the transmembrane influx of calcium into vascular smooth muscle and cardiac muscle, resulting in dilation of arterioles. The drug has greater potency on vascular smooth muscle than on cardiac muscle. Chronic use of nisoldipine results in a sustained decrease in vascular resistance and small increases in SI and LV ejection fraction. It has a weak diuretic effect and has no clinically important chronotropic effects. Nisoldipine is well absorbed following PO use; however, absolute bioavailability is low due to presystemic metabolism in the gut wall. Foods high in fat result in a significant increase in peak plasma levels. **Maximum plasma levels:** 6–12 hr. **t½, terminal:** 7–12 hr. The drug is almost completely bound to plasma proteins. The drug is metabolized in the liver and excreted through the urine. **Uses:** Treatment of hypertension alone or in combination with other antihypertensive drugs.

Contraindications: Nisoldipine should not be taken with grapefruit juice as it interferes with metabolism, resulting in a significant increase in plasma levels of the drug. Use in those with known hypersensitivity to dihydropyridine calcium channel blockers. Lactation.

Special Concerns: Geriatric clients may show a two- to threefold higher plasma concentration; therefore caution should be used in dosing. Use with caution and at lower doses in those with hepatic insufficiency. Use with caution in clients with CHF or compromised ventricular function, especially in combination with a beta blocker.

Side Effects: *CV:* Increased angina and/or MI in clients with CAD. Initially, excessive hypotension, especially in those taking other antihypertensive drugs. Vasodilation, palpitation, atrial fibrillation, ***CVA, MI,*** CHF, first-degree AV block, hypertension, hypotension, jugular venous distension, migraine, postural hypotension, ventricular extrasystoles, SVT, syncope, systolic ejection murmur, T-wave abnormalities on ECG, venous insufficiency. *Body as a whole:* Peripheral edema, cellulitis, chills, facial edema, fever, flu syndrome, malaise. *GI:* Anorexia, nausea, colitis, diarrhea, dry mouth, dyspepsia, dysphagia, flatulence, gastritis, ***GI hemorrhage,*** gingival hyperplasia, glossitis, hepatomegaly, increased appetite, melena, mouth ulceration.

CNS: Headache, dizziness, abnormal dreams, abnormal thinking and confusion, amnesia, anxiety, ataxia, cerebral ischemia, decreased libido, depression, hypesthesia, hypertonia, insomnia, nervousness, paresthesia, somnolence, tremor, vertigo. *Musculoskeletal:* Arthralgia, arthritis, leg cramps, myalgia, myasthenia, myositis, tenosynovitis. *Hematologic:* Anemia, ecchymoses, leukopenia, petechiae. *Respiratory:* Pharyngitis, sinusitis, asthma, dyspnea, end-inspiratory wheeze and fine rales, epistaxis, increased cough, laryngitis, pleural effusion, rhinitis. *Dermatologic:* Acne, alopecia, dry skin, exfoliative dermatitis, fungal dermatitis, herpes simplex, herpes zoster, maculopapular rash, pruritus, pustular rash, skin discoloration, skin ulcer, sweating, urticaria. *GU:* Dysuria, hematuria, impotence, nocturia, urinary frequency, vaginal hemorrhage, vaginitis. *Metabolic:* Gout, hypokalemia, weight gain or loss. *Ophthalmic:* Abnormal vision, amblyopia, blepharitis, conjunctivitis, glaucoma, itchy eyes, keratoconjunctivitis, retinal detachment, temporary unilateral loss of vision, vitreous floater, watery eyes. *Miscellaneous:* Diabetes mellitus, thyroiditis, chest pain, ear pain, otitis media, tinnitus, taste disturbance.

OD **Overdose Management:** *Symptoms:* Pronounced hypotension. *Treatment:* Active CV support, including monitoring of CV and respiratory function, elevation of extremities, judicious use of calcium infusion, pressor agents, and fluids. Dialysis is not likely to be beneficial, although plasmapheresis may be helpful.

Drug Interactions: Cimetidine significantly ↑ the plasma levels of nisoldipine.

Laboratory Test Interferences: ↑ Serum creatine kinase, NPN, BUN, serum creatinine. Abnormal liver function tests.

Dosage
- **Tablets, Extended-Release**
  Hypertension.

Dose must be adjusted to the needs of each person. **Initial:** 20 mg once daily; **then,** increase by 10 mg/week or longer intervals to reach adequate BP control. **Usual maintenance:** 20–40 mg once daily. Doses beyond 60 mg once daily are not recommended. **Initial dose, clients over 65 years and those with impaired renal function:** 10 mg once daily.

RESPIRATORY CARE CONSIDERATIONS

See also *Respiratory Care Considerations* for *Calcium Channel Blocking Agents.*

Administration/Storage

1. Tablets should be swallowed whole and should not be chewed, divided, or crushed.
2. Tablets should not be given with grapefruit juice or a high-fat meal.
3. Closely monitor dosage adjustments in clients over 65 years of age and those with impaired liver function.

Assessment

1. Document indications for therapy, onset and duration of symptoms, other agents trialed, and the outcome.
2. Anticipate reduced dosage in the elderly and those with impaired liver function.
3. Obtain baseline ECG and note any history or evidence of CHF or compromised LV function.
4. List other drugs currently prescribed to ensure none interact unfavorably.

Evaluate: Desired reduction in BP

Nitroglycerin IV

(nye-troh-**GLIH**-sir-in)
Pregnancy Category: C
Nitro-Bid IV, Nitroglycerin in 5% Dextrose, Tridil **(Rx)**
Classification: Antianginal agent (coronary vasodilator)

See also *Antianginal Drugs, Nitrates/Nitrites.*

Action/Kinetics: Onset: 1–2 min; **duration:** 3–5 min (dose-dependent).

Uses: Hypertension associated with surgery (e.g., associated with ET intubation, skin incision, sternotomy, anesthesia, cardiac bypass, immediate postsurgical period). CHF associated with acute MI. Angina unresponsive to usual doses of organic nitrate or beta-adrenergic blocking agents. Cardiac-load reducing agent. Produce controlled hypotension during surgical procedures.

Special Concerns: Dosage has not been established in children.

Dosage
• **IV Infusion Only**
Initial: 5 mcg/min delivered by precise infusion pump. May be increased by 5 mcg/min q 3–5 min until response is seen. If no response seen at 20 mcg/min, dose can be increased by 10–20 mcg/min until response noted. Monitor titration continuously until client reaches desired level of response.

RESPIRATORY CARE CONSIDERATIONS

See also *Respiratory Care Considerations* for *Antianginal Drugs, Nitrates/Nitrites.*

Administration/Storage

1. Dilute with 5% dextrose USP, or 0.9% sodium chloride injection. Nitroglycerin injection is not for direct IV use; it must first be diluted.
2. Use only a glass IV bottle and administration set provided by the manufacturer because nitroglycerin is readily adsorbed onto many plastics. Avoid adding unnecessary plastic to IV system.
3. Aspirate medication into a syringe and then inject immediately into a glass bottle (or polyolefin bottle) to minimize contact with plastic.
4. Do not administer with any other medications in the IV system.
5. Do not interrupt IV nitroglycerin for administration of a bolus of any other medication.

6. To provide correct dosage, remove 15 mL of solution from the IV tubing if concentration of solution is changed.

7. Administer IV solution with an electronic infusion device (volumetric) and in a closely monitored environment.

8. Have emergency drugs readily available.

Assessment

1. Document indications and goals of therapy.

2. Assess and rate pain, noting location, onset, duration, and any precipitating factors.

Interventions

1. Obtain written parameters for BP and pulse and monitor closely throughout drug therapy.

2. Be prepared to monitor CVP and/or PA pressure as ordered.

3. Monitor VS and ECG. Note any evidence of hypotension, client complaint of nausea, sweating, and/or vomiting. Document presence of tachycardia or bradycardia. These symptoms may indicate that the dosage of drug is more than the client can tolerate.

• Elevate the legs to restore BP.

• Be prepared to reduce the rate of flow of the solution or to administer additional IV fluids.

4. Assess for thrombophlebitis at the IV site and remove IV if reddened.

5. Anticipate that after the initial positive response to therapy the dosage increments will be smaller. Adjustments in dosage will also be made at longer intervals.

6. Sinus tachycardia may occur in a client with angina pectoris who is receiving a maintenance dose of nitroglycerin (HR of 80 beats/min or less reduces myocardial demand).

7. Check that topical, PO, or sublingual doses are adjusted or held if client is on concomitant therapy with IV nitroglycerin.

8. Anticipate that client will be weaned from IV nitroglycerin by gradually decreasing doses to avoid posttherapy or CV distress. Tapering off is usually initiated when the client is receiving the peak effect from PO

or topical vasodilators. The IV flow is usually reduced, and the client is monitored for hypertension and angina, which would require increased titration.

9. Obtain an order for a nonnarcotic analgesic (usually acetaminophen) because headache is a common side effect of drug therapy.

Evaluate

• Resolution or control of angina

• ↓ BP

• Improvement in S&S of CHF (↑ output, ↓ rales, ↓ CVP)

• ↑ Activity tolerance

Nitroglycerin sublingual
(nye-troh-**GLIH**-sir-in)
Pregnancy Category: C
Nitrostat **(Rx)**
Classification: Antianginal agent
(coronary vasodilator)

See also *Antianginal Drugs, Nitrates/Nitrites.*

Action/Kinetics: Sublingual. Onset: 1–3 min; **duration:** 30–60 min.

Uses: Agents of choice for prophylaxis and treatment of angina pectoris.

Special Concerns: Dosage has not been established in children.

Dosage ———————

• **Sublingual Tablets**

150–600 mcg under the tongue or in the buccal pouch at first sign of attack; may be repeated in 5 min if necessary (no more than 3 tablets should be taken within 15 min). For prophylaxis, tablets may be taken 5–10 min prior to activities that may precipitate an attack.

RESPIRATORY CARE CONSIDERATIONS

See also *Respiratory Care Considerations* for *Antianginal Drugs, Nitrates/Nitrites.*

Administration/Storage

1. Sublingual tablets should be placed under the tongue and allowed to dissolve; they should not be swallowed.

2. Sublingual tablets should be stored in the original container at

room temperature protected from moisture. Unused tablets should be discarded if 6 months has elapsed since the original container was opened.

Evaluate
• Angina prophylaxis prior to strenuous activities
• Termination of anginal attack

Nitroglycerin sustained-release capsules
(nye-troh-**GLIH**-sir-in)
Pregnancy Category: C
Nitroglyn **(Rx)**

Nitroglycerin sustained-release tablets
(nye-troh-**GLIH**-sir-in)
Pregnancy Category: C
Nitrogard-SR ✿, Nitrong, Nitrong SR ✿ **(Rx)**
Classification: Antianginal agent (coronary vasodilator)

See also *Antianginal Drugs, Nitrates/Nitrites.*
Action/Kinetics: Sustained-release. Onset: 20–45 min; **duration:** 3–8 hr.
Uses: To prevent anginal attacks. "Possibly effective" for the prophylaxis or treatment of anginal attacks.
Special Concerns: Dosage has not been established in children.

Dosage —————
• **Sustained-Release Capsules**
2.5, 6.5, or 9 mg q 8–12 hr.
• **Sustained-Release Tablets**
1.3, 2.6, or 6.5 mg q 8–12 hr.

RESPIRATORY CARE CONSIDERATIONS

See also *Respiratory Care Considerations* for *Antianginal Drugs, Nitrates/Nitrites.*
Administration/Storage
1. Sustained-release tablets and capsules should not be chewed and are not intended for sublingual use.
2. The smallest effective dose should be given 2–4 times/day.

3. Tolerance may develop.
Evaluate: Desired angina prophylaxis

Nitroglycerin topical ointment
(nye-troh-**GLIH**-sir-in)
Pregnancy Category: C
Nitro-Bid, Nitrol, Nitrol TSAR Kit ✿, Nitrong ✿ **(Rx)**
Classification: Antianginal agent (coronary vasodilator)

See also *Antianginal Drugs, Nitrates/Nitrites.*
Action/Kinetics: Onset: 30–60 min; **duration:** 2–12 hr (depending on amount used per unit of surface area).
Uses: Prophylaxis and treatment of angina pectoris due to CAD.
Special Concerns: Dosage has not been established in children.

Dosage —————
• **Topical Ointment (2%)**
1–2 in. (15–30 mg) q 8 hr; up to 4–5 in. (60–75 mg) q 4 hr may be necessary. One inch equals approximately 15 mg nitroglycerin. Determine optimum dosage by starting with ½ in./8 hr and increasing by ½ in. with each successive dose until headache occurs; then, decrease to largest dose that does not cause headache. When ending treatment, reduce both the dose and frequency of administration over 4–6 weeks to prevent sudden withdrawal reactions.

RESPIRATORY CARE CONSIDERATIONS

See also *Respiratory Care Considerations* for *Antianginal Drugs, Nitrates/Nitrites.*
Administration/Storage
1. Squeeze ointment carefully onto dose-measuring application papers, which are packaged with the medicine. Use applicator to spread ointment or fold paper in half and rub back and forth.
2. Use the paper to spread the oint-

N

ment onto a nonhairy area of skin. Many clients find application to the chest psychologically helpful, but ointment may be applied to other nonhairy areas.

3. Rotate sites to prevent irritation. Keep a record of areas used to avoid unnecessary repetitive use of sites.

4. Apply ointment in a thin, even layer covering an area of skin 5–6 in. in diameter. Remember to remove last dose.

5. Tape the application paper over the area, or cover the area with a piece of plastic wrap-type material. A clear plastic cover causes less leakage of ointment, decreases skin irritation, increases the amount absorbed, and prevents clothing stains. Date, time, and initial tape at site.

6. Once the dose is established, use the same type of covering to ensure that the same amount of drug is absorbed during each application.

7. Clean around tube opening and tightly cap tube after use.

8. To prevent systemic absorption into nurse's system, the nurse should protect her own skin from contact with the ointment. Wash hands thoroughly after application to prevent headache.

9. Remove at bedtime or as directed to prevent tolerance or loss of drug effect. Remember to reapply upon awakening the next morning.

Evaluate: Termination and prevention of acute anginal episodes

Nitroglycerin transdermal system

(nye-troh-**GLIH**-sir-in)
Pregnancy Category: C
Deponit 0.2 mg/hr and 0.4 mg/hr, Minitran 0.1 mg/hr, 0.2 mg/hr, 0.4 mg/hr, and 0.6 mg/hr, Nitrocine 0.6 mg/hr, Nitrodisc 0.2 mg/hr, 0.3 mg/hr, and 0.4 mg/hr, Nitro-Dur 0.1 mg/hr, 0.2 mg/hr, 0.3 mg/hr, 0.4 mg/hr, 0.6 mg/hr, and 0.8 mg/hr, Transderm-Nitro 0.1 mg/hr, 0.2 mg/hr, 0.4 mg/hr, and 0.6 mg/hr **(Rx)**
Classification: Antianginal agent (coronary vasodilator)

See also *Antianginal Drugs, Nitrates/Nitrites*.
Action/Kinetics: Onset: 30–60 min; **duration:** 8–24 hr. The amount released each hour is indicated in the name.

Uses: Prophylaxis of angina pectoris due to CAD. *NOTE:* There is some evidence that nitroglycerin patches stop preterm labor.

Special Concerns: Dosage has not been established in children.

Dosage

• **Topical Patch**
Initial: 0.2–0.4 mg/hr (initially the smallest available dose in the dosage series) applied each day to skin site free of hair and free of excessive movement (e.g., chest, upper arm).
Maintenance: Additional systems or strengths may be added depending on the clinical response.

RESPIRATORY CARE CONSIDERATIONS

See also *Respiratory Care Considerations* for *Antianginal Drugs, Nitrates/Nitrites*.
Administration/Storage

1. Follow instructions for specific products on package insert.

2. To avoid skin irritation, the application site should be slightly different each day.

3. Do not apply to distal areas of extremities.

4. If the pad loosens, apply a new pad.

5. It is important to note that there is a wide variety between clients in the actual amount of nitroglycerin absorbed each day. Physical exercise and increased ambient temperatures may increase the amount absorbed.

6. When terminating therapy, the dose and frequency of application should be gradually reduced over 4–6 weeks.

7. Tolerance is a significant factor affecting efficacy if the system is used continuously for more than 12 hr/day. Thus, a dosage regimen would include a daily period where the patch is on for 12–14 hr and a pe-

riod of 10–12 hr when the patch is off (i.e., while asleep).

8. Remove patch before defibrillating as patch may explode.

9. The various products differ in the mechanism for the delivery system; the most important factor is the amount of drug released per hour. A wide range of client variability will be noted. Variables in the rate of absorption include the skin, physical exercise, and elevated ambient temperature.

Evaluate: Control and prevention of anginal episodes

Nitroglycerin translingual spray

(nye-troh-**GLIH**-sir-in)
Pregnancy Category: C
Nitrolingual **(Rx)**
Classification: Antianginal agent (coronary vasodilator)

See also *Antianginal Drugs, Nitrates/Nitrites.*
Action/Kinetics: Onset: 2 min; **duration:** 30–60 min.
Uses: Coronary artery disease to relieve an acute attack or used prophylactically 10–15 min before beginning activities that can cause an acute anginal attack.
Special Concerns: Dosage has not been established in children.

Dosage —————————
• **Spray**
  Termination of acute attack.
One to two metered doses (400–800 mcg) on or under the tongue q 5 min as needed; no more than three metered doses should be administered within a 15-min period.
  Prophylaxis.
One to two metered doses 5–10 min before beginning activities that might precipitate an acute attack.

RESPIRATORY CARE CONSIDERATIONS

See also *Respiratory Care Considerations* for *Antianginal Drugs, Nitrates/Nitrites.*
Administration/Storage
1. The spray should *not* be inhaled. Spray under the tongue.
2. Immediate medical attention should be sought if chest pain persists.
Evaluate: Control and prevention of acute anginal episodes

Nitroglycerin transmucosal

(nye-troh-**GLIH**-sir-in)
Pregnancy Category: C
Nitrogard, Nitrogard-SR ✿ **(Rx)**
Classification: Antianginal agent (coronary vasodilator)

See also *Antianginal Drugs, Nitrates/Nitrites.*
Action/Kinetics: Onset: 1–2 min; **duration:** 3–5 hr.
Uses: Treatment and prophylaxis of angina.
Special Concerns: Dosage has not been established in children.

Dosage —————————
• **Tablets, Extended Release**
Initial: 1 mg q 3–5 hr during time client is awake. Dose may be increased if necessary.

RESPIRATORY CARE CONSIDERATIONS

See also *Respiratory Care Considerations* for *Antianginal Drugs, Nitrates/Nitrites.*
Administration/Storage
1. Tablet should be placed either between the lip and gum above the upper incisors or between the gum and cheek in the buccal area.
2. Allow tablet to dissolve in the mouth. The client should be warned not to swallow the tablet.
3. From 3 to 5 hr is required for tablet dissolution.
4. Store properly to maintain potency.
• Do not expose to light, heat, or air.

N

• Keep in a tightly closed container below 30°C (86°F).
• *Do not* keep cotton in the container once the bottle has been opened.
Evaluate: ↓ Frequency and ↓ intensity of anginal episodes

Nitroprusside sodium
(nye-troh-**PRUS**-eyed)
Pregnancy Category: C
Nitropress **(Rx)**
Classification: Antihypertensive, direct action on vascular smooth muscle

Action/Kinetics: Direct action on vascular smooth muscle, leading to peripheral vasodilation of arteries and veins. The drug acts on excitation-contraction coupling of vascular smooth muscle by interfering with both influx and intracellular activation of calcium. Nitroprusside has no effect on smooth muscle of the duodenum or uterus and is more active on veins than on arteries. The drug may also improve CHF by decreasing systemic resistance, preload and afterload reduction, and improved CO. **Onset** (drug must be given by IV infusion): 0.5–1 min; **peak effect:** 1–2 min; **t½:** 2 min; **duration:** Up to 10 min after infusion stopped. Nitroprusside reacts with hemoglobin to produce cyanmethemoglobin and cyanide ion. Caution must be exercised as nitroprusside injection can result in toxic levels of cyanide. However, when used briefly or at low infusion rates, the cyanide produced reacts with thiosulfate to produce thiocyanate, which is excreted in the urine.
Uses: Hypertensive crisis to reduce BP immediately. To produce controlled hypotension during anesthesia to reduce bleeding. Acute CHF. *Investigational:* In combination with dopamine for acute MI. Left ventricular failure with coadministration of oxygen, morphine, and a loop diuretic.
Contraindications: Compensatory hypertension where the primary hemodynamic lesion is aortic coarctation or AV shunting. Use to produce controlled hypotension during surgery in clients with known inadequate cerebral circulation or in moribund clients. Clients with congenital optic atrophy or tobacco amblyopia (both of which are rare). Acute CHF associated with decreased peripheral vascular resistance (e.g., high-output heart failure that may be seen in endotoxic sepsis). Lactation.
Special Concerns: Use with caution in hypothyroidism, liver or kidney impairment, during lactation, and in the presence of increased ICP. Geriatric clients may be more sensitive to the hypotensive effects of nitroprusside; also, a decrease in dose may be necessary in these clients due to age-related decreases in renal function.
Side Effects: Excessive hypotension. *Large doses may lead to cyanide toxicity. Following rapid BP reduction:* Dizziness, nausea, restlessness, headache, sweating, muscle twitching, palpitations, abdominal pain, apprehension, retching, retrosternal discomfort. *Other side effects:* Bradycardia, tachycardia, ECG changes, venous streaking, rash, methemoglobinemia, decreased platelet aggregation, flushing, hypothyroidism, ileus, irritation at injection site, hypothyroidism. *Symptoms of thiocyanate toxicity:* Blurred vision, tinnitus, confusion, hyperreflexia, seizures. *CNS symptoms (transitory):* Restlessness, agitation, increased ICP, and muscle twitching. Vomiting or skin rash.
OD **Overdose Management:** *Symptoms:* Excessive hypotension, cyanide toxicity, thiocyanate toxicity. *Treatment:*
• Measure cyanide levels and blood gases to determine venous hyperoxemia or acidosis.
• To treat cyanide toxicity, discontinue nitroprusside and give sodium nitrite, 4–6 mg/kg (about 0.2 mL/kg) over 2–4 min (to convert hemoglobin into methemoglobin); follow by sodium thiosulfate, 150–200 mg/kg (about 50 mL of the 25% solution). This regimen can be given again, at half the original doses, after 2 hr.

Drug Interactions: Concomitant use of other antihypertensives, volatile liquid anesthetics, or certain depressants ↑ response to nitroprusside.

Dosage
- **IV Infusion Only**
  Hypertensive crisis.
  Adults: average, 3 mcg/kg/min. **Range:** 0.3–10 mcg/kg/min. Smaller dose is required for clients receiving other antihypertensives. **Pediatric:** 1.4 mcg/kg/min adjusted slowly depending on the response.

Monitor BP and use as guide to regulate rate of administration to maintain desired antihypertensive effect. Rate of administration should not exceed 10 mcg/kg/min.

RESPIRATORY CARE CONSIDERATIONS

See also *Respiratory Care Considerations* for *Antihypertensive Agents.*

Administration/Storage
1. Protect drug from heat, light, and moisture. The drug should be stored at 15°C–30°C (59°F–86°F).
2. Protect dilute solutions during administration by wrapping flask with opaque material, such as aluminum foil.
3. The contents of the vial (50 mg) should be dissolved in 2–3 mL of D5W. This stock solution must be diluted further in 250–1,000 mL D5W.
4. If properly protected from light, the reconstituted solution is stable for 24 hr.
5. Discard solutions that are any color but light brown.
6. Do not add any other drug or preservative to solution.

7. Cover IV bag and tubing with aluminum foil or foil-lined bags and change setup every 24 hr, unless otherwise indicated. Explain that covering the IV bag protects the medication from light and maintains drug stability. Administer IV solution with an electronic infusion device in a monitored environment.
8. Cyanide toxicity is possible if more than 500 mcg/kg nitroprusside is given faster than 2 mcg/kg/min. To reduce this possibility, sodium thiosulfate can be co-infused with nitroprusside at rates of 5–10 times that of nitroprusside.

Assessment
1. Document indications for therapy, onset of symptoms, and other therapies used unsuccessfully.
2. Note any history of hypothyroidism or vitamin B_{12} deficiency.
3. Obtain baseline CBC, electrolytes, ABGs, PACWP, and liver and renal function studies.

Interventions
1. Monitor VS, I&O, and ECG. Obtain written parameters for BP and monitor closely throughout drug therapy. Titrate infusion accordingly.
2. Observe for symptoms of thiocyanate toxicity listed under side effects. Evaluate lab values for thiocyanate levels q 24–48 hr or as directed. Levels should be less than 100 mcg thiocyanate/mL or 3 μmol cyanide/mL.
3. Metabolic acidosis may be an early indicator of cyanide toxicity. Interrupt infusion and report if evident.

Evaluate
- ↓ BP to within desired range
- Improvement in S&S of refractory CHF

Ofloxacin
(oh-**FLOX**-ah-zeen)
Pregnancy Category: C

Floxin, Floxin I.V., Ocuflox **(Rx)**
Classification: Antibacterial, fluoroquinolone

See also *Anti-Infectives*.

Action/Kinetics: Ofloxacin has activity against a wide range of gram-positive and gram-negative aerobic and anaerobic bacteria. The production of penicillinase should have no effect on the activity of ofloxacin. The drug is widely distributed to body fluids. **Maximum serum levels:** 1–2 hr. t½, **first phase:** 5–7 hr; **second phase:** 20–25 hr. **Peak serum levels at steady state, after PO doses:** 1.5 mcg/mL after 200-mg doses, 2.4 mcg/mL after 300-mg doses, and 2.9 mcg/mL after 400-mg doses. **Peak serum levels after IV doses:** 2.7 mcg/mL after 200-mg dose and 4 mcg/mL after 400-mg dose. Between 70% and 80% is excreted unchanged in the urine.

Uses: Systemic: Pneumonia or acute bacterial exacerbations of chronic bronchitis or community-acquired pneumonia due to *Haemophilus influenzae* or *Streptococcus pneumoniae*. Not a drug of first choice in the treatment of presumed or confirmed pneumococcal pneumonia. Not effective for syphilis.

Acute, uncomplicated urethral and cervical gonorrhea due to *Neisseria gonorrhoeae;* nongonococcal urethritis, and cervicitis due to *Chlamydia trachomatis*. Mixed infections of the urethra and cervix due to *N. gonorrhoeae* and *C. trachomatis*.

Mild to moderate skin and skin structure infections due to *Staphylococcus aureus, Streptococcus pyogenes,* or *Proteus mirabilis*.

Uncomplicated cystitis due to *Citrobacter diversus, Enterobacter aerogenes, E. coli, Klebsiella pneumoniae, Proteus mirabilis,* or *Pseudomonas aeruginosa*. Complicated UTIs due to *Escherichia coli, K. pneumoniae, P. mirabilis, C. diversus,* or *P. aeruginosa*. Prostatitis due to *E. coli*.

IV therapy is indicated when the client is unable to take PO medication.

Ophthalmic: Treatment of conjunctivitis caused by *S. aureus, Staphylococcus epidermidis, S. pneumoniae, Enterobacter cloacae, H. influenzae, P. mirabilis,* and *P. aeruginosa*. Corneal ulcers caused by susceptible organisms.

Contraindications: Hypersensitivity to quinolone antibacterial agents. Use during lactation. Use for syphilis (ineffective). Ophthalmic use in dendritic keratitis, vaccinia, varicella, mycobacterial infections of the eye, fungal diseases of the eye, and with steroid combinations after uncomplicated removal of a corneal foreign body.

Special Concerns: Safety and effectiveness of the systemic forms have not been established in children, adolescents under the age of 18 years, pregnant women, and lactating women. Safety and effectiveness of the ophthalmic form have not been established in children less than 1 year of age. Use with caution in clients with known or suspected CNS disorders such as severe cerebral atherosclerosis, epilepsy, or factors that predispose to seizures. The effectiveness of the IV dosage form in treating severe infections has not been determined.

Side Effects: See also *Side Effects* for *Fluroquinolones*.

GI: Nausea, diarrhea, vomiting, abdominal pain or discomfort, dry or painful mouth, dyspepsia, flatulence, constipation, pseudomembranous colitis, dysgeusia, decreased appetite. *CNS:* Headache, dizziness, fatigue, malaise, somnolence, depression, insomnia, seizures, sleep disorders, nervousness, anxiety, cognitive change, dream abnormality, euphoria, hallucinations, vertigo. *CV:* Chest pain, edema, hypertension, palpitations, vasodilation. *Hypersensitivity reactions:* Dyspnea, **anaphylaxis.** *GU:* External genital pruritus in women, vaginitis, vaginal discharge; burning, irritation, pain, and rash of the female genitalia; glucosuria, proteinuria, hematuria, pyuria, dysmenorrhea, menorrhagia, metrorrhagia, urinary frequency or pain. *Respiratory:* Cough, rhinorrhea. *Dermatologic:* Diaphoresis, vasculitis, photosensitivity, rash, pruritus. *Hematologic:* Leukocytosis, lymphocytopenia, eosinophilia. *Musculoskeletal:* Asthenia, extremity pain, arthralgia, myalgia, possibility of osteochondrosis. *Miscellaneous:* Chills, malaise, syncope, hyperglycemia or hypoglycemia, whole body pain, thirst, weight loss, photophobia, trunk pain, paresthesia, visual disturbances, hypersensitivity, hearing loss, fever.

After ophthalmic use: Transient ocular burning or discomfort, stinging, redness, itching, photophobia, tearing, and dryness.

Laboratory Test Interferences: ↑ ALT, AST.

Dosage ————————————
• **Tablets, IV**
Pneumonia, exacerbation of chronic bronchitis.
400 mg q 12 hr for 10 days.
Acute uncomplicated gonorrhea.
One 400-mg dose. The Centers for Disease Control also recommend adding doxycycline.
Cervicitis/urethritis due to C. trachomatis or N. gonorrhoeae.
300 mg q 12 hr for 7 days.
Mild to moderate skin and skin structure infections.
400 mg q 12 hr for 10 days.
Cystitis due to E. coli or K. pneumoniae.
200 mg q 12 hr for 3 days.
Cystitis due to other organisms.
200 mg q 12 hr for 7 days.
Complicated UTIs.
200 mg q 12 hr for 10 days.
Prostatitis.
300 mg q 12 hr for 6 weeks.
Chlamydia.
300 mg PO b.i.d. for 7 days.
Epididymitis.
300 mg PO b.i.d. for 10 days.
Pelvic inflammatory disease, outpatient.
400 mg PO b.i.d. for 14 days plus clindamycin or metronidazole.

NOTE: The dose should be adjusted in clients with a creatinine clearance of 50 mL/min or less. If the creatinine clearance is 10–50 mL/min, the dosage interval should be q 24 hr, and if creatinine clearance is

less than 10 mL/min, the dose should be half the recommended dose given q 24 hr.
• **Ophthalmic Solution (0.3%)**
Conjunctivitis.
Initial: 1–2 gtt in the affected eye(s) q 2–4 hr for the first 2 days; **then,** 1–2 gtt q.i.d. for five additional days.

RESPIRATORY CARE CONSIDERATIONS

See also *Respiratory Care Considerations* for *Fluoroquinolones* and *Anti-Infectives.*

Administration/Storage
1. The drug should not be taken with food.
2. The drug should be stored in tightly closed containers at a temperature below 30°C (86°F).
3. The ophthalmic solution should not be injected subconjunctivally and it should not be introduced directly into the anterior chamber of the eye.
4. Care should be taken so that the ophthalmic applicator tip does not get contaminated with material from the eye, fingers, or other sources.
5. For IV use, give slowly over a period of time not less than 60 min; not to be given by rapid or bolus IV infusion.
6. The IV product must be diluted prior to use to a final concentration of 4 mg/mL. The following solutions may be used for dilution: 0.9% sodium chloride; 5% dextrose; 5% dextrose and 0.9% sodium chloride; 5% dextrose in lactated Ringer's; 5% sodium bicarbonate; Plasma-Lyte 56 in 5% dextrose; 5% dextrose, 0.45% sodium chloride, and 0.15% KCl; sodium lactate (M/6); water for injection. Infuse slowly, over 1 hr.
7. Oflaxacin in premixed bottles or flexible containers does not have to be diluted further as it is already premixed in 5% dextrose. The premixed product should be stored at 25°C or less (77°F).
8. The drug should be protected from excessive heat, freezing, and light.

Assessment
1. Note any client history of hypersensitivity to quinolone derivatives.
2. Document indications for therapy and type and onset of symptoms.
3. Determine that baseline CBC and liver and renal function studies as well as necessary cultures have been performed prior to administering drug.
4. Assess client and history carefully and document any evidence of CNS disorders.

Interventions
1. Anticipate reduced dosage with altered renal function. Review other prescribed agents; probenecid may block tubular excretion.
2. Perform C&S studies throughout therapy to assess for any evidence of bacterial resistance.
3. Observe client with CNS disorders closely. Document and report any evidence of CNS effects such as tremors, restlessness, confusion, and hallucinations as drug therapy may need to be discontinued.

Evaluate
• Negative culture reports
• Reports of symptomatic improvement

Oxacillin sodium
(ox-ah-**SILL**-in)
Bactocill, Prostaphlin **(Rx)**
Classification: Antibiotic, penicillin

See also *Anti-Infectives* and *Penicillins*.

Action/Kinetics: This is a penicillinase-resistant, acid-stable drug used for resistant staphylococcal infections. **Peak plasma levels: PO,** 1.6–10 mcg after 30–60 min; **IM,** 5–11 mcg/mL after 30 min. **t½:** 30 min.

Uses: Infections caused by penicillinase-producing staphylococci; also certain pneumococci and streptococci.

Dosage
• **Capsules, Oral Solution**
Mild to moderate infections of the upper respiratory tract, skin, soft tissue.

Adults and children (over 20 kg): 500 mg q 4–6 hr for at least 5 days. **Children less than 20 kg:** 50 mg/kg/day in equally divided doses q 6 hr for at least 5 days.
Septicemia, deep-seated infections.
Parenteral therapy (see below) followed by PO therapy. **Adults:** 1 g q 4–6 hr; **children:** 100 mg/kg/day in equally divided doses q 4–6 hr.
• **IM, IV**
General infections.
Adults and children over 40 kg: 250–500 mg q 4–6 hr. **Children less than 40 kg:** 50 mg/kg/day in equally divided doses q 6 hr.
Severe infections of the lower respiratory tract or disseminated infections.
Adults and children over 40 kg: Up to 1 g q 4–6 hr. **Children less than 40 kg:** Up to 100 mg/kg/day. **Neonates and premature infants, less than 2,000 g:** 50 mg/kg/day divided q 12 hr if less than 7 days of age and 100 mg/kg/day divided q 8 hr if more than 7 days of age. **Neonates and premature infants, more than 2,000 g:** 75 mg/kg/day divided q 8 hr if less than 7 days of age and 150 mg/kg/day divided q 6 hr if more than 7 days of age. Maximum daily dose: **Adults,** 12 g; **children,** 100–300 mg/kg.

RESPIRATORY CARE CONSIDERATIONS

See also *Respiratory Care Considerations* for *Penicillins*.

Administration/Storage
1. Administer IM by deep intragluteal injection, rotate injection sites, and observe for pain and swelling at IM injection site.
2. Reconstitution: Add sterile water for injection or sodium chloride injection in amount indicated on vial. Shake until solution is clear. For parenteral use, reconstituted solution may be kept for 3 days at room temperature or 1 week in refrigerator. Discard outdated solutions.
3. IV administration (two methods):

• For rapid, direct administration, add an equal amount of sterile water or isotonic saline to reconstituted dosage (usually 250- to 500-mg vial with 5 mL of solution) and administer over a period of 10 min.

• For IV infusion, add reconstituted solution to either dextrose, saline, or invert sugar solution for a concentration of 0.5–40 mg/mL and administer over a 6-hr period, during which time drug remains potent.

• Observe for pain, redness, and edema at the site of IV injection and along the course of the vein.

4. Treatment of osteomyelitis may require several months of intensive PO therapy.

Evaluate

• Clinical evidence and reports of improvement in S&S of infection
• Negative lab culture reports

Oxycodone hydrochloride
(ox-ee-**KOH**-dohn)
Pregnancy Category: C
OxyContin, Roxicodone, Roxicodone Intensol, Supeudol ✤ **(C-II) (Rx)**

Oxycodone terephthalate
(ox-ee-**KOH**-dohn teh-ref-**THAL**-ayt)
Pregnancy Category: C
(C-II) (Rx)
Classification: Narcotic analgesic, morphine type

See also *Narcotic Analgesics.*
Action/Kinetics: A semisynthetic opiate, oxycodone produces mild sedation with little or no antitussive effect. It is most effective in relieving acute pain. **Onset:** 15–30 min. **Peak effect:** 60 min. **Duration:** 4–6 hr. t½: 3.2 hr for immediate-release product and 4.5 hr for extended-release. Dependence liability is moderate. Oxycodone terephthalate is only available in combination with aspirin (e.g., Percodan) or acetaminophen.
Uses: Moderate to severe pain. The extended-release product (OxyContin)

is indicated for moderate to severe pain, including that due to cancer, injuries, arthritis, lower back problems, and other musculoskeletal conditions that require treatment for more than a few days.
Additional Contraindications: Use in children.
Additional Drug Interactions: Clients with gastric distress, such as colitis or gastric or duodenal ulcer, and clients who have glaucoma should not receive Percodan, which also contains aspirin.

Dosage ——————
• **Capsule, Oral Solution, Concentrated Solution, Tablet, Extended Release Tablet**
   Analgesia.
Adults: 5 mg q 6 hr.
• **Extended Release Tablet**
   Analgesia.
Adults, opioid-naive: 10 mg q 12 hr. **Adults, with prior narcotic therapy:** 10–30 mg b.i.d.

RESPIRATORY CARE CONSIDERATIONS

See also *Respiratory Care Considerations* for *Narcotic Analgesics.*
Administration/Storage: The extended-release tablets must be swallowed whole. Ingesting broken, crushed, or chewed extended-release tablets may lead to rapid release and absorption and the possibility of toxic effects.
Assessment: Document indications for therapy, noting onset, location, and duration of pain and characteristics of symptoms. Use a pain-rating scale to rate pain levels.
Evaluate: Reports of relief of pain

Oxymorphone hydrochloride
(ox-ee-**MOR**-fohn)
Pregnancy Category: C
Numorphan **(C-I) (Rx)**
Classification: Narcotic analgesic, morphine type

See also *Narcotic Analgesics*.
Action/Kinetics: Oxymorphone, on a weight basis, is said to be 2–10 times more potent as an analgesic than morphine although potency depends on the route of administration. It produces mild sedation and moderate depression of the cough reflex. **Onset:** 5–10 min. **Peak effect:** 30–60 min. **Duration:** 3–6 hr.
Uses: Moderate to severe pain. **Parenteral:** Preoperative analgesia, to support anesthesia, obstetrics, relief of anxiety in clients with dyspnea associated with acute LV failure and pulmonary edema.

Dosage ————————
• **SC, IM**
Analgesia.
Adults, initial: 1–1.5 mg q 4–6 hr; dose can be increased carefully until analgesic response obtained.
Analgesia during labor.
Adults: 0.5–1.0 mg IM.
• **IV**
Analgesia.
Adults, initial: 0.5 mg.
• **Suppositories**
Analgesia.
Adults: 5 mg q 4–6 hr. **Not recommended for children under 12 years of age.**

RESPIRATORY CARE CONSIDERATIONS

See also *Respiratory Care Considerations* for *Narcotic Analgesics*.
Administration/Storage
1. If the drug is to be administered IV, dilute the dosage in 5 mL of sterile water or NSS and administer over 2–3 min.
2. Suppositories should be stored in the refrigerator.
Assessment: Document indications for therapy and when indicated, including onset, location, **and** duration of pain and rate pain on rating scale to evaluate drug's effectiveness.
Interventions
1. Encourage to C&DB several times each hour while awake to prevent atelectasis; incentive spirometry may be useful.
2. This particular drug may aggravate gallbladder conditions so carefully assess any client complaint that resembles gallbladder pain.
3. Use safety precautions and assist client with activities as drug causes drowsiness and dizziness.
Evaluate: Relief of pain and control of anxiety

Pancuronium bromide
(pan-kyou-**ROH**-nee-um)
Pregnancy Category: C
Pavulon **(Rx)**
Classification: Neuromuscular blocking agent, nondepolarizing

See also *Neuromuscular Blocking Agents*.
Action/Kinetics: Effects similar to *d*-tubocurarine although pancuronium is 5 times as potent. Drug effects can be reversed by anticholinesterase agents. Pancuronium possesses vagolytic activity although it is not likely to cause histamine release. **Onset:** Within 45 sec. **Time to peak effect:** 3–4.5 min (depending on the dose). **Duration:** 35–45 min (increased with multiple doses). **t½, elimination:** 89–161 min. Forty percent of the total dose is excreted through the urine either unchanged or as metabolites; 10% is excreted through the bile. In clients with renal failure, the t½ is doubled. Significantly bound to plasma protein.
Uses: Adjunct to anesthesia to produce relaxation of skeletal muscle. Facilitate ET intubation. Facilitate management of clients undergoing mechanical ventilation.
Special Concerns: Children up to 1 month of age may be more sensitive

to the effects of atracurium. Clients with myasthenia gravis or Eaton-Lambert syndrome may have profound effects from small doses.

Additional Side Effects: *Respiratory:* ***Apnea, respiratory insufficiency.*** *CV:* Increased HR and MAP. *Miscellaneous:* Salivation, skin rashes, ***hypersensitivity reactions (e.g., bronchospasm,*** flushing, hypotension, redness, tachycardia).

Additional Drug Interactions:

Azathioprine / Reverses effects of pancuronium

Bacitracin / Additive muscle relaxation

Enflurane / ↑ Muscle relaxation

Isoflurane / ↑ Muscle relaxation

Metocurine / ↑ Muscle relaxation but duration is not prolonged

Quinine / ↑ Effect of pancuronium

Sodium colistimethate / ↑ Muscle relaxation

Succinylcholine / ↑ Intensity and duration of action of pancuronium

Tetracyclines / Additive muscle relaxation

Theophyllines / ↓ Effects of pancuronium; also, possible cardiac arrhythmias

Tricyclic antidepressants with halothane / Administration of pancuronium may cause severe arrhythmias

Tubocurarine / ↑ Muscle relaxation but duration is not prolonged

Dosage ⎯⎯⎯⎯⎯⎯⎯⎯⎯

• **IV Only**

Muscle relaxation during anesthesia.

Adults and children over 1 month of age, initial: 0.04–0.1 mg/kg. Additional doses of 0.01 mg/kg may be administered as required (usually q 20–60 min). **Neonates:** A test dose of 0.02 mg/kg should be administered first to determine responsiveness.

ET intubation.

0.06–0.1 mg/kg as a bolus dose. Can undertake intubation in 2 to 3 min.

RESPIRATORY CARE CONSIDERATIONS

See also *Respiratory Care Considerations* for *Neuromuscular Blocking Agents.*

Administration/Storage:

1. Additional doses of pancuronium significantly increase the duration of skeletal muscle relaxation.

2. The drug may be mixed with 5% dextrose, 5% dextrose and sodium chloride, lactated Ringer's injection, and 0.9% sodium chloride injection. When mixed with any of these solutions, the drug is stable with no change in pH or potency for 2 days in glass or plastic containers.

3. Anticipate the medication will act within 3 min upon administration and last 35–45 min.

4. Administer IV drug in a continuously monitored environment.

5. Have appropriate anticholinesterase agents available to reverse drug effects. These include pyridostigmine bromide, neostigmine, or edrophonium and are usually administered with atropine or glycopyrrolate.

Interventions:

1. Provide ventilatory support.

2. Monitor and record VS, ECG, and I&O. Drug can cause vagal stimulation resulting in bradycardia, hypotension, and cardiac arrhythmias.

3. A peripheral nerve stimulator should be used to evaluate neuromuscular response and recovery.

4. Consciousness is not affected by pancuronium. Explain all procedures and provide emotional support. Do not conduct any discussions that should not be overheard.

5. With short-term therapy, reassure clients that they will be able to talk and move once the drug effects are reversed.

6. Muscle fasciculations may cause the client to be sore or injured after recovery. Administer prescribed nondepolarizing agent and reassure that the soreness is likely caused by the unsynchronized contractions of ad-

P

jacent muscle fibers just before the onset of paralysis.

7. Position the client for comfort and so that the body is in proper alignment. Turn and perform mouth care and eye care frequently (protect eyes; blink reflex is suppressed).

8. Assess the client's airway at frequent intervals. Have a suction machine at the bedside.

9. Check to be certain that the ventilator alarms are set and on at all times. *Never* leave client unmonitored.

10. Determine client need and administer medications for anxiety, pain, and/or sedation regularly.

Evaluate:

• Skeletal muscle relaxation with desired level of paralysis

• Facilitation of endotracheal intubation and tolerance of mechanical ventilation

---

Papaverine

(pah-**PAV**-er-een)
Pregnancy Category: C
Genabid, Pavabid HP Capsulet, Pavabid Plateau Caps, Pavacap, Pavacen, Pavagen, Pavarine Spancaps, Pavatine, Paverolan Lanacaps **(Rx)**
Classification: Peripheral vasodilator

Action/Kinetics: Direct spasmolytic effect on smooth muscle, possibly by inhibiting cyclic nucleotide phosphodiesterase, thus increasing levels of cyclic AMP. This effect is seen in the vascular system, bronchial muscle, and in the GI, biliary, and urinary tracts. Large doses produce CNS sedation and sleepiness as well as depressing AV nodal and intraventricular conduction. The drug may also directly relax cerebral vessels as it increases cerebral blood flow and decreases cerebral vascular resistance. Absorbed fairly rapidly. Localized in fat tissues and liver. Steady plasma concentration maintained when drug is given q 6 hr. **Peak plasma levels:** 1–2 hr. **t½:** 30–120 min. Sustained-release products may be poorly and erratically absorbed. Metabolized in the liver and inactive metabolites excreted in the urine.

Uses: PO. Cerebral and peripheral ischemia due to arterial spasm and myocardial ischemia complicated by arrhythmias.Smooth muscle relaxant. **Parenteral.** Various conditions in which muscle spasm is observed including AMI, angina pectoris, peripheral vascular disease (with a vasospastic element), peripheral and pulmonary embolism, certain cerebral angiospastic states; ureteral, biliary, and GI colic. *Investigational:* Alone or with phentolamine as an intracavernous injection for impotence.

NOTE: The FDA has determined that papaverine is not effective for its claimed indications.

Contraindications: Complete AV block; administer with extreme caution in presence of coronary insufficiency and glaucoma.

Special Concerns: Safe use during lactation or for children not established.

Side Effects: *CV:* Flushing of face, hypertension, increase in HR. *GI:* Nausea, anorexia, abdominal distress, constipation or diarrhea, dry mouth and throat. *CNS:* Headache, drowsiness, sedation, vertigo. *Miscellaneous:* Sweating, malaise, pruritus, skin rashes, increase in depth of respiration, hepatitis, jaundice, eosinophilia, altered liver function tests.

OD **Overdose Management:** *NOTE:* Both acute and chronic poisoning may result from use of papaverine. Symptoms are extensions of side effects.

Symptoms (Acute Poisoning): Nystagmus, diplopia, drowsiness, weakness, lassitude, incoordination, coma, cyanosis, ***respiratory depression.*** *Treatment (Acute Poisoning):* Delay absorption by giving tap water, milk, or activated charcoal followed by gastric lavage or induction of vomiting and then a cathartic. BP should be maintained and measures taken to treat respiratory depression and coma. Hemodialysis is effective.

Symptoms (Chronic Poisoning): Ataxia, blurred vision, drowsiness, anxiety, headache, GI upset, depression, urticaria, erythematous macular eruptions, blood dyscrasias, hypotension. *Treatment (Chronic Poisoning):* Discontinue medication. Monitor and treat blood dyscrasias. Provide symptomatic treatment. Treat hypotension by IV fluids, elevation of legs, and a vasopressor with inotropic effects.

Drug Interactions:
Diazoxide IV / Additive hypotensive effect
Levodopa / Papaverine ↓ effect of levodopa by blocking dopamine receptors
Laboratory Test Interferences: ↑ AST, ALT, and bilirubin.

Dosage ⸻
- **Capsules, Extended-Release**
  Vasospastic therapy.
  150 mg q 12 hr up to 150 mg q 8 hr or 300 mg q 12 hr for severe cases.
- **Tablets**
  Vasospastic therapy.
  100–300 mg 3–5 times/day.
- **IM, IV**
  Vasospastic therapy.
  30–120 mg given slowly (over 1–2 min, if IV) q 3 hr.
  Cardiac extrasystoles.
  30–120 mg. Two doses 10 min apart either IM or IV (given slowly over 2 min). **Pediatric:** 6 mg/kg.
- **Intra-arterial**
  Vasospastic therapy.
  40 mg given slowly over 1–2 min.
- **Intracavernosal**
  Impotence therapy.
  30 mg (of the injectable) mixed with 0.5–1 mg phentolamine mesylate for injection.

RESPIRATORY CARE CONSIDERATIONS
Administration/Storage:
1. IV injections must be given by the physician or under physician's immediate supervision.
2. Do not mix with Ringer's lactate solution because a precipitate will form.
Assessment:
1. Document indications for therapy

and type, onset, and duration of symptoms.
2. Note any drugs prescribed that would interact unfavorably with papaverine.
3. Determine any evidence of cardiac dysfunction; obtain baseline VS, ECG, and liver function tests.
4. Document baseline mental status and assess all extremities for color, warmth, and pulses.
Interventions:
1. Monitor VS closely for at least 30 min after IV injection.
2. Report any symptoms of autonomic nervous system distress such as nystagmus, diplopia, or blurred vision.
3. Assess for GI reactions such as nausea or anorexia as these may be symptoms of acute poisoning and require the immediate withdrawal of the drug and institution of emergency measures.
Evaluate:
- ↓ Pain symptoms
- Improvement in extremity color, warmth, and pulse quality
- ↑ Levels of mental alertness

Penbutolol sulfate
(pen-**BYOU**-toe-lohl)
Pregnancy Category: C
Levatol **(Rx)**
Classification: Beta-adrenergic blocking agent

P

See also *Beta-Adrenergic Blocking Agents.*
Action/Kinetics: Penbutolol has both beta-1- and beta-2-receptor blocking activity. It has no membrane-stabilizing activity but does possess minimal intrinsic sympathomimetic activity. High lipid solubility. **t½:** 5 hr. 80%–98% protein bound. Penbutolol is metabolized in the liver and excreted through the urine.
Uses: Mild to moderate arterial hypertension.
Contraindications: Bronchial asthma or bronchospasms, including severe COPD.

Special Concerns: Dosage has not been established in children. Geriatric clients may manifest increased or decreased sensitivity to the usual adult dose.

Dosage
- **Tablets**

Hypertension.

Initial: 20 mg/day either alone or with other antihypertensive agents.
Maintenance: Same as initial dose. Doses greater than 40 mg/day do not result in a greater antihypertensive effect.

RESPIRATORY CARE CONSIDERATIONS

See also Respiratory Care *Considerations* for *Antihypertensive Agents.*
Administration/Storage:
1. The full effect of a 20- to 40-mg dose may not be observed for 2 weeks.
2. Doses of 10 mg/day are effective but full effects are not evident for 4–6 weeks.
Evaluate: ↓ BP with desired control of hypertension

————COMBINATION DRUG————

Penicillin G benzathine and Procaine combined
(pen-ih-**SILL**-in, **BEN**-zah-theen, **PROH**-kain)
Pregnancy Category: B
Bicillin C-R, Bicillin C-R 900/300 **(Rx)**
Classification: Antibiotic, penicillin

See also *Anti-Infectives* and *Penicillins.*
Content: The injection contains the following: *300,000 units/dose:* 150,000 units each of penicillin G benzathine and penicillin G procaine. *600,000 units/dose:* 300,000 units each of penicillin G benzathine and penicillin G procaine. *1,200,000 units/dose:* 600,000 units each of penicillin G benzathine and penicillin G procaine. *2,400,000 units/dose:* 1,200,000 units each of penicillin G benzathine and penicillin G procaine. *Injection, 900/300 per dose.* 900,000 units of penicillin G

benzathine and 300,000 units of penicillin G procaine.
Uses: Streptococcal infections (A, C, G, H, L, and M) without bacteremia, of the upper respiratory tract, skin, and soft tissues. Scarlet fever, erysipelas, pneumococcal infections, and otitis media.
Contraindications: Use to treat syphilis, gonorrhea, yaws, bejel, and pinta.

Dosage
- **IM Only**

Streptococcal infections.

Adults and children over 27 kg: 2,400,000 units, given at a single session using multiple injection sites or, alternatively, in divided doses on days 1 and 3; **children 13.5–27 kg:** 900,000–1,200,000 units; **infants and children under 13.5 kg:** 600,000 units.

Pneumococcal infections, except meningitis.

Adults: 1,200,000 units; **pediatric:** 600,000 units. Give q 2–3 days until temperature is normal for 48 hr.

RESPIRATORY CARE CONSIDERATIONS

See also *Respiratory Care Considerations* for *Penicillins.*
Administration/Storage:
1. For adults, administer by deep IM injection in the upper outer quadrant of the buttock. For infants and children, use the midlateral aspect of the thigh.
2. Injection sites should be rotated for repeated doses.
Evaluate: Resolution of infection

Penicillin G benzathine, parenteral
(pen-ih-**SILL**-in, **BEN**-zah-theen)
Pregnancy Category: B
Bicillin 1200 L-A ✹, Bicillin L-A, Megacillin Suspension ✹, Permapen **(Rx)**
Classification: Antibiotic, penicillin

See also *Anti-Infectives* and *Penicillins.*
Action/Kinetics: Penicillin G is neither penicillinase resistant nor acid

stable. The product is a long-acting (repository) form of penicillin in an aqueous vehicle; it is administered as a sterile suspension. **Peak plasma levels: IM** 0.03–0.05 unit/mL.

Uses: Most gram-positive (streptococci, staphylococci, pneumococci) and some gram-negative (gonococci, meningococci) organisms. Syphilis. Prophylaxis of glomerulonephritis and rheumatic fever. Surgical infections, secondary infections following tooth extraction, tonsillectomy.

Dosage

• Parenteral Suspension (IM Only)

Upper respiratory tract infections, erysipeloid, yaws.

Adults: 1,200,000 units as a single dose; **older children:** 900,000 units as a single dose; **children under 27 kg:** 300,000–600,000 units as a single dose; **neonates:** 50,000 units/kg as a single dose.

Early syphilis.

Adults: 2,400,000 units as a single dose.

Late syphilis.

Adults: 2,400,000 units q 7 days for 3 weeks.

Neurosyphilis.

Adults: Penicillin G, 12,000,000–24,000,000 units IV/day for 10–14 days followed by penicillin G benzathine, 2,400,000 units IM q week for 3 weeks.

Congenital syphilis, older children.

50,000 units/kg IM (up to adult dose of 2,400,000 units).

Prophylaxis of rheumatic fever.

Adults and children over 27.3 kg: 1,200,000 units/ q 4 weeks; **children and infants less than 27.3 kg:** 50,000 units/kg as a single dose.

RESPIRATORY CARE CONSIDERATIONS

See also *Respiratory Care Considerations* for *Penicillins.*

Administration/Storage:

1. Shake multiple-dose vial vigorously before withdrawing the de-

sired dose because medication tends to clump on standing. Check that all medication is dissolved and that no residue is present at bottom of bottle.

2. Use a 20-gauge needle and do not allow medication to remain in the syringe and needle for long periods of time before administration because the needle may become plugged and the syringe "frozen."

3. Inject slowly and steadily into the muscle and *do not massage* injection site.

4. For adults, use the upper outer quadrant of the buttock; for infants and small children, the midlateral aspect of the thigh should be used. Benzathine penicillin should not be administered in the gluteal region in children less than 2 years of age.

5. *Do not administer IV.* Before injection of medication, aspirate needle to ascertain that needle is not in a vein.

6. Rotate and chart site of injections.

7. Divide between two injection sites if dose is large or available muscle mass is small.

Evaluate:

• Effective prophylaxis of poststreptococcal rheumatic fever

• Resolution of symptoms of infection

• Negative serologic tests for syphilis

Penicillin G potassium for injection

(pen-ih-**SILL**-in)
Pregnancy Category: B
Pfizerpen **(Rx)**

Penicillin G (Aqueous) sodium for injection

(pen-ih-**SILL**-in)
Pregnancy Category: B
(Rx)
Classification: Antibiotic, penicillin

See also *Anti-Infectives* and *Penicillins.*

Action/Kinetics: The low cost of penicillin G still makes it the first choice for treatment of many infec-

P

tions. Rapid onset makes it especially suitable for fulminating infections. Penicillin G is neither penicillinase resistant nor acid stable. **Peak plasma levels: IM or SC,** 6–20 units/mL after 15–30 min t½: 30 min.

Uses: Streptococci of groups A, C, G, H, L, and M are sensitive to penicillin G. High serum levels are effective against streptococci of the D group.

Additional Side Effects: Rapid IV administration may cause hyperkalemia and cardiac arrhythmias. Renal damage occurs rarely.

Dosage

• **Penicillin G Potassium and Sodium Injections (IM, Continuous IV Infusion)**

Streptococcal infections.
Adults: 300,000–30 million units/day, depending on the use. **Pediatric:** 100,000–250,000 units/kg/day (given in divided doses q 4 hr). **Infants over 7 days of age weighing more than 2 kg:** 100,000 units/kg/day (given in divided doses q 6 hr). **Infants over 7 days of age weighing less than 2 kg:** 75,000 units/day (given in divided doses q 8 hr). **Infants less than 7 days of age weighing more than 2 kg:** 50,000 units/kg/day (given in divided doses q 8 hr). **Infants less than 7 days of age weighing less than 2 kg:** 50,000 units/kg/day (given in divided doses q 12 hr).

Meningitis.
Infants over 7 days of age weighing more than 2 kg: 200,000 units/kg. **Infants over 7 days of age weighing less than 2 kg:** 150,000 units/kg. **Infants less than 7 days of age weighing more than 2 kg:** 150,000 units/kg. **Infants less than 7 days of age weighing less than 2 kg:** 100,000 units/kg/day for 14 days.

Gram-negative bacillary bacteremia.
20 million or more units daily.

Anthrax.
A minimum of 5 million units/day (up to 12–20 million units have been used).

Clostridial infections.
20 million units/day used with an antitoxin.

Actinomycosis, cervicofacial.
1–6 million units/day; *thoracic and abdominal disease:* **initial,** 12–20 million units/day IV for 6 weeks followed by penicillin V, PO, 500 mg q.i.d. for 2–3 months.

Rat-bite fever, Haverhill fever.
12–20 million units/day for 3–4 weeks.

Endocarditis due to Listeria.
15–20 million units/day for 4 weeks (in adults).

Endocarditis due to Erysipelothrix rhusiopathiae.
12–20 million units/day for 4–6 weeks.

Meningitis due to Listeria.
15–20 million units/day for 2 weeks (in adults).

Pasteurella infections causing bacteremia and meningitis.
4–6 million units/day for 2 weeks.

Severe fusospirochetal infections of the oropharynx, lower respiratory tract, and genital area.
5–10 million units/day.

Pneumococcal infections causing empyema.
5–24 million units/day in divided doses q 4–6 hr.

Pneumococcal infections causing meningitis.
20–24 million units/day for 14 days.

Pneumococcal infections causing endocarditis, pericarditis, peritonitis, suppurative arthritis, osteomyelitis, mastoiditis.
12–20 million units/day for 2–4 weeks.

Adjunct with antitoxic to prevent diphtheria.
2–3 million units/day in divided doses for 10–12 days.

Meningococcal meningitis.
20–30 million units/day by continuous IV drip for 14 days (or until there is no fever for 7 days) or 200,000–300,000 units/kg/day q 2–4 hr in divided doses for a total of 24 doses.

Neurosyphilis.
12–24 million units/day for 10–14 days (can be followed by benza-

thine penicillin G, 2.4 million units IM weekly for 3 weeks).

Congenital syphilis in newborns. 50,000 units/kg/day (IV) in divided doses q 8–12 hr for 10–14 days; *in infants after newborn period:* 50,000 units/kg q 4–6 hr for 10–14 days.

Gonococcal infections in infants. 100,000 units/kg/day in two equal doses.

• **Oral Solution, Tablets**
General use.
Adults: 200,000–500,000 units q 6–8 hr; **pediatric under 12 years of age:** 25,000–90,000 units/kg/day in three to six divided doses. *NOTE:* 250 mg Penicillin G potassium, PO, is equivalent to 400,000 units.

Upper respiratory tract infections due to streptococci.
200,000–250,000 units q 6–8 hr for 10 days (for severe infections, use 400,000–500,000 units q 8 hr for 10 days or 800,000 units q 12 hr).

Infections of the respiratory tract due to pneumococci.
400,000–500,000 units q 6 hr until client has no fever for 48 hr.

Infections of the skin and skin structures due to staphylococci.
200,000–500,000 units q 6–8 hr until cured.

Infections of the oropharynx due to fusospirochetes.
400,000–500,000 units q 6–8 hr.

Prophylaxis of rheumatic fever and/or chorea.
200,000–250,000 units b.i.d. chronically.

RESPIRATORY CARE CONSIDERATIONS

See also *Respiratory Care Considerations* for *Penicillins.*

Administration/Storage:
1. IM administration is preferred; discomfort is minimized by using solutions of up to 100,000 units/mL.
2. Use sterile water, isotonic saline USP, or 5% D5W and mix with recommended volume for desired strength.
3. Loosen powder by shaking bottle before adding diluent.

4. Hold vial horizontally and rotate slowly while directing the stream of the diluent against the wall of the vial.
5. Shake vigorously after addition of diluent.
6. Solutions may be stored at room temperature for 24 hr or in refrigerator for 1 week. Discard remaining solution.
7. Use 1%–2% lidocaine solution as diluent for IM (if ordered) to lessen pain at injection site. Do not use procaine as diluent for aqueous penicillin.
8. The PO products should be taken at least 1 hr before or 2 hr after meals.
9. Note the drugs that should *not* be mixed with penicillin during IV administration: aminophylline, amphotericin B, ascorbic acid, chlorpheniramine, chlorpromazine, gentamicin, heparin, hydroxyzine, lincomycin, metaraminol, novobiocin, oxytetracycline, phenylephrine, phenytoin, polymyxin B, prochlorperazine, promazine, promethazine, sodium bicarbonate, sodium salts of barbiturates, sulfadiazine, tetracycline, tromethamine, vancomycin, vitamin B complex.
10. For intermittent IV administration (q 6 hr) drug may be reconstituted with 100 mL of dextrose or saline solution and infused over 1 hr.
11. Electrolyte contents: Penicillin G Sodium (1 mg =1,600 units) contains 2 mEq sodium/1 million units; Penicillin G Potassium (1 mg =1,600 units) contains 1.7 mEq potassium and 0.3 mEq sodium/1 million units.

Assessment:
1. Document indications for therapy and type and onset of symptoms.
2. List other agents prescribed and the outcome.
3. Obtain baseline CBC and liver and renal function studies.
4. Ensure that appropriate cultures have been obtained before initiating therapy.

P

Interventions:

1. Order drug by specifying sodium or potassium salt.

2. Monitor I&O. Dehydration decreases excretion of the drug and may raise the blood level of penicillin G to dangerously high levels that can cause kidney damage.

3. Assess client for GI disturbances, which may lead to dehydration.

4. Very high doses (>20 million units) may cause seizures or platelet dysfunction, especially in clients with impaired renal function.

Evaluate:

• Clinical evidence and reports of symptomatic improvement

• Negative lab culture reports

• Prophylaxis of rheumatic fever or chorea

Penicillin G Procaine Suspension, Sterile

(pen-ih-**SILL**-in, **PROH**-caine)
Pregnancy Category: B
Ayercillin ✲, Crysticillin 300 A.S. and 600 A.S., Pfizerpen-AS, Wycillin **(Rx)**
Classification: Antibiotic, penicillin

See also *Anti-Infectives* and *Penicillins.*

Action/Kinetics: Long-acting (repository) form in aqueous or oily vehicle. Destroyed by penicillinase. Because of slow onset, a soluble penicillin is often administered concomitantly for fulminating infections.

Uses: Penicillin-sensitive staphylococci, pneumococci, streptococci, and bacterial endocarditis (for *Streptococcus viridans* and *S. bovis* infections). Gonorrhea, all stages of syphilis. *Prophylaxis:* Rheumatic fever, pre- and postsurgery. Diphtheria, anthrax, fusospirochetosis (Vincent's infection), erysipeloid, rat-bite fever.

Dosage ————
• **IM Only**

Pneumococcccal, staphylococcal, streptococcal infections; erysipeloid, rat-bite fever, anthrax, fusospirochetosis.
Adults, usual: 600,000–1,200,000 units/day for 10–14 days. **New-**

borns, usual: 50,000 units/kg/day in a single dose.

Bacterial endocarditis.
Adults: 1,200,000 units penicillin G procaine q.i.d. for 2–4 weeks with streptomycin, 500 mg b.i.d. for the first 14 days.

Diphtheria carrier state.
300,000 units/day for 10 days.

Diphtheria, adjunct with antitoxin.
300,000–600,000 units/day.

Gonococcal infections.
4.8 million units divided into at least two doses and given with 1 g PO probenecid (given 30 min before the injections).

Neurosyphilis.
2.4 million units/day for 10 days (given at two sites) with probenecid 500 mg PO q.i.d.; **then,** benzathine penicillin G, 2.4 million units/week for 3 weeks.

Congenital syphilis in infants, symptomatic and asymptomatic.
50,000 units/kg/day for 10–14 days.

Syphilis: primary, secondary, latent with negative spinal fluid.
Adults and children over 12 years: 600,000 units/day for 8 days (total of 4.8 million units).

RESPIRATORY CARE CONSIDERATIONS

See also *Respiratory Care Considerations* for *Penicillins.*
Administration/Storage:

1. Note on package whether medication is to be refrigerated, since some brands require this to maintain stability.

2. Shake multiple-dose vial thoroughly to ensure uniform suspension before injection. If the medication is clumped at the bottom of the vial, it must be shaken until clump dissolves.

3. Use a 20-gauge needle and aspirate immediately after withdrawing medication from the vial; otherwise needle may become clogged and syringe may "freeze."

4. Administer into two sites if dose is large or available muscle mass is small.

5. Aspirate to check that the needle is not in a vein.

6. Inject deep into muscle at a slow rate.

7. Do not massage after injection.

8. Rotate and chart injection sites.

9. Drug is for IM use only.

Assessment:

1. Document indications for therapy, onset of symptoms, and any other treatments prescribed.

2. Obtain appropriate pretreatment cultures.

Evaluate: Laboratory confirmation of successful treatment of underlying pathogenic agent

---

Penicillin V potassium (Phenoxymethyl-penicillin potassium)

[pen-ih-**SILL**-in]

Pregnancy Category: B

Apo-Pen-VK ✿, Beepen-VK, Betapen-VK, Ledercillin VK, Nadopen-V ✿, Novo–Pen-VK ✿, Nu-Pen-VK ✿, Penicillin VK, Pen-V, Pen-Vee K, PVF K ✿, Robicillin VK, V-Cillin K, Veetids 125, 250, and 500 **(Rx)**

Classification: Antibiotic, penicillin

See also *Anti-Infectives* and *Penicillins.*

Action/Kinetics: These preparations are related closely to penicillin G. They are not penicillinase resistant but are acid stable and resist inactivation by gastric secretions. They are well absorbed from the GI tract and are not affected by foods. **Peak plasma levels:** Penicillin V, **PO:** 2.7 mcg/mL after 30–60 min; penicillin V potassium, **PO:** 1–9 mcg/mL after 30–60 min. **t½:** 30 min.

Periodic blood counts and renal function tests are indicated during long-term usage.

Uses: Penicillin-sensitive staphylococci, pneumococci, streptococci, gonococci. Vincent's infection of the oropharynx. Lyme disease. *Prophylaxis:* Rheumatic fever, chorea, bacterial endocarditis, pre- and postsurgery. Should *not* be used as prophylaxis for GU instrumentation or surgery, sigmoidoscopy, or childbirth or during the acute stage of severe pneumonia, bacteremia, arthritis, empyema, pericarditis, and meningitis. Penicillin G, IV, should be used for treating neurologic complications due to Lyme disease.

Special Concerns: More and more strains of staphylococci are resistant to penicillin V, necessitating culture and sensitivity studies.

Additional Drug Interactions:

Contraceptives, oral / ↓ Effectiveness of oral contraceptives

Neomycin, oral / ↓ Absorption of penicillin V

Dosage ————
• **Oral Solution, Tablets**
Streptococcal infections.
Adults and children over 12 years: 125–250 mg q 6–8 hr for 10 days. **Children, usual:** 25–50 mg/kg/day in divided doses q 6–8 hr.

Pneumococcal or staphylococcal infections, fusospirochetosis of oropharynx.
Adults and children over 12 years: 250–500 mg q 6–8 hr.

Prophylaxis of rheumatic fever/chorea.
125–250 mg b.i.d.

Prophylaxis of bacterial endocarditis.
Adults and children over 27 kg: 2 g 30–60 min prior to procedure; then, 1 g q 6 hr. **Pediatric:** 1 g 30–60 min prior to procedure; then, 500 mg/ q 6 hr.

Anaerobic infections.
250 mg q.i.d. See also *Penicillin G, Procaine, Aqueous, Sterile.*

Prophylaxis of septicemia caused by Staphylococcus pneumoniae in children with sickle cell anemia.
125 mg b.i.d.

Streptococcal pharyngitis in children.
250 mg b.i.d. for 10 days.

Streptococcal otitis media and sinusitis.
250–500 mg q 6 hr for 14 days.

Lyme disease.

P

250–500 mg q.i.d. for 10–20 days (for children less than 2 years of age, 50 mg/kg/day in four divided doses for 10–20 days).

NOTE: 250 mg penicillin V is equivalent to 400,000 units.

RESPIRATORY CARE CONSIDERATIONS

See also *Respiratory Care Considerations* for *Penicillins.*

Administration/Storage:
1. Administer without regard to meals. Blood levels may be slightly higher when administered on an empty stomach, however.
2. Do not administer at the same time as neomycin because malabsorption of penicillin V may occur.

Evaluate:
• Reports of symptomatic improvement
• Negative lab C&S reports
• Endocarditis and/or rheumatic fever prophylaxis during invasive medical and/or dental procedures

---

Pentaerythritol tetranitrate sustained-release capsules

(pen-tah-er-**ITH**-rih-toll)
Pregnancy Category: C
Duotrate, Duotrate 45 **(Rx)**

Pentaerythritol tetranitrate sustained-release tablets

(pen-tah-er-**ITH**-rih-toll)
Pregnancy Category: C
Peritrate SA **(Rx)**

Pentaerythritol tetranitrate tablets

(pen-tah-er-**ITH**-rih-toll)
Pregnancy Category: C
Pentylan, Peritrate, Peritrate Forte ✦ **(Rx)**
Classification: Coronary vasodilator

See also *Antianginal Drugs, Nitrates/Nitrites.*

Action/Kinetics: Onset, Tablets: 20–60 min; **Sustained-release Capsules/Tablets:** 30 min. **Duration, Tablets:** 4–6 hr; **Sustained-release**

Capsules/Tablets: 12 hr. Excreted in urine and feces.

Uses: Prophylaxis of anginal attacks but is not to be used to terminate acute attacks.

Special Concerns: Dosage has not been established in children.

Additional Side Effects: Severe rash, exfoliative dermatitis.

Additional Drug Interactions:
Acetylcholine / Pentaerythritol antagonizes the effect of acetylcholine
Norepinephrine / Pentaerythritol antagonizes the effect of norepinephrine

Dosage —————
• **Tablets**
Initial: 10–20 mg t.i.d.–q.i.d.; **then,** up to 40 mg q.i.d.
• **Sustained-Release Capsules or Tablets**
1 capsule or tablet (30, 45, or 80 mg) q 12 hr.

RESPIRATORY CARE CONSIDERATIONS

See also *Respiratory Care Considerations* for *Antianginal Drugs, Nitrates/Nitrites.*

Assessment: Document indications for therapy, noting onset, location, duration, and characteristics of symptoms.

Evaluate: ↓ Frequency and severity of anginal attacks

Pentamidine isethionate

(pen-**TAM**-ih-deen)
Pregnancy Category: C
NebuPent, Pentacarinate ✦, Pentam, Pneumopent ✦ **(Rx)**
Classification: Antibiotic, miscellaneous (antiprotozoal)

Action/Kinetics: The drug inhibits synthesis of DNA, RNA, phospholipids, and proteins, thereby interfering with cell metabolism. It may interfere also with folate transformation. About one-third of the dose may be excreted unchanged in the urine. Plasma levels following inhalation are significantly lower than after a comparable IV dose.

P

Uses: Parenteral.   Pneumonia caused by *Pneumocystis carinii.* **Inhalation.** Prophylaxis of *P. carinii* in high-risk HIV-infected clients defined by one or both of the following: (a) a history of one or more cases of pneumonia caused by *P. carinii* and/or (b) a peripheral CD4+ lymphocyte count less than 200/mm³. *Investigational:* Trypanosomiasis, visceral leishmaniasis.

Contraindications: Clients manifesting anaphylaxis to inhaled or parenteral pentamidine.

Special Concerns: Use with caution in clients with hepatic or kidney disease, hypertension or hypotension, hyperglycemia or hypoglycemia, hypocalcemia, leukopenia, thrombocytopenia, anemia, ventricular tachycardia, pancreatitis, Stevens-Johnson syndrome.

Side Effects: Parenteral. C*V:* Hypotension, ***ventricular tachycardia,*** phlebitis. *GI:* Nausea, anorexia, bad taste in mouth. *Hematologic:* Leukopenia, thrombocytopenia, anemia. *Electrolytes/glucose:* Hypoglycemia, hypocalcemia, hyperkalemia. *CNS:* Dizziness without hypotension, confusion, hallucinations. *Miscellaneous:* Acute renal failure, ***Stevens-Johnson syndrome,*** elevated serum creatinine, elevated liver function tests, pain or induration at IM injection site, sterile abscess at injection site, rash, neuralgia.

Inhalation. Most frequent include the following. *GI:* Decreased appetite, N&V, metallic taste, diarrhea, abdominal pain. *CNS:* Fatigue, dizziness, headache. *Respiratory:* SOB, cough, pharyngitis, chest pain, chest congestion, ***bronchospasm,*** pneumothorax. *Miscellaneous:* Rash, night sweats, chills, myalgia, headache, anemia, edema.

Dosage ————————
• **IV, Deep IM**
Adults and children: 4 mg/kg/day for 14 days. Dosage should be reduced in renal disease.
• **Aerosol**

Prevention of P. carinii pneumonia.
300 mg q 4 weeks given via the Respirgard II nebulizer.

RESPIRATORY CARE CONSIDERATIONS

See also *General Respiratory Care Considerations for All Anti-Infectives.*

Administration/Storage:
1. To prepare IM solution, dissolve one vial in 3 mL of sterile water for injection.
2. To prepare IV solution, dissolve one vial in 3–5 mL of sterile water for injection or 5% dextrose injection. The drug is then further diluted in 50–250 mL of 5% dextrose solution. This solution then can be infused slowly over 60 min.
3. IV solutions in concentrations of 1 and 2.5 mg/mL in 5% dextrose injection are stable for 48 hr at room temperature.
4. The dose using the nebulizer should be delivered until the chamber is empty (30–45 min). The suggested flow rate is 5–7 L/min from a 40- to 50-psi (pounds per square inch) air or oxygen source.
5. Reconstitution for use in the nebulizer is accomplished by dissolving the contents of the vial in 6 mL sterile water for injection. Saline solution cannot be used because it causes the drug to precipitate.
6. When used for nebulization, pentamidine should not be mixed with any other drug.
7. The solution for nebulization is stable at room temperature for 48 hr if protected from light.

Assessment:
1. Document indications for therapy and assess extent of infection.
2. Determine history of kidney disease, hypertension, and past blood disorders. Ensure that appropriate baseline lab studies have been performed (cultures, CBC, electrolytes, blood sugar, calcium, CD₄ counts, liver and renal function) and monitor as needed.

3. Note results of tuberculosis screening tests.

4. Auscultate lung sounds and document CXR and respiratory assessment findings.

Interventions:

1. Observe for symptoms of hypoglycemia, hypocalcemia, and/or hyperkalemia.

2. During IV therapy monitor BP frequently (q 15 min during therapy and q 2 hr following therapy until stable).

3. Monitor and record VS and I&O.

4. Obtain apical pulse and auscultate for any evidence of arrhythmia if client not monitored.

5. During administration of aerosolized pentamidine, appropriate precautions should be followed to protect the health care worker. Do not administer if pregnant; remove contact lenses. Wear:

• Eye protection with side shields

• Disposable gowns

• Respiratory protective equipment such as an organic dust-mist respirator unless client is under hood stalls or in a ventilated booth

• Gloves

• Administer with the Respirgard II nebulizer

• Document worker exposure(s) and report any persistent or unusual symptoms, especially chronic URIs

6. Follow appropriate institutional guidelines and Occupational Safety and Health Association (OSHA) standards for administration of drug.

7. Incorporate Universal Precautions to protect immunocompromised clients.

Client/Family Teaching:

1. Advise client to report any adverse effects such as bruising, hematuria, blood in stools, or other evidence of bleeding.

2. Avoid aspirin-containing compounds, alcohol, IM injections, or rectal thermometers.

3. Advise to use a soft toothbrush, electric razor, and night light to prevent injury and falls.

4. Be alert for S&S of hypoglycemia (which may be severe) and report

immediately after consuming juice with sugar.

5. Report early signs of Stevens-Johnson syndrome (characterized by high fever, severe headaches, stomatitis, conjunctivitis, rhinitis, urethritis, and balanitis), all of which may necessitate the discontinuation of drug therapy.

6. Intake of fluids should be increased to 2–3 L/day during drug therapy.

7. Rise from a prone position slowly and dangle legs before standing as drug may cause dizziness and postural hypotension.

8. During inhalation, advise that a metallic taste may be experienced.

9. Stress the importance of completing the prescribed course of therapy.

Evaluate:

• (Parenterally) Radiographic evidence and reports of improvement in symptoms of *P. carinii* pneumonia

• (Inhalation) Evidence of prophylaxis of *P. carinii* pneumonia in HIV-infected at-risk individuals

---COMBINATION DRUG---

Pentazocine hydrochloride with Naloxone hydrochloride

(pen-**TAZ**-oh-seen, nah-**LOX**-ohn)

Pregnancy Category: C

Talwin NX **(C-IV) (Rx)**

Pentazocine lactate

(pen-**TAZ**-oh-seen)

Pregnancy Category: C

Talwin **(C-IV) (Rx)**

Classification: Narcotic agonist/antagonist

See also *Narcotic Analgesics*.

General Statement: When administered preoperatively for pain, pentazocine is approximately one-third as potent as morphine. It is a weak antagonist of the analgesic effects of meperidine, morphine, and other narcotic analgesics. It also manifests sedative effects.

Pentazocine has been abused by combining it with the antihistamine tripelennamine (a combination known as *T's and Blues*). This combination has been injected IV as a substitute for heroin. To reduce this possibility, the PO dosage form of pentazocine has been combined with naloxone (Talwin NX), which will prevent the effects of IV administered pentazocine but will not affect the efficacy of pentazocine when taken PO. If pentazocine with naloxone is used IV, fatal reactions may occur, which include vascular occlusion, pulmonary emboli, ulceration, and abscesses, and withdrawal in narcotic-dependent individuals.

Content: Each tablet of pentazocine HCl with naloxone HCl contains: pentazocine HCl, 50 mg, and naloxone HCl, 0.5 mg.

Action/Kinetics: Pentazocine manifests both narcotic agonist and antagonist properties. It exerts its agonist effects by an action on kappa and sigma opioid receptors and its antagonistic effect by an action on mu opioid receptors. The drug also elevates systemic and pulmonary arterial pressure, systemic vascular resistance, and LV end-diastolic pressure, which results in an increased cardiac workload. **Onset: IM,** 15–20 min; **PO,** 15–30 min; **IV,** 2–3 min. **Peak effect: IM,** 15–60 min; **PO,** 60–180 min. **Duration, all routes:** 3 hr. However, onset, duration, and degree of relief depend on both dose and severity of pain. **t½:** 2–3 hr. Extensive first-pass metabolism in the liver.

Uses: PO: Moderate to severe pain. **Parenteral:** Preoperative or preanesthetic medication, obstetrics, supplement to surgical anesthesia. Moderate to severe pain.

Additional Contraindications: Increased ICP or head injury. Not recommended for use in children under 12 years of age. Avoid using methadone or other narcotics for pentazocine withdrawal.

Special Concerns: Use with caution in impaired renal or hepatic function, as well as after MI, when

N&V are present. Use with caution in women delivering premature infants and in clients with respiratory depression. Safety and efficacy in children less than 12 years of age have not been determined.

Additional Side Effects: *CNS:* Syncope, dysphoria, nightmares, hallucinations, disorientation, paresthesias, confusion, **_seizures. Miscellaneous;_** Decreased WBCs, edema of the face, chills. Both psychologic and physical dependence are possible, although the addiction liability is thought to be no greater than for codeine. Multiple parenteral doses may cause severe sclerosis of the skin, SC tissues, and underlying muscle.

Dosage

PENTAZOCINE HYDROCHLORIDE WITH NALOXONE
• **Tablets**
  Analgesia.
Adults: 50 mg q 3–4 hr, up to 100 mg. Daily dose should not exceed 600 mg.
PENTAZOCINE LACTATE
• **IM, IV, SC**
  Analgesia.
Adults: 30 mg q 3–4 hr; doses exceeding 30 mg IV or 60 mg IM not recommended. Total daily dosage should not exceed 360 mg.
  Obstetric analgesia.
Adults: 30 mg IM given once; or, 20 mg IV q 2–3 hr for two or three doses.

RESPIRATORY CARE CONSIDERATIONS

See also Respiratory Care *Considerations* for *Narcotic Analgesics.*
Administration/Storage:
1. Do not mix soluble barbiturates in the same syringe with pentazocine. It will form a precipitate.
2. IV pentazocine may be administered undiluted. However, if the drug is to be diluted, place 5 mg of drug into 5 mL of sterile water for injection. Administer each 5 mg or less over a 1-min period.

3. Review the list of drugs with which the medication interacts.

Assessment:

1. Document indications for therapy and any other agents used and the outcome.

2. Note characteristics of pain and rate using a pain-rating scale.

3. Note any evidence of head injury or increased ICP; document mental status.

4. Determine any history of hepatic, renal, or cardiac dysfunction.

Evaluate: Relief of pain

———COMBINATION DRUG———
Phenergan VC with Codeine syrup
(**FEN**-er-gan, **KOH**-deen)
Pregnancy Category: C
(C-V) (Rx)

Phenergan VC syrup
(**FEN**-er-gan)
Pregnancy Category: C
(Rx)
Classification: Anthistamine, decongestant, antitussive

See also *Antihistamines, Phenylephrine,* and *Codeine.*

Content: Phenergan VC contains the following: *Antihistamine:* Promethazine HCl, 6.25 mg/5 mL. *Decongestant:* Phenylephrine HCl, 5 mg/5 mL. Phenergan VC with Codeine contains the preceding plus: *Narcotic antitussive:* Codeine phosphate, 10 mg/5 mL.

Uses: Phenergan VC: Nasal congestion accompanying allergy or the common cold. Phenergan VC with Codeine: Cough and nasal congestion accompanying allergy or the common cold.

Contraindications: Use for lower respiratory tract symptoms, including asthma. Use in children less than 2 years of age.

Special Concerns: Use with caution during lactation.

Dosage ——————————
• **Phenergan VC Syrup, Phenergan VC with Codeine Syrup**

Adults: 5 mL q 4–6 hr, not to exceed 30 mL/day. **Pediatric, 6–12 years:** 2.5–5 mL q 4–6 hr, not to exceed 30 mL/day; **2–6 years:** 1.25–2.5 mL q 4–6 hr (the maximum daily dose of Phenergan VC with Codeine ranges from 6 to 9 mL depending on the body weight).

RESPIRATORY CARE CONSIDERATIONS

See also *Respiratory Care Considerations* for *Phenylephrine,* and *Codeine.*

Administration/Storage: The maximum daily dose of medication for children between 2 and 6 years of age depends on body weight. The amount of drug administered should not exceed:
• 9 mL for 18 kg of body weight, or
• 8 mL for 16 kg of body weight, or
• 7 mL for 14 kg of body weight, or
• 6 mL for 12 kg of body weight

Assessment: Note onset, duration, and characteristics of symptoms. Document ENT and pulmonary assessment findings.

Evaluate: Control of cough and related congestion with fewer night time awakenings

———COMBINATION DRUG———
Phenergan with Codeine syrup
(**FEN**-er-gan, **KOH**-deen)
Pregnancy Category: C
(C-V) (Rx)
Classification: Antihistamine, antitussive

See also *Antihistamines* and *Codeine.*

Content: *Antihistamine:* Promethazine HCl, 6.25 mg/5 mL. *Antitussive, narcotic:* Codeine phosphate, 10 mg/5 mL.

Uses: Relief of coughs and other upper respiratory tract problems associated with the common cold or with allergy.

Contraindications: Clients with lower respiratory tract symptoms, including asthma. Use in children less than 2 years of age.

Special Concerns: Use with caution during lactation.

Dosage
• **Syrup**
Adults: 5 mL q 4–6 hr, not to exceed 30 mL/day; **pediatric, 6–12 years:** 2.5–5 mL q 4–6 hr, not to exceed 30 mL/day; **pediatric, 2–6 years:** 1.25–2.5 mL q 4–6 hr.

RESPIRATORY CARE CONSIDERATIONS

See also *Respiratory Care Considerations* for and *Narcotics*.
Administration/Storage: The maximum daily dose of medication for children between 2 and 6 years of age depends on body weight. The amount of drug administered should not exceed:
• 9 mL for 18 kg of body weight, or
• 8 mL for 16 kg of body weight, or
• 7 mL for 14 kg of body weight, or
• 6 mL for 12 kg of body weight.
Assessment
1. Take a thorough history to determine how long the client has had the symptoms and assess whether or not the problem may be related to an allergy.
2. Document ENT and pulmonary assessment findings.
Evaluate: Control of cough and congestion

————COMBINATION DRUG————
Phenergan with Dextromethorphan syrup
(**FEN**-er-gan, dex-troh-meth-**OR**-fan)
(Rx)
Pregnancy Category: C
Classification: Antihistamine, antitussive

See also *Antihistamines* and *Dextromethorphan*.
Content: *Antihistamine:* Promethazine HCl, 6.25 mg/5 mL. *Nonnarcotic antitussive:* Dextromethorphan HCl, 15 mg/5 mL.
Uses: To treat symptoms of cough and upper respiratory problems observed with the common cold and allergies.
Contraindications: Use in children less than 2 years of age.
Special Concerns: Use with caution during lactation.

Dosage
• **Syrup**
Adults: 5 mL q 4–6 hr, not to exceed 30 mL/day. **Pediatric, 6–12 years:** 2.5–5 mL q 4–6 hr, not to exceed 20 mL/day; **2–6 years:** 1.25–2.5 mL q 4–6 hr, not to exceed 10 mL/day.

RESPIRATORY CARE CONSIDERATIONS

See also *Respiratory Care Considerations* for *Dextromethorphan*.
Assessment:
1. Determine type, onset, and characteristics of symptoms.
2. List any other agents used and the outcome.
3. Auscultate lungs and document respiratory findings.
Evaluate: Control of cough and relief of congestion

Phenoxybenzamine hydrochloride
(fen-ox-ee-**BEN**-zah-meen)
Pregnancy Category: C
Dibenzyline **(Rx)**
Classification: Alpha-adrenergic blocking agent

Action/Kinetics: Phenoxybenzamine is an irreversible alpha-adrenergic blocking agent. The drug increases blood flow to the skin, mucosa, and abdominal viscera and lowers BP. Beneficial effects may not be noted for 2–4 weeks. **Onset:** gradual. **Peak effect:** 4–6 hr. **Duration:** 3–4 days after one dose. **t½:** 24 hr. Metabolized slowly and excreted in urine and feces.
Uses: To control hypertension and sweating in pheochromocytoma before surgery, when surgery is contraindicated, or in malignant pheochromocytoma.

Contraindications: Conditions in which a decrease in BP is not desired. Essential hypertension.

Special Concerns: Geriatric clients may be more sensitive to the hypotensive hypothermic effects. Use with caution in coronary or cerebral arteriosclerosis, respiratory infections, and renal disease.

Side Effects: Due to adrenergic blockade and include miosis, postural hypotension, tachycardia, nasal congestion, and inhibition of ejaculation. Also, drowsiness, fatigue, GI upset.

OD **Overdose Management:** *Symptoms:* Dizziness or fainting due to postural hypotension. Also, tachycardia, GI irritation, drowsiness, fatigue, vomiting, lethargy, and shock. *Treatment:* Discontinue the drug and consider one or more of the following:

- Have client lie down with legs elevated to restore cerebral circulation.
- In severe overdose, institute measures to treat shock.
- Leg bandages and an abdominal binder may shorten the time the client needs to lie down.
- Severe hypotension may be helped by IV norepinephrine.

Dosage
- **Capsules**
  Pheochromocytoma.

Adults, initial: 10 mg b.i.d.; may be increased every other day until desired effect is obtained. **Maintenance:** 20–40 mg b.i.d.–t.i.d. **Pediatric, initial:** 0.2 mg/kg (6 mg/m²) up to a maximum of 10 mg/day; dose may be increased q 4 days until desired effect is reached. **Maintenance:** 0.4 mg (1.2 mg/m²) daily in three to four divided doses.

RESPIRATORY CARE CONSIDERATIONS

Administration/Storage:
1. Observe the client closely before increasing the dosage of drug.
2. Because phenoxybenzamine is irreversible, the drug is usually started in low doses and gradually increased.
3. It may take 2 weeks to titrate the medication to the optimum dosage.

Interventions:
1. Obtain renal function studies and monitor.
2. Take BP with the client in both supine and erect positions to check for excessive hypotension.
3. Note the quality of peripheral pulses, and assess the extremities for increased warmth for 4 days after a change in drug dosage. The results may help determine whether the client needs an adjustment in dosage.
4. If the client has a preexisting respiratory infection, it may be aggravated by the drug. Increased pulmonary supportive care may be required.

Evaluate: Control of hypertension and ↓ sweating in clients with pheochromocytoma

Phentolamine mesylate
(fen-**TOLL**-ah-meen)
Pregnancy Category: C
Regitine, Rogitine ✦ **(Rx)**
Classification: Alpha-adrenergic blocking agent

Action/Kinetics: Phentolamine competitively blocks both presynaptic (alpha-2) and postsynaptic (alpha-1) adrenergic receptors producing vasodilation and a decrease in peripheral resistance. The drug has little effect on BP. In CHF, phentolamine reduces afterload and pulmonary arterial pressure as well as increases CO. **Onset** (parenteral): Immediate. **Duration:** Short. Poorly absorbed from the GI tract. About 10% excreted unchanged in the urine after parenteral use.

Uses: Treatment of hypertension caused by pheochromocytoma prior to or during surgery. Dermal necrosis and sloughing following IV use or extravasation of norepinephrine. To test for pheochromocytoma (not the method of choice). *Investigational:* Hypertensive crisis secondary to MAO inhibitor/sympathomimetic amine interactions, as well as rebound hypertension due to withdrawal of clonidine, propranolol, or other antihypertensive drugs. In combination with papaverine as an intracavernous injection for impotence.

Contraindications: Coronary artery disease including angina, MI, or coronary insufficiency.

Special Concerns: Use during pregnancy and lactation only if benefits clearly outweigh risks. Geriatric clients may have a greater risk of developing hypothermia. Use with great caution in the presence of gastritis, ulcers, and clients with a history thereof. Use of cardiac glycosides should be deferred until cardiac rhythm returns to normal.

Side Effects: *CV:* Acute and prolonged hypotension, tachycardia, and arrhythmias, especially after parenteral administration. Orthostatic hypotension, flushing. *GI:* N&V, diarrhea. *Other:* Dizziness, weakness, nasal stuffiness.

OD **Overdose Management:** *Symptoms:* **Hypotension, shock.** *Treatment:* Maintain BP by giving IV norepinephrine (DO NOT USE EPINEPHRINE).

Drug Interactions:

Ephedrine / Phentolamine antagonizes vasoconstrictor and hypertensive effect

Epinephrine / Phentolamine antagonizes vasoconstrictor and hypertensive effect

Norepinephrine / Suitable antagonist to treat overdosage induced by phentolamine

Propranolol / Concomitant use during surgery for pheochromocytoma is indicated

Dosage —————————
• **IV, IM**

Prevent hypertension in pheochromocytoma, preoperative.

Adults, IV: 5 mg 1–2 hr before surgery; dose may be repeated if needed. **Pediatric, IV, IM:** 1 mg (or 0.1 mg/kg) 1–2 hr before surgery; dose may be repeated if needed.

Prevent or control hypertension during surgery.

Adults, IV: 5 mg. **IV infusion:** 0.5–1 mg/min. **Pediatric, IV:** 0.1 mg/kg (3 mg/m²). May be repeated, if necessary. During surgery 5 mg for adults and 1 mg for children may be given to prevent or control symptoms of epinephrine intoxication (e.g., paroxysms of hypertension, respiratory depression, seizures, tachycardia).

Dermal necrosis/sloughing following IV or extravasation of norepinephrine.

Prevention: 10 mg/1,000 mL norepinephrine solution; *treatment:* 5–10 mg/10 mL saline injected into area of extravasation within 12 hr. **Pediatric:** 0.1–0.2 mg/kg to a maximum of 10 mg.

CHF.

Adults, IV infusion: 0.17–0.4 mg/min.

Diagnosis of pheochromocytoma.

Adults, rapid IV, initial: 2.5 mg (if response is negative, a 5-mg test should be undertaken before concluding the test is negative); **children, rapid IV:** 1 mg. **Adults, IM:** 5 mg; **children, IM:** 3 mg.

• **Intracavernosal**

Impotence.

Adults: Papaverine, 30 mg, and 0.5–1 mg phentolamine; adjust dose according to response.

RESPIRATORY CARE CONSIDERATIONS

Administration/Storage:

1. For IV administration reconstitute 5 mg with 1 mL sterile water or 0.9% NaCl and inject over 1 min.

2. Drug may also be further diluted: 5–10 mg in 500 mL of D5W and titrated to desired response.

3. When the IV administration of norepinephrine or dopamine results in infiltration, administer solutions of phentolamine SC at the site and within 12 hr for beneficial effects. Use 5–10 mg of phentolamine in 10–15 mL of 0.9% NaCl.

P

Assessment:
1. Note any history of CAD. Obtain VS and ECG.
2. Determine any evidence of gastritis or PUD.

Interventions:
1. Monitor the BP and pulse frequently during parenteral administration and until stabilized.
2. To avoid postural hypotension, keep clients supine for at least 30 min after injection. Then have clients dangle their legs over the side of the bed and rise slowly to avoid orthostatic hypotension.
3. If clients show signs of drug overdose, place them in the Trendelenburg position. Assist with the administration of parenteral fluids. Have levarterenol available to minimize hypotension. *Do not use epinephrine.*

For the diagnosis of pheochromocytoma:
1. The test for pheochromocytoma should not be undertaken on normotensive clients.
2. Sedatives, analgesics, and other nonessential medication should be withheld for 24 hr (and preferably 72 hr) prior to the test.
3. When testing for pheochromocytoma, the client should be kept in a supine position, preferably in a dark, quiet room.
4. If the IV test is used, BP should be measured immediately after the injection, at 30-sec intervals for the first 3 min and at 60-sec intervals for the next 7 min. If the IM test is used, BP should be measured every 5 min for 30–45 min.
5. The pheochromocytoma test is most reliable in clients with sustained hypertension and least reliable in clients with paroxysmal hypertension.
6. A positive response for pheochromocytoma is a drop in BP of more than 35 mm Hg systolic and 25 mm Hg diastolic pressure. Maximal decreases in BP usually occur within 2 min after injection of phentolamine and return to preinjection pressure within 15–30 min. A negative response is indicated when the BP is unchanged, elevated, or reduced less than 35 mm Hg systolic and 25 mm Hg diastolic pressure.

Evaluate:
• Control of hypertension
• Prevention of local tissue necrosis following extravasation with norepinephrine or dopamine
• Positive response with test for pheochromocytoma

Phenylephrine hydrochloride
(fen-ill-**EF**-rin)

Pregnancy Category: C
Nasal: Alconefrin 12, 25, and 50, Children's Nostril, Doktors, Duration, Neo-Synephrine Solution, Nostril, Rhinall, Vicks Sinex. **Ophthalmic:** AK-Dilate, Dionephrine ✦, Mydfrin 2.5%, Neo-Synephrine, Neo-Synephrine Viscous, Phenoptic, Prefrin Liquifilm, Relief. **Parenteral:** Neo-Synephrine. (Rx: Parenteral and Ophthalmic Solutions 2.5% or greater; OTC: Nasal products and ophthalmic solutions 0.12% or less)
Classification: Alpha-adrenergic agent (sympathomimetic)

See also *Sympathomimetic Drugs* and *Nasal Decongestants.*

Action/Kinetics: Phenylephrine stimulates alpha-adrenergic receptors, producing pronounced vasoconstriction and hence an increase in both SBP and DBP; reflex bradycardia results from increased vagal activity. The drug also acts on alpha receptors producing vasoconstriction in the skin, mucous membranes, and the mucosa as well as mydriasis by contracting the dilator muscle of the pupil. It resembles epinephrine, but it has more prolonged action and few cardiac effects. **IV: Onset,** immediate; **duration,** 15–20 min. **IM, SC: Onset,** 10–15 min; **duration:** 0.5–2 hr for IM and 50–60 min for SC. *Nasal decongestion (topical):* **Onset:** 15–20 min; **duration,** 30 min–4 hr. *Ophthalmic:* **Time to peak effect for mydriasis,** 15–60 min for 2.5% solution and 10–90 min for 10% solution. **Duration:** 0.5–1.5 hr for 0.12%, 3 hr for 2.5%, and 5–7 hr with 10% (when used for mydriasis). Excreted in urine.

Phenylephrine is also found in Chlor-Trimetron Expectorant, Naldecon, Dimetane, and Dimetapp.

Uses: Systemic: Vascular failure in shock, shock-like states, drug-induced hypotension or hypersensitivity. To maintain BP during spinal and inhalation anesthesia; to prolong spinal anesthesia. As a vasoconstrictor in regional analgesia. Paroxysmal SVT. **Nasal:** Nasal congestion due to allergies, sinusitis, common cold, or hay fever. **Ophthalmologic: 0.12%:** Temporary relief of redness of the eye associated with colds, hay fever, wind, dust, sun, smog, smoke, contact lens. **2.5% and 10%:** Decongestant and vasoconstrictor, treatment of uveitis with posterior synechiae, open-angle glaucoma, refraction without cycloplegia, ophthalmoscopic examination, funduscopy, prior to surgery.

Contraindications: Severe hypertension, ventricular tachycardia.

Special Concerns: Use with caution in geriatric clients, in severe arteriosclerosis, and during pregnancy and lactation. Nasal and ophthalmic use of phenylephrine may be systemically absorbed. Use of the 2.5% or 10% ophthalmic solutions in children may cause hypertension and irregular heart beat. In geriatric clients, chronic use of the 2.5% or 10% ophthalmic solutions may cause rebound miosis and a decreased mydriatic effect.

Side Effects: *CV:* Reflex bradycardia. *CNS:* Headache, excitability, restlessness. *Ophthalmologic:* Rebound miosis and decreased mydriatic response in geriatric clients, blurred vision.

OD **Overdose Management:** *Symptoms:* Ventricular extrasystoles, short paroxysms of ventricular tachycardia, sensation of fullness in the head, tingling of extremities. *Treatment:* Administer an alpha-

adrenergic blocking agent (e.g., phentolamine).

Additional Drug Interactions: Bretylium may ↑ the effect of phenylephrine → possible arrhythmias.

Dosage
• **IM, IV, SC**
Vasopressor, mild to moderate hypotension.
Adults: 2–5 mg (range: 1–10 mg), not to exceed an initial dose of 5 mg IM or SC repeated no more often than q 10–15 min; or, 0.2 mg (range: 0.1–0.5 mg), not to exceed an initial dose of 0.5 mg IV repeated no more often than q 10–15 min. **Pediatric:** 0.1 mg/kg (3 mg/m²) IM or SC repeated in 1–2 hr if needed.

Vasopressor, severe hypotension and shock.
Adults: 10 mg by continuous IV infusion using 250–500 mL 5% dextrose injection or 0.9% sodium chloride injection given at a rate of 0.1–0.18 mg/min initial; **then,** give at a rate of 0.04–0.06 mg/min.

Prophylaxis of hypotension during spinal anesthesia.
Adults: 2–3 mg IM or SC 3–4 min before anesthetic given; subsequent doses should not exceed the previous dose by more than 0.1–0.2 mg. No more than 0.5 mg should be given in a single dose. **Pediatric:** 0.044–0.088 mg/kg IM or SC.

Hypotensive emergencies during spinal anesthesia.
Adults, initial: 0.2 mg IV; dose can be increased by no more than 0.2 mg for each subsequent dose not to exceed 0.5 mg/dose.

Prolongation of spinal anesthesia.
2–5 mg added to the anesthetic solution increases the duration of action up to 50% without increasing side effects or complications.

Vasoconstrictor for regional anesthesia.
Add 1 mg to every 20 mL of local anesthetic solution. If more than 2 mg phenylephrine is used, pressor reactions can be expected.

Paroxysmal SVT.

Initial: 0.5 mg (maximum) given by rapid IV injection (over 20–30 seconds). Subsequent doses are determined by BP and should not exceed the previous dose by more than 0.1–0.2 mg and should never be more than 1 mg.

• **Nasal Solution, Nasal Spray**
Adults and children over 12 years of age: 2–3 gtt of the 0.25% or 0.5% solution into each nostril q 3–4 hr as needed. In resistant cases, the 1% solution can be used but no more often than q 4 hr. **Children, 6–12 years of age:** 2–3 gtt of the 0.25% solution q 3–4 hr as needed. **Infants, greater than 6 months of age:** 1–2 gtt of the 0.16% solution into each nostril q 3–4 hr.

• **Ophthalmic Solution, 0.12%, 2.5%, 10%**

Vasoconstriction, pupillary dilation.
1 gtt of the 2.5% or 10% solution on the upper limbus a few minutes following 1 gtt of topical anesthetic (prevents stinging and dilution of solution by lacrimation). An additional drop may be needed after 1 hr.

Uveitis.
1 gtt of the 2.5% or 10% solution with atropine. To free recently formed posterior synechiae, 1 gtt of the 2.5% or 10% solution to the upper surface of the cornea. Treatment should be continued the following day, if needed. In the interim, hot compresses should be applied for 5–10 min t.i.d. using 1 gtt of 1% or 2% atropine sulfate before and after each series of compresses.

Glaucoma.
1 gtt of 10% solution on the upper surface of the cornea as needed. Both the 2.5% and 10% solutions may be used with miotics in clients with open-angle glaucoma.

Surgery.
2.5% or 10% solution 30–60 min before surgery for wide dilation of the pupil.

Refraction.
Adults: 1 gtt of a cycloplegic (homatropine HBr, atropine sulfate, cyclopentolate, tropicamide HCl, or a combination of homatropine and co-caine HCl) in each eye followed in 5 min with 1 gtt of 2.5% phenylephrine solution and in 10 min with another drop of cycloplegic. The eyes are ready for refraction in 50–60 min.
Children: 1 gtt of atropine sulfate, 1%, in each eye followed in 10–15 min with 1 gtt of phenylephrine solution, 2.5%, and in 5–10 min with a second drop of atropine sulfate, 1%. The eyes are ready for refraction in 1–2 hr.

Ophthalmoscopic examination.
1 gtt of 2.5% solution in each eye. The eyes are ready for examination in 15–30 min and the effect lasts for 1–3 hr.

Minor eye irritations.
1–2 gtt of the 0.12% solution in the eye(s) up to q.i.d. as needed.

RESPIRATORY CARE CONSIDERATIONS

See also *Respiratory Care Considerations* for *Sympathomimetic Drugs* and *Nasal Decongestants.*

Administration/Storage:
1. Store drug in a brown bottle and away from light.
2. Anticipate that before administering the 10% ophthalmic solution, instillation of a drop of local anesthetic willbe necessary.
3. When the drug is used as a nasal decongestant, instruct clients to blow their noses before administration.
4. For IV administration, dilute each 1 mg with 9 mL of sterile water and administer over 1 min. Further dilution of 10 mg in 500 mL of dextrose, Ringer's, or saline solution may be titrated to client response.
5. When drug is used parenterally, monitor infusion site closely to avoid extravasation. If evident, local SC administration of phentolamine should be performed to prevent tissue necrosis.
6. Prolonged exposure to air or strong light may result in oxidation and discoloration. Solution should not be used if it changes color, becomes cloudy, or contains a precipitate.

Assessment:

1. Document indications for therapy, type and onset of symptoms; note goals of therapy.

2. During IV administration monitor cardiac rhythm and BP continuously until stabilized, noting any evidence of bradycardia or arrhythmias.

Client/Family Teaching:

1. Demonstrate and review the appropriate method for drug administration.

2. Advise that ophthalmic instillations and nasal decongestants may produce systemic sympathomimetic effects. Stress that chronic excessive use may cause rebound congestion. Provide with printed material explaining how to identify these effects and instruct to report should they occur.

3. Wear sunglasses in bright light. Symptoms of photosensitivity and blurred vision should be reported if they persist after 12 hr. Advise that blurred vision should decrease with repeated use.

4. When using ophthalmic solution, report if there is no relief of symptoms within 2 days.

5. When using the drug for nasal decongestion, report if there is no relief of symptoms within 3 days. Rebound nasal congestion may occur with longer therapy.

Evaluate:

- ↑ BP
- Termination of PSVT
- Relief of nasal congestion
- ↓ Conjunctivitis and allergic manifestations
- Dilatation of pupils

Phenylpropanolamine hydrochloride

(fen-ill-**proh**-pah-**NOHL**-ah-meen)
Acutrim 16 Hour, Acutrim Late Day, Acutrim II Maximum Strength, Control, Dexatrim, Dexatrim Maximum Strength and Maximum Strength Caplets, Dexatrim Maximum Strength Pre-Meal Caplets, Efed II Yellow, Maigret-50, Phenyldrine, Propagest,

Unitrol (OTC except Maigret-50 and Rhindecon)
Classification: Sympathomimetic decongestant, appetite suppressant

---

See also *Stimulants,* and *Sympathomimetic Drugs.*

Action/Kinetics: Phenylpropanolamine is thought to stimulate both alpha and beta receptors as well as to act indirectly through release of norepinephrine from storage sites. Increases in BP are due mainly to increased CO rather than to vasoconstriction; has minimal CNS effects. The drug acts on alpha-adrenergic receptors to produce a decongestant effect in the nasal mucosa. **Onset, decongestant:** 15–30 min; **peak plasma levels:** 1–2 hr; **duration, capsules and tablets:** 3 hr; **extended-release tablets:** 12–16 hr. **Peak plasma levels:** 100 ng. **t½:** 3–4 hr. Eighty percent to 90% excreted in the urine unchanged.

Uses: Nasal congestion due to colds, hay fever, allergies. Short-term (8–12 weeks) treatment of exogenous obesity in conjunction with a weight reduction program including reduced caloric intake, exercise, and behavior modification. *Investigational:* Mild to moderate stress incontinence in women.

Contraindications: Arteriosclerosis, depression, glaucoma, hypertension, diabetes, kidney disease, hyperthyroidism, during or within 14 days of use of MAO inhibitors, hypersensitivity to sympathomimetics. Not recommended as an anorexiant for children less than 12 years of age. Sustained-release forms during lactation and in children less than 12 years of age.

Special Concerns: Safety and efficacy during pregnancy and lactation and for children not established. Children less than 6 years of age may be at greater risk for developing psychiatric disorders when using phenylpropanolamine. The anorexiant dose must be individualized for children 12–18 years of age.

P

Side Effects: *CNS:* Dizziness, headache, insomnia, restlessness, bizarre behavior. Serious effects due to abuse include: agitation, tremor, increased motor activity, hallucinations, *seizures, stroke, and death. CV:* Palpitations, *hypertension (may be severe and lead to crisis),* tachycardia. *Miscellaneous:* Dry mouth, dysuria, renal failure, nausea, nasal dryness.

Additional Drug Interactions:
Bromocriptine / Worsening of side effects of bromocriptine; possibility of ventricular tachycardia and cardiac dysfunction
Caffeine / ↑ Serum caffeine levels, ↑ risk of pharmacologic and toxic effects
Indomethacin / Possibility of severe hypertensive episode

Dosage ————————
• **Capsules, Tablets**
Decongestant.
Adults: 25 mg q 4 hr or 50 mg q 6–8 hr (not to exceed 150 mg/day); **Children, 2–6 years:** 6.25 mg q 4 hr, not to exceed 37.5 mg in 24 hr; **6–12 years:** 12.5 mg q 4 hr, not to exceed 75 mg in 24 hr.
Anorexiant.
Adults: 25 mg t.i.d. 30 min before meals, not to exceed 75 mg in 24 hr.
• **Extended-Release   Capsules, Extended-Release Tablets**
Decongestant.
Adults: 75 mg q 12 hr.
Anorexiant.
Adults: 75 mg once daily in the morning.

RESPIRATORY CARE CONSIDERATIONS

See also *Respiratory Care Considerations* for *Sympathomimetic Drugs.*
Client/Family Teaching:
1. Stress the importance of regular exercise, reduced caloric intake, and behavorial modification programs in the overall management of obesity.
2. Caution older men to report difficulties in voiding because they are more susceptible to drug-induced urinary retention.
3. Advise caution as drug may cause dizziness and tremors.

4. Avoid any caffeine-containing products or foods.
Evaluate:
• ↓ Symptoms of nasal congestion
• ↓ Appetite and evidence of desired weight loss

Phenytoin (Diphenylhydantoin)
(**FEN**-ih-toyn, dye-**fen**-ill-hy-**DAN**-toyn)
Dilantin Infatab, Dilantin-125, Novo-Phenytoin ✿ **(Rx)**

Phenytoin sodium, extended
(**FEN**-ih-toyn)
Dilantin Kapseals **(Rx)**

Phenytoin sodium, parenteral
(**FEN**-ih-toyn)
Dilantin Sodium **(Rx)**

Phenytoin sodium prompt
(**FEN**-ih-toyn)
Diphenylan Sodium **(Rx)**
Classification: Anticonvulsant, hydantoin type; antiarrhythmic (type I)

See also *Antiarrhythmic Agents.*
Action/Kinetics: Phenytoin acts in the motor cortex of the brain to reduce the spread of electrical discharges from the rapidly firing epileptic foci in this area. This is accomplished by stabilizing hyperexcitable cells possibly by affecting sodium efflux. Also, phenytoin decreases activity of centers in the brain stem responsible for the tonic phase of grand mal seizures. This drug has few sedative effects.

Serum levels must be monitored because the serum concentrations of phenytoin increase disproportionately as the dosage is increased. Phenytoin extended is designed for once-a-day dosage. It has a slow dissolution rate—no more than 35% in 30 min, 30%–70% in 60 min, and less than 85% in 120 min. Absorption is variable following PO dosage. **Peak**

serum levels: PO, 4–8 hr. Since the rate and extent of absorption depend on the particular preparation, the same product should be used for a particular client. **Peak serum levels (following IM):** 24 hr (wide variation). **Therapeutic serum levels:** 5–20 mcg/mL. **t½:** 8–60 hr (average: 20–30 hr). Steady state attained 7–10 days after initiation. Phenytoin is biotransformed in the liver. Both inactive metabolites and unchanged drug are excreted in the urine.

As an antiarrhythmic, phenytoin increases the electrical stimulation threshold of heart muscle, although it is less effective than quinidine, procainamide, or lidocaine. **Onset:** 30–60 min. **Duration:** 24 hr or more. **t½:** 22–36 hr. **Therapeutic serum level:** 10–20 mcg/mL.

Uses: Chronic epilepsy, especially of the tonic-clonic, psychomotor type. Not effective against absence seizures and may even increase the frequency of seizures in this disorder. Parenteral phenytoin is sometimes used to treat status epilepticus and to control seizures during neurosurgery.

PO for certain PVCs and IV for PVCs and tachycardia. The drug is particularly useful for arrhythmias produced by digitalis overdosage.

Investigational: Paroxysmal choreoathetosis; to treat blistering and erosions in clients with recessive dystrophic epidermolysis bullosa; episodic dyscontrol; trigeminal neuralgia; as a muscle relaxant in neuromyotonia, myotonia congenita, or myotonic muscular dystrophy; to treat cardiac symptoms in overdosage of tricyclic antidepressants. Severe preeclampsia.

Contraindications: Hypersensitivity to hydantoins, exfoliative dermatitis, sinus bradycardia, second- and third-degree AV block, clients with Adams-Stokes syndrome, SA block. Lactation.

Special Concerns: Use with caution in acute, intermittent porphyria. Administer with extreme caution to clients with a history of asthma or other allergies, impaired renal or hepatic function, and heart disease (hypotension, severe myocardial insufficiency). Abrupt withdrawal may cause status epilepticus. Combined drug therapy is required if petit mal seizures are also present.

Side Effects: *CNS:* Most commonly, drowsiness, ataxia, dysarthria, confusion, insomnia, nervousness, irritability, depression, tremor, numbness, headache, psychoses, *increased seizures.* Choreoathetosis following IV use. *GI:* Gingival hyperplasia, N&V, either diarrhea or constipation. *Dermatologic:* Various dermatoses including a measles-like rash (common), scarlatiniform, maculopapular, and urticarial rashes. Rarely, drug-induced lupus erythematosus, *Stevens-Johnson syndrome,* exfoliative or purpuric dermatitis, and *toxic epidermal necrolysis.* Alopecia, hirsutism. Skin reactions may necessitate withdrawal of therapy. *Hematopoietic:* Leukopenia, granulocytopenia, thrombocytopenia, pancytopenia, *agranulocytosis,* macrocytosis, megaloblastic anemia, leukocytosis, monocytosis, eosinophilia, simple anemia, *aplastic anemia, hemolytic anemia.* *Hepatic:* Liver damage, toxic hepatitis, hypersensitivity reactions involving the liver including hepatocellular degeneration and *fatal hepatocellular necrosis.* *Ophthalmic:* Diplopia, nystagmus, conjunctivitis. *Miscellaneous:* Hyperglycemia, chest pain, edema, fever, photophobia, weight gain, *pulmonary fibrosis,* lymph node hyperplasia, gynecomastia, periarteritis nodosa, depression of IgA, soft tissue injury at injection site, coarsening of facial features, Peyronie's disease, enlarged lips.

Rapid parenteral administration may cause serious CV effects, including hypotension, arrhythmias, CV collapse, and heart block, as well as CNS depression.

Many clients have a partial deficiency in the ability of the liver to degrade phenytoin, and as a result, toxicity may develop after a small PO dose. Liver and kidney function tests and hematopoietic studies are indicated prior to and periodically during drug therapy.

OD **Overdose Management:**
Symptoms: Initially, ataxia, dysarthria, and nystagmus followed by unresponsive pupils, hypotension, and *coma.* Plasma levels greater than 40 mcg/mL result in significant decreases in mental capacity. *Treatment:* Treat symptoms. Hemodialysis may be effective. In children, total-exchange transfusion has been used.

Drug Interactions:
Acetaminophen / ↓ Effect of acetaminophen due to ↑ breakdown by liver; however, hepatotoxicity may be ↑

Alcohol, ethyl / In alcoholics, ↓ effect of phenytoin due to ↑ breakdown by liver

Allopurinol / ↑ Effect of phenytoin due to ↓ breakdown in liver

Amiodarone / ↑ Effect of phenytoin or amiodarone due to ↓ breakdown by liver

Antacids / ↓ Effect of phenytoin due to ↓ GI absorption

Anticoagulants, oral / ↑ Effect of phenytoin due to ↓ breakdown by liver. Also, possible ↑ anticoagulant effect due to ↓ plasma protein binding

Antidepressants, tricyclic / May ↑ incidence of epileptic seizures or ↑ effect of phenytoin by ↓ plasma protein binding

Barbiturates / Effect of phenytoin may be ↑ , ↓ , or not changed; possible ↑ effect of barbiturates

Benzodiazepines / ↑ Effect of phenytoin due to ↓ breakdown by liver

Carbamazepine / ↓ Effect of phenytoin or carbamazepine due to ↑ breakdown by liver

Charcoal / ↓ Effect of phenytoin due to ↓ absorption from GI tract

Chloramphenicol / ↑ Effect of phenytoin due to ↓ breakdown by liver

Chlorpheniramine / ↑ Effect of phenytoin

Cimetidine / ↑ Effect of phenytoin due to ↓ breakdown by liver

Clonazepam / ↓ Plasma levels of clonazepam or phenytoin; or, ↑ risk of phenytoin toxicity

Contraceptives, oral / Estrogen-induced fluid retention may precipitate seizures; also, ↓ effect of contraceptives due to ↑ breakdown by liver

Corticosteroids / Effect of corticosteroids ↓ due to ↑ breakdown by liver; also, corticosteroids may mask hypersensitivity reactions due to phenytoin

Cyclosporine / ↓ Effect of cyclosporine due to ↑ breakdown by liver

Diazoxide / ↓ Effect of phenytoin due to ↑ breakdown by liver

Dicumarol / Phenytoin ↓ effect of dicumarol due to ↑ breakdown by liver

Digitalis glycosides / ↓ Effect of digitalis glycosides due to ↑ breakdown by liver

Disopyrimide / ↓ Effect of disopyramide due to ↑ breakdown by liver

Disulfiram / ↑ Effect of phenytoin due to ↓ breakdown by liver

Dopamine / IV phenytoin results in hypotension and bradycardia; also, ↓ effect of dopamine

Doxycycline / ↓ Effect of doxycycline due to ↑ breakdown by liver

Estrogens / See *Contraceptives, oral*

Fluconazole / ↑ Effect of phenytoin due to ↓ breakdown by liver

Folic acid / ↓ Effect of phenytoin

Furosemide / ↓ Effect of furosemide due to ↓ absorption

Haloperidol / ↓ Effect of haloperidol due to ↑ breakdown by liver

Ibuprofen / ↑ Effect of phenytoin

Isoniazid / ↑ Effect of phenytoin due to ↓ breakdown by liver

Levodopa / Phenytoin ↓ effect of levodopa

Levonorgestrel / ↓ Effect of norgestrel

Lithium / ↑ Risk of lithium toxicity

Loxapine / ↓ Effect of phenytoin

Mebendazole / ↓ Effect of mebendazole

Meperidine / ↓ Effect of meperidine due to ↑ breakdown by liver; toxic effects of meperidine may ↑ due to accumulation of active metabolite (normeperidine)

Methadone / ↓ Effect of methadone due to ↑ breakdown by liver

Metronidazole / ↑ Effect of phenytoin due to ↓ breakdown by liver

Metyrapone / ↓ Effect of metyrapone due to ↑ breakdown by liver

Mexiletine / ↓ Effect of mexiletine due to ↑ breakdown by liver

Miconazole / ↑ Effect of phenytoin due to ↓ breakdown by liver

Nitrofurantoin / ↓ Effect of phenytoin

Omeprazole / ↑ Effect of phenytoin due to ↓ breakdown by liver

Phenacemide / ↑ Effect of phenytoin due to ↓ breakdown by liver

Phenothiazines / ↑ Effect of phenytoin due to ↓ breakdown by liver

Phenylbutazone / ↑ Effect of phenytoin due to ↓ breakdown by liver and ↓ plasma protein binding

Primidone / Possible ↑ effect of primidone

Pyridoxine / ↓ Effect of phenytoin

Quinidine / ↓ Effect of quinidine due to ↑ breakdown by liver

Rifampin / ↓ Effect of phenytoin due to ↑ breakdown by liver

Salicylates / ↑ Effect of phenytoin by ↓ plasma protein binding

Sucralfate / ↓ Effect of phenytoin due to ↓ absorption from GI tract

Sulfonamides / ↑ Effect of phenytoin due to ↓ breakdown in liver

Sulfonylureas / ↓ Effect of sulfonylureas

Theophylline / ↓ Effect of both drugs due to ↑ breakdown by liver

Trimethoprim / ↑ Effect of phenytoin due to ↓ breakdown by liver

Valproic acid / ↑ Effect of phenytoin due to ↓ breakdown by liver and ↓ plasma protein binding; phenytoin may also ↓ effect of valproic acid due to ↑ breakdown by liver

Laboratory Test Interferences: Alters liver function tests, ↑ blood glucose values, and ↓ PBI values. ↑ Gamma globulins. Phenytoin ↓ immunoglobulins A and G. False + Coombs' test.

Dosage ———————
• **Oral Suspension, Chewable Tablets**
Seizures.
Adults, initial: 100 mg (125 mg of the suspension) t.i.d.; adjust dosage at 7- to 10-day intervals until seizures are controlled; **usual, maintenance:** 300–400 mg/day, although 600 mg/day (625 mg of the suspension) may be required in some. **Pediatric, initial:** 5 mg/kg/day in two to three divided doses; **maintenance,** 4–8 mg/kg (up to maximum of 300 mg/day). Children over 6 years may require up to 300 mg/day. **Geriatric:** 3 mg/kg initially in divided doses; **then,** adjust dosage according to serum levels and response. Once dosage level has been established, the extended capsules may be used for once-a-day dosage.

• **Capsules, Extended-Release Capsules**
Seizures.
Adults, initial: 100 mg t.i.d.; adjust dose at 7- to 10-day intervals until control is achieved. An initial loading dose of 12–15 mg/kg divided into two to three doses over 6 hr followed by 100 mg t.i.d. on subsequent days may be preferred if seizures are frequent. **Pediatric:** See dose for Oral Suspension and Chewable Tablets.

Arrhythmias.
Adults: 200–400 mg/day.

• **IV**
Status epilepticus.
Adults, loading dose: 10–15 mg/kg at a rate not to exceed 50 mg/min; **then,** 100 mg PO or IV q 6–8 hr. **Pediatric, loading dose:** 15–20 mg/kg in divided doses of 5–10 mg/kg given at a rate of 1–3 mg/kg/min.

Arrhythmias.
Adults: 100 mg q 5 min up to maximum of 1 g.

• **IM**
Dose should be 50% greater than the PO dose.

Neurosurgery.
100–200 mg q 4 hr during and after surgery (during first 24 hr, no more

than 1,000 mg should be administered; after first day, give maintenance dosage).

RESPIRATORY CARE CONSIDERATIONS

See also *Respiratory Care Considerations* for *Antiarrhythmic Agents*.

Administration/Storage

1. Ful l effectiveness of PO administered hydantoins is delayed and may take 6–9 days to be fully established. A similar period of time will elapse before effects disappear completely.

2. When hydantoins are substituted for or added to another anticonvulsant medication, their dosage is gradually increased, while dosage of the other drug is decreased proportionally.

3. For parenteral preparations:

• Only a clear solution of the drug may be used.

• Dilute with special diluent supplied by manufacturer.

• Shake the vials until the solution is clear. It may take about 10 min for the drug to dissolve.

• To hasten the process, warm the vial in warm water after adding the diluent.

• The drug is incompatible with acid solutions.

4. Use of IV infusion is not recommended, as the drug is poorly soluble and may form a precipitate. Inject slowly and directly into a large vein through a large-gauge needle or IV catheter.

5. If IV infusion is used, a rate of 50 mg/min should not be exceeded in adults or 1–3 mg/kg/min in neonates.

6. Following the IV administration of the drug, administer sodium chloride injection through the same needle or IV catheter to avoid local irritation of the vein due to alkalinity of the solution. Do not use dextrose solutions.

7. *Do not* add phenytoin to an already running IV solution.

8. Avoid IM, SC, or perivascular injections. Pain, inflammation, and necrosis may be caused by the highly alkaline solutions.

9. For treatment of status epilepticus, inject the IV slowly at a rate not to exceed 50 mg/min. If necessary, the dose may be repeated 30 min after the initial administration.

10. If the client is receiving tube feedings of Isocal or Osmolite, there may be interference with the absorption of PO phenytoin. Therefore, do not administer them together.

11. Due to potential differences in bioavailability between PO products, brand interchange is not recommended. Also, when switching from extended to prompt products, dosage adjustments may be required.

Assessment:

1. Document indications for therapy and type and onset of symptoms.

2. Note the history and nature of the client's seizures, addressing location, frequency, duration, causes, and characteristics.

3. Determine if the client is hypersensitive to hydantoins or has exfoliative dermatitis.

4. If the client is female and pregnant, note that she should not breast-feed the baby following delivery.

5. Obtain baseline ECG hematologic, liver, and renal function studies and monitor throughout therapy.

6. Consider fosphenytoin in those unable to tolerate phenytoin.

Interventions:

1. During IV administration, monitor BP closely for hypotension.

2. Monitor serum drug levels on a routine basis:

• Seven to 10 days may be required to achieve recommended serum levels. Drug is highly protein bound; may consider requesting free and bound drug levels to better assess response. The drug is metabolized much more slowly by elderly clients; thus most may be managed with once a day dosing.

• If the client is receiving drugs that interact with hydantoins or has impaired liver function, the level should be done more frequently. Dilantin induces hepatic microsomal enzymes for drug metabolism.

3. Oral form has variable absorption; do not administer with tube feedings. Administer separately, flush, and clamp tube for 20 min to ensure absorption.

Evaluate:
• Control of seizures
• Termination of ventricular arrhythmias
• Restoration of stable cardiac rhythm
• Therapeutic serum drug levels (5–20 mcg/mL) depending on condition being managed

Physostigmine salicylate
(fye-zoh-**STIG**-meen)
Pregnancy Category: C
Antilirium **(Rx)**

Physostigmine sulfate
(fye-zoh-**STIG**-meen)
Pregnancy Category: C
Eserine Sulfate **(Rx)**
Classification: Indirectly acting cholinergic-acetylcholinesterase inhibitor

See also *Neostigmine.*
Action/Kinetics: Physostigmine is a reversible acetylcholinesterase inhibitor, resulting in an increased concentration of acetylcholine at nerve endings, which can antagonize anticholinergic drugs. It produces miosis, increased accommodation, and a decrease in intraocular pressure with decreased resistance to outflow of aqueous humor. When used for chronic open-angle glaucoma, ciliary muscle contraction may open the intertrabecular spaces, facilitating aqueous humor outflow. **Onset, IV:** 3–5 min. **Duration, IV:** 1–2 hr. **t½:** 1–2 hr. No dosage alteration is necessary in clients with renal impairment. **Onset, miosis:** 20–30 min; **duration, miosis:** 12–36 hr. **Reduction of intraocular pressure, peak:** 2–6 hr; **duration:** 12–36 hr.
Uses: Overdosage due to cholinergic blocking drugs (e.g., atropine) and tricyclic antidepressant overdosage. Reduce intraocular pressure in open-angle glaucoma. Friedreich's and other inherited ataxias (FDA has granted orphan status for this use). *Investigational:* Angle-closure glaucoma during or after iridectomy, secondary glaucoma if no inflammation present. Treat delirium tremens and Alzheimer's disease. May also antagonize the CNS depressant effect of diazepam.
Contraindications: Active uveal inflammation, any inflammatory disease of the iris or ciliary body, glaucoma associated with iridocyclitis. Asthma, gangrene, diabetes, CV disease, GI or GU tract obstruction, any vagotonic state, in those receiving choline esters or depolarizing neuromuscular blocking drugs.
Special Concerns: Use with caution during lactation, in clients with chronic angle-closure glaucoma, or in clients with narrow angles. Safety and efficacy have not been established for ophthalmic use in children. Systemic use in children should be reserved for life-threatening situations only. Benzyl alcohol, found in the parenteral product, may cause a fatal "gasping syndrome" in premature infants. The parenteral form also contains sulfites that may cause allergic reactions.
Additional Side Effects: If IV administration is too rapid, bradycardia, hypersalivation, breathing difficulties, and *seizures* may occur. Conjunctivitis when used for glaucoma.
OD **Overdose Management:** *Symptoms:* Cholinergic crisis. *Treatment:* IV atropine sulfate: **Adults:** 0.4–0.6 mg; **infants and children up to 12 years of age:** 0.01 mg/kg q 2 hr as needed (maximum single dose should not exceed 0.4 mg). A short-acting barbiturate may be used for seizures not relieved by atropine.
Drug Interactions:
Anticholinesterases, systemic / Additive effects → toxicity
Succinylcholine / ↑ Risk of respiratory and CV collapse

Dosage ─────────────
• **IM, IV**
   Anticholinergic drug overdose.
Adults, IM, IV: 0.5–2 mg at a rate of 1 mg/min; may be repeated if necessary. **Pediatric, IV:** 0.02 mg/kg IM or by slow IV injection (0.5 mg given over a period of at least 1 min). Dose may be repeated at 5–10 min if needed to a maximum of 2 mg if no toxic effects are manifested.
   Postanesthesia.
0.5–1 mg given IM or by slow IV (less than 1 mg/min). May be repeated at 10- to 30-min intervals to attain desired response.
• **Ophthalmic Ointment**
   Glaucoma.
Adults and children: 1 cm of the 0.25% sulfate ointment applied to the lower fornix up to t.i.d.

RESPIRATORY CARE CONSIDERATIONS

See also *Respiratory Care Considerations* for *Neostigmine, Cholinergic Blocking Agents.*
Administration/Storage:
1. The ophthalmic ointment may be used at night for prolonged effect of the medication.
2. The ophthalmic ointment should be stored tightly closed and protected from heat.
3. May administer IV undiluted: 1 mg/min (0.5 mg/min for children).
Assessment:
1. Document indications for therapy and onset and duration of symptoms.
2. Determine cause of overdosage (drug or plant ingestion), amount, and time ingested.
Interventions:
1. During IV administration, monitor ECG and record VS; report any evidence of bradycardia, hypersalivation, respiratory difficulty, or seizure activity.
2. Have the client void prior to administering the medication. If the client develops incontinence, it may be caused by too high a dose.
Evaluate:
• Reversal of toxic CNS symptoms

R/T overdosage with cholinergic blocking agents or tricyclic antidepressants or from ingestion of poisonous plants
• ↓ Intraocular pressures
• Control of symptoms R/T delirium tremens and/or Alzheimer's disease

Pindolol
(**PIN**-doh-lohl)
Pregnancy Category: B
Apo-Pindol ✤, Gen-Pindolol ✤, Novo–Pindol ✤, Nu-Pindol ✤, Syn-Pindolol ✤, Visken **(Rx)**
Classification: Beta-adrenergic blocking agent

See also *Beta-Adrenergic Blocking Agents.*
Action/Kinetics: Manifests both beta-1 and beta-2 adrenergic blocking activity. Pindolol also has significant intrinsic sympathomimetic effects and minimal membrane-stabilizing activity. Moderate lipid solubility. $t^{1/2}$: 3–4 hr; however, geriatric clients have a variable half-life ranging from 7 to 15 hr, even with normal renal function. The drug is metabolized by the liver, and the metabolites and unchanged (35%–40%) drug are excreted through the kidneys.
Uses: Hypertension (alone or in combination with other antihypertensive agents as thiazide diuretics). *Investigational:* Ventricular arrhythmias and tachycardias, antipsychotic-induced akathisia, situational anxiety.
Contraindications: Bronchial asthma or bronchospasm, including severe COPD.
Special Concerns: Dosage has not been established in children.
Laboratory Test Interferences: ↑ AST and ALT. Rarely, ↑ LDH, uric acid, alkaline phosphatase.

Dosage ─────────────
• **Tablets**
   Hypertension.
Initial: 5 mg b.i.d. (alone or with other antihypertensive drugs). If no response in 3–4 weeks, increase by 10 mg/day q 3–4 weeks to a maximum of 60 mg/day.

Antipsychotic-induced akathisia.
5 mg/day.

RESPIRATORY CARE CONSIDERATIONS

See also *Respiratory Care Considerations* for *Beta-Adrenergic Blocking Agents* and Antihypertensive Agents, .

Assessment:

1. Document indications for therapy, onset and duration of symptoms, and any other agents trialed.

2. Assess diet, sodium consumption, weight, exercise regimens, and lifestyle.

3. Document VS and note cardiopulmonary assessment findings.

Evaluate:

- ↓ BP
- ↓ Agitation and anxiety

Pipecuronium bromide

(pih-peh-kyour-**OHN**-ee-um)

Pregnancy Category: C

Arduan **(Rx)**

Classification: Neuromuscular blocking agent, nondepolarizing

See also *Neuromuscular Blocking Agents.*

Action/Kinetics: Pipecuronium is similar to tubocurarine in that it competes for cholinergic receptors at the motor end-plate and is antagonized by acetylcholinesterase inhibitors. It has no effect on consciousness, pain threshold, or cerebration; thus, use must be accompanied by adequate anesthesia. **Maximum time for blockade:** 5 min following single doses of 70–85 mcg/kg. **Time to recovery to 25% of control:** 30–175 min under balanced anesthesia following single doses of 70 mcg/kg. **t½, distribution:** 6.22 min (4.33 min in renal transplant clients); **t½, elimination:** 1.7 hr (4 hr in renal transplant clients). Increased plasma levels are seen in clients with impaired renal function. The drug is metabolized in the liver and metabolites as well as unchanged drug are eliminated in the urine.

Uses: Adjunct to general anesthesia to provide relaxation of skeletal muscle during surgery. Skeletal muscle relaxation for ET intubation. Recommended for procedures lasting 90 or more minutes.

Contraindications: Due to the long duration of action, the drug should not be used in myasthenia gravis or Eaton-Lambert syndrome, as low doses can lead to a profound effect. Clients undergoing cesarean section. Use of pipecuronium before succinylcholine in order to reduce side effects of succinylcholine. In those requiring prolonged mechanical ventilation in the ICU or prior to or following other nondepolarizing neuromuscular blocking agents.

Special Concerns: Although the drug is used in infants and children, no information is available on maintenance dosing. Also, children 1–14 years of age under balanced or halothane anesthesia may be less sensitive to the drug than adults. Use with caution in clients with impaired renal function. The drug should be administered only if there are adequate facilities for intubation, artificial respiration, oxygen therapy, and administration of an antagonist. Obesity may prolong the duration of action. Conditions resulting in an increased volume of distribution (e.g., old age, edematous states, slower circulation time in CV disease) may cause a delay in the time of onset.

Side Effects: *Neuromuscular: Prolongation of blockade including skeletal muscle paralysis resulting in respiratory insufficiency or apnea.* Muscle atrophy, difficult intubation. *CV:* Hypotension, bradycardia, hypertension, CVA, thrombosis, myocardial ischemia, atrial fibrillation, ventricular extrasystole. *CNS:* Hypesthesia, CNS depression. *Respiratory:* Dyspnea, respiratory insufficiency, laryngismus, atelectasis. *Metabolic:* Hypoglycemia, hyperkalemia, increased creatinine. *Miscellaneous:* Rash, urticaria, anuria.

P

OD **Overdose Management:** *Symptoms:* **Skeletal muscle paralysis including depressed respiration.** *Treatment:* Artificial respiration until effects of drug have worn off. Antagonize neuromuscular blockade by administration of neostigmine, 0.04 mg/kg. Use of edrophonium is not recommended.

Drug Interactions:
Aminoglycosides / ↑ Intensity and duration of neuromuscular blockade
Bacitracin / ↑ Intensity and duration of neuromuscular blockade
Colistin/Sodium colistimethate / ↑ Intensity and duration of neuromuscular blockade
Enflurane / ↑ Duration of action of pipecuronium
Halothane / ↑ Duration of action of pipecuronium
Isoflurane / ↑ Duration of action of pipecuronium
Magnesium salts / ↑ Intensity of neuromuscular blockade when used for toxemia of pregnancy
Polymyxin B / ↑ Intensity and duration of neuromuscular blockade
Quinidine / ↑ Risk of recurrent paralysis
Tetracyclines / ↑ Intensity and duration of neuromuscular blockade

Dosage ————————————————
• **IV Only**
Adjunct to general anesthesia.
Adults: Initial dose may be based on the creatinine clearance and the ideal body weight (see information provided by manufacturer). Dose is individualized. The dose range is 50–100 mcg/kg.
ET intubation using balanced anesthesia.
70–85 mcg/kg with halothane, isoflurane, or enflurane in clients with normal renal function who are not obese; duration of muscle relaxation is 1–2 hr using this dosage range.
Use following recovery from succinylcholine.
50 mcg/kg in clients with normal renal function who are not obese; duration of muscle relaxation using this dose is 45 min. *Maintenance.*
Adults: 10–15 mcg/kg given at 25%

recovery of control T_1 will provide muscle relaxation for an average of 50 min using balanced anesthesia; lower doses should be used in clients receiving inhalation anesthetics. **Pediatric:** The duration of action in infants following a dose of 40 mcg/kg ranged from 10 to 44 min while the duration in children following a dose of 57 mcg/kg ranged from 18 to 52 min.

RESPIRATORY CARE CONSIDERATIONS

See also *Respiratory Care Considerations* for *Neuromuscular Blocking Agents.*

Administration/Storage:
1. Pipecuronium should be administered only under the supervision of individuals experienced with the use of neuromuscular blocking agents.
2. Pipecuronium can be reconstituted using 0.9% sodium chloride, 5% dextrose in saline, D5W, lactated Ringer's, sterile water for injection, and bacteriostatic water for injection.
3. If used in newborns, the drug should not be reconstituted with bacteriostatic water for injection because it contains benzyl alcohol.
4. When reconstituted with bacteriostatic water for injection, the solution may be stored at room temperature or in the refrigerator; it should be used within 5 days.
5. When reconstituted with sterile water for injection or other IV solutions, the vial should be refrigerated and used within 24 hr.
6. Pipecuronium should not be diluted with or administered from large volumes of IV solutions.
7. The drug should be s tored at 2°C–30°C (35°F–86°F) and protected from light.

Assessment:
1. Document indications for therapy and anticipated duration of use and review the expected loss of muscle control.
2. Document height and weight and note any evidence of obesity; drug dose should be correlated for *ideal* body weight.

3. Review client history for evidence of myasthenia gravis or Eaton-Lambert syndrome because drug is not recommended with these conditions.

4. List drugs client currently prescribed because many interact unfavorably with pipecuronium.

5. Determine if diarrhea is present and the duration because this may alter desired neuromuscular blockade.

6. Obtain baseline ECG, VS, electrolytes, and renal function studies.

Interventions:

1. The twitch response should be used to evaluate neuromuscular response and recovery and to minimize overdosage potential. Use a peripheral nerve stimulator to assess the height of the twitch wave. This device will assist to monitor drug response, to assess the need for additional doses of the drug, and to evaluate the adequacy of spontaneous recovery or antagonism.

2. Allow more time for pipecuronium to achieve maximum effect in older clients with slowed circulation, CV diseases, and/or edematous states. *Do not* increase drug dose because this will produce a longer duration of action.

3. Monitor BP and pulse closely and observe postrecovery for adequate clinical evidence of antagonism:

• 5-sec head lift
• Adequate pronation
• Effective airway and ventilatory patterns

4. Monitor VS and ECG. Drug can cause vagal stimulation resulting in bradycardia, hypotension, and cardiac arrhythmias.

5. Muscle fasciculations may cause the client to be sore or injured after recovery. Administer prescribed nondepolarizing agent and reassure that the soreness is likely caused by the unsynchronized contractions of adjacent muscle fibers just before the onset of paralysis.

6. Document length of time client is receiving the drug. It should be used only on a short-term basis and in a continuously monitored environment.

7. Remember client is fully conscious and aware of surroundings and conversations.

8. Drug does not affect pain or anxiety so administer analgesics and antianxiety agents as indicated.

9. Prolonged use, as in an ICU setting, may lead to skeletal muscle weakness and symptoms consistent with muscle disuse atrophy. This may complicate ventilator weaning and some clients may require extensive physical therapy.

Evaluate:

• Desired level of skeletal muscle relaxation
• Suppression of twitch response when tested with a peripheral nerve stimulator

Piperacillin sodium

(pie-**PER**-ah-sill-in)
Pregnancy Category: B
Pipracil **(Rx)**
Classification: Antibiotic, penicillin

See also *Penicillins*.

Action/Kinetics: Piperacillin is a semisynthetic, broad-spectrum penicillin for parenteral use. It is not penicillinase resistant. The drug penetrates CSF in the presence of inflamed meninges. **Peak serum level:** 244 mcg/mL. **t½:** 36–72 min. Excreted unchanged in urine and bile.

Uses: Intra-abdominal infections, gynecologic infections, septicemia, skin and skin structure infections, bone and joint infections, UTIs, lower respiratory tract infections, gonococcal infections, streptococcal infections. Mixed infections prior to the identification of the causative organisms. Prophylaxis in surgery including GI, biliary, hysterectomy, cesarean section.

Aminoglycosides have been used with ampicillin sodium, especially in clients with impaired host defenses.

P

Additional Side Effects: Rarely, prolonged muscle relaxation.
Laboratory Test Interferences: Positive Coombs' test; ↑ (especially in infants) AST, ALT, LDH, bilirubin.

Dosage

• **IM, IV**
  Serious infections.
IV: 3–4 g q 4–6 hr (12–18 g/day) as a 20- to 30-min infusion.
  Complicated UTIs.
IV: 8–16 g/day (125–200 mg/kg/day) in divided doses q 6–8 hr.
  Uncomplicated UTIs and most community-acquired pneumonias.
IM, IV: 6–8 g/day (100–125 mg/kg/day) in divided doses q 6–12 hr.
  Uncomplicated gonorrhea infections.
2 g **IM** with 1 g probenecid **PO** 30 min before injection (both given as single dose).
  Prophylaxis in surgery.
First dose: IV, 2 g prior to surgery; **second dose:** 2 g either during surgery (abdominal) or 4–6 hr after surgery (hysterectomy, cesarean); **third dose:** 2 g at an interval depending on use. Dosage should be decreased in renal impairment.

Dosages have not been established in infants and children under 12 years of age although the following doses have been suggested: **Neonates,** 100 mg/kg q 12 hr; **children,** 200–300 mg/kg/day (up to a maximum of 24 g/day) divided q 4–6 hr.
  For cystic fibrosis.
350–500 mg/kg/day divided q 4–6 hr.

RESPIRATORY CARE CONSIDERATIONS

See also *Respiratory Care Considerations* for *Penicillins* and *Zosyn.*
Administration/Storage:
1. No more than 2 g should be administered IM at any one site.
2. For IM administration, use upper, outer quadrant of gluteus or well-developed deltoid muscle. Do not use lower or mid-third of upper arm.
3. For IV administration reconstitute each gram with at least 5 mL diluent, such as sterile or bacteriostatic water

for injection, sodium chloride for injection, or bacteriostatic sodium chloride for injection. Shake until dissolved.
4. Inject IV slowly over a period of 3–5 min to avoid vein irritation.
5. Administer by intermittent IV infusion in at least 50 mL of dextrose or saline solutions over a period of 20–30 min.
6. After reconstitution, solution may be stored at room temperature for 24 hr, refrigerated for 1 week, or frozen for 1 month.
Assessment:
1. Document indications for therapy and type and onset of symptoms.
2. Ensure that appropriate pretreatment cultures have been sent.
3. Obtain baseline electrolytes, hematologic, liver, and renal function studies and monitor throughout therapy.
4. Assess for diarrhea or any other evidence of superinfection.
Evaluate:
• Infection prophylaxis during surgery
• Clinical evidence and reports of symptomatic improvement
• Negative lab C&S reports

Pirbuterol acetate

(peer-**BYOU**-ter-ohl)
Pregnancy Category: C
Maxair Autohaler **(Rx)**
Classification: Sympathomimetic, bronchodilator

See also *Sympathomimetic Drugs.*
Action/Kinetics: Pirbuterol causes bronchodilation by stimulating beta-2-adrenergic receptors. It has minimal effects on beta-1 receptors. The drug also inhibits histamine release from mast cells, causes vasodilation, and increases ciliary motility. It has minimal beta-1 activity. **Onset, inhalation:** Approximately 5 min. **Time to peak effect:** 30–60 min. **Duration:** 5 hr.
Uses: Alone or with theophylline or steroids, for prophylaxis and treatment of bronchospasm in asthma and other conditions with reversible

bronchospasms, including bronchitis, emphysema, bronchiectasis, obstructive pulmonary disease. May be used with or without theophylline or steroids.

Contraindications: Cardiac arrhythmias due to tachycardia; tachycardia caused by digitalis toxicity.

Special Concerns: Safety and efficacy have not been determined in children less than 12 years of age.

Additional Side Effects: *CV:* PVCs, hypotension. *CNS:* Hyperactivity, hyperkinesia, anxiety, confusion, depression, fatigue, syncope. *GI:* Diarrhea, dry mouth, anorexia, loss of appetite, bad taste or taste change, abdominal pain, abdominal cramps, stomatitis, glossitis. *Dermatologic:* Rash, edema, pruritus, alopecia. *Miscellaneous:* Flushing, numbness in extremities, weight gain.

Dosage ⎯⎯⎯⎯⎯⎯⎯⎯
• **Inhalation Aerosol**
Adults and children over 12 years: 0.2–0.4 mg (1–2 inhalations) q 4–6 hr, not to exceed 12 inhalations (2.4 mg) daily.

RESPIRATORY CARE CONSIDERATIONS

See also *Respiratory Care Considerations* for *Sympathomimetic Drugs*.
Assessment: Document indications for therapy, noting onset, duration, and characteristics of symptoms. Perform cardiopulmonary assessment.
Evaluate: Improved pulmonary function

Potassium Salts Potassium acetate, parenteral
Pregnancy Category: C
(Rx)

Potassium acetate, Potassium bicarbonate, and Potassium citrate (Trikates)
Oral Solution: Tri-K **(Rx)**

Potassium bicarbonate
K + Care ET **(Rx)**

Potassium bicarbonate and Citric acid
Effervescent Tablets: K+ Care ET, Klor-Con/EF **(Rx)**

Potassium bicarbonate and Potassium chloride
Effervescent Granules: Neo-K ✿ **(Rx)**.
Effervescent Tablets: Klorvess, K-Lyte/Cl, K-Lyte/Cl 50, Potassium-Sandoz ✿ **(Rx)**

Potassium bicarbonate and Potassium citrate
Effervescent Tablets: Effer-K, Effervescent Potassium, K-Lyte **(Rx)**

Potassium chloride
Extended-Release Capsules: K-Lease, K-Norm, Micro-K Extencaps, Micro-K 10 Extencaps **(Rx)**. **Injection:** Potassium Chloride for Injection Concentrate **(Rx)**. **Oral Solution:** Cena-K 10% and 20%, K-10 ✿, Kaochlor-10 and -20 ✿, Kaochlor 10%, Kaochlor S-F 10%, Kaon-Cl 20% Liquid, Kay Ciel, KCl 5% ✿, Klorvess 10% Liquid, Potasalan, Rum-K **(Rx)**. **Powder for Oral Solution:** Gen-K, Kay Ciel, K+ Care, K-Lor, Klor-Con Powder, Klor-Con/25 Powder, K-Lyte/Cl Powder, Micro-K LS **(Rx)**. , **Extended-Release Tablets:** Apo-K ✿, K+ 10, Kalium Durules ✿, Kaon-Cl, Kaon-Cl-10, K-Dur 10 and 20, K-Long ✿, Klor-Con 8 and 10, Klotrix, K-Tab, Novolente-K ✿, Slow-K, Slo-Pot 600 ✿, Slow-K ✿, Ten-K **(Rx)**

Potassium chloride, Potassium bicarbonate, and Potassium citrate
Effervescent Granules: Klorvess Effervescent Granules **(Rx)**

Potassium gluconate
Elixir: Kaon, Kaylixir, K-G Elixir, Potassium-Rougier ✿, Royonate ✿ **(Rx)**.
Tablets: Kaon ✿ **(Rx)**

P

✿ = Available in Canada   ***bold italic*** = life threatening side effect

Potassium gluconate and Potassium chloride
Oral Solution and Powder for Oral Solution: Kolyum **(Rx)**

Potassium gluconate and Potassium citrate
Oral Solution: Twin-K **(Rx)**
Classification: Electrolyte

General Statement: Potassium is the major cation of the body's intracellular fluid. It is essential for the maintenance of important physiologic processes, including cardiac, smooth, and skeletal muscle function, acid-base balance, gastric secretions, renal function, protein and carbohydrate metabolism. Symptoms of hypokalemia include weakness, cardiac arrhythmias, fatigue, ileus, hyporeflexia or areflexia, tetany, polydipsia, and, in severe cases, flaccid paralysis and inability to concentrate urine. Loss of potassium is usually accompanied by a loss of chloride resulting in hypochloremic metabolic alkalosis.

The usual adult daily requirement of potassium is 40–80 mg. In adults, the normal extracellular concentration of potassium ranges from 3.5 to 5 mEq/L with the intracellular levels being 150–160 mEq/L. Extracellular concentrations of up to 5.6 mEq/L are normal in children.

Both hypokalemia and hyperkalemia, if uncorrected, can be fatal; thus, potassium must always be administered cautiously.

Potassium is readily and rapidly absorbed from the GI tract. Though a number of salts can be used to supply the potassium cation, potassium chloride is the agent of choice since hypochloremia frequently accompanies potassium deficiency. Dietary measures can often prevent and even correct potassium deficiencies. Potassium-rich foods include most meats (beef, chicken, ham, turkey, veal), fish, beans, broccoli, brussels sprouts, lentils, spinach, potatoes, milk, bananas, dates, prunes, raisins, avocados, watermelon, cantaloupe, apricots, and molasses.

From 80% to 90% of potassium intake is excreted by the kidney and is partially reabsorbed from the glomerular filtrate.

Uses: PO. Treat hypokalemia due to digitalis intoxication, diabetic acidosis, diarrhea and vomiting, familial periodic paralysis, certain cases of uremia, hyperadrenalism, starvation and debilitation, and corticosteroid or diuretic therapy. Also, hypokalemia with or without metabolic acidosis and following surgical conditions accompanied by nitrogen loss, vomiting and diarrhea, suction drainage, and increased urinary excretion of potassium. Prophylaxis of potassium depletion when dietary intake is not adequate in the following conditions: clients on digitalis and diuretics for CHF, hepatic cirrhosis with ascites, excess aldosterone with normal renal function, significant cardiac arrhythmias, potassium-losing nephropathy, and certain states accompanied by diarrhea. *Investigational:* Mild hypertension.

NOTE: Potassium chloride should be used when hypokalemia is associated with alkalosis; potassium bicarbonate, citrate, acetate, or gluconate should be used when hypokalemia is associated with acidosis.

IV. Prophylaxis and treatment of moderate to severe potassium loss when PO therapy is not feasible. Potassium acetate is used as an additive for preparing specific IV formulas when client needs cannot be met by usual nutrient or electrolyte preparations. Potassium acetate is also used in the following conditions: marked loss of GI secretions due to vomiting, diarrhea, GI intubation, or fistulas; prolonged parenteral use of potassium-free fluids (e.g., dextrose or NSS); diabetic acidosis, especially during treatment with insulin and dextrose infusions; prolonged diuresis; metabolic alkalosis; hyperadrenocorticism; primary aldosteronism; overdose of adrenocortical steroids, testosterone, or corticotropin; attacks of hereditary or familial periodic paralysis; during the healing phase of burns or scalds; and cardiac arrhythmias, especially due to digitalis glycosides.

Contraindications: Severe renal function impairment with azotemia or oliguria, postoperatively before urine flow has been reestablished. Crush syndrome, Addison's disease, hyperkalemia from any cause, anuria, heat cramps, acute dehydration, severe hemolytic reactions, adynamia episodica hereditaria, clients receiving potassium-sparing diuretics or aldosterone-inhibiting drugs. Solid dosage forms in clients in whom there is a reason for delay or arrest in passage of tablets through the GI tract.

Special Concerns: Safety during lactation and in children has not been established. Geriatric clients are at greater risk of developing hyperkalemia due to age-related changes in renal function. Administer with caution in the presence of cardiac and renal disease. Potassium loss is often accompanied by an obligatory loss of chloride resulting in hypochloremic metabolic alkalosis; thus, the underlying cause of the potassium loss should be treated.

Side Effects: Hypokalemia. *CNS:* Dizziness, mental confusion. *CV:* Arrhythmias; weak, irregular pulse; hypotension, *heart block,* ECG abnormalities, *cardiac arrest.* *GI:* Abdominal distention, anorexia, N&V, *Neuromuscular:* Weakness, paresthesia of extremities, flaccid paralysis, areflexia, muscle or *respiratory paralysis,* weakness and heaviness of legs. *Other:* Malaise.

Hyperkalemia. *CV:* Bradycardia, then tachycardia, *cardiac arrest.* *GI:* N&V, diarrhea, abdominal cramps, GI bleeding or obstruction. Ulceration or perforation of the small bowel from enteric-coated potassium chloride tablets. *GU:* Oliguria, anuria. *Neuromuscular:* Weakness, tingling, paralysis. *Other:* Skin rashes, hyperkalemia.

Effects due to solution or IV technique used. Fever, infection at injection site, venous thrombosis, phlebitis extending from injection site, extravasation, venospasm, hypervolemia, hyperkalemia.

OD **Overdose Management:** *Symptoms:* Mild (5.5–6.5 mEq/L) to moderate (6.5–8 mEq/L) hyperkalemia (may be asymptomatic except for ECG changes). ECG changes include progression in height and peak of T waves, lowering of the R wave, decreased amplitude and eventually disappearance of P waves, prolonged PR interval and QRS complex, shortening of the QT interval, *ventricular fibrillation, death. Muscle weakness that may progress to flaccid quadriplegia and respiratory failure,* although dangerous cardiac arrhythmias usually occur before onset of complete paralysis. *Treatment (plasma potassium levels greater than 6.5 mEq/L):* All measures must be monitored by ECG. Measures consist of actions taken to shift potassium ions from plasma into cells by.
• **Sodium bicarbonate:** IV infusion of 50–100 mEq over period of 5 min. May be repeated after 10–15 minutes if ECG abnormalities persist.
• **Glucose and insulin:** IV infusion of 3 g glucose to 1 unit regular insulin to shift potassium into cells.
• **Calcium gluconate—or other calcium salt** (only for clients not on digitalis or other cardiotonic glycosides): IV infusion of 0.5–1 g (5–10 mL of a 10% solution) over period of 2 min. Dosage may be repeated after 1–2 min if ECG remains abnormal. When ECG is approximately normal, the excess potassium should be removed from the body by administration of polystyrene sulfonate, hemodialysis or peritoneal dialysis (clients with renal insufficiency), or other means.
• **Sodium polystyrene sulfonate, hemodialysis, peritoneal dialysis:** To remove potassium from the body.

Drug Interactions:
ACE inhibitors / May cause potassium retention → hyperkalemia

Digitalis glycosides / Cardiac arrhythmias
Potassium-sparing diuretics / Severe hyperkalemia with possibility of cardiac arrhythmias or arrest

Dosage ⎯⎯⎯⎯⎯⎯⎯⎯⎯
Highly individualized. Oral administration is preferred because the slow absorption from the GI tract prevents sudden, large increases in plasma potassium levels. Dosage is usually expressed as mEq/L of potassium. The bicarbonate, chloride, citrate, and gluconate salts are usually administered PO. The chloride, acetate, and phosphate may be administered by **slow IV** infusion.

• **IV Infusion**
Serum K less than 2.0 mEq/L.
400 mEq/day at a rate not to exceed 40 mEq/hr. A maximum concentration of 80 mEq/L should be used.
Serum K more than 2.5 mEq/L.
200 mEq/day at a rate not to exceed 20 mEq/hr. A maximum concentration of 40 mEq/L should be used.
Pediatric: Up to 3 mEq potassium/kg (or 40 mEq/m^2) daily. The volume administered should be adjusted depending on the body size.

• **Effervescent Granules, Effervescent Tablets, Elixir, Extended-Release Capsules, Extended Release Granules, Extended-Release Tablets, Oral Solution, Powder for Oral Solution, Tablets**
Prophylaxis of hypokalemia.
16–24 mEq/day.
Potassium depletion.
40–100 mEq/day.
NOTE: Usual dietary intake of potassium is 40–250 mEq/day.
For clients with accompanying metabolic acidosis, an alkalizing potassium salt (potassium bicarbonate, potassium citrate, or potassium acetate) should be selected.

RESPIRATORY CARE CONSIDERATIONS
Administration/Storage:
Oral
1. Dilute or dissolve PO liquids, effervescent tablets, or soluble powders in 3–8 oz of cold water, fruit or vegetable juice, or other suitable liquid and drink slowly.
2. Chill to increase palatability.
3. Instruct client to swallow enteric-coated tablets and extended-release capsules and tablets and not to dissolve them in the mouth.
4. Give PO doses 2–4 times/day. Hypokalemia should be corrected slowly over a period of 3–7 days to minimize the development of hyperkalemia.
5. Salt substitutes should not be used concomitantly with potassium preparations.
6. Administer dilute liquid solutions of potassium rather than tablets to clients with esophageal compression.
7. If GI upset occurs, products can be taken after meals or with food with a full glass of water.
Parenteral
1. All parenteral products must be diluted with a suitable large volume of parenteral solution, mixed well, and given by slow IV infusion. The usual concentration of potassium chloride is 40 mEq/L of IV fluid (up to a maximum of 80 mEq/L).
2. "Layering" of potassium should be avoided by properly agitating the prepared IV solution. Potassium should never be added to an IV bottle that is hanging.
3. Potassium should not be administered IV undiluted. Usual method is to administer by slow IV infusion in dextrose solution at a concentration of 40–80 mEq/L and at a rate not to exceed 10–20 mEq/hr.
4. Ensure uniform distribution of potassium by inverting container during addition of potassium solution and then by agitating container. Squeezing the plastic container will not prevent potassium chloride from settling to the bottom.
5. Check site of administration frequently for pain and redness because drug is extremely irritating.
6. In critical clients, potassium chloride may be given slow IV in a solution of saline (unless contraindicated) since dextrose may lower serum potassium levels by producing an intracellular shift.

7. Administer all concentrated potassium infusions and riders with an infusion control device.

8. Have sodium polystyrene sulfonate (Kayexalate) available for oral or rectal administration in the event of hyperkalemia.

Assessment:

1. Note indications for therapy; document baseline serum electrolytes and ECG.

2. Note any prior history of impaired renal function.

3. Assess for adequate urinary flow before administering potassium. Impaired renal function can lead to hyperkalemia.

Interventions:

1. Once parenteral potassium administration is initiated, discontinue administering potassium-rich foods and potassium supplements.

2. If the client develops abdominal pain, distention, or GI bleeding, withhold PO potassium medication and report.

3. Note any complaints of weakness, fatigue, or the presence of cardiac arrhythmias. These may be symptoms of hypokalemia indicating a low *intracellular* potassium level, although the serum potassium level may appear to be within normal limits.

4. Monitor I&O. If the client develops oliguria, anuria, or azoturia, withhold the drug and report.

5. Observe carefully for symptoms of adrenal insufficiency or extensive tissue breakdown.

6. Report complaints of weakness or heaviness of the legs, the presence of a gray pallor, cold skin, listlessness, mental confusion, flaccid paralysis, hypotension, or cardiac arrhythmias. These are symptoms of hyperkalemia and the medication should be stopped immediately as the client may go into CV collapse.

7. Monitor serum potassium levels while the client is receiving parenteral potassium. The normal level is 3.5–5.0 mEq/L; any variation should be reported.

Evaluate:

• Correction of potassium deficiency
• Serum potassium levels within desired range

Prazosin hydrochloride
(**PRAY**-zoh-sin)
Pregnancy Category: C
Apo-Prazo ✦, Minipress, Novo-Prazin ✦, Nu-Prazo ✦ **(Rx)**
Classification: Antihypertensive, alpha-1-adrenergic blocking agent

See also *Alpha-1-Adrenergic Blocking Agents* and *Antihypertensive Agents.*

Action/Kinetics: Produces selective blockade of postsynaptic alpha-1-adrenergic receptors. Dilates arterioles and veins, thereby decreasing total peripheral resistance and decreasing DBP more than SBP. CO, HR, and renal blood flow are not affected. Can be used to initiate antihypertensive therapy and is most effective when used with other agents (e.g., diuretics, beta-adrenergic blocking agents). **Onset:** 2 hr. Absorption is not affected by food. **Maximum effect:** 2–3 hr; **duration:** 6–12 hr. **t½:** 2–3 hr. Full therapeutic effect: 4–6 weeks. Metabolized extensively; excreted primarily in feces.

Uses: Mild to moderate hypertension alone or in combination with other antihypertensive drugs. *Investigational:* CHF refractory to other treatment. Raynaud's disease, benign prostatic hypertrophy.

Special Concerns: Safe use in children has not been established. Use with caution during lactation. Geriatric clients may be more sensitive to the hypotensive and hypothermic effects of prazosin; also, it may be necessary to decrease the dose in these clients due to age-related decreases in renal function.

Side Effects: First-dose effect: *Marked hypotension* and syncope 30–90 min after administration of initial dose (usually 2 or more mg), increase of dosage, or addition of other antihypertensive agent. *CNS:* Dizziness, drowsiness, headache, fatigue, paresthesias, depression, vertigo, nervousness, hallucinations. *CV:* Palpitations, syncope, tachycardia, orthostatic hypotension, aggravation of angina. *GI:* N&V, diarrhea or constipation, dry mouth, abdominal pain, pancreatitis. *GU:* Urinary frequency or incontinence, impotence, priapism. *Respiratory:* Dyspnea, nasal congestion, epistaxis. *Dermatologic:* Pruritus, rash, sweating, alopecia, lichen planus. *Miscellaneous:* Asthenia, edema, symptoms of lupus erythematosus, blurred vision, tinnitus, arthralgia, myalgia, reddening of sclera, eye pain, conjunctivitis, edema, fever.

OD **Overdose Management:**
Symptoms: Hypotension, **shock.** *Treatment:* Keep client supine to restore BP and HR. If shock is manifested, use volume expanders and vasopressors; maintain renal function.

Drug Interactions:
Antihypertensives (other) / ↑ Antihypertensive effect
Beta-adrenergic blocking agents / Enhanced acute postural hypotension following the first dose of prazosin
Clonidine / ↓ Antihypertensive effect of clonidine
Diuretics / ↑ Antihypertensive effect
Indomethacin / ↓ Effect of prazosin
Nifedipine / ↑ Hypotensive effect
Propranolol / Especially pronounced additive hypotensive effect
Verapamil / ↑ Hypotensive effect; ↑ sensitivity to prazosin-induced postural hypotension

Laboratory Test Interferences: ↑ Urinary metabolites of norepinephrine, VMA.

Dosage ——————
• **Capsules**
Hypertension.
Individualized: Initial, 1 mg b.i.d.–t.i.d.; **maintenance:** if necessary, increase gradually to 6–15 mg/day in two to three divided doses. Daily dose should not exceed 20 mg, although some clients have benefitted from doses of 40 mg daily. If

used with diuretics or other antihypertensives, reduce dose to 1–2 mg t.i.d. **Pediatric, less than 7 years of age, initial:** 0.25 mg b.i.d.–t.i.d. adjusted according to response. **Pediatric, 7–12 years of age, initial:** 0.5 mg b.i.d.–t.i.d. adjusted according to response.

RESPIRATORY CARE CONSIDERATIONS

See also *Respiratory Care Considerations* for *Antihypertensive Agents* and *Alpha-1-Adrenergic Blocking Agents.*

Administration/Storage:
1. The first dose should be taken at bedtime. Also, the first dose of each increment should be given at bedtime to reduce the incidence of syncope.
2. Due to the first-dose effect, clients should not drive or operate machinery for 24 hr after the first dose.
3. The dose should be reduced to 1 or 2 mg t.i.d. if a diuretic or other antihypertensive agent is added to the regimen. The client can then be retitrated.

Evaluate:
• ↓ BP
• Improvement in symptoms of refractory CHF

Prednisolone
(pred-**NISS**-oh-lohn)
Syrup: Prelone. **Tablets:** Delta-Cortef **(Rx)**

Prednisolone acetate
(pred-**NISS**-oh-lohn)
Parenteral: Articulose-50, Key-Pred 25 and 50, Predalone 50, **Ophthalmic Suspension:**, Diopred ✿, Econopred Ophthalmic, Econopred Plus, Ophtho-Tate ✿, Pred Forte Ophthalmic, Pred Mild Ophthalmic **(Rx)**

Prednisolone acetate and Prednisolone sodium phosphate
(pred-**NISS**-oh-lohn)
(Rx)

Prednisolone sodium phosphate

(pred-**NISS**-oh-lohn)

Pregnancy Category: C

Oral Solution: Pediapred **(Rx)**. **Ophthalmic Solution:** AK-Pred Ophthalmic, Inflamase Forte Ophthalmic, Inflamase Mild Ophthalmic, Inflamase Forte Ophthalmic **(Rx)**. **Parenteral:** Hydeltrasol, Key-Pred-SP **(Rx)**

Prednisolone tebutate

(pred-**NISS**-oh-lohn)

Hydeltra-T.B.A., Prednisol TPA **(Rx)**

Classification: Corticosteroid, synthetic

See also *Corticosteroids.*

Action/Kinetics: Intermediate-acting. Prednisolone is five times more potent than hydrocortisone and cortisone. Side effects are minimal except for GI distress. Has moderate mineralocorticoid activity. **Plasma t½:** over 200 min.

Contraindications: Lactation.

Special Concerns: Use during pregnancy only if benefits outweigh risks. Use with particular caution in diabetes.

Dosage ――――――――――――

PREDNISOLONE

- **Tablets, Syrup**
  Most uses.
5–60 mg/day, depending on disease being treated.
  Multiple sclerosis (exacerbation).
200 mg/day for 1 week; **then,** 80 mg on alternate days for 1 month.
  Pleurisy of tuberculosis.
0.75 mg/kg/day (then taper) given concurrently with antituberculosis therapy.

PREDNISOLONE ACETATE

- **IM**
4–60 mg/day. **Not for IV use.**
  Multiple sclerosis (exacerbation).
See *Prednisolone.*

- **Intralesional,   Intra-articular, Soft Tissue Injection**
4–100 mg (larger doses for large joints).

- **Ophthalmic   Suspension (0.12%, 0.125%, 1%)**

1–2 gtt in the conjunctival sac q hr during the day and q 2 hr during the night; **then,** after response obtained, decrease dose to 1 gtt/ q 4 hr and then later 1 gtt t.i.d.–q.i.d.

PREDNISOLONE ACETATE AND PREDNISOLONE SODIUM PHOSPHATE

- **IM Only**
20–80 mg acetate and 5–20 mg sodium phosphate every few days for 3–4 weeks.

- **Intra-articular, Intrasynovial**
20–40 mg prednisolone acetate and 5–10 mg prednisolone sodium phosphate.

PREDNISOLONE SODIUM PHOSPHATE

- **PO Solution**
  Most uses.
5–60 mg/day in single or divided doses.
  Adrenocortical insufficiency.
Pediatric: 0.14 mg/kg (4 mg/m²) daily in three to four divided doses.
  Other pediatric uses.
0.5–2 mg/kg (15–60 mg/m²) daily in three to four divided doses.

- **IM, IV**
4–60 mg/day.
  Multiple sclerosis (exacerbation).
See *Prednisolone.*

- **Intralesional,   Intra-articular, Soft Tissue Injection**
2–30 mg, depending on site and severity of disease.

- **Ophthalmic Solution (0.125%, 1%)**
See *Prednisolone acetate.*

PREDNISOLONE TEBUTATE

- **Intra-articular,   Intralesional, Soft Tissue Injection**
4–30 mg, depending on site and severity of disease. Doses higher than 40 mg are not recommended.

RESPIRATORY CARE CONSIDERATIONS

See also *Respiratory Care Considerations* for *Corticosteroids.*

Administration/Storage:

1. Before administering prednisolone, check spelling and dose carefully; this drug is frequently confused with prednisone.

2. Check to see if provider wants

PO form of drug administered with an antacid.

3. Prednisolone sodium phosphate oral solution produces a 20% higher peak plasma level of prednisolone than is seen with tablets.

4. The IV form (sodium phosphate) may be administered at a rate not to exceed 10 mg/min.

Assessment:

1. Document indications for therapy and type and onset of symptoms.

2. Note any previous experiences with this drug and the outcome.

3. Obtain baseline VS, CBC, electrolytes, blood sugar, weight, and mental status.

Evaluate:

• Desired replacement therapy during adrenocortical hypofunction

• Symptomatic relief of allergic, immune, and inflammatory manifestations

Prednisone

(**PRED**-nih-sohn)

Oral Solution: Prednisone Intensol Concentrate **(Rx). Syrup:** Liquid Pred **(Rx). Tablets:** Apo-Prednisone ✦, Deltasone, Jaa Prednisone ✦, Meticorten, Novo-Prednisone ✦, Orasone 1, 5, 10, 20, and 50, Panasol-S, Sterapred DS, Winpred ✦ **(Rx)**
Classification: Corticosteroid, synthetic

See also *Corticosteroids*.
Action/Kinetics: Drug is three to five times as potent as cortisone or hydrocortisone. May cause moderate fluid retention. Prednisone is metabolized in the liver to prednisolone, the active form.
Special Concerns: Use during pregnancy only if benefits outweigh risks. Dose must be highly individualized.

Dosage ———————————
• **Oral Concentrate, Syrup, Tablets**
   Acute, severe conditions.
Initial: 5–60 mg/day in four equally divided doses after meals and at bedtime. Decrease gradually by 5–10 mg q 4–5 days to establish min-

imum maintenance dosage (5–10 mg) or discontinue altogether until symptoms recur.
   Replacement.
Pediatric: 0.1–0.15 mg/kg/day.
   COPD.
30–60 mg/day for 1–2 weeks; then taper.
   Ophthalmopathy due to Graves' disease.
60 mg/day; **then,** taper to 20 mg/day.
   Duchenne's muscular dystrophy.
0.75–1.5 mg/kg/day (used to improve strength).

RESPIRATORY CARE CONSIDERATIONS

See also *Respiratory Care Considerations* for *Corticosteroids*.
Assessment:

1. Document indications for therapy and type, onset, and duration of symptoms.

2. List other agents prescribed and the outcome.

3. Obtain baseline CBC, electrolytes, blood sugar, weights, and mental status.

Client/Family Teaching

1. Take with food to decrease GI upset.

2. With long-term therapy, advise not to stop abruptly.

3. Report any S&S of adrenal insufficiency or loss of effectiveness.

4. Avoid ethanol and all OTC agents without provider approval.

Evaluate: Symptomatic relief of allergic, immune, and inflammatory manifestations

Procainamide hydrochloride

(proh-**KAYN**-ah-myd)
Pregnancy Category: C
Apo-Procainamide ✦, Procanbid, Pronestyl, Pronestyl-SR **(Rx)**
Classification: Antiarrhythmic, class IA

See also *Antiarrhythmic Agents*.
Action/Kinetics: Procainamide produces a direct cardiac effect to prolong the refractory period of the

atria and to a lesser extent the bundle of His-Purkinje system and ventricles. Large doses may cause AV block. It has some anticholinergic and local anesthetic effects. Antiarrhythmic drugs have not been shown to increase the rate of survival in clients with ventricular arrhythmias. **Onset: PO,** 30 min; **IV,** 1–5 min. **Time to peak effect, PO:** 90–120 min; **IM,** 15–60 min; **IV,** immediate. **Duration:** 3 hr. **t½:** 2.5–4.7 hr. **Therapeutic serum level:** 4–8 mcg/mL. **Protein binding:** 15%. From 40% to 70% excreted unchanged. The drug may be metabolized in the liver (16%–21% by slow acetylators and 24%–33% by fast acetylators) to the active N-acetylprocainamide (NAPA).

Uses: Documented ventricular arrhythmias (e.g., sustained ventricular tachycardia) that may be life threatening in clients where benefits of treatment clearly outweigh risks. Antiarrhythmic drugs have not been shown to improve survival in clients with ventricular arrhythmias.

Contraindications: Hypersensitivity to drug, complete AV heart block, lupus erythematosus, torsades de pointes, asymptomatic ventricular premature contractions. Lactation.

Special Concerns: With use of procainamide there is an increased risk of death in those with non-life-threatening arrhythmias. Although used in children, safety and efficacy have not been established. Use with extreme caution in clients for whom a sudden drop in BP could be detrimental, in CHF, acute ischemic heart disease, or cardiomyopathy. Also, use with caution in clients with liver or kidney dysfunction, preexisting bone marrow failure or cytopenia of any type, development of first-degree heart block while on procainamide, myasthenia gravis, and those with bronchial asthma or other respiratory disorders. Procainamide may cause more hypotension in geriatric clients; also, in this population, the

dose may have to be decreased due to age-related decreases in renal function.

Side Effects: *Body as a whole:* Lupus erythematosus–like syndrome especially in those on maintenance therapy and who are slow acetylators. Symptoms include arthralgia, pleural or abdominal pain, arthritis, pleural effusion, pericarditis, fever, chills, myalgia, skin lesions, hematologic changes. *CV:* Following IV use: Hypotension, *ventricular asystole or fibrillation, partial or complete heart block.* Rarely, second-degree heart block after PO use. *GI:* N&V, diarrhea, anorexia, bitter taste, abdominal pain. *Hematologic:* Thrombocytopenia, *agranulocytosis,* neutropenia. *Rarely, hemolytic anemia. Dermatologic:* Urticaria, pruritus, angioneurotic edema, flushing, maculopapular rash. *CNS:* Depression, dizziness, weakness, giddiness, psychoses, hallucinations. *Other:* Granulomatous hepatitis, weakness, fever, chills.

OD **Overdose Management:** *Symptoms:* Plasma levels of 10–15 mcg/mL are associated with toxic symptoms. Progressive widening of the QRS complex, prolonged QT or PR intervals, lowering of R and T waves, increased AV block, increased ventricular extrasystoles, *ventricular tachycardia or fibrillation. IV overdose may result in hypotension, CNS depression, tremor, respiratory depression. Treatment:*
• Induce emesis or perform gastric lavage followed by administration of activated charcoal.
• To treat hypotension, give IV fluids and/or a vasopressor (dopamine, phenylephrine, or norepinephrine).
• Infusion of ⅙ molar sodium lactate reduces the cardiotoxic effects.
• Hemodialysis (but not peritoneal dialysis) is effective in reducing serum levels.
• Renal clearance can be enhanced by acidification of the urine and with high flow rates.
• A ventricular pacing electrode can

P

be inserted as a precaution in the event AV block develops.

Drug Interactions:

Acetazolamide / ↑ Effect of procainamide due to ↓ excretion by kidney

Anticholinergic agents, atropine / Additive anticholinergic effects

Antihypertensive agents / Additive hypotensive effect

Cholinergic agents / Anticholinergic activity of procainamide antagonizes effect of cholinergic drugs

Cimetidine / ↑ Effect of procainamide due to ↑ bioavailability

Disopyramide / ↑ Risk of enhanced prolongation of conduction or depression of contractility and hypotension

Ethanol / Effect of procainamide may be altered, but because the main metabolite is active as an antiarrhythmic, specific outcome not clear

Kanamycin / Procainamide ↑ muscle relaxation produced by kanamycin

Lidocaine / Additive cardiodepressant effects

Magnesium salts / Procainamide ↑ muscle relaxation produced by magnesium salts

Neomycin / Procainamide ↑ muscle relaxation produced by neomycin

Propranolol / ↑ Serum procainamide levels

Quinidine / ↑ Risk of enhanced prolongation of conduction or depression of contractility and hypotension

Ranitidine / ↑ Effect of procainamide due to ↑ bioavailability

Sodium bicarbonate / ↑ Effect of procainamide due to ↓ excretion by the kidney

Succinylcholine / Procainamide ↑ muscle relaxation produced by succinylcholine

Trimethoprim / ↑ Effect of procainamide due to ↑ serum levels

Laboratory Test Interferences: May affect liver function tests. False + ↑ in serum alkaline phosphatase. Positive ANA test. High levels of lidocaine and meprobamate may inhib-

it fluorescence of procainamide and NAPA.

Dosage ─────────────────

• **Capsules, Extended-Release Tablets, Tablets**

Adults, initial: 50 mg/kg/day in divided doses q 3 hr. **Usual, 40–50 kg:** 250 mg q 3 hr of standard formulation or 500 mg q 6 hr of sustained-release; **60–70 kg:** 375 mg q 3 hr of standard formulation or 750 mg q 6 hr of sustained-release; **80–90 kg:** 500 mg q 3 hr of standard formulation or 1 g q 6 hr of sustained-release; **over 100 kg:** 625 mg q 3 hr of standard formulation or 1.25 g q 6 hr of sustained-release. **Pediatric:** 15–50 mg/kg/day divided q 3–6 hr (up to a maximum of 4 g/day).

• **Procanbid Extended-Release Tablets**

Life-threatening arrhythmias.
500 or 1,000 mg b.i.d.

• **IM**

Ventricular arrhythmias.

Adults, initial: 50 mg/kg/day divided into fractional doses of ⅛–¼ given q 3–6 hr until PO therapy is possible. **Pediatric:** 20–30 mg/kg/day divided q 4–6 hr (up to a maximum of 4 g/day).

Arrhythmias associated with surgery or anesthesia.

Adults: 100–500 mg.

• **IV**

Initial loading infusion: 20 mg/min (for up to 25–30 min). **Maintenance infusion:** 2–6 mg/min. **Pediatric, initial loading dose:** 3–5 mg/kg/dose over 5 min (maximum of 100 mg); **maintenance:** 20–80 mcg/kg/min continuous infusion (maximum of 2 g/day).

RESPIRATORY CARE CONSIDERATIONS

See also *Respiratory Care Considerations* for *Antiarrhythmic Agents.*

Administration/Storage:

1. IV use should be reserved for emergency situations.

2. IM therapy may be used as an alternative to PO for clients with less threatening arrhythmias but who are nauseated or vomiting, who cannot

take anything PO (e.g., preoperatively), or who have malabsorptive problems.

3. If more than three IM injections are required, the age and renal function of the client should be assessed as well as blood levels of procainamide and NAPA; adjust dosage accordingly.

4. For IV initial therapy, the drug should be diluted with 5% dextrose solution and a maximum of 1 g administered slowly to minimize side effects by one of the following methods:

• Direct injection into a vein or into tubing of an established infusion line at a rate not to exceed 50 mg/min. Dilute either the 100- or 500-mg/mL vials prior to injection to facilitate control of the dosage rate. Doses of 100 mg may be given q 5 min until arrhythmia is suppressed or until 500 mg has been given (then wait 10 or more min before resuming administration).

• Loading infusion containing 20 mg/mL (1 g diluted with 50 mL of 5% dextrose injection) given at a constant rate of 1 mL/min for 25–30 min to deliver 500–600 mg.

5. For IV maintenance infusion, the dose is usually 2–6 mg/min. Drug solutions should be administered with an electronic infusion device for safety and accuracy.

6. Discard solutions of drug that are darker than light amber or otherwise colored. Solutions that have turned slightly yellow on standing may be used. Consult with pharmacist for clarification.

7. Extended-release tablets are not recommended for use in children or for initiating treatment.

8. Procainamide metabolite NAPA also has antiarrhythmic properties with a longer half-life than procainamide.

Assessment:

1. Document indications for therapy and type, onset, and duration of symptoms.

2. List other agents prescribed and the outcome.

3. Assess cardiopulmonary status and note findings.

4. Obtain baseline ECG, CBC, electrolytes, ANA titers, and liver and renal function studies and monitor throughout therapy.

Interventions:

1. Place client in a supine position during IV infusion and monitor SBP frequently. Be prepared to discontinue infusion if SBP falls 15 mm Hg or more during administration or if increased SA or AV block is noted on cardiac monitor or EKG.

2. Assess clients on PO drug maintenance for symptoms of lupus erythematosus, as manifested by polyarthralgia, arthritis, pleuritic pain, fever, myalgia, and skin lesions.

3. Weigh clients and assess GI symptoms. If severe and persistent the provider may permit the client to take the medication with meals or with a snack to ensure compliance with drug therapy.

Evaluate:

• Termination of arrhythmias with restoration of stable cardiac rhythm

• Therapeutic serum drug levels (4–8 mcg/mL)

Promethazine hydrochloride
(proh-**METH**-ah-zeen)

Syrup, Tablets: Histanil ✦, Phenergan Fortis, Phenergan Plain, PMS Promethazine ✦, Prothazine Plain. **Parenteral:** Anergan 50, K-Phen, Mallergan, Pentazine, Phenazine 50, Phenergan, Phenoject-50, Pro-50, Prometh-25 and -50, Prorex-25 and -50, Prothazine, **Rectal:** Phenergan, Promethagan. **(Rx)**

Classification: Antihistamine, phenothiazine-type

See also *Antihistamines* and *Antiemetics*.

Action/Kinetics: Promethazine is a potent antihistamine with prolonged action. It may cause severe drowsiness. The antiemetic effects are likely due to inhibition of the CTZ. The drug is effective in vertigo by its central anticholinergic effect which inhibits the vestibular apparatus and the integrative vomiting center as well as the CTZ. **Onset, PO, IM, PR:** 20 min; **IV:**3–5 min. **Duration, antihistaminic:** 6–12 hr; **sedative:** 2–8 hr. Slowly eliminated through urine and feces.

Uses: Treatment and prophylaxis of motion sickness. N&V due to anesthesia or surgery. Pre- or postoperative sedative, obstetric sedative. Treatment of pruritus, urticaria, angioedema, dermographism, nasal and ophthalmic allergies. Adjunct in the treatment of anaphylaxis or anaphylactoid reactions. Adjunct to analgesics for postoperative pain. IV with meperidine or other narcotics in special surgical procedures as bronchoscopy, ophthalmic surgery, or in poor-risk clients.

Contraindications: Lactation. Children up to 2 years of age.

Special Concerns: Safe use during pregnancy has not been established. Use in children may cause paradoxical hyperexcitability and nightmares. Injection not recommended for children less than 2 years of age. Geriatric clients are more likely to experience confusion, dizziness, hypotension, and sedation.

Additional Side Effects: Leukopenia and *agranulocytosis (especially if used with cytotoxic agents)*.

Dosage ⸺⸺⸺⸺
• **Syrup, Tablets**
  Antihistaminic.
Adults: 12.5 mg q.i.d. before meals and at bedtime (or 25 mg at bedtime if needed). **Pediatric,** 0.125 mg/kg (3.75 mg/m²) q 4–6 hr; 0.5 mg/kg (15 mg/m²) at bedtime if needed; or, 6.26–12.6 mg t.i.d. (or 25 mg at bedtime if needed).
  Vertigo.
Adults: 25 mg b.i.d.; **pediatric,** 0.5 mg/kg (15 mg/m²) q 12 hr or 12.5–25 mg b.i.d.
  Antiemetic.
Adults: 25 mg b.i.d. as needed; **pediatric,** 0.25–0.5 mg/kg (7.5–15

mg/m²) q 4–6 hr as needed (or 12.5–25 mg q 4–6 hr).
  Sedative-hypnotic.
Adults: 25–50 mg; **pediatric,** 0.5–1 mg/kg (15–30 mg/m²) or 12.5–25 mg as needed.
• **IM, IV, Suppositories**
  Antihistaminic.
Adults, IM, IV, Rectal: 25 mg repeated in 2 hr if needed; **pediatric, IM, Rectal:** 0.125 mg/kg q 4–6 hr (or 0.5 mg/kg at bedtime).
  Antiemetic.
Adults, IM, IV, Rectal: 12.5–25 mg q 4 hr; **pediatric, IM, Rectal,** 0.25–0.5 mg/kg q 4–6 hr (or 12.5–25 mg q 4–6 hr).
  Sedative-hypnotic.
Adults, IM, IV, Rectal: 25–50 mg; **pediatric, IM, Rectal,** 0.5–1 mg/kg (or 12.5–25 mg).
  Vertigo.
Adults, Rectal: 25 mg b.i.d.; **pediatric, Rectal:** 0.5 mg/kg q 12 hr (or 12.5–25 mg b.i.d.)

⸺⸺⸺⸺⸺⸺⸺⸺⸺⸺

RESPIRATORY CARE CONSIDERATIONS

See also *Respiratory Care Considerations* for *Antihistamines,* and *Antiemetics.*

Administration/Storage:
1. Drug may be taken with food or milk to lessen GI irritation.
2. Dosage should be decreased in dehydrated clients or those with oliguria.
3. When used to prevent motion sickness, the medication should be taken 30 min, and preferably 1–2 hr, before travel.

Assessment:
1. Document indications for therapy and type and onset of symptoms.
2. Note age because older client may manifest more adverse side effects.

Client/Family Teaching
1. Take only as directed and do not exceed dose, as arrhythmias may occur. May take with food or milk to decrease GI upset.
2. Avoid activities that require mental alertness until drug effects realized.

3. Do not consume alcohol or any OTC agents without provider approval.

4. Advise that drug may alter skin testing; stop 72 hr before procedure, with provider knowledge.

Evaluate:
- Prevention of vertigo
- Control of N&V
- Promotion of sleep
- Control of allergic manifestations

Propafenone hydrochloride

(proh-pah-**FEN**-ohn)
Pregnancy Category: C
Rythmol **(Rx)**
Classification: Antiarrhythmic, class IC

Action/Kinetics: Propafenone manifests local anesthetic effects and a direct stabilizing action on the myocardium. The drug reduces upstroke velocity (Phase O) of the monophasic action potential, reduces the fast inward current carried by sodium ions in the Purkinje fibers, increases diastolic excitability threshold, and prolongs the effective refractory period. Also, spontaneous activity is decreased. The drug slows AV conduction and causes first-degree heart block. The drug has slight beta-adrenergic blocking activity. **Peak plasma levels:** 3.5 hr. **Therapeutic plasma levels:** 0.5–3 mcg/mL. Significant first-pass effect. Most clients metabolize propafenone rapidly (**t½:** 2–10 hr) to two active metabolites: 5-hydroxypropafenone and N-depropylpropafenone. However, approximately 10% of clients (as well as those taking quinidine) metabolize the drug more slowly (**t½:** 10–32 hr). However, because the 5-hydroxy metabolite is not formed in slow metabolizers and because steady-state levels are reached after 4–5 days in all clients, the recommended dosing regimen is the same for all clients.

Uses: Documented life-threatening ventricular arrhythmias such as sustained ventricular tachycardia where the benefits outweigh the risks. Should not be used in less severe ventricular arrhythmias even if the client is symptomatic. Antiarrhythmic drugs have not been shown to improve survival in clients with ventricular arrhythmias. *Investigational:* SVTs including atrial fibrillation or flutter and arrhythmias associated with Wolff-Parkinson-White syndrome.

Contraindications: Uncontrolled CHF, cardiogenic shock, sick sinus node syndrome or AV block in the absence of an artificial pacemaker, bradycardia, marked hypotension, bronchospastic disorders, electrolyte disorders, hypersensitivity to the drug. MI more than 6 days but less than 2 years previously. Lactation.

Special Concerns: With use of procainamide there is an increased risk of death in those with non-life-threatening arrhythmias. Use with caution during labor and delivery. The safety and effectiveness have not been determined in children. Use with caution in clients with impaired hepatic or renal function. Geriatric clients may require lower dosage.

Side Effects: *CV: New or worsened arrhythmias.* First-degree AV block, intraventricular conduction delay, palpitations, PVCs, proarrhythmia, bradycardia, atrial fibrillation, angina, syncope, CHF, *ventricular tachycardia, second-degree AV block,* increased QRS duration, chest pain, hypotension, bundle branch block. Less commonly, atrial flutter, AV dissociation, flushing, hot flashes, sick sinus syndrome, sinus pause or arrest, SVT, *cardiac arrest. CNS:* Dizziness, headache, anxiety, drowsiness, fatigue, loss of balance, ataxia, insomnia. Less commonly, abnormal speech, abnormal dreams, abnormal vision, confusion, depression, memory loss, *apnea,* psychosis/mania, vertigo, *seizures, coma,* numbness, paresthesias. *GI:* Unusual taste, con-

P

stipation, nausea and/or vomiting, dry mouth, anorexia, flatulence, abdominal pain, cramps, diarrhea, dyspepsia. Less commonly, gastroenteritis and liver abnormalities (cholestasis, hepatitis, elevated enzymes, hepatitis). *Hematologic:* **Agranulocytosis,** increased bleeding time, anemia, granulocytopenia, bruising, leukopenia, purpura, anemia, thrombocytopenia. *Miscellaneous:* Blurred vision, dyspnea, weakness, rash, edema, tremors, diaphoresis, joint pain, possible decrease in spermatogenesis. Less commonly, tinnitus, unusual smell sensation, alopecia, eye irritation, hyponatremia, inappropriate ADH secretion, impotence, increased glucose, kidney failure, lupus erythematosus, muscle cramps or weakness, nephrotic syndrome, pain, pruritus.

OD **Overdose Management:** *Symptoms:* Bradycardia, hypotension, IA and intraventricular conduction disturbances, somnolence. *Rarely, high-grade ventricular arrhythmias and seizures. Treatment:* To control BP and cardiac rhythm, defibrillation and infusion of dopamine or isoproterenol. If seizures occur, diazepam, IV, can be given. External cardiac massage and assisted ventilation may be required.

Drug Interactions:
Beta-adrenergic blockers / Propafenone ↑ plasma levels of beta blockers metabolized by the liver
Cimetidine / Cimetidine ↓ plasma levels of propafenone
Cyclosporine / ↑ Blood trough levels of cyclosporine; ↓ renal function
Digoxin / Propafenone ↑ plasma levels of digoxin necessitating a ↓ in the dose of digoxin
Local anesthetics / May ↑ risk of CNS side effects
Quinidine / ↑ Serum levels of propafenone in rapid metabolizers → possible ↑ effect
Rifampin / ↓ Effect of propafenone due to ↑ clearance
Warfarin / Propafenone may ↑ plasma levels of warfarin necessitating ↓ dose of warfarin

Laboratory Test Interferences: ↑ ANA titers.

Dosage ————————————
• **Tablets**
Adults, initial: 150 mg q 8 hr; dose may be increased at a minimum of q 3–4 days to 225 mg q 8 hr and, if necessary, to 300 mg q 8 hr.

RESPIRATORY CARE CONSIDERATIONS

See also *Respiratory Care Considerations* for *Antiarrhythmic Agents.*
Administration/Storage:
1. Initiation of propafenone therapy should always be undertaken in a hospital setting.
2. The effectiveness and safety of doses exceeding 900 mg/day have not been determined.
3. There is no evidence that the use of propafenone affects the survival or incidence of sudden death in clients with recent MI or SVT.
Assessment:
1. Assess ECG and monitor; document baseline arrhythmias and note any client history of cardiac problems.
2. Determine if there is any history of renal or hepatic disease. Propafenone must be used with caution in these clients.
3. Obtain baseline CBC, electrolytes, and liver and renal function studies and monitor during therapy.
Interventions:
1. Propafenone may induce new or more severe arrhythmias. Document ECG strips and monitor client response closely, as the dose of propafenone should be titrated in each client on the basis of response and tolerance.
2. Report any significant widening of the QRS complex or any evidence of second- or third-degree AV block.
3. Anticipate that the dose of propafenone will be increased more gradually in elderly clients as well as in clients with previous myocardial damage.
4. Monitor VS. Weigh client and place on strict I&O.
5. Evaluate hematologic studies dur-

P

ing drug therapy to determine the presence of anemia, agranulocytosis, leukopenia, thrombocytopenia, or altered prothrombin and coagulation times.

6. Client may complain of an unusual taste in the mouth. This may interfere with eating and nutritional status, so observe closely.

Evaluate:
• Termination of life-threatening ventricular tachycardia
• Therapeutic serum drug levels (0.5–3 mcg/mL)

Propoxyphene hydrochloride
(proh-**POX**-ih-feen)
Pregnancy Category: C
642 Tablets ✦, Darvon, Dolene, Doloxene, Doraphen, Doxaphene, Novo-Propoxyn ✦, Profene, Progesic, Pro Pox, Propoxycon **(C-IV) (Rx)**

Propoxyphene napsylate
(proh-**POX**-ih-feen)
Pregnancy Category: C
Darvon-N **(C-IV) (Rx)**
Classification: Analgesic, narcotic, miscellaneous

Action/Kinetics: Propoxyphene resembles the narcotics with respect to its mechanism and analgesic effect; it is one-half to one-third as potent as codeine. It is devoid of antitussive, anti-inflammatory, or antipyretic activity. When taken in excessive doses for long periods, psychologic dependence and occasionally physical dependence and tolerance will be manifested. **Peak plasma levels:** hydrochloride: 2–2.5 hr; napsylate: 3–4 hr. **Analgesic onset:** 30–60 min. **Peak analgesic effect:** 2–2.5 hr. **Duration:** 4–6 hr. **Therapeutic serum levels:** 0.05–0.12 mcg/mL. **t½, propoxyphene:** 6–12 hr; **norpropoxyphene:** 30–36 hr. Extensive first-pass effect; metabolites are excreted in the urine.

Propoxyphene is often prescribed in combination with salicylates. In such instances, the information on

salicylates should also be consulted. Propoxyphene hydrochloride is found in Darvon Compound and Wygesic, while propoxyphene napsylate is found in Darvocet-N.

Uses: To relieve mild to moderate pain. Propoxyphene napsylate has been used experimentally to suppress the withdrawal syndrome from narcotics.

Contraindications: Hypersensitivity to drug. Not recommended for use in children.

Special Concerns: Safe use during pregnancy has not been established. Use with caution during lactation. Safety and efficacy have not been established in children.

Side Effects: *GI:* N&V, constipation, abdominal pain. *CNS:* Sedation, dizziness, lightheadedness, headache, weakness, euphoria, dysphoria. *Other:* Skin rashes, visual disturbances. Propoxyphene can produce psychologic dependence, as well as physical dependence and tolerance.

OD **Overdose Management:** *Symptoms:* Stupor, respiratory depression, apnea, hypotension, pulmonary edema, ***circulatory collapse, cardiac arrhythmias,*** conduction abnormalities, ***coma, seizures,*** respiratory-metabolic acidosis. *Treatment:* Maintain an patent airway, assisted ventilation, and naloxone, 0.4–2 mg IV (repeat at 2- to 3-min intervals) to combat respiratory depression. Gastric lavage or administration of activated charcoal may be helpful. Correct acidosis and electrolyte imbalance. Acidosis due to lactic acid may require IV sodium bicarbonate.

Drug Interactions:
Alcohol, antianxiety drugs, antipsychotic agents, narcotics, sedative-hypnotics / Concomitant use may lead to drowsiness, lethargy, stupor, respiratory, depression, and coma
Carbamazepine / ↑ Effect of carbamazepine due to ↓ breakdown by liver
CNS depressants / Additive CNS depression

Orphenadrine / Concomitant use may lead to confusion, anxiety, and tremors

Phenobarbital / ↑ Effect of phenobarbital due to ↓ breakdown by liver

Skeletal muscle relaxants / Additive respiratory depression

Warfarin / ↑ Hypoprothrombinemic effects of warfarin

Dosage
- **Capsules (Hydrochloride)**
  Analgesia.
  Adults: 65 mg q 4 hr, not to exceed 390 mg/day.
- **Tablets (Napsylate)**
  Analgesia.
  Adults: 100 mg q 4 hr, not to exceed 600 mg/day. Dose of propoxyphene should be reduced in clients with renal or hepatic impairment.

RESPIRATORY CARE CONSIDERATIONS

See also *Respiratory Care Considerations* for *Narcotic Analgesics.*

Assessment:

1. Document indications for therapy; note onset, duration, location, and characteristics of pain. Use a pain-rating scale to assess pain. Note other agents prescribed, and the outcome.

2. Note any history of opiate or alcohol dependency.

3. Obtain baseline liver and renal function studies. Anticipate reduced dose with renal and liver dysfunction.

4. Determine if client smokes. Smoking reduces drug effect by increasing metabolism.

5. Use with caution in the elderly and review drug profile to ensure other prescribed agents do not cause additive CNS effects.

Evaluate: Relief of pain

Propranolol hydrochloride
(proh-**PRAN**-oh-lohl)
Pregnancy Category: C
Apo-Propranolol ✦, Detensol ✦, Inderal, Inderal 10, 20, 40, 60, 80, and 90, Inderal LA, Novo-Pranol ✦, Nu-Propranolol ✦, PMS Propranolol ✦, Propranolol Intensol **(Rx)**
Classification: Beta-adrenergic blocking agent; antiarrhythmic (type II)

See also *Beta-Adrenergic Blocking Agents.*

Action/Kinetics: Propranolol manifests both beta-1- and beta-2-adrenergic blocking activity. The antiarrhythmic action results from both beta-adrenergic receptor blockade and a direct membrane-stabilizing action on the cardiac cell. Propranolol has no intrinsic sympathomimetic activity and has high lipid solubility. **PO: Onset,** 30 min. **Maximum effect:** 1–1.5 hr. **Duration:** 3–5 hr. **t½:** 2–3 hr (8–11 hr for long-acting). **Therapeutic serum level, antiarrhythmic:** 0.05–0.1 mcg/mL. Onset after IV administration is almost immediate. Completely metabolized by liver and excreted in urine. Although food increases bioavailability of the drug, absorption may be decreased.

Uses: Hypertension (alone or in combination with other antihypertensive agents). Angina pectoris, hypertrophic subaortic stenosis, prophylaxis of MI, pheochromocytoma, prophylaxis of migraine, essential tremor. Cardiac arrhythmias including ventricular tachycardias and arrhythmias, tachycardias due to digitalis intoxication, supraventricular arrhythmias, PVCs, resistant tachyarrhythmias due to anesthesia/catecholamines.

Investigational: Schizophrenia, tremors due to parkinsonism, aggressive behavior, antipsychotic-induced akathisia, rebleeding due to esophageal varices, situational anxiety, acute panic attacks, gastric bleeding in portal hypertension, vaginal contraceptive, anxiety, alcohol withdrawal syndrome, winter depression.

Contraindications: Bronchial asthma, bronchospasms including severe COPD.

Special Concerns: It is dangerous to use propranolol for pheochromocytoma unless an alpha-adrenergic blocking agent is already in use.

Additional Side Effects: Psoriasis-like eruptions, skin necrosis, SLE (rare).

Additional Drug Interactions:

Haloperidol / Severe hypotension
Hydralazine / ↑ Effect of both agents
Methimazole / May ↑ effects of propranolol
Phenobarbital / ↓ Effect of propranolol due to ↑ breakdown by liver
Propylthiouracil / May ↑ the effects of propranolol
Rifampin / ↓ Effect of propranolol due to ↑ breakdown by liver
Smoking / ↓ Serum levels and ↑ clearance of propranolol

Laboratory Test Interferences: ↑ Blood urea, serum transaminase, alkaline phosphatase, LDH. Interference with glaucoma screening test.

Dosage

• **Tablets, Sustained-Release Capsules, Oral Solution, Concentrate**

Hypertension.
Initial: 40 mg b.i.d. or 80 mg of sustained-release/day; **then,** increase dose to maintenance level of 120–240 mg/day given in two to three divided doses or 120–160 mg of sustained-release medication once daily. Maximum daily dose should not exceed 640 mg. **Pediatric, initial:** 0.5 mg/kg b.i.d.; dose may be increased at 3- to 5-day intervals to a maximum of 1 mg/kg b.i.d. The dosage range should be calculated by weight and not by body surface area.

Angina.
Initial: 80–320 mg b.i.d., t.i.d., or q.i.d.; or, 80 mg of sustained-release once daily; **then,** increase dose gradually to maintenance level of 160 mg/day of sustained-release capsule. The maximum daily dose should not exceed 320 mg.

Arrhythmias.
10–30 mg t.i.d.–q.i.d. given after meals and at bedtime.

Hypertrophic subaortic stenosis.
20–40 mg t.i.d.–q.i.d. before meals and at bedtime or 80–160 mg of sustained-release medication given once daily.

MI prophylaxis.
180–240 mg/day given in three to four divided doses. Total daily dose should not exceed 240 mg.

Pheochromocytoma, preoperatively.
60 mg/day for 3 days before surgery, given concomitantly with an alpha-adrenergic blocking agent.

Inoperable tumors.
30 mg/day in divided doses.

Migraine.
Initial: 80 mg sustained-release medication given once daily; **then,** increase dose gradually to maintenance of 160–240 mg/day in divided doses. If a satisfactory response has not been observed after 4–6 weeks, the drug should be discontinued and withdrawn gradually.

Essential tremor.
Initial: 40 mg b.i.d.; **then,** 120 mg/day up to a maximum of 320 mg/day.

Aggressive behavior.
80–300 mg/day.

Antipsychotic-induced akathisia.
20–80 mg/day.

Tremors associated with Parkinson's disease.
160 mg/day.

Rebleeding from esophageal varices.
20–180 mg b.i.d.

Schizophrenia.
300–5,000 mg/day.

Acute panic symptoms.
40–320 mg/day.

Anxiety.
80–320 mg/day.

Intermittent explosive disorder.
50–1,600 mg/day.

Nonvariceal gastric bleeding in portal hypertension.
24–480 mg/day.

• **IV**
Life-threatening arrhythmias or those occurring under anesthesia.
1–3 mg not to exceed 1 mg/min; a second dose may be given after 2

min, with subsequent doses q 4 hr. Clients should begin PO therapy as soon as possible. Although use in pediatrics is not recommended, investigational doses of 0.01–0.1 mg/kg/dose, up to a maximum of 1 mg/dose (by slow push), have been used for arrhythmias.

RESPIRATORY CARE CONSIDERATIONS

See also *Respiratory Care Considerations* for *Beta-Adrenergic Blocking Agents* and *Antihypertensive Agents*.
Administration/Storage:
1. Do not administer for a minimum of 2 weeks in client who has discontinued MAO inhibitor drugs.
2. If signs of serious myocardial depression occur following propranolol administration, isoproterenol (Isuprel) should be slowly infused IV.
3. For IV use, dilute 1 mg in 10 mL of D5W and administer IV over at least 1 min. May be further reconstituted in 50 mL of dextrose or saline solution and infused IVPB over 10–15 min.
4. After IV administration, have available emergency drugs and equipment to combat hypotension or circulatory collapse.
Assessment:
1. Document indications for therapy, type, onset, and duration of symptoms, and other agents prescribed.
2. Note ECG, VS, and cardiopulmonary assessment. Determine any evidence or history of pulmonary disease, bronchospasms, or depression.
Interventions:
1. Observe client for evidence of a rash, fever, and/or purpura. These may be symptoms of a hypersensitivity reaction.
2. Monitor I&O. Observe for S&S of CHF (e.g., SOB, rales, edema, and weight gain).
3. Monitor VS. Pronounced hypotension, bradycardia, or reports of PND may necessitate discontinuation of therapy.
Evaluate:
• ↓ BP, ↓ HR

• ↓ Frequency and intensity of angina episodes
• Effective migraine prophylaxis
• Control of tachyarrhythmias
• Desired behavioral changes
• Prevention of myocardial reinfarction
• Relief/control of chronic pain
• Therapeutic serum drug levels as an antiarrhythmic (0.05–0.1 mcg/mL)

Pseudoephedrine hydrochloride
(soo-doh-eh-**FED**-rin)
Pregnancy Category: B
Allermed, Balminil Decongestant Syrup ✚, Cenafed, Children's Congestion Relief, Children's Sudafed Liquid, Congestion Relief, Decofed Syrup, DeFed-60, Dorcol Children's Decongestant Liquid, Efidac/24, Eltor 120 ✚, Genaphed, Halofed, Maxenal ✚, PediaCare Infants' Oral Decongestant Drops, PMS-Pseudoephedrine ✚, Pseudo, Pseudo-Gest, Robidrine ✚, Seudotabs, Sinustop Pro, Sudafed, Sudafed 12 Hour **(OTC)**

Pseudoephedrine sulfate
(soo-doh-eh-**FED**-rin)
Pregnancy Category: B
Afrin Extended-Release Tablets, Drixoral N.D. ✚, Drixoral Non-Drowsy Formula **(OTC)**
Classification: Direct- and indirect-acting sympathomimetic, nasal decongestant

See also *Sympathomimetic Drugs*.
Action/Kinetics: Pseudoephedrine produces direct stimulation of both alpha-(pronounced) and beta-adrenergic receptors, as well as indirect stimulation through release of norepinephrine from storage sites. These actions produce a decongestant effect on the nasal mucosa. Systemic administration eliminates possible damage to the nasal mucosa. **Onset:** 15–30 min. **Time to peak effect:** 30–60 min. **Duration:** 3–4 hr. **Extended-release: duration,** 8–12 hr. Urinary excretion slowed by alkalinization, causing reabsorption of drug. Pseudoephedrine is also found

in Actifed, Chlor-Trimeton, and Drixoral.

Uses: Nasal congestion associated with sinus conditions, otitis, allergies. Relief of eustachian tube congestion.

Additional Contraindications: Lactation. Use of sustained-release products in children less than 12 years of age.

Special Concerns: Use with caution in newborn and premature infants due to a higher risk of side effects. Geriatric clients may be more prone to age-related prostatic hypertrophy.

Dosage ——————————
HYDROCHLORIDE
- **Oral Solution, Syrup, Tablets**
  Decongestant.
Adults: 60 mg q 4–6 hr, not to exceed 240 mg in 24 hr. **Pediatric, 6–12 years:** 30 mg using the oral solution or syrup q 4–6 hr, not to exceed 120 mg in 24 hr; **2–6 years:** 15 mg using the oral solution or syrup q 4–6 hr, not to exceed 60 mg in 24 hr. For children less than 2 years of age, the dose must be individualized.
- **Extended-Release Capsules, Tablets**
  Decongestant.
Adults and children over 12 years: 120 mg q 12 hr or 240 mg q 24 hr. Use is not recommended for children less than 12 years of age.
SULFATE
- **Extended-Release Tablets**
  Decongestant.
Adults and children over 12 years: 120 mg q 12 hr. Use is not recommended for children less than 12 years of age.

RESPIRATORY CARE CONSIDERATIONS

See also *Respiratory Care Considerations* for *Sympathomimetic Drugs.*
Client/Family Teaching:
1. Avoid taking the drug at bedtime. Pseudoephedrine causes stimulation that can produce insomnia.
2. Advise clients with hypertension to report symptoms such as headache, dizziness, or increased BP readings.
3. Stress that extended-release products should not be crushed or chewed.
4. Notify provider if symptoms do not improve after 3–5 days.
Evaluate: Symptomatic relief of nasal, sinus, or eustachian tube congestion and associated allergic manifestations

Pyridostigmine bromide
(peer-id-oh-**STIG**-meen)
Mestinon, Mestinon-SR ✦, Regonol
(Rx)
Classification: Indirectly acting cholinergic-acetylcholinesterase inhibitor

For all information, see also *Neostigmine.*
Action/Kinetics: Has a slower onset, longer duration of action, and fewer side effects than neostigmine. **Onset, PO:** 30–45 min for syrup and tablets and 30–60 min for extended-release tablets; **IM:** 15 min; **IV:** 2–5 min. **Duration, PO:** 3–6 hr for syrup and tablets and 6–12 hr for extended-release tablets; **IM, IV:** 2–4 hr. Poorly absorbed from the GI tract; excreted in urine up to 72 hr after administration.
Uses: Myasthenia gravis. Antidote for nondepolarizing muscle relaxants (e.g., tubocurarine).
Additional Contraindications: Sensitivity to bromides.
Special Concerns: Safe use during pregnancy and during lactation has not been established. May cause uterine irritability and premature labor if given IV to pregnant women near term. In geriatric clients, the duration of action may be increased.
Additional Side Effects: Skin rash. Thrombophlebitis after IV use.
OD Overdose Management: *Symptoms:* Abdominal cramps, vomiting, diarrhea, epigastric distress, excessive salivation, cold sweating, pallor, blurred vision, urinary urgen-

cy, fasciculation and *paralysis of voluntary muscles* (including the tongue), miosis, increased BP (may be accompanied by bradycardia), sensation of internal trembling, panic, severe anxiety. *Treatment:* Discontinue medication temporarily. Give atropine, 0.5–1 mg IV (up to 5–10 mg or more may be needed to get HR to 80 beats/min). Supportive treatment including assisted ventilation and oxygen.

Dosage
• **Syrup, Tablets**
  Myasthenia gravis.
Adults: 60–120 mg q 3–4 hr with dosage adjusted to client response. **Maintenance:** 600 mg/day (range: 60 mg–1.5 g). **Pediatric:** 7 mg/kg (200 mg/m²) daily in five to six divided doses.
• **Sustained-Release Tablets**
  Myasthenia gravis.
Adults: 180–540 mg 1–2 times/day with at least 6 hr between doses. Sustained-release tablets not recommended for use in children.
• **IM, IV**
  Myasthenia gravis.
Adults, IM, IV: 2 mg (about 1/30 the adult dose) q 2–3 hr.
  Neonates of myasthenic mothers.
IM: 0.05–0.15 mg/kg q 4–6 hr.
  Antidote for nondepolarizing drugs.
Adults, IV: 10–20 mg with 0.6–1.2 mg atropine sulfate given IV.

RESPIRATORY CARE CONSIDERATIONS

See also *Respiratory Care Considerations* for *Neostigmine.*
Administration/Storage:
1. During dosage adjustment, administer the drug to the client in a closely monitored environment.
2. Parenteral medication dosage is 1/30 of the PO dose. May give undiluted at a rate of 0.5 mg IV over 1 min for myasthenia and at a rate of 5 mg IV over 1 min (with atropine) for reversal of nondepolarizing drug effects.
3. After PO administration, onset of action occurs in 30–45 min and lasts for 3–6 hr. When administered IM, the onset of action occurs within 15 min. When administered IV, the onset of action occurs within 2–5 min.
Interventions:
1. Monitor VS and observe client for toxic reactions demonstrated by generalized cholinergic stimulation.
2. Assess for muscular weakness. This may be a sign of impending myasthenic crisis and cholinergic overdose.
3. Work with the client to determine the best individualized medication administration schedule according to client's routines and lifestyle.
Evaluate:
• Improvement in muscle strength and function with multiple sclerosis
• Reversal of nondepolarizing muscle relaxants

Quinapril hydrochloride
(**KWIN**-ah-prill)
Pregnancy Category: D
Accupril **(Rx)**
Classification: Angiotensin-converting enzyme inhibitor

See also *Angiotensin-Converting Enzyme Inhibitors.*
Action/Kinetics: Onset: 1 hr. **Time to peak serum levels:** 1 hr. The peak reduction of BP occurs within 2–4 hr after dosing. Quinapril is metabolized to quinaprilat, the active metabolite. **t½, quinaprilat:** 2 hr. **Duration:** 24 hr. Significantly bound to plasma proteins. The drug is metabolized with approximately 60% excreted through the urine and 37% excreted in the feces. The drug also appears to improve endothelial function, which is an early marker of coronary atherosclerosis.
Uses: Alone or in combination with

a thiazide diuretic for the treatment of hypertension. Adjunct with a diuretic or digitalis to treat CHF in those not responding adequately to diuretics or digitalis.

Special Concerns: Use with caution during lactation. Safety and effectiveness have not been determined in children. Geriatric clients may be more sensitive to the effects of quinapril and manifest higher peak quinaprilat blood levels.

Side Effects: *CV:* Vasodilation, tachycardia, *heart failure,* palpitations, *MI, CVA, hypertensive crisis,* angina pectoris, orthostatic hypotension, *cardiac rhythm disturbances, cardiogenic shock.* *GI:* Dry mouth or throat, constipation, N&V, abdominal pain, *GI hemorrhage.* *CNS:* Somnolence, vertigo, nervousness, depression, headache, dizziness, fatigue. *Hematologic:* *Agranulocytosis,* bone marrow depression, thrombocytopenia. *Dermatologic:* *Angioedema of the lips, tongue, glottis, and larynx;* sweating, pruritus, exfoliative dermatitis, photosensitivity, dermatopolymyositis. *Body as a whole:* Malaise, back pain. *GU:* Oliguria and/or progressive azotemia and rarely *acute renal failure and/or death in severe heart failure.* Worsening renal failure. *Respiratory:* Pharyngitis, cough, asthma, bronchospasm. *Miscellaneous:* Oligohydramnios in fetuses exposed to the drug in utero. Abnormal liver function tests, pancreatitis, syncope, hyperkalemia, amblyopia, viral infections.

OD **Overdose Management:** *Symptoms:* Commonly, hypotension. *Treatment:* IV infusion of normal saline to restore blood pressure.

Drug Interactions:
Potassium-containing salt substitutes / ↑ Risk of hyperkalemia
Potassium-sparing diuretics / ↑ Risk of hyperkalemia
Potassium supplements / ↑ Risk of hyperkalemia
Tetracyclines / ↓ Absorption of tetracycline due to high magnesium content of quinapril tablets

Dosage —————
• **Tablets**
Hypertension.
Initial: 10 mg/day; **then,** adjust dosage based on BP response at peak (2–6 hr) and trough (predose) blood levels. The dose should be adjusted at 2-week intervals. **Maintenance:** 20, 40, or 80 mg daily as a single dose or in two equally divided doses. In clients with impaired renal function, the initial dose should be 10 mg if the creatinine clearance is greater than 60 mL/min, 5 mg if the creatinine clearance is between 30 and 60 mL/min, and 2.5 mg if the creatinine clearance is between 10 and 30 mL/min. If the initial dose is well tolerated, the drug may be given the following day as a b.i.d.regimen.

CHF.
Initial: 5 mg b.i.d. If this dose is well tolerated, titrate clients at weekly intervals until an effective dose, usually 20–40 mg daily in two equally divided doses, is attained. Undesirable hypotension, orthostasis, or azotemia may prevent this dosage level from being reached.

RESPIRATORY CARE CONSIDERATIONS

See also *Angiotensin-Converting Enzyme Inhibitors* and *Antihypertensive Agents.*

Administration/Storage:
1. If the client is taking a diuretic, the diuretic should be discontinued 2–3 days prior to beginning quinapril therapy. If the BP is not controlled, the diuretic should be reinstituted. If the diuretic cannot be discontinued, an initial dose of quinapril should be 1.25 mg.
2. If the antihypertensive effect decreases at the end of the dosing interval in clients taking the medication once daily, either twice daily administration should be considered or the dose should be increased.
3. The antihypertensive effect may not be observed for 1–2 weeks.

Assessment:
1. Obtain   baseline   electrolytes,

Q

CBC, and renal function studies and monitor throughout therapy. Agranulocytosis and bone marrow depression are seen more often in clients with renal impairment, especially if they also have a collagen vascular disease (e.g., SLE, scleroderma).

2. Clients with unilateral or bilateral renal artery stenosis may manifest increase BUN and serum creatinine if given quinapril. Thus, renal function should be monitored closely the first few weeks of therapy.

Interventions:

1. Monitor VS, I&O, and weights.

2. If angioedema occurs, the drug should be discontinued immediately and the client observed until the swelling disappears. Antihistamines may be useful in relieving symptoms.

3. Infants exposed to quinapril *in utero* should be closely observed for the development of hypotension, oliguria, and hyperkalemia and managed symptomatically.

Evaluate: ↓ BP to within desired range

Quinidine bisulfate

(**KWIN**-ih-deen)
Pregnancy Category: D
Biquin Durules ✦ **(Rx)**

Quinidine gluconate

(**KWIN**-ih-deen)
Pregnancy Category: C
Quinaglute Dura-Tabs, Quinalan, Quinate ✦ **(Rx)**

Quinidine polygalacturonate

(**KWIN**-ih-deen)
Pregnancy Category: C
Cardioquin **(Rx)**

Quinidine sulfate

(**KWIN**-ih-deen)
Pregnancy Category: C
Apo-Quinidine ✦, Quinidex Extentabs, Quinora **(Rx)**
Classification: Antiarrhythmic, class IA

See also *Antiarrhythmic Agents.*

Action/Kinetics: Quinidine reduces the excitability of the heart and depresses conduction velocity and contractility. The drug prolongs the refractory period and increases conduction time. It also decreases CO and possesses anticholinergic, antimalarial, antipyretic, and oxytocic properties. **PO: Onset:** 0.5–3 hr. **Maximum effects, after IM:** 30–90 min. **t½:** 6–7 hr. **Time to peak levels, PO:** 3–5 hr for gluconate salt, 1–1.5 hr for sulfate salt, and 6 hr for polygalacturonate salt; **IM:** 1 hr. **Therapeutic serum levels:** 2–6 mcg/mL. **Protein binding:** 60%–80%. **Duration:** 6–8 hr for tablets/capsules and 12 hr for extended-release tablets. Metabolized by liver. Rate of urinary excretion (10%–50% excreted unchanged) is affected by urinary pH.

Uses: Premature atrial, AV junctional, and ventricular contractions. Treatment and control of atrial flutter, established atrial fibrillation, paroxysmal atrial tachycardia, paroxysmal AV junctional rhythm, paroxysmal and chronic atrial fibrillation, paroxysmal ventricular tachycardia not associated with complete heart block, maintenance therapy after electrical conversion of atrial flutter or fibrillation. The parenteral route is indicated when PO therapy is not feasible or immediate effects are required. *Investigational:* Gluconate salt for life-threatening *Plasmodium falciparum* malaria.

Contraindications: Hypersensitivity to drug or other cinchona drugs. Myasthenia gravis, history of thrombocytopenic purpura associated with quinidine use, digitalis intoxication evidenced by arrhythmias or AV conduction disorders. Also, complete heart block, left bundle branch block, or other intraventricular conduction defects manifested by marked QRS widening or bizarre complexes. Complete AV block with an AV nodal or idioventricular pacemaker, aberrant ectopic impulses and abnormal rhythms due to escape mechanisms. History of drug-induced torsades de pointes or long QT syndrome.

Special Concerns: Safety in children and during lactation has not been established. Quinidine should be used with extreme caution in clients in whom a sudden change in BP might be detrimental or in those suffering from extensive myocardial damage, subacute endocarditis, bradycardia, coronary occlusion, disturbances in impulse conduction, chronic valvular disease, considerable cardiac enlargement, frank CHF, and renal or hepatic disease. Cautious use is also recommended in clients with acute infections, hyperthyroidism, muscular weakness, respiratory distress, and bronchial asthma. The dose in geriatric clients may have to be reduced due to age-related changes in renal function.

Side Effects: *CV:* Widening of QRS complex, hypotension, cardiac asystole, ectopic ventricular beats, ***ventricular tachycardia or fibrillation, torsades de pointes,*** paradoxical tachycardia, ***arterial embolism,*** ventricular extrasystoles (one or more every 6 beats), prolonged QT interval, complete AV block, ventricular flutter. *GI:* N&V, abdominal pain, anorexia, diarrhea, urge to defecate as well as urinate, esophagitis (rare). *CNS:* Syncope, headache, confusion, excitement, vertigo, apprehension, delirium, dementia, ataxia, depression. *Dermatologic:* Rash, urticaria, exfoliative dermatitis, photosensitivity, flushing with intense pruritus, eczema, psoriasis, pigmentation abnormalities. *Allergic:* Acute asthma, angioneurotic edema, ***respiratory arrest,*** dyspnea, fever, ***vascular collapse,*** purpura, vasculitis, hepatic dysfunction (including granulomatous hepatitis), hepatic toxicity. *Hematologic:* Hypoprothrombinemia, acute hemolytic anemia, thrombocytopenic purpura, ***agranulocytosis,*** thrombocytopenia, leukocytosis, neutropenia, shift to left in WBC differential. *Ophthalmologic:* Blurred vision, mydriasis, alterations in color perception, decreased field of vision, double vision, photophobia, optic neuritis, night blindness, scotomata. *Other:* Liver toxicity including hepatitis, lupus nephritis, tinnitus, decreased hearing acuity, arthritis, myalgia, increase in serum skeletal muscle CPK, lupus erythematosus.

OD **Overdose Management:** *Symptoms: CNS:* Lethargy, confusion, ***coma, seizures, respiratory depression or arrest,*** headache, paresthesia, vertigo. CNS symptoms may be seen after onset of CV toxicity. *GI:* Vomiting, diarrhea, abdominal pain, hypokalemia, nausea. *CV:* Sinus tachycardia, ***ventricular tachycardia or fibrillation, torsades de pointes, depressed automaticity and conduction*** (including bundle branch block, sinus bradycardia, SA block, prolongation of QRS and QTc, sinus arrest, AV block, ST depression, T inversion), syncope, ***heart failure.*** Hypotension due to decreased conduction and CO and vasodilation. *Miscellaneous:* Cinchonism, visual and auditory disturbances, hypokalemia, tinnitus, acidosis. *Treatment:*
• Perform gastric lavage, induce vomiting, and administer activated charcoal if ingestion is recent.
• Monitor ECG, blood gases, serum electrolytes, and BP.
• Institute cardiac pacing, if necessary.
• Acidify the urine.
• Use assisted ventilation and other supportive measures.
• Infusions of ⅙ molar sodium lactate IV may decrease the cardiotoxic effects.
• Treat hypotension with metaraminol or norepinephrine after fluid volume replacement.
• Use phenytoin or lidocaine to treat tachydysrhythmias.
• Hemodialysis is effective but not often required.

Drug Interactions:
Acetazolamide, Antacids / ↑ Effect of quinidine due to ↓ renal excretion
Amiodarone / ↑ Quinidine levels with possible fatal cardiac dysrhythmias

Anticholinergic agents, Atropine / Additive effect on blockade of vagus nerve action

Anticoagulants, oral / Additive hypoprothrombinemia with possible hemorrhage

Barbiturates / ↓ Effect of quinidine due to ↑ breakdown by liver

Cholinergic agents / Quinidine antagonizes effect of cholinergic drugs

Cimetidine / ↑ Effect of quinidine due to ↓ breakdown by liver

Digoxin, Digitoxin / ↑ Symptoms of digoxin or digitoxin toxicity

Disopyramide / Either ↑ disopyramide levels or ↓ quinidine levels

Guanethidine / Additive hypotensive effect

Methyldopa / Additive hypotensive effect

Metoprolol / ↑ Effect of propranolol in fast metabolizers

Neuromuscular blocking agents / ↑ Respiratory depression

Nifedipine / ↓ Effect of quinidine

Phenobarbital, Phenytoin / ↓ Effect of quinidine by ↑ rate of metabolism in liver

Potassium / ↑ Effect of quinidine

Procainamide / ↑ Effects of procainamide with possible toxicity

Propafenone / ↑ Serum propafenone levels in rapid metabolizers

Propranolol / ↑ Effect of propranolol in fast metabolizers

Reserpine / Additive cardiac depressant effects

Rifampin / ↓ Effect of quinidine due to ↑ breakdown by liver

Skeletal muscle relaxants / ↑ Skeletal muscle relaxation

Sodium bicarbonate / ↑ Effect of quinidine due to ↓ renal excretion

Sucralfate / ↓ Serum levels of quinidine → ↓ effect

Thiazide diuretics / ↑ Effect of quinidine due to ↓ renal excretion

Tricyclic antidepressants / ↑ Effect of antidepressant due to ↓ clearance

Verapamil / ↓ Clearance of verapamil → ↑ hypotension, bradycardia, AV block, ventricular tachycardia, and pulmonary edema

Laboratory Test Interferences: False + or ↑ PSP, 17-ketosteroids, PT.

Dosage ⸺
- **Quinidine Bisulfate Controlled-Release Tablets**

  Antiarrhythmic.

  Initial: Test dose of 200 mg in the morning (to ascertain hypersensitivity). In the evening, administer 500 mg. **Then,** beginning the next day, 500–750 mg/12 hr. **Maintenance:** 0.5–1.25 g morning and evening.
- **Quinidine Polygalacturonate Tablets, Quinidine Sulfate Tablets**

  Premature atrial and ventricular contractions.

  Adults: 200–300 mg t.i.d.–q.i.d.

  Paroxysmal SVTs.

  Adults: 400–600 mg q 2–3 hr until the paroxysm is terminated.

  Conversion of atrial flutter.

  Adults: 200 mg q 2–3 hr for five to eight doses; daily doses can be increased until rhythm is restored or toxic effects occur.

  Conversion of atrial flutter, maintenance therapy.

  Adults: 200–300 mg t.i.d.–q.i.d. Large doses or more frequent administration may be required in some clients.
- **Quinidine Gluconate Sustained-Release Tablets, Quinidine Sulfate Sustained-Release Tablets**

  All uses.

  Adults: 300–600 mg q 8–12 hr.
- **Quinidine Gluconate Injection (IM or IV)**

  Acute tachycardia.

  Adults, initial: 600 mg IM; **then,** 400 mg IM repeated as often as q 2 hr.

  Arrhythmias.

  Adults: 330 mg IM or less IV (as much as 500–750 mg may be required).

  P. falciparum malaria.

  Two regimens may be used. (1) *Loading dose:* 15 mg/kg in 250 mL NSS given over 4 hr; 24 hr after beginning the loading dose, institute 7.5 mg/kg infused over 4 hr and given q 8 hr for 7 days or until PO therapy can be started. (2) *Loading dose:* 10 mg/kg in 250 mL NSS infused over 1–2 hr followed immediately by 0.02 mg/kg/min for up to 72 hr or until parasitemia decreases to less than 1% or PO therapy can be started.

RESPIRATORY CARE CONSIDERATIONS

See also *Respiratory Care Considerations* for *Antiarrhythmic Agents*.

Administration/Storage:
1. A preliminary test dose may be given before instituting quinidine therapy. **Adults:** 200 mg quinidine sulfate or quinidine gluconate administered PO or IM. **Children:** Test dose of 2 mg of quinidine sulfate per kilogram of body weight.
2. The sustained-release forms cannot be considered interchangeable.
3. IV solution can be prepared by diluting 10 mL of quinidine gluconate injection (800 mg) with 50 mL of 5% glucose solution; this should be given at a rate of 1 mL/min.
4. Use only colorless clear solution for injection because light may cause quinidine to crystallize, which turns solution brownish.

Assessment:
1. Note any history of allergic reactions to antiarrhythmic drugs or tartrazine, which is found in some formulations. A test dose may be performed by administering one regular PO tablet before therapy is instituted. Observe client for hypersensitivity reactions and check for any intolerance.
2. Document indications for therapy and type, onset, and duration of symptoms.
3. Determine that pretreatment glucose, CBC, liver and renal function studies and CXR have been performed. Monitor serum electrolytes, CBC, and liver and renal function studies during prolonged therapy with quinidine.
4. Obtain VS and ECG and carefully assess heart and lung sounds.

Interventions:
1. Evaluate ECG and report any evidence of increased AV block, cardiac irritability, or rhythm suppression during IV administration.
2. Monitor I&O and VS; observe closely for evidence of hypotension. The drug induces urinary alkalization.
3. Observe and report any neurologic deficits or sensory impairment (i.e., numbness, confusion, pyschosis, depression, or involuntary movements) .
4. Report any persistent diarrhea.
5. Among the elderly, there is a higher risk of toxicity, reduced CO, and unpredictable effects from drug therapy.
6. Clients with long-standing atrial fibrillation or CHF with atrial fibrillation run a risk of embolization from mural thrombi when converting to sinus rhythm.

Evaluate:
• Control of arrhythmia with restoration of stable cardiac rhythm
• Therapeutic serum drug levels (2–6 mcg/mL)

Ramipril
(**RAM**-ih-prill)
Pregnancy Category: D
Altace **(Rx)**
Classification: Angiotensin-converting enzyme inhibitor

See also *Angiotensin-Converting Enzyme Inhibitors*.

Action/Kinetics: Onset: 1–2 hr. **Time to peak serum levels:** 1 hr (1–2 hr for ramiprilat, the active metabolite). Ramiprilat has approximately six times the ACE inhibitory activity than ramipril. t½: 1–2 hr (13–17 hr for ramiprilat); prolonged in impaired renal function. **Duration:** 24 hr. Metabolized in the liver with

60% excreted through the urine and 40% in the feces. Food decreases the rate, but not the extent, of absorption of ramipril.

Uses: Alone or in combination with other antihypertensive agents (especially thiazide diuretics) for the treatment of hypertension. Treatment of CHF following MI to decrease risk of CV death and decrease the risk of failure-related hospitalization and progression to severe or resistant heart failure.

Contraindications: Use during lactation.

Special Concerns: Geriatric clients may manifest higher peak blood levels of ramiprilat.

Side Effects: *CV:* Hypotension, chest pain, palpitations, angina pectoris, *MI, arrhythmias. GI:* N&V, abdominal pain, diarrhea, dysgeusia, anorexia, constipation, dry mouth, dyspepsia, enzyme changes suggesting pancreatitis, dysphagia, gastroenteritis, increased salivation. *CNS:* Headache, dizziness, fatigue, insomnia, sleep disturbances, somnolence, depression, nervousness, malaise, vertigo, anxiety, amnesia, *convulsions,* tremor. *Respiratory:* Cough, dyspnea, upper respiratory tract infection, asthma, *bronchospasm. Hematologic:* Leukopenia, eosinophilia. Rarely, decreases in hemoglobin or hematocrit. *Dermatologic:* Diaphoresis, photosensitivity, pruritus, rash, dermatitis, purpura. *Body as a whole:* Paresthesias, angioedema, asthenia, syncope, fever, muscle cramps, myalgia, arthralgia, arthritis, neuralgia, neuropathy, influenza, edema. *Miscellaneous:* Impotence, tinnitus, hearing loss, vision disturbances, epistaxis, weight gain, proteinuria.

Laboratory Test Interferences: ↓ H&H.

Dosage ————————
• **Capsules**
  Hypertension.
Initial: 2.5 mg once daily in clients not taking a diuretic; **maintenance:** 2.5–20 mg/day as a single dose or two equally divided doses. *Clients*

taking diuretics or who have a creatinine clearance less than 40 mL/min/1.73 m²: initially 1.25 mg/day; dose may then be increased to a maximum of 5 mg/day.
  CHF following MI.
Initial: 2.5 mg b.i.d. Clients intolerant of this dose may be started on 1.25 mg b.i.d. The target maintenance dose is 5 mg b.i.d.

RESPIRATORY CARE CONSIDERATIONS

See also *Respiratory Care Considerations* for *Angiotensin-Converting Enzyme Inhibitors* and *Antihypertensive Agents.*

Administration/Storage:
1. The contents of the capsule can be mixed with water, apple juice, or apple sauce to make the medication easier to swallow.
2. If the antihypertensive effect decreases at the end of the dosing interval in clients taking the medication once daily, either twice daily administration should be considered or the dose should be increased.
3. If the client is taking a diuretic, the diuretic should be discontinued 2–3 days prior to beginning ramipril therapy. If the BP is not controlled, the diuretic should be reinstituted. If the diuretic cannot be discontinued, an initial dose of ramipril should be 1.25 mg.

Evaluate:
• ↓ BP to within desired range
• Resolution of S&S of CHF

Remifentanil hydrochloride
((rem-ih-**FEN**-tah-nil))
Pregnancy Category: C
Ultiva **(Rx)**
Classification: Narcotic analgesic

See also *Narcotic Analgesics.*
Action/Kinetics: Remifentanil is a narcotic analgesic that binds with mu-opioid receptors. It has rapid onset and peak effect and a short duration of action. Remifentanil depresses respiration in a dose-depen-

dent manner, causes muscle rigidity, and is an analgesic. The drug is rapidly metabolized by nonspecific blood and tissue esterases; it is not metabolized appreciably by the liver or lung. **t½, elimination:** 3–10 min. Recovery from the effects of remifentanil occurs within 5–10 min.

Uses: As an analgesic during the induction and maintenance of general anesthesia and for continuation as an analgesic in the immediate postoperative period. It is also an analgesic component of monitored anesthesia care.

Contraindications: Epidural or intrathecal use due to the presence of glycine in the formulation. Hypersensitivity to fentanyl analogues. Not to be used as the sole agent in general anesthesia because LOC cannot be ensured and due to a high incidence of apnea, muscle rigidity, and tachycardia.

Special Concerns: Use with caution in obese clients. Respiratory depression and other narcotic effects may be seen in newborns whose mothers are given remifentanil shortly before delivery. Geriatric clients are twice as sensitive as younger clients to the effects of the drug. Use with caution during lactation. Remifentanil has not been studied in children less than 2 years of age.

Side Effects: *GI:* N&V, constipation, abdominal discomfort, xerostomia, gastroesophageal reflux, dysphagia, diarrhea, heartburn, ileus. *CNS:* Shivering, fever, dizziness, headache, agitation, chills, warm sensation, anxiety, involuntary movement, prolonged emergence from anesthesia, tremors, disorientation, dysphoria, nightmares, hallucinations, paresthesia, nystagmus, twitch, sleep disorder, seizures, amnesia. *CV:* Hypotension, bradycardia, tachycardia, hypertension, atrial and ventricular arrhythmias, heart block, ECG change consistent with myocardial ischemia, syncope. *Musculoskeletal:* Muscle rigidity, muscle stiffness, musculoskeletal chest pain, delayed recovery from neuromuscular block. *Respiratory:* Respiratory depression, apnea, hypoxia, cough, dyspnea, bronchospasm, laryngospasm, rhonchi, stridor, nasal congestion, pharyngitis, pleural effusion, hiccoughs, pulmonary edema, rales, bronchitis, rhinorrhea. *Dermatologic:* Pruritus, rash, urticaria, erythema, sweating, flushing, pain at IV site. *GU:* Urine retention, oliguria, dysuria, urine incontinence. *Hematologic:* Anemia, lymphopenia, leukocytosis, thrombocytopenia. *Metabolic:* Abnormal liver function, hyperglycemia, electrolyte disorders. *Miscellaneous:* Decreased body temperature, **anaphylactic reaction,** visual disturbances, postoperative pain.

OD **Overdose Management:** *Symptoms:* Apnea, chest-wall rigidity, seizures, hypoxemia, hypotension, bradycardia. *Treatment:* Discontinue administration, maintain a patent airway, initiate assisted or controlled ventilation with oxygen, and maintain adequate CV function. A neuromuscular blocking agent or a mu-opiate receptor antagonist may be used to treat muscle rigidity. IV fluids, vasopressors, and other supportive measures are indicated to treat hypotension. Bradycardia or hypotension may also be treated with atropine or glycopyrrolate. IV naloxone is used to treat respiratory depression or muscle rigidity. Reversal of the opioid effects may lead to acute pain and sympathetic hyperactivity.

Drug Interactions: Remifentanil is synergistic with other anesthetics. Doses of thiopental, propofol, isoflurane, and midazolam have been reduced by up to 75% with the coadministration of remifentanil.

Laboratory Test Interferences: CPK-MB levels.

Dosage
• **Continuous IV Infusion Only**
   Induction of anesthesia through intubation.
0.5–1 mcg/kg/min given with a hypnotic or volatile agent. If endotra-

R

bold italic = life threatening side effect

cheal intubation is to occur less than 8 min after the start of the infusion of remifentanil, the initial dose of 1 mcg/kg may be given over 30 to 60 sec.

Maintenance of nitrous oxide (66%) anesthesia.

The dose of remifentanil is 0.4 mcg/kg/min (range of 0.1–2 mcg/kg/min). A supplemental IV bolus dose of 1 mcg/kg may be given.

Maintenance of isoflurance (0.4 to 1.5 MAC) or propofol (100–200 mcg/kg/min) anesthesia.

The dose of remifentanil is 0.25 mcg/kg/min (range of 0.05–2 mcg/kg/min). A supplemental IV bolus dose of 1 mcg/kg may be given.

Continuation as an analgesic into the immediate postoperative period.

The dose of remifentanil is 0.1 mcg/kg/min (range of 0.025–0.2 mcg/kg/min). The infusion rate may be adjusted every 5 min in 0.025-mcg/kg/min increments to balance the client's level of analgesia and respiratory rate.

Analgesic component of monitored anesthesia care.

Single IV dose: 1 mcg/kg administered over 30 to 60 sec and given 90 sec before the local anesthetic. If remifentanil is given with midazolam (2 mg), the dose should be 0.5 mcg/kg.

Continuous IV infusion: 0.1 mcg/kg beginning 5 min before the local anesthetic. After the local anesthetic, the dose of remifentanil is 0.05 mcg/kg/min (range 0.025–0.2 mcg/kg/min) at 5-min intervals in order to balance the level of analgesia and respiratory rate. If remifentanil is given with midazolam (2 mg), the dose should be 0.025 mcg/kg/min (range 0.025–0.2 mcg/kg/min).

RESPIRATORY CARE CONSIDERATIONS

See also *Respiratory Care Considerations* for *Narcotic Analgesics.*

Administration/Storage

1. Continuous infusions of remifentanil are given only by an infusion device. The injection site should be close to the venous cannula.

2. Due to the rapid onset and short duration of remifentanil, the administration during anesthesia can be titrated upward in 25%- to 100%-increments or downward in 25%- to 50%-decrements every 2 to 5 min to attain the desired level of opiate effect. In response to light anesthesia or transient periods of intense surgical stress, supplemental bolus doses of 1 mcg/kg may be given every 2 to 5 min.

3. Administration of remifentanil into the immediate postoperative period should be under the supervision of an anesthesia practitioner. Infusion rates greater than 0.2 mcg/kg/min are associated with respiratory depression.

4. When remifentanil infusion is discontinued, the IV tubing should be cleared to prevent inadvertant administration at a later time.

5. Due to its duration, no opioid activity will be present within 5–10 min of discontinuation.

6. The starting dose of remifentanil should be decreased by 50% in clients over 65 years of age. Cautiously titrate to the desired effect.

7. Use the adult dose for pediatric clients 2 years of age and older.

8. The starting dose in obese clients (i.e., greater than 30% over their ideal body weight) should be based on ideal body weight.

9. The need for preanesthetic drugs and the choice of anesthetic must be individualized.

10. Remifentanil is stable for 24 hr at room temperature after reconstitution and further dilution to concentrations of 20–250 mcg/mL. Dilution may be with sterile water for injection, 5% dextrose injection, 5% dextrose and 0.9% sodium chloride injection, 0.9% sodium chloride injection, or 0.45% sodium chloride injection.

11. Remifentanil is compatible with propofal when coadministered into a running IV administration set.

12. Remifentanil should be stored at 2°C–25°C (36°F–77°F).

Assessment

1. Document indications for therapy, noting onset, location, and duration of symptoms, and any other agents prescribed and the outcome.

2. Determine if pain is acute or chronic in nature; describe any distinguishing characteristics and use a pain-rating scale to rate pain level.

3. Obtain baseline liver and renal function studies.

Evaluate: Desired level of pain control and analgesia

Respiratory Syncytial Virus Immune Globulin Intravenous (Human) (RSV-IGIV)

Pregnancy Category: C
RespiGam **(Rx)**
Classification: Immunosuppressant

Action/Kinetics: Respiratory Syncytial Virus Immune Globulin Intravenous (RSV-IGIV) is an IgG containing neutralizing antibody to respiratory syncytial virus (RSV). The immunoglobulin is obtained and purified from pooled adult human plasma that has been selected for high titers of neutralizing antibody against RSV. Each milliliter contains 50 mg of immunoglobulin, primarily IgG with trace amounts of IgA and IgM.

Uses: Prevention of serious lower respiratory tract infection caused by RSV in children less than 24 months old with bronchopulmonary dysplasia or a history of premature birth (less than 35 weeks gestation).

Contraindications: History of a severe prior reaction associated with administration of RSV-IGIV or other human immunoglobulin products. Clients with selective IgA deficiency who have the potential for developing antibodies to IgA and which could cause anaphylaxis or allergic reactions to blood products that contain IgA.

Special Concerns: The safety and efficacy of RSV-IGIV has not been determined in children with congenital heart disease. Side effects may be related to the rate of administration; thus, close attention should be given to the infusion rate. Since RSV-IGIV is made from human plasma, there is the possibility for transmission of blood-borne pathogenic organisms, although the risk is considered to be low due to screening of donors and viral inactivation and removal steps in the manufacturing process.

Side Effects: Infusion of RSV-IGIV may cause fluid overload, especially in children with bronchopulmonary dysplasia. Aseptic meningitis syndrome has been reported within several hours to 2 days following RSV-IGIV treatment. Symptoms include severe headache, drowsiness, fever, photophobia, painful eye movements, muscle rigidity, nausea, and vomiting. The CSF shows pleocytosis, predominately granulocytic, as well as elevated protein levels.

Allergic: Hypotension, ***anaphylaxis, angioneurotic edema,*** respiratory distress. *CNS:* Fever, pyrexia, sleepiness. *Respiratory:* Respiratory distress, wheezing, rales, tachypnea, cough. *GI:* Vomiting, diarrhea, gagging, gastroenteritis. *CV:* Tachycardia, increased pulse rate, hypertension, hypotension, heart murmur. *Dermatologic:* Rash, pallor, cyanosis, eczema, cold and clammy skin. *Miscellaneous:* Hypoxia, hypoxemia, inflammation at injection site, edema, rhinorrhea, conjunctival hemorrhage.

Reactions similar to other immunoglobulins may occur as follows. *Body as a whole:* Dizziness, flushing, ***immediate allergic, anaphylactic, or hypersensitivity reactions.*** *CV:* Blood pressure changes, palpitations, chest tightness. *Miscellaneous:* Anxiety, dyspnea, abdominal cramps, pruritus, myalgia, arthralgia.

OD **Overdose Management:** *Symptoms:* Symptoms due to fluid volume overload. *Treatment:* Ad-

R

ministration of diuretics and modification of the infusion rate.

Drug Interactions: Antibodies found in immunoglobulin products may interfere with the immune response to live virus vaccines, including those for mumps, rubella, and measles. Also, the antibody response to diphtheria, tetanus, pertussis, and *Haemophilus influenzae b* may be lower in RSV-IGIV recipients.

Dosage
• **IV Injection**
Prevention of RSV infections.
1.5 mL/kg/hr for 15 min. If the clinical condition of the client allows, the rate can be increased to 3 mL/kg/hr for the next 15-min period and, finally, increased to a maximum rate of 6 mL/kg/hr from 30 min to the end of the infusion.

RESPIRATORY CARE CONSIDERATIONS
Administration/Storage
1. The single-use vial should be entered only once for drug administration. Infusion of the drug should be initiated within 6 hr and completed within 12 hr of removal from the vial.
2. The drug should not be used if the solution is turbid.
3. The rate of infusion listed above *must not* be exceeded.
4. RSV-IGIV should be given separately from other drugs or medications.
5. RSV-IGIV is to be given through an IV line (preferably a separate line) using a constant infusion pump. Administration may be "piggy-backed" into an existing line if that line contains one of the following dextrose solutions (with or without sodium chloride): 2.5%, 5%, 10%, or 20% dextrose in water. If a preexisting line must be used, the RSV-IGIV should not be diluted more than 1:2 with one of the above solutions. Predilution of RSV-IGIV before infusion is not recommended.
6. Although use of filters is not necessary, an in-line filter with a pore size greater than 15 μm may be used.
7. The injection should be stored at 2°C–8°C (35.6°F–46.4°F). The product should not be frozen or shaken (to prevent foaming).

Assessment
1. Document indications for therapy and any previous experiences with this drug and the outcome.
2. Note any evidence of IgA deficiency.
3. The client's VS and cardiopulmonary status must be assessed prior to infusion, before each rate increase, and thereafter at 30-min intervals until 30 min following completion of the infusion.

Interventions
1. Monitor VS and I&O. Observe for evidence of fluid overload (increased HR, increased respiratory rate, rales, retractions), especially in infants with bronchopulmonary dysplasia.
2. The drug should be administered cautiously. A loop diuretic (e.g., furosemide or bumetanide) should be available for management of fluid overload.
3. Observe and report any evidence of severe headache, painful eye movements, drowsiness, fever, N&V, muscle rigidity (symptoms of aseptic meningitis) following therapy.
4. Clients showing symptoms of aseptic meningitis syndrome should be evaluated in order to rule out other causes of meningitis.
5. If virus vaccines are given during or within 10 months after RSV-IGIV infusion, reimmunization is recommended.

Client/Family Teaching
1. Advise that the first dose of RSV-IGIV should be given prior to the beginning of the RSV season and monthly throughout the RSV season (in the Northern Hemisphere, this is from November through April) in order to maintain protection.
2. Caution that drug is derived from human plasma and review the potential risks related to blood-borne pathogenic agents.

Evaluate
- RSV disease prophylaxis
- ↓ Severity of RSV illness with ↓ incidence and duration of RSV hospitalizations

Ribavirin

(rye-bah-**VYE**-rin)
Pregnancy Category: X
Virazole, Virazole (Lyophilized) ✦ **(Rx)**
Classification: Antiviral agent

See also *Antiviral Drugs.*

Action/Kinetics: Ribavirin has antiviral activity against respiratory syncytial virus, influenza virus, and herpes simplex virus. Although the precise mechanism is not known, ribavirin may act as a competitive inhibitor of cellular enzymes that act on guanosine and xanthosine. Ribavirin is distributed to the plasma, respiratory tract, and RBCs and is rapidly taken up by cells. **t½:** 9.5 hr. Eliminated through both the urine and feces.

Uses: Hospitalized pediatric clients (including infants) with severe lower respiratory tract infections (viral pneumonia including bronchiolitis) due to respiratory syncytial virus (RSV). Underlying conditions, such as prematurity or cardiopulmonary disease, may increase the severity of the RSV infection. Ribavirin is intended to be used along with standard treatment (including fluid management) for such clients with severe lower respiratory tract infections. *Investigational:* Ribavirin aerosol has been used against influenza A and B. Oral ribavirin has been used against herpes genitalis, acute and chronic hepatitis, measles, and Lassa fever.

Contraindications: Children with mild RSV lower respiratory tract infections who require a shorter hospital stay than required for a full course of ribavirin therapy. Pregnancy or women who may become pregnant during drug therapy (the drug may cause fetal harm and is known to be teratogenic). Lactation.

Special Concerns: If given to infants receiving mechanical ventilation, special cautions must be taken to place filters in the ventilator circuit to prevent residue from causing malfunction. Use with caution in adults with asthma or chronic obstructive lung disease (deterioration of respiratory function may occur). Deterioration of respiratory function in infants and adults with COPD or asthma.

Side Effects: *Pulmonary:* Worsening of respiratory status, pneumothorax, apnea, bacterial pneumonia, dependence on ventilator, ***bronchospasm,*** pulmonary edema, hypoventilation, cyanosis, dyspnea, pneumothorax, atelectasis. *CV:* Hypotension, ***cardiac arrest,*** manifestations of digitalis toxicity, bradycardia, bigeminy, tachycardia. *Hematologic:* Anemia (with IV or PO ribavirin), reticulocytosis. *Other:* Conjunctivitis and rash (with the aerosol).

NOTE: The following symptoms have been noted in health care workers: headache, conjunctivitis, rhinitis, nausea, rash, dizziness, pharyngitis, lacrimation, bronchospasm, chest pain. Also, damage to contact lenses after prolonged close exposure to the aerosolized product.

Dosage
- **Aerosol Only, to an Infant Oxygen Hood Using the Small Particle Aerosol Generator-2 (SPAG-2)**
The concentration administered is 20 mg/mL and the average aerosol concentration for a 12-hr period is 190 mcg/L of air. See *Administration/Storage.*

RESPIRATORY CARE CONSIDERATIONS
Administration/Storage:
1. Administration of the drug should be carried out for 12–18 hr/day for 3 (minimum)–7 (maximum) days.
2. Treatment is most effective if initiated within the first 3 days of the res-

R

piratory syncytial virus, which causes lower respiratory tract infections.

3. Ribavirin aerosol should only be administered using the SPAG-2 aerosol generator.

4. Therapy should *not* be instituted in clients requiring mechanical ventilation without a thorough understanding of appropriate safeguards.

5. No other aerosolized medications should be given if ribavirin aerosol is being used.

6. The drug may be solubilized with sterile water (USP) for injection or inhalation in the 100-mL vial. The solution is then transferred to the SPAG-2 reservoir utilizing a sterilized 500-mL wide-mouth Erlenmeyer flask and further diluted to a final volume of 300 mL with sterile water.

7. Solutions in the SPAG-2 reservoir should be replaced daily. Also, if the liquid level is low, it should be discarded before new drug solution is added.

8. Reconstituted solutions of ribavirin may be stored at room temperature for 24 hr.

9. Drug is not to be administered by women of childbearing age. *Post* this advisement so they do not come in contact with the drug.

Interventions:

1. Health care workers administering drug should use goggles and respirator to protect mucous membranes; remove contact lens, and monitor exposure times. Review list of side effects related to drug administration.

2. It is essential that constant monitoring be undertaken for both the fluid and respiratory status of the client.

3. Assess frequently for evidence of respiratory distress; stop therapy and report if distress occurs. Do not leave child unattended and unstimulated in the tent for long periods during therapy.

4. Monitor and record VS and I&O.

5. Anticipate limited use in infants and adults with COPD or asthma.

6. With prolonged therapy (more than 7 days), observe for S&S of anemia; monitor CBC values.

Evaluate:

• Auscultatory and radiographic evidence of improved airway exchange

• Clinical and lab evidence of resolution of RSV pneumonia

Rifabutin

(**rif**-ah-**BYOU**-tin)
Pregnancy Category: B
Mycobutin **(Rx)**
Classification: Antitubercular drug

Action/Kinetics: Rifabutin is an antimycobacterial drug derived from rifamycin. It inhibits DNA-dependent RNA polymerase in susceptible strains of *Escherichia coli* and *Bacillus subtilis.* The drug is rapidly absorbed from the GI tract. **Peak plasma levels after a single dose:** 3.3 hr. **Mean terminal t½:** 45 hr. About 85% is bound to plasma proteins. High-fat meals slow the rate, but not the extent, of absorption. About 30% of a dose is excreted in the feces and 53% excreted in the urine, primarily as metabolites. The 25-O-desacetyl metabolite is equal in activity to rifabutin.

Uses: Prevention of disseminated *Mycobacterium avium* complex (MAC) disease in clients with advanced HIV infection.

Contraindications: Hypersensitivity to rifabutin or other rifamycins (e.g., rifampin). Use in clients with active tuberculosis. Lactation.

Special Concerns: Safety and efficacy have not been determined in children, although the drug has been used in HIV-positive children.

Side Effects: *GI:* Anorexia, abdominal pain, diarrhea, dyspepsia, eructation, flatulence, N&V, taste perversion. *Respiratory:* Chest pain, chest pressure or pain with dyspnea. *CNS:* Insomnia, *seizures,* paresthesia, aphasia, confusion. *Musculoskeletal:* Asthenia, myalgia, arthralgia, myositis. *Body as a whole:* Fever, headache, generalized pain, flu-like syndrome. *Dermatologic:* Rash, skin discoloration. *Hematologic:* Neutropenia, leukopenia, anemia, eosinophilia, thrombocytopenia. *Miscella-*

neous: Discolored urine, nonspecific T wave changes on ECG, hepatitis, hemolysis, uveitis.

OD **Overdose Management:** *Symptoms:* Worsening of side effects. *Treatment:* Gastric lavage followed by instillation into the stomach of an activated charcoal slurry.

Drug Interactions: Rifabutin has liver enzyme-inducing properties and may be expected to have similar interactions as does rifampin. However, rifabutin is a less potent enzyme inducer than rifampin.

AZT / ↓ Steady-state plasma levels of AZT after repeated rifabutin dosing

Oral contraceptives / Rifabutin may ↓ the effectiveness of oral contraceptives

Laboratory Test Interferences: ↑ AST, ALT, alkaline phosphatase.

Dosage
• **Capsules**
Prophylaxis of MAC disease in clients with advanced HIV infection.
Adults: 300 mg/day.

RESPIRATORY CARE CONSIDERATIONS

See also *General Respiratory Care Considerations for All Anti-Infectives.*

Administration/Storage:
1. The drug can be given at doses of 150 mg b.i.d. with food if clients experience N&V or other GI upset.
2. Urine, feces, saliva, sputum, perspiration, tears, and skin may be colored brown-orange. Soft contact lenses may be permanently stained.
Assessment:
1. Document indications for therapy, noting type, onset, and characteristics of symptoms.
2. Obtain baseline CBC and monitor for neutropenia.
3. Ensure that CXR, PPD, and sputum AFB cultures have been performed to rule outactive tuberculosis. Clients who develop active tuberculosis during therapy must be covered

with appropriate antituberculosis medications.

Evaluate: Prevention of disseminated MAC disease in clients with advanced HIV

Rifampin
(rih-**FAM**-pin)
Pregnancy Category: C
Rifadin, Rimactane, Rofact ✱ **(Rx)**
Classification: Primary antitubercular agent

Action/Kinetics: Semisynthetic antibiotic derived from *Streptomyces mediterranei.* Rifampin suppresses RNA synthesis by binding to the beta subunit of DNA-dependent RNA polymerase. This prevents attachment of the enzyme to DNA and blockade of RNA transcription. The drug is both bacteriostatic and bactericidal and is most active against rapidly replicating organisms. The drug is well absorbed from the GI tract and is widely distributed in body tissues. **Peak plasma concentration:** 4–32 mcg/mL after 2–4 hr. **t½:** 1.5–5 hr (higher in clients with hepatic impairment). In normal clients t½ decreases with usage. The drug is metabolized in liver; 60% is excreted in feces.

Uses: All types of tuberculosis. Must be used in conjunction with at least one other tuberculostatic drug (such as isoniazid, ethambutol, pyrazinamide) but is the drug of choice for retreatment. Also for treatment of asymptomatic meningococcal carriers to eliminate *Neisseria meningitidis. Investigational:* Used in combination for infections due to *Staphylococcus aureus* and *S. epidermidis* (endocarditis, osteomyelitis, prostatitis); Legionnaire's disease; in combination with dapsone for leprosy; prophylaxis of meningitis due to *Haemophilus influenzae* and gram-negative bacteremia in infants.

Contraindications: Hypersensitivity; not recommended for intermittent therapy.

R

Special Concerns: Safe use during lactation has not been established. Safety and effectiveness not determined in children less than 5 years of age. Use with extreme caution in clients with hepatic dysfunction.

Side Effects: *GI:* N&V, diarrhea, anorexia, gas, pseudomembranous colitis, pancreatitis, sore mouth and tongue, cramps, heartburn, flatulence. *CNS:* Headache, drowsiness, fatigue, ataxia, dizziness, confusion, generalized numbness, fever, difficulty in concentrating. *Hepatic:* Jaundice, hepatitis. Increases in AST, ALT, bilirubin, alkaline phosphatase. *Hematologic:* Thrombocytopenia, eosinophilia, hemolysis, leukopenia, hemolytic anemia. *Allergic:* Flu-like symptoms, dyspnea, wheezing, SOB, purpura, pruritus, urticaria, skin rashes, sore mouth and tongue, conjunctivitis. *Renal:* Hematuria, hemoglobinuria, renal insufficiency, acute renal failure. *Miscellaneous:* Visual disturbances, muscle weakness or pain, arthralgia, decreased BP, osteomalacia, menstrual disturbances, edema of face and extremities, adrenocortical insufficiency, increases in BUN and serum uric acid. *NOTE:* Body fluids and feces may be red-orange.

OD **Overdose Management:** *Symptoms:* Shortly after ingestion, N&V, and lethargy will occur. Followed by severe hepatic involvement (liver enlargement with tenderness, increased direct and total bilirubin, change in hepatic enzymes) with unconsciousness. Also, brownish red or orange discoloration of urine, saliva, tears, sweat, skin, and feces. *Treatment:* Gastric lavage followed by activated charcoal slurry introduced into the stomach. Antiemetics to control N&V. Forced diuresis to enhance excretion. If hepatic function is seriously impaired, bile drainage may be required. Extracorporeal hemodialysis may be necessary.

Drug Interactions:
Acetaminophen / ↓ Effect of acetaminophen due to ↑ breakdown by liver

Aminophylline / ↓ Effect of aminophylline due to ↑ breakdown by liver

Anticoagulants, oral / ↓ Effect of anticoagulants due to ↑ breakdown by liver

Antidiabetics, oral / ↓ Effect of oral antidiabetic due to ↑ breakdown by liver

Barbiturates / ↓ Effect of barbiturates due to ↑ breakdown by liver

Benzodiazepines / ↓ Effect of benzodiazepines due to ↑ breakdown by liver

Beta-adrenergic blocking agents / ↓ Effect of beta-blocking agents due to ↑ breakdown by liver

Chloramphenicol / ↓ Effect of chloramphenicol due to ↑ breakdown by liver

Clofibrate / ↓ Effect of clofibrate due to ↑ breakdown by liver

Contraceptives, oral / ↓ Effect of oral contraceptives due to ↑ breakdown by liver

Corticosteroids / ↓ Effect of corticosteroids due to ↑ breakdown by liver

Cyclosporine / ↓ Effect of cyclosporine due to ↑ breakdown by liver

Digitoxin / ↓ Effect of digitoxin due to ↑ breakdown by liver

Digoxin / ↓ Serum levels of digoxin

Disopyramide / ↓ Effect of disopyramide due to ↑ breakdown by liver

Estrogens / ↓ Effect of estrogens due to ↑ breakdown by liver

Halothane / ↑ Risk of hepatotoxicity and hepatic encephalopathy

Hydantoins / ↓ Effect of hydantoins due to ↑ breakdown by liver

Isoniazid / ↑ Risk of hepatotoxicity

Ketoconazole / ↓ Effect of either ketoconazole or rifampin

Methadone / ↓ Effect of methadone due to ↑ breakdown by liver

Mexiletine / ↓ Effect of mexiletine due to ↑ breakdown by liver

Quinidine / ↓ Effect of quinidine due to ↑ breakdown by liver

Sulfones / ↓ Effect of sulfones due to ↑ breakdown by liver

Theophylline / ↓ Effect of theophylline due to ↑ breakdown by liver

Tocainide / ↓ Effect of tocainide due to ↑ breakdown by liver

Verapamil / ↓ Effect of verapamil due to ↑ breakdown by liver

Laboratory Test Interferences: ↑ AST, ALT, alkaline phosphatase, BUN, bilirubin, uric acid, BSP retention values. False + Coombs' test.

Dosage ————————
- **Capsules, IV**
  Pulmonary tuberculosis.
  Adults: Single dose of 600 mg/day; **children over 5 years:** 10–20 mg/kg/day, not to exceed 600 mg/day.
  Meningococcal carriers.
  Adults: 600 mg b.i.d. for 2 days; **children:** 10–20 mg/kg q 12 hr for four doses. Dosage should not exceed 600 mg/day.

RESPIRATORY CARE CONSIDERATIONS

See also *General Respiratory Care Considerations for All Anti-Infectives.*

Administration/Storage:

1. Administer capsules once daily 1 hr before or 2 hr after meals to ensure maximum absorption.
2. Check to be sure that there is a desiccant in the bottle containing capsules of rifampin because these are relatively moisture sensitive.
3. If administered concomitantly with PAS, drugs should be given 8–12 hr apart because the acid interferes with the absorption of rifampin.
4. When used for tuberculosis, therapy should continue for 6–9 months.
5. Reconstitute 600-mg vial using 10 mL of sterile water for injection. Gently swirl vial to dissolve. The resultant solution contains 60 mg/mL rifampin; it is stable at room temperature for 24 hr.
6. Add the volume of reconstituted solution needed to 500 mL of D5W and infuse over 3 hr, or it may be added to 100 mL D5W and infused over 30 min. Sterile saline may be used when dextrose is contraindicated; however, the stability of rifampin is slightly less.

7. The dilution solution must be used within 4 hr or drug may precipitate from solution.
8. Injectable solution appears dark reddish brown.
9. A PO suspension (10 mg/mL) may be prepared as follows: The contents of either four 300-mg rifampin capsules or eight 150-mg capsules are emptied into a 4-oz amber glass bottle. To this is added 20 mL of simple syrup; shake vigorously. Add 100 mL of simple syrup and shake again. The suspension is stable for 4 weeks when stored at room temperature or in the refrigerator.

Assessment:

1. Document indications for therapy and type, onset, and duration of symptoms.
2. List any previous therapy, the duration, and the outcome.
3. Obtain baseline CBC, liver and renal function studies, and cultures. Evaluate for impaired liver or renal function and blood dyscrasias.
4. Assess and document any GI disturbances or auditory nerve impairment.
5. Obtain baseline CXR; auscultate and document lung sounds and characteristics of sputum. Note PPD skin test results.

Evaluate:

- Effectiveness as a combination agent in treating tuberculosis based on radiographic and lab evidence
- Prophylaxis of meningitis due to *H. influenzae* and gram-negative bacteremia in infants

R

Rocuronium bromide
(**roh**-kyou-**ROH**-nee-um)
Pregnancy Category: B
Zemuron **(Rx)**
Classification: Neuromuscular blocking agent

See also *Neuromuscular Blocking Agents.*
Action/Kinetics: Rocuronium is a nondepolarizing neuromuscular blocking agent that acts by competing with acetylcholine for receptors at

the motor end-plate. In a small number of clients, the drug causes histamine release. Use of rocuronium must be accompanied by adequate anesthesia or sedation, as the drug has no effect on consciousness, pain threshold, or cerebration. Depending on the dose, it has a rapid to intermediate onset and an intermediate duration of action. **t½, rapid distribution phase:** 1–2 min; **t½, slower distribution phase:** 14–18 min. The drug is metabolized by the liver.

Uses: As an adjunct to general anesthesia to facilitate rapid sequence and routine tracheal intubation; also, to cause relaxation of skeletal muscle during surgery or mechanical ventilation.

Special Concerns: Use with caution in clients with pulmonary hypertension, valvular heart disease, or significant hepatic disease. Burn clients may develop resistance to nondepolarizing neuromuscular blocking agents. Elderly clients may exhibit a slightly prolonged medical clinical duration of action. Use in children less than 3 months of age has not been studied.

Side Effects: *CV:* Arrhythmias, abnormal ECG, transient hypotension and hypertension, tachycardia. *GI:* N&V. *Respiratory:* Symptoms of asthma, including **bronchospasm,** wheezing, rhonchi; hiccup. *Dermatologic:* Rash, edema at injection site, pruritus.

OD **Overdose Management:** *Symptoms:* Neuromuscular blockade longer than needed for anesthesia and surgery. *Treatment:* Careful monitoring of client. Assisted ventilation may be required.

Dosage
• **IV Only**
Rapid sequence intubation.
0.6–1.2 mg/kg in appropriately premedicated and adequately anesthetized clients will result in good intubating conditions in less than 2 min.
Tracheal intubation.
Initial, regardless of anesthetic technique: 0.6 mg/kg. Maximum

blockade is noted in less than 3 min with a mean duration of 31 min. However, a dose of 0.45 mg/kg may also be used with maximum blockade in less than 4 min with a mean duration of 22 min. Initial doses of 0.6 mg/kg in children under halothane anesthesia produce good intubating conditions within 1 min with a mean duration of 41 min in children 3 months to 1 year and 27 min in children 1–2 years of age. Maintenance doses in children of 0.075–0.125 mg/kg, given upon return of T_1 of 25% of control provide muscle relaxation for 7–10 min.

Maintenance doses.
0.1, 0.15, and 0.2 mg/kg, given at 25% recovery of control T_1 (defined as three twitches of train-of-four), provide a median of 12, 17, and 24 min of duration under opioid/nitrous oxide/oxygen anesthesia. The dose should not be administered until recovery of neuromuscular function is evident.

Continuous infusion.
Initial: 0.01–0.02 mg/kg/min only after early evidence of spontaneous recovery from an intubating dose. Upon reaching the desired level of neuromuscular blockade, the infusion must be individualized for each client; the rate should be adjusted based on the twitch response (monitored with the use of a peripheral nerve stimulator) of the client. **Maintenance, usual:** 0.004–0.016 mg/kg/min.

RESPIRATORY CARE CONSIDERATIONS

See also *Respiratory Care Considerations* for *Neuromuscular Blocking Agents.*
Administration/Storage:
1. Inhalation anesthetics (especially enflurane or isoflurane) may enhance the effects of rocuronium. When inhalation anesthetics are used, it may be necessary to reduce the rate of infusion by 30%–50% 45–60 min after the intubating dose.
2. Solutions for infusion can be prepared by mixing rocuronium with

D5W or lactated Ringer's solution. However, the drug is also compatible with 0.9% sodium chloride solution, sterile water for injection, and 5% dextrose in saline. The solution should be used within 24 hr after mixing and any unused portions of infusion solutions should be discarded.

3. Spontaneous recovery occurs at about the same rate in children 3 months–1 year as in adults, but is more rapid in children 1–12 years of age.

4. Rocuronium, which has an acid pH, should not be mixed with alkaline solutions (e.g., barbiturates) in the same syringe or given at the same time during IV infusion through the same needle.

5. The drug should be stored from 2°C–8°C (36°F–46°F) and should not be frozen.

Assessment:

1. Ensure that appropriate baseline ECG and liver and renal function studies are available.

2. In the critically ill, client should be intubated prior to administration of rocuronium.

3. A peripheral nerve stimulator should be used to assess neuromuscular function and to confirm recovery from neuromuscular blockade.

Evaluate:

• Desired level of skeletal muscle relaxation

• Control of breathing during mechanical ventilation

Salmeterol xinafoate

(sal-**MET**-er-ole)
Pregnancy Category: C
Serevent **(Rx)**
Classification: Beta-2 adrenergic agonist

See also *Sympathomimetic Drugs.*

Action/Kinetics: Salmeterol is selective for beta-2 adrenergic receptors; these receptors are located in the bronchi and heart. The drug is thought to act by stimulating intracellular adenyl cyclase, the enzyme that converts ATP to cyclic AMP. Increased AMP levels cause relaxation of bronchial smooth muscle and inhibition of release of mediators of immediate hypersensitivity, especially from mast cells. Salmeterol is significantly bound to plasma proteins. The drug is cleared by hepatic metabolism.

Uses: Long-term maintenance treatment of asthma. Prevention of bronchospasms in clients over 12 years of age with reversible obstructive airway disease, including nocturnal asthma. Prevention of exercise-induced bronchospasms.

Contraindications: Use in clients who can be controlled by short-acting, inhaled beta-2 agonists. Use to treat acute symptoms of asthma or in those who have worsening or deteriorating asthma. Lactation.

Special Concerns: Use with caution in clients with impaired hepatic function. The drug is not a substitute for PO or inhaled corticosteroids. The safety and efficacy of using salmeterol with a spacer or other devices has not been studied adequately. Use with caution in clients with cardiovascular disorders, including coronary insufficiency, cardiac arrhythmias, and hypertension; in clients with convulsive disorders or thyrotoxicosis; and in clients who respond unusually to sympathomimetic amines. Because of the potential of the drug interfering with uterine contractility, use of salmeterol during labor should be restricted to those in whom benefits clearly outweigh risks. Safety and efficacy in children

---

less than 12 years of age have not been determined.

Side Effects: *Respiratory:* Paradoxical bronchospasms, upper or lower respiratory tract infection, nasopharyngitis, disease of nasal cavity/sinus, cough, pharyngitis, allergic rhinitis, laryngitis, tracheitis, bronchitis. *Allergic:* ***Immediate hypersensitivity reactions,*** including urticaria, rash, and ***bronchospasm.*** *CV:* Palpitations, chest pain, increased BP, tachycardia. *CNS:* Headache, sinus headache, tremors, nervousness, malaise, fatigue, dizziness, giddiness. *GI:* Stomachache. *Musculoskeletal:* Joint pain, back pain, muscle cramps, muscle contractions, myalgia, myositis, muscle soreness. *Miscellaneous:* Flu, dental pain, rash, skin eruption, dysmenorrhea.

OD **Overdose Management:** *Symptoms:* Tachycardia, arrhythmia, tremors, headache, muscle cramps, hypokalemia, hyperglycemia. *Treatment:* Supportive therapy. Consideration can be given to the judicious use of a beta-adrenergic blocking agent, although these drugs can cause bronchospasms. Cardiac monitoring is necessary. Dialysis is not an appropriate treatment of overdosage.

Drug Interactions:
MAO Inhibitors / Potentiation of the effect of salmeterol
Tricyclic antidepressants / Potentiation of the effect of salmeterol
Laboratory Test Interferences: ↓ Serum potassium.

S

Dosage —————————————
• **Metered Dose Inhaler**
Maintenance of bronchodilation, prevention of symptoms of asthma, including nocturnal asthma.
Adults and children over 12 years of age: Two inhalations (42 mcg) b.i.d. (morning and evening, approximately 12 hr apart).
Prevention of exercise-induced bronchospasms.
Adults and children over 12 years of age: Two inhalations (42 mcg) at least 30–60 min before exercise. Additional doses should not be used for 12 hr.

RESPIRATORY CARE CONSIDERATIONS

See also *Respiratory Care Considerations* for *Sympathomimetic Drugs.*
Administration/Storage:
1. The bronchodilator activity of salmeterol lasts for 12 hr; thus, doses should be spaced q 12 hr.
2. The safety of concomitant use of more than 8 inhalations per day of short-acting beta-2 agonists with salmeterol has not been established.
3. If a previously effective dose fails to provide the usual response, contact provider immediately.
4. Clients using salmeterol twice daily should not use additional doses to prevent exercise-induced bronchospasms.
5. Salmeterol should only be used with the actuator provided. The actuator should not be used with other aerosol medications.
6. The drug should be stored between 2°C and 30°C (36°F and 86°F). The canister should be stored nozzle end down and should be protected from freezing temperatures and direct sunlight.
7. Caution should be exercised so the drug is not sprayed in the eyes.
8. The canister should be shaken well before using and should be at room temperature, as the therapeutic effect may diminish if the canister is cold.
Assessment:
1. Document onset and duration of symptoms, other agents prescribed, and the outcome.
2. Determine any evidence or history of cardiac or liver dysfunction, thyrotoxicosis, hypertension, or convulsive disorders.
3. Document pulmonary function status and lung sounds.
4. Obtain baseline VS, liver enzymes, and pulmonary function tests (ABGs, peak expiratory flow rate, and forced expiratory volume at 1 sec) and assess periodically.
Client/Family Teaching:
1. Demonstrate proper use (with actuator) and observe client self-administer.

2. Use only as prescribed and do not exceed prescribed dosage and administration frequency (drug effects last 12 hr).

3. Reinforce not to use this drug during an acute asthma attack.

4. Review the procedure for use of the short-acting beta-2 agonist prescribed to treat symptoms of asthma that occur between the salmeterol dosing schedule. Advise that increased utilization warrants medical evaluation (e.g., when used more than 4 times/day or more than one canister of 200 inhalations/8 weeks).

5. Client may experience palpitations, chest pain, headaches, tremors, and nervousness as side effects of drug therapy.

6. If client experiences chest pain, fast pounding irregular heart beat, hives, increased wheezing, or difficulty breathing, advise to notify provider immediately.

7. Instruct to take the drug 30–60 min before activity in order to prevent acute bronchospasms.

8. Stress that salmeterol does not replace inhaled or systemic steroids and to not stop prescribed steroid therapy abruptly without medical supervision.

9. Refer to appropriate support groups that may assist client to cope and live a normal life with this disorder.

10. Stress the importance of not smoking and avoiding a smokey environment. Avoid any other triggers that may aggravate condition.

Evaluate:
• Prevention and control of asthmatic symptoms (e.g., decreased wheezing, dyspnea, orthopnea, and cough)
• Prevention of exercise-induced bronchospasms

Scopolamine hydrobromide
(scoh-**POLL**-ah-meen)
Pregnancy Category: C

Hyoscine Hydrobromide, Isopto Hyoscine Ophthalmic **(Rx)**

Scopolamine transdermal therapeutic system
(scoh-**POLL**-ah-meen)
Pregnancy Category: C
Transderm-Scop, Transderm-V ✿ **(Rx)**
Classification: Anticholinergic, antiemetic

See also *Cholinergic Blocking Agents.*

Action/Kinetics: Scopolamine is an anticholinergic with CNS depressant effects. It produces amnesia when given with morphine or meperidine. In the presence of pain, delirium may be produced. Scopolamine dilates the pupil and paralyzes the muscle required to accommodate for close vision (cycloplegia). This enables the physician to examine the inner structure of the eye, including the retina, as well as to examine refractive errors of the lens without automatic accommodation by the client. Tolerance may develop if scopolamine is used alone. When used for refraction: **peak for mydriasis,** 20–30 min; **peak for cycloplegia,** 30–60 min; **duration:** 24 hr (residual cycloplegia and mydriasis may last for 3–7 days). Recovery time can be reduced by using 1–2 gtt pilocarpine (1% or 2%). To reduce absorption, pressure should be applied over the nasolacrimal sac for 2–3 min.

The transdermal therapeutic system contains 1.5 mg scopolamine, which is slowly released from a mineral oil–polyisobutylene matrix. Approximately 0.5 mg is released from the system per day.

Uses: Ophthalmic: For cycloplegia and mydriasis in diagnostic procedures. Preoperatively and postoperatively in the treatment of iridocyclitis. Dilate the pupil in treatment of uveitis or posterior synechiae. *Investigational:* Prophylaxis of synechaie, treatment of iridocyclitis. **Parenteral:** Antiemetic, antivertigo. Preanesthetic sedation and obstetric amnesia.

S

Antiarrhythmic during anesthesia and surgery. **Transdermal:** Antiemetic, antivertigo. Prevention of motion sickness.

Additional Contraindications: For transdermal therapeutic system: Children, lactating women. Ophthalmic use contraindicated in glaucoma, infants less than 3 months of age.

Special Concerns: Use with caution in children, infants, geriatric clients, diabetes, hypo- or hyperthyroidism, narrow anterior chamber angle. Use for prophylaxis of excess secretions is not recommended for children less than 4 months of age. The transdermal system is not recommended for children.

Additional Side Effects: Disorientation, delirium, increased HR, decreased respiratory rate. *Ophthalmologic:* Blurred vision, stinging, increased intraocular pressure. Long-term use may cause irritation, photophobia, conjunctivitis, hyperemia, or edema.

Dosage ────────────
• **Ophthalmic Solution**
Cycloplegia/mydriasis.
Adults: 1–2 gtt of the 0.25% solution in the conjunctiva 1 hr prior to refraction; **children:** 1 gtt of the 0.25% solution b.i.d. for 2 days prior to refraction.
Uveitis.
Adults and children: 1 gtt of the 0.25% solution in the conjunctiva 1–4 times/day, depending on the severity of the condition.
Treatment of posterior synechiae.
Adults and children: 1 gtt of the 0.25% solution q min for 5 min. (1 gtt of either a 2.5% or 10% solution of phenylephrine instilled q min for 3 min will enhance the effect of scopolamine.)
Postoperative mydriasis.
Adults: 1 gtt of the 0.25% solution once daily. For dark brown irides, administration 2 or 3 times/day may be required.
Pre- or Postoperative iridocyclitis.
Adults and children: 1 gtt of the 0.25% solution 1–4 times/day as re-

quired. The pediatric dose should be individualized based on age, weight, and severity of the inflammation.
• **Injection (IM, IV, SC)**
Anticholinergic, antiemetic.
Adults: 0.3–0.6 mg (single dose).
Pediatric: 0.006 mg/kg (0.2 mg/m²) as a single dose.
Prophylaxis of excessive salivation and respiratory tract secretions in anesthesia.
Adults: 0.2–0.6 mg 30–60 min before induction of anesthesia. **Pediatric (given IM): 8–12 years:** 0.3 mg; **3–8 years:** 0.2 mg; **7 months–3 years:** 0.15 mg; **4–7 months:** 0.1 mg. Not recommended for children less than 4 months of age.
Adjunct to anesthesia, sedative-hypnotic.
Adults: 0.6 mg t.i.d–q.i.d.
Adjunct to anesthesia, amnesia.
Adults: 0.32–0.65 mg.
• **Transdermal System**
Antiemetic, antivertigo.
Adults: 1 transdermal system placed on the postauricular skin to deliver 0.5 mg over 3 days (apply at least 4 hr before antiemetic effect is required). The Canadian product delivers 1 mg over a 3-day period; it should be applied about 12 hr before the antiemetic effect is desired.

RESPIRATORY CARE CONSIDERATIONS

See also *Respiratory Care Considerations* for *Cholinergic Blocking Agents.*
Administration/Storage:
1. Drops are instilled into the conjunctival sac followed by digital pressure for 2–3 min after instillation.
2. Scopolamine should not be administered alone for pain because it may cause delirium. Use an analgesic or sedative in this event.
3. The solution should be protected from light.
4. With the transdermal system:
• Wash hands before and after application
• Apply at least 4 hr before desired effect

• Apply to a clean, nonhairy site, behind the ear
• Use pressure to apply the patch to ensure contact with the skin
• Replace with a new system if patch becomes dislodged
• System is water-proof so bathing and swimming are permitted
• System effects last for 3 days

Assessment:
1. Document indications for therapy and type and onset of symptoms. List other agents prescribed and the outcome.
2. Assess for additional side effects and for tolerance after a long course of therapy.
3. Before administering eyedrops, check for any history of angle-closure glaucoma because the drug may precipitate an acute glaucoma crisis.
4. Observe closely during initial therapy. Some clients experience toxic delirium with therapeutic doses. Have physostigmine available to reverse drug effects.

Evaluate:
• Effective control of vomiting
• Preoperative sedation; postoperative amnesia
• Desired amount of mydriasis
• Prevention of motion sickness

Sodium bicarbonate
(**SO**-dee-um bye-**KAR**-bon-ayt)
Pregnancy Category: C
Arm and Hammer Pure Baking Soda, Bell/ans, Citrocarbonate, Neut, Soda Mint (Rx and OTC)
Classification: Alkalinizing agent, antacid, electrolyte

Action/Kinetics: The antacid action is due to neutralization of hydrochloric acid by forming sodium chloride and carbon dioxide (1 g of sodium bicarbonate neutralizes 12 mEq of acid). Provides temporary relief of peptic ulcer pain and of discomfort associated with indigestion. Although widely used by the public, sodium bicarbonate is rarely prescribed as an antacid because of its high sodium content, short duration of action, and ability to cause alkalosis (sometimes desired). Sodium bicarbonate is also a systemic and urinary alkalinizer by increasing plasma and urinary bicarbonate, respectively.

Uses: Treatment of hyperacidity, severe diarrhea (where there is loss of bicarbonate). Alkalization of the urine to treat drug toxicity (e.g., due to barbiturates, salicylates, methanol). Treatment of acute mild to moderate metabolic acidosis due to shock, severe dehydration, anoxia, uncontrolled diabetes, renal disease, cardiac arrest, extracorporeal circulation of blood, severe primary lactic acidosis. Prophylaxis of renal calculi in gout. During sulfonamide therapy to prevent renal calculi and nephrotoxicity. Neutralizing additive solution to decrease chemical phlebitis and client discomfort due to vein irritation at or near the site of infusion of IV acid solutions. *Investigational:* Sickle cell anemia.

Contraindications: Chloride loss due to vomiting or from continuous GI suction. With diuretics known to produce a hypochloremic alkalosis. Metabolic and respiratory alkalosis. Hypocalcemia in which alkalosis may cause tetany. Hypertension, convulsions, CHF, and other situations where administration of sodium can be dangerous. As a systemic alkalinizer when used as a neutralizing additive solution. Do not use as an antidote for strong mineral acids because carbon dioxide is formed, which may cause discomfort and even perforation.

Special Concerns: Use with caution in impaired renal function, in clients with oliguria or anuria, and during lactation. Also use with caution in geriatric or postoperative clients with renal or CV insufficiency with or without CHF.

Side Effects: *GI:* Acid rebound, gastric distention. *Milk-alkali syndrome:* Hypercalcemia, metabolic alkalosis (dizziness, cramps, thirst, anorexia, N&V, hyperexcitability, tetany, di-

S

minished breathing, **seizures**), renal dysfunction. *Following rapid infusion:* Hypernatremia, alkalosis, hyperirritability, tetany, fluid or solute overload. Extravasation following IV use may manifest ulceration, sloughing, cellulitis, or tissue necrosis at the site of injection.

OD **Overdose Management:** *Symptoms:* Severe alkalosis that may be accompanied by tetany or hyperirritability. *Treatment:* Discontinue sodium bicarbonate. Symptoms of alkalosis can be reversed by rebreathing expired air from a paper bag or using a rebreathing mask. An IV infusion of ammonium chloride solution, 2.14%, can be used to control severe cases. Hypokalemia may be treated by IV sodium chloride or potassium chloride. Calcium gluconate will control tetany.

Drug Interactions:
Amphetamines / ↑ Effect of amphetamines by ↑ renal tubular reabsorption
Antidepressants, tricyclic / ↑ Effect of tricyclics by ↑ renal tubular reabsorption
Benzodiazepines / ↓ Effect due to ↑ alkalinity of urine
Chlorpropamide / ↑ Rate of excretion due to alkalinization of the urine
Ephedrine / ↑ Effect of ephedrine by ↑ renal tubular reabsorption
Erythromycin / ↑ Effect of erythromycin in urine due to ↑ alkalinity of urine
Flecainide / ↑ Effect due to ↑ alkalinity of urine
Iron products / ↓ Effect due to ↑ alkalinity of urine
Ketoconazole / ↓ Effect due to ↑ alkalinity of urine
Lithium carbonate / Excretion of lithium is proportional to amount of sodium ingested. If client on sodium-free diet, may develop lithium toxicity because less lithium is excreted
Mecamylamine / ↓ Excretion due to alkalinization of the urine
Methenamine compounds / ↓ Effect of methenamine due to ↑ alkalinity of urine

Methotrexate / ↑ Renal excretion due to alkalinization of the urine
Nitrofurantoin / ↓ Effect of nitrofurantoin due to ↑ alkalinity of urine
Procainamide / ↑ Effect of procainamide due to ↓ excretion by kidney
Pseudoephedrine / ↑ Effect of pseudoephedrine due to ↑ tubular reabsorption
Quinidine / ↑ Effect of quinidine by ↑ renal tubular reabsorption
Salicylates / ↑ Rate of excretion due to alkalinization of the urine
Sulfonylureas / ↓ Effect due to ↑ alkalinity of urine
Sympathomimetics / ↓ Renal excretion due to alkalinization of the urine
Tetracyclines / ↓ Effect of tetracyclines due to ↑ excretion by kidney

Dosage ⎯⎯⎯⎯⎯⎯⎯⎯
• **Effervescent Powder**
  Antacid.
Adults: 3.9–10 g in a glass of cold water after meals. **Geriatric and pediatric, 6–12 years:** 1.9–3.9 g after meals.
• **Oral Powder**
  Antacid.
Adults: ½ teaspoon in a glass of water q 2 hr; adjust dosage as required.
  Urinary alkalinizer.
Adults: 1 teaspoon in a glass of water q 4 hr; adjust dosage as required. Dosage not established for this form for children.
• **Tablets**
  Antacid.
Adults: 0.325–2 g 1–4 times/day; pediatric, 6–12 years: 520 mg; may be repeated once after 30 min.
  Urinary alkalinizer.
Adults, initial: 4 g; then, 1–2 g q 4 hr. Pediatric: 23–230 mg/kg/day; adjust dosage as needed.
• **IV**
  Cardiac arrest.
Adults: 200–300 mEq given rapidly as a 7.5% or 8.4% solution. In emergencies, 300–500 mL of a 5% solution given as rapidly as possible without overalkalinizing the client. Infants, less than 2 years of age, initial: 1–2 mEq/kg/min given over 1–2 min;

then, 1 mEq/kg q 10 min of arrest. Do not exceed 8 mEq/kg/day.

Severe metabolic acidosis.
90–180 mEq/L (about 7.5–15 g) at a rate of 1–1.5 L during the first hour. Adjust to needs of client.

Less severe metabolic acidosis.
Add to other IV fluids. **Adults and older children:** 2–5 mEq/kg given over a 4- to 8-hr period.

Neutralizing additive solution.
One vial of neutralizing additive solution added to 1 L of commonly used parenteral solutions, including dextrose, sodium chloride, and Ringer's.

RESPIRATORY CARE CONSIDERATIONS
Administration/Storage:
1. Hypertonic solutions must be administered by trained personnel. Avoid extravasation as tissue irritation or cellulitis may result.
2. IV dose should be determined by arterial blood pH, pCO_2, and base deficit and may be given IV push in an arrest situation or may be diluted in dextrose or saline solution and administered over 4–8 hr.
3. Isotonic solutions should be administered slowly as ordered. Too-rapid administration may result in death due to cellular acidity. Therefore, check rate of flow frequently.
4. If only the 7.5% or 8.4% solution is available, it should be diluted 1:1 with 5% dextrose in water when used in infants for cardiac arrest.
5. The rate of administration in infants with cardiac arrest should not exceed 8 mEq/kg/day to guard against hypernatremia, induction of intracranial hemorrhage, and decreasing CSF pressure.
6. Have available a parenteral solution of calcium gluconate and 2.14% solution of ammonium chloride in the event of severe alkalosis or tetany.
7. Sodium bicarbonate should not be added to calcium-containing solutions, except where the compatibility has been established.
8. Norepinephrine and dobutamine are incompatible with sodium bicarbonate.

Assessment:
1. Note any history of renal impairment, CHF, or if prescribed a sodium-restricted diet.
2. Assess for evidence of edema that may indicate the inability to utilize sodium bicarbonate.
3. If the client is on low continuous or intermittent NG suctioning or is vomiting, assess for evidence of excessive loss of chloride.
4. List other medications prescribed and determine any potential interactive effects.
5. If prescribed to counteract metabolic acidosis, obtain baseline serum electrolytes and ABGs (pH, pCO_2, and HCO_3).

Interventions:
1. Record I&O. Observe the client for dry skin and mucous membranes, polydipsia, polyuria, and air hunger. These are indications of a reversal of symptoms of metabolic acidosis and need to be documented.
2. Monitor serum pH and electrolyte values to ensure that the client is not developing an alkalosis.
3. Observe acidotic clients for the relief of dyspnea and hyperpnea.
4. Report if edema develops and anticipate a change to potassium bicarbonate since the sodium content of the drug is 27%.
5. Test urine periodically with nitrazine paper to determine if the urine is becoming alkaline and adjust dosage accordingly.

Evaluate:
- Reversal of metabolic acidosis
- ↑ Urinary and serum pH
- ↓ Gastric discomfort

Sodium chloride
(**SO**-dee-um **KLOR**-eyed)
Pregnancy Category: C
Topical: Ayr Saline, HuMIST Saline Nasal, Muro-128 ✤, NaSal Saline Nasal, Ocean Mist, Otrivin Saline ✤, Salinex Nasal Mist. **Ophthalmic:** Adsorbonac Ophthalmic, AK-NaCl, Cordema ✤, Hypersal 5%, Muro-128 Ophthalmic,

S

Muroptic-5, **Parenteral:** Sodium Chloride IV Infusions (0.45%, 0.9%, 3%, 5%), Sodium Chloride Injection for Admixtures (50, 100, 625 mEq/vial), Sodium Chloride Diluent (0.9%), Concentrated Sodium Chloride Injection (14.6%, 23.4%) (parenteral is Rx; topical and ophthalmic are OTC)

Classification: Electrolyte

Action/Kinetics: Sodium is the major cation of the body's extracellular fluid. It plays a crucial role in maintaining the fluid and electrolyte balance. Excess retention of sodium results in overhydration (edema, hypervolemia), which is often treated with diuretics. Abnormally low levels of sodium result in dehydration. Normally, the plasma contains 136–145 mEq sodium/L and 98–106 mEq chloride/L. The average daily requirement of salt is approximately 5 g.

Uses: PO: Prophylaxis of heat prostration or muscle cramps, chloride deficiency due to diuresis or salt restriction, prevention or treatment of extracellular volume depletion.

Parenteral:

0.9% (Isotonic) Sodium Chloride. To restore sodium and chloride losses; to dilute or dissolve drugs for IV, IM, or SC use; flushing of IV catheters; extracellular fluid replacement; priming solution for hemodialysis; initiate and terminate blood transfusions so RBCs will not hemolyze; metabolic alkalosis when there is fluid loss and mild sodium depletion.

0.45% (Hypotonic) Sodium Chloride. Fluid replacement when fluid loss exceeds depletion of electrolytes; hyperosmolar diabetes when dextrose should not be used (need for large volume of fluid but without excess sodium ions).

3% or 5% (Hypertonic) Sodium Chloride. Hyponatremia and hypochloremia due to electrolyte losses; to dilute body water significantly following excessive fluid intake; emergency treatment of severe salt depletion.

Concentrated Sodium Chloride. Additive in parenteral therapy for clients with special needs for sodium intake.

Bacteriostatic Sodium Chloride. Used only to dilute or dissolve drugs for IM, IV, or SC injection.

Topical: Relief of inflamed, dry, or crusted nasal membranes; irrigating solution. **Ophthalmic:** Use hypertonic solutions to decrease corneal edema due to bullous keratitis; as an aid to facilitate ophthalmoscopic examination in gonioscopy, biomicroscopy, and funduscopy.

Contraindications: Congestive heart failure, severely impaired renal function, hypernatremia, fluid retention. The 3% or 5% solutions are contraindicated in elevated, normal, or only slightly depressed levels of plasma sodium and chloride. Use of bacteriostatic sodium chloride injection in newborns.

Special Concerns: Administer with caution to clients with CV, cirrhotic, or renal disease; in presence of hyperproteinemia, hypervolemia, urinary tract obstruction, and CHF; in those with concurrent edema and sodium retention and in clients receiving corticosteroids or corticotropin; and during lactation. Use with caution in geriatric or postoperative clients with renal or CV insufficiency with or without CHF.

Side Effects: Hypernatremia. Excessive sodium chloride may lead to hypopotassemia and acidosis. Fluid and solute overload leading to dilution of serum electrolyte levels, CHF, overhydration, *acute pulmonary edema* (especially in clients with CV disease or in those receiving corticosteroids or other drugs that cause sodium retention). Too rapid administration may cause local pain and venous irritation.

Postoperative intolerance of sodium chloride: Cellular dehydration, weakness, asthenia, disorientation, anorexia, nausea, oliguria, increased BUN levels, distention, deep respiration.

Symptoms due to solution or administration technique: Fever, abscess, tissue necrosis, infection at injection site, venous thrombosis or phlebitis extending from injection site, local tenderness, extravasation, hypervolemia.

Inadvertent administration of concentrated sodium chloride (i.e., without dilution) will cause sudden hypernatremia with the possibility of CV shock, extensive hemolysis, CNS problems, necrosis of the cortex of the kidneys, local tissue necrosis (if given extravascularly). **OD** **Overdose Management:** *Symptoms:* Irritation of GI mucosa, N&V, abdominal cramps, diarrhea, edema. Hypernatremia–symptoms include, irritability, restlessness, weakness, seizures, coma, tachycardia, hypertension, fluid accumulation, *pulmonary edema, respiratory arrest. Treatment:* Supportive measures, including gastric lavage, induction of vomiting, provide adequate airway and ventilation, maintain vascular volume and tissue perfusion. Magnesium sulfate given as a cathartic.

Dosage ——————————————
• **Tablets (Including Extended-Release and Enteric-Coated)**
Heat cramps/dehydration.
0.5–1 g with 8 oz water up to 10 times/day; total daily dose should not exceed 4.8 g.
• **IV**
Individualized. Daily requirements of sodium and chloride can be met by administering 1 L of 0.9% sodium chloride.
To calculate sodium deficit. Amount of sodium to be given to raise serum sodium to the desired level:
Total body water (TBW): sodium deficit (mEq) = TBW × (desired plasma Na – observed plasma Na).
• **Ophthalmic Solution 2% or 5%**
1–2 gtt in eye q 3–4 hr.
• **Ophthalmic Ointment 5%**
A small amount (approximately ¼ in.) to the inside of the affected eye(s) (i.e., by pulling down the lower eyelid) q 3–4 hr.

RESPIRATORY CARE CONSIDERATIONS
Administration/Storage:
1. Hypertonic injections of NaCl must be given slowly through a small-bore needle placed well within the lumen of a large vein (to minimize irritation). Infiltration should be avoided.
2. Concentrated NaCl injection must be diluted before use.
3. If the fluid is given using a pumping device, it should be disconnected before the container runs dry or an air embolism may occur.
4. IV catheters should be flushed before and after the medication is given using 0.9% NaCl for injection.
5. Incompatibilities may occur when mixing NaCl injection with other additives; the final product should be inspected for cloudiness or a precipitate immediately after mixing, before administration, and periodically during administration. These mixtures should not be stored.

Assessment:
Note indications for therapy and document baseline electrolytes, liver and renal function studies, and ECG.

Interventions:
1. Observe client for S&S of hypernatremia including flushed skin, elevated temperature, rough dry tongue, and edema.
2. Symptoms of hyponatremia may include N&V, muscle cramps, dry mucous membranes, increased HR, and headaches.
3. Monitor VS and I&O. Assess urine specific gravity and serum sodium levels. If the urine specific gravity is above 1.020 and serum sodium level is above 146 mEq/L, report and anticipate that the drug will be discontinued.
4. Monitor electrolyte levels and hepatic and renal function studies.
5. Note level of consciousness and periodically assess heart and lung sounds.
6. When administering IV the 0.45% NaCl is hypotonic, the 0.9% NaCl is

S

isotonic, and the 3% and 5% NaCl solutions are hypertonic.

Evaluate:

• Prophylaxis of heat prostration during exposure to high temperatures or during increased activity

• Prevention of chloride deficiency R/T excessive diuresis or salt restriction or excessive sweating

• Correction of sodium and/or chloride deficiency

Sodium polystyrene sulfonate

(**SO**-dee-um pol-ee-**STY**-reen **SUL**-fon-ayt)

Kayexalate, K-Exit ✶, PMS Sodium Polystyrene Sulfonate ✶, SPS **(Rx)**

Classification: Potassium ion exchange resin

Action/Kinetics: Sodium polystyrene sulfonate is a resin that exchanges sodium ions for potassium ions primarily in the large intestine. Thus, excess amounts of potassium (as well as calcium and magnesium) may be removed. Therapy is governed by daily monitoring of serum potassium levels. Discontinue therapy when serum potassium levels have reached 4–5 mEq/L. Clients should also be monitored for serum calcium and magnesium levels. **Onset, PO:** 2–12 hr.

Uses: Hyperkalemia.

Special Concerns: Use with caution in geriatric clients because they are more likely to develop fecal impaction. Use with caution in clients sensitive to sodium overload (e.g., in CV disease) or for those receiving digitalis preparations because the action of these agents is potentiated by hypokalemia. Effective decreases in potassium may take several hours to accomplish; other treatment (e.g., IV calcium or sodium bicarbonate or glucose and insulin) may be considered in states of severe hyperkalemia (e.g., burns, renal failure).

Side Effects: *GI:* N&V, constipation, anorexia, gastric irritation, diarrhea (rarely). Fecal impaction in geriatric clients. *Electrolyte:* Sodium retention,

hypokalemia, hypocalcemia, hypomagnesemia. *Other:* Overhydration, **pulmonary edema.**

Drug Interactions:

Aluminum hydroxide / ↑ Risk of intestinal obstruction

Calcium- or magnesium-containing antacids or laxatives / ↑ Risk of metabolic alkalosis

Dosage ———————

• **Powder for Suspension, Suspension**

Hyperkalemia.

Adults: 15 g resin suspended in 20–100 mL water or syrup (to increase palatability) 1–4 times/day. Up to 40 g/day has been used. **Pediatric:** To calculate dose, use an exchange ratio of 1 mEq potassium/g resin (usually, 1 g/kg dose).

• **Enema**

Hyperkalemia.

Adults: 30–50 g suspended in 100 mL sorbitol or 20% dextrose in water q 6 hr.

RESPIRATORY CARE CONSIDERATIONS

Administration/Storage:

1. To treat or to prevent constipation, 10–20 mL of 70% sorbitol may be given PO q 2 hr (or as necessary) to produce 1–2 watery stools each day.

2. For PO administration, give the resin suspended in water or sorbitol syrup (3–4 mL/g resin). If necessary, the resin can be administered through a NGT, either as an aqueous suspension, mixed with dextrose, or as a peanut or olive oil emulsion.

3. Rectal administration:

• First, administer a cleansing enema.

• To administer medication, insert a large-size rubber tube (e.g., French 28) into the rectum for a distance of 20 cm until it is well into the sigmoid colon and tape in place.

• Suspend resin in appropriate vehicle (see *Dosage*) at body temperature. Administer by gravity while stirring suspension.

• Flush suspension that remains in the container with 50–100 mL fluid, clamp the tube, and leave in place.

- Elevate client's hips or ask the client to assume a knee-chest position for a short time if there is back leakage.
- The enema should be kept in the colon as long as possible (3–4 hr).
- Resin is removed by colonic irrigation with 2 quarts of a *non-sodium*-containing solution warmed to body temperature. Returns are drained constantly through a Y tube.
4. Retention enemas of the resin are less effective than PO administration.
5. Use freshly prepared solutions within 24 hr. Do not heat resin.
6. Oral suspension products contain sorbitol and sodium.
7. Orders for the drug should designate the grams of powder and the percent sorbitol and volume to be used or the amount of premixed suspension. The frequency and route of administration should also be specified.
8. Avoid inhaling the powder for suspension when admixing.

Assessment:
1. Document serum potassium levels. Attempt to identify cause for increased levels.
2. Determine if the client has a history of CV disease and/or is taking any digitalis preparations.

Interventions:
1. Monitor renal function studies and the level of serum potassium, sodium, magnesium, and calcium. Observe for symptoms of electrolyte imbalance.
2. Assess clients on sodium restrictions closely; drug contains 100 mg Na/g.
3. The administration of calcium- or magnesium-containing antacids during PO administration of sodium polystyrene sulfonate may predispose the client to metabolic alkalosis. Therefore, administer antacids cautiously.
4. Monitor VS and I&O. Report any increase in urinary output or constipation.
5. Encourage clients receiving the

medication PR to retain the solution for several hours to ensure effectiveness of drug therapy.

Evaluate: Reduction of high serum potassium levels to within desired range (4.0–5.5 mEq/L)

Sotalol hydrochloride
(**SOH**-tah-lol)
Pregnancy Category: B
Betapace, Sotacor ✤ **(Rx)**
Classification: Beta-adrenergic blocking agent

See also *Beta-Adrenergic Blocking Agents*.

Action/Kinetics: Sotalol blocks both beta-1 and beta-2 adrenergic receptors and has no membrane-stabilizing activity or intrinsic sympathomimetic activity. It has both Group II and Group III antiarrhythmic properties (dose dependent). Sotalol significantly increases the refractory period of the atria, His-Purkinje fibers, and ventricles. It also prolongs the QTc and JT intervals. **t½:** 12 hr. The drug is not metabolized and is excreted unchanged in the urine.

Uses: Treatment of documented ventricular arrhythmias such as life-threatening sustained ventricular tachycardia.

Contraindications: Use in asymptomatic PVCs or supraventricular arrhythmias due to the proarrhythmic effects of sotalol. Congenital or acquired long QT syndromes. Use in clients with hypokalemia or hypomagnesemia until the imbalance is corrected, as these conditions aggravate the degree of QT prolongation and increase the risk for torsades de pointes.

Special Concerns: Clients with sustained ventricular tachycardia and a history of CHF appear to be at the highest risk for serious proarrhythmia. Dose, presence of sustained ventricular tachycardia, females, excessive prolongation of the QTc interval, and history of cardiomegaly or CHF are risk factors for torsades de pointes. Use with caution in clients with chronic bronchitis or emphysema and in those with asthma if an IV agent is required. Use with extreme caution in clients with sick sinus syndrome associated with symptomatic arrhythmias due to the increased risk of sinus bradycardia, sinus pauses, or sinus arrest. The dosage should be reduced in clients with impaired renal function. Safety and efficacy in children have not been established.

Additional Side Effects: *CV: New or worsened ventricular arrhythmias, including sustained ventricular tachycardia or ventricular fibrillation that might be fatal. Torsades de pointes.*

Dosage ⸺⸺⸺⸺⸺⸺
- **Tablets**
  Ventricular arrhythmias.
Adults, initial: 80 mg b.i.d. The dose may be increased to 240 or 320 mg/day after appropriate evaluation. **Usual:** 160–320 mg/day given in two or three divided doses. Clients with life-threatening refractory ventricular arrhythmias may require doses ranging from 480 to 640 mg/day (due to potential proarrhythmias, these doses should only be used if the potential benefit outweighs the increased risk of side effects).

RESPIRATORY CARE CONSIDERATIONS

See also *Respiratory Care Considerations* for *Beta-Adrenergic Blocking Agents.*

Administration/Storage:
1. Food decreases the absorption of sotalol; thus, the drug should be taken on an empty stomach.
2. Dosage should be adjusted gradually, allowing 2–3 days between increments in dosage. This allows steady-state plasma levels to be reached and QT intervals to be monitored.
3. Initiation of and increases in dosage should be undertaken in a hospital with facilities for cardiac rhythm monitoring and assessment. The dose for each client must be individualized only after appropriate clinical assessment.

4. Proarrhythmias can occur during initiation of therapy and with each increment in dosage.
5. In clients with impaired renal function, the dosing interval should be altered as follows: if creatinine clearance is 30–60 mL/min, the dosing interval is 24 hr; if creatinine clearance is 10–30 mL/min, the dosing interval should be 36–48 hr. The dose in clients with creatinine clearance less than 10 mL/min must be individualized. Dosage adjustments in clients with impaired renal function should only be undertaken after five to six doses at the intervals described.
6. Before initiating sotalol, previous antiarrhythmic therapy should be withdrawn with careful monitoring for a minimum of 2–3 plasma half-lives if the client's condition permits.
7. After amiodarone is discontinued, do not initiate sotalol until the QT interval is normalized.

Assessment:
1. Perform a thorough nursing history. Document any evidence of cardiomegaly or CHF.
2. Obtain baseline electrolytes, magnesium level, and liver and renal function studies.
3. List all medications used for treatment of arrhythmia and the outcome.
4. Document baseline ECG and note symptoms associated with the ventricular arrhythmia.

Interventions:
1. Client should be in a closely monitored environment with VS and ECG monitored during initiation and adjustment of sotalol.
2. Monitor VS and I&O frequently and assess serum potassium and magnesium levels.
3. Document QT interval and report any prolongation or altered cardiac rhythm.
4. Report any symptoms of CHF (increased fatigue, dyspnea, or bradycardia).

Evaluate: ECG evidence of control or conversion of life-threatening ventricular arrhythmias to a stable cardiac rhythm

Sparfoxacin
(spar–**FOX**-ih-sin)
Pregnancy Category:
Zagam **(Rx)**
Classification: Fluoroquinolone antibiotic

See also Fluoroquinolones.
Uses: Community acquired pneumonia due to *Chlamydia pneumoniae, Haemophilus influenzae, Haemophilus parainfluenzae, Moraxella catarrhalis, Mycoplasma pneumoniae,* or *Streptococcus pneumoniae.* Acute bacterial exacerbations of chronic bronchitis caused by *C. pneumoniae, Enterobacter cloacae, H. influenzae, H. parainfluenzae, Klebsiella pneumoniae, M. catarrhalis, Staphylococcus aureus,* or S. pneumoniae.
Special Concerns: Safety and efficacy have not been determined in children less than 18 years of age.

Dosage
• **Tablets**
Community-acquired pneumonia, acute bacterial exacerbations of chronic bronchitis.
Adults over 18 years of age: Two - 200 mg tablets taken on the first day as a loading dose. Then, one - 200 mg tablet q 24 hr for a total of 10 days of therapy (i.e., a total of 11 tablets). For clients with a creatinine clearance less than 50 mL/min, the loading dose is two - 200 mg tablets taken on the first day. Then, one - 200 mg tablet q 48 hr for a total of 9 days (i.e., a total of 6 tablets).

RESPIRATORY CARE CONSIDERATIONS

See also *Respiratory Care Considerations* for *Fluoroquinolones.*
Administration/Storage: The drug may be taken with or without food.
Assessment
1. Document indications for therapy, noting onset, location, duration, and characteristics of symptoms.
2. Obtain baseline CBC, cultures, and renal function studies. Antici-

pate reduced dosage with impaired renal function.
Evaluate
• Reports of symptomatic improvement
• Resolution of infective organism

Spironolactone
(speer-oh-no-**LAK**-tohn)
Aldactone, Novo-Spiroton ✦ **(Rx)**
Classification: Diuretic, potassium-sparing

See also *Diuretics, Thiazides.*
Action/Kinetics: Spironolactone is a mild diuretic that acts on the distal tubule to inhibit sodium exchange for potassium, which results in increased secretion of sodium and water and conservation of potassium. It is also an aldosterone antagonist. The drug manifests a slight antihypertensive effect. It also interferes with synthesis of testosterone and may increase formation of estradiol from testosterone, thus leading to endocrine abnormalities. **Onset:** Urine output increases over 1–2 days. **Peak:** 2–3 days. **Duration:** 2–3 days, and declines thereafter. It is metabolized to an active metabolite (canrenone). **t½:** 13–24 hr for canrenone. Canrenone is excreted through the urine (primary) and the bile. The drug is almost completely bound to plasma protein. Spironolactone is also found in Aldactazide.
Uses: Primary hyperaldosteronism, including diagnosis, short-term preoperative treatment, long-term maintenance therapy for those who are poor surgical risks and those with bilateral micronodular or macronodular adrenal hyperplasia. To treat edema when other approaches are inadequate or ineffective (e.g., CHF, cirrhosis of the liver, nephrotic syndrome). Essential hypertension (usually in combination with other drugs). Prophylaxis of hypokalemia in clients taking digitalis. *Investigational:* Hirsutism, treat symptoms of PMS, with testolactone to treat famil-

ial male precocious puberty (short-term treatment), acne vulgaris.

Contraindications: Acute renal insufficiency, progressive renal failure, hyperkalemia, and anuria. Clients receiving potassium supplements, amiloride, or triamterene.

Special Concerns: Use during pregnancy only if benefits clearly outweigh risks. Use with caution in impaired renal function. Geriatric clients may be more sensitive to the usual adult dose.

Side Effects: *Electrolyte:* Hyperkalemia, hyponatremia (characterized by lethargy, dry mouth, thirst, tiredness). *GI:* Diarrhea, cramps, ulcers, gastritis, gastric bleeding, vomiting. *CNS:* Drowsiness, ataxia, lethargy, mental confusion, headache. *Endocrine:* Gynecomastia, menstrual irregularities, impotence, bleeding in postmenopausal women, deepening of voice, hirsutism. *Dermatologic:* Maculopapular or erythematous cutaneous eruptions, urticaria. *Miscellaneous:* Drug fever, breast carcinoma, gynecomastia, hyperchloremic metabolic acidosis in hepatic cirrhosis (decompensated), **agranulocytosis.** *NOTE:* Spironolactone has been shown to be tumorigenic in chronic rodent studies.

Drug Interactions:

Anesthetics, general / Additive hypotension

ACE inhibitors / Significant hyperkalemia

Anticoagulants, oral / Inhibited by spironolactone

Antihypertensives / Potentiation of hypotensive effect of both agents. Reduce dosage, especially of ganglionic blockers, by one-half

Captopril / ↑ Risk of significant hyperkalemia

Digitalis / ↑ Half-life of digoxin → ↓ clearance. Spironolactone may ↓ inotropic effect of digoxin. Spironolactone both ↑ and ↓ elimination t½ of digitoxin

Diuretics, others / Often administered concurrently because of potassium-sparing effect of spironolactone. Severe hyponatremia may occur. Monitor closely

Lithium / ↑ Chance of lithium toxicity due to ↓ renal clearance

Norepinephrine / ↓ Responsiveness to norepinephrine

Potassium salts / Since spironolactone conserves potassium excessively, hyperkalemia may result. Rarely used together

Salicylates / Large doses may ↓ effects of spironolactone

Triamterene / Hazardous hyperkalemia may result from combination

Laboratory Test Interferences: Interference with radioimmunoassay for digoxin. False + plasma cortisol (as determined by fluorometric assay of Mattingly).

Dosage ————————————

• **Tablets**

Treat edema.

Adults, initial: 100 mg/day (range: 25–200 mg/day) in two to four divided doses for at least 5 days; **maintenance:** 75–400 mg/day in two to four divided doses. **Pediatric:** 3.3 mg/kg/day as a single dose or as two to four divided doses.

Antihypertensive.

Adults, initial: 50–100 mg/day as a single dose or as two to four divided doses—give for at least 2 weeks; **maintenance:** adjust to individual response. **Pediatric:** 1–2 mg/kg in a single dose or in two to four divided doses.

Treat hypokalemia.

Adults: 25–100 mg/day as a single dose or two to four divided doses.

Diagnosis of primary hyperaldosteronism.

Adults: 400 mg/day for either 4 days (short-test) or 3–4 weeks (long-test).

Hyperaldosteronism, prior to surgery.

Adults: 100–400 mg/day in two to four doses prior to surgery.

Hyperaldosteronism, chronic-therapy.

Use lowest possible dose.

Hirsutim.

50–200 mg/day.

Symptoms of PMS.

25 mg q.i.d. beginning on day 14 of the menstrual cycle.

Familial male precocious puberty, short-term.

Spironolactone, 2 mg/kg/day, and testolactone, 20–40 mg/kg/day, for at least 6 months.

Acne vulgaris.

100 mg/day.

RESPIRATORY CARE CONSIDERATIONS

See also *Respiratory Care Considerations* for *Diuretics, Thiazides.*

Administration/Storage:

1. When used as the sole drug to treat edema, the initial dose should continue for at least 5 days. After that, adjustments may be made. If the dosage is not effective, a second diuretic may be added, especially one that acts in the proximal tubules.

2. When administered to small children, the tablets may be crushed and given as a suspension in cherry syrup.

3. Food may increase the absorption of spironolactone.

4. Protect the drug from light.

Assessment:

1. Document indications for therapy, type and onset of symptoms, other agents prescribed, and the outcome.

2. Obtain baseline ECG, ABGs, and serum electrolyte levels prior to starting therapy. If the serum potassium level is greater than 5.5 mEq/L, withhold the medication and report.

3. If the client has a history of cardiac disease, be alert for cardiac irregularities R/T hypokalemia.

Interventions:

1. Monitor ABGs, CBC, blood sugar, uric acid, serum electrolytes, and liver and renal function studies. Compare with the baseline data and report any abnormalities.

2. If the client develops deep, rapid respirations, complains of headaches, or appears to be slower mentally, document and report as this may indicate hyperchloremic metabolic acidosis.

3. Monitor and record VS, I&O, and weights.

4. Note if the client develops dysuria, urinary frequency, or renal spasm. Request a urinalysis and urine culture and check for sensitivity.

5. Assess client for tolerance to the drug, which may be characterized by edema and reduced urine output.

6. Report if the client develops jaundice or tremors or appears mentally confused. If hepatic disease already exists, clients may develop hepatic encephalopathy. Drug is metabolized in the liver.

7. Administer the drug with a snack or meals to relieve the symptoms of gastric distress. Report if nausea, bloating, anorexia, vomiting, or diarrhea persist. The dosage of drug may need to be changed or the drug may need to be discontinued.

Evaluate:

• Enhanced diuresis with ↓ edema
• ↓ BP
• Antagonism of high levels of aldosterone
• Prevention of hypokalemia in those taking digitalis and/or other diuretics

Streptomycin sulfate

(strep-toe-**MY**-sin)

Pregnancy Category: D

(Rx)

Classification: Antibiotic, aminoglycoside

See also *Aminoglycosides.*

Action/Kinetics: Like other aminoglycoside antibiotics, streptomycin is distributed rapidly throughout most tissues and body fluids, including necrotic tubercular lesions. **Therapeutic serum levels:** 20–30 mcg/mL. **t½:** 2–3 hr. Toxic serum levels: >50 mcg/mL (peak).

Uses: With other drugs to treat *Mycobacterium tuberculosis* infections. Used in the following infections when less potentially hazardous drugs are either ineffective or contraindicated. UTIs due to *Escherichia* *coli, Proteus, Enterobacter aerogenes, Klebsiella pneumoniae,* and *Enterococcus faecalis.* With penicillin to treat endocardial infections due to *Streptoccus viridans* and *E. faecalis.* With other drugs to treat bacteremia. With another agent to treat respiratory, endocardial, and meningeal infections due to *H. influenzae.* Infections due to *Brucella, Haemophilus ducreyi* (chancroid), *Francisella tularensis* (tularemia), *Pasturella pestis* (plague), and granuloma inguinale. *Investigational:* As part of multiple-drug regimen to treat *Mycobacterium avium* complex in AIDS clients.

Additional Contraindications: Hypersensitivity, contact dermatitis, and exfoliative dermatitis. Do not give to clients with myasthenia gravis.

Special Concerns: Use during pregnancy only if benefits clearly outweigh risks.

OD **Overdose Management:** *Symptoms:* Extension of side effects. *Treatment:* Hemodialysis (preferred) or peritoneal dialysis.

Additional Laboratory Test Interference: False urine glucose determinations with Benedict's solution and Clinitest.

Dosage ⎯⎯⎯⎯⎯⎯⎯⎯
• **IM Only**
Tuberculosis (adjunct).
The usual regimen for treating drug-susceptible tuberculosis has been 2 months of isoniazid, rifampin, and pyrazinamide, followed by 4 months of isoniazid and rifampin. When streptomycin is added to the drug regimen, the following doses are recommended. **Adults:** 15 mg/kg/day (maximum of 1 g/day), 25–30 mg/kg twice weekly (maximum of 1.5 g), or 25–30 mg/kg thrice weekly (maximum of 1.5 g). The total period of drug treatment is a minimum of 1 year. **Pediatric:** 20–40 mg/kg/day (not to exceed 1 g/day), 25–30 mg/kg twice weekly (maximum of 1.5 g), or 25–30 mg/kg thrice weekly (maximum of 1.5 g). Older, debilitated clients should receive lower dosages.

Bacterial endocarditis due to penicillin-sensitive alpha-hemolytic and nonhemolytic streptococci (with penicillin).
1 g b.i.d. for 1 week; **then,** 0.5 g b.i.d. for second week.
Enterococcal endocarditis (with penicillin).
1 g b.i.d. for 2 weeks; **then,** 0.5 g b.i.d. for 4 weeks.
Plague.
1 g q 12 hr for at least 10 days.
Tularemia.
0.25–0.5 g q 6 hr for 7–10 days or until client is afebrile for 5–7 days.
Moderate to severe fulminating infections.
Adults: 1–2 g in divided doses q 6–12 hr, depending on severity of infections; **pediatric:** 20–40 mg/kg/day in divided doses q 6–12 hr.
Less severe infections.
Adults: 1–2 g/day.
Mycobacterium avium *complex in AIDS clients.*
11–13 mg/kg/day IV or 15 mg/kg/day IM used with three to five agents as part of a multiple-drug regimen.

RESPIRATORY CARE CONSIDERATIONS

See also *Respiratory Care Considerations* for *Aminoglycosides.*
Administration/Storage:
1. Protect hands when preparing drug. Wear gloves if drug is prepared often because it is irritating.
2. In a dry form, the drug is stable for at least 2 years at room temperature.
3. Aqueous solutions prepared without preservatives are stable for at least 1 week at room temperature and for at least 3 months under refrigeration.
4. Use only solutions prepared freshly from dry powder for intrathecal, subarachnoid, and intrapleural administration because commercially prepared solutions contain preservatives harmful to tissues of the CNS and pleural cavity.
5. Commercially prepared, ready-to-inject solutions are for IM use only.

These solutions are prepared with phenol and are stable at room temperature for prolonged periods of time.

6. When injection into the subarachnoid space is required for treatment of meningitis, only solutions made freshly from the dry powder should be used. Commercial solutions may contain preservatives toxic to the CNS.

7. Administer deep into muscle mass to minimize pain and local irritation.

8. Solutions may darken after exposure to light, but this does not necessarily cause a loss in potency. Check with pharmacist if unsure of potency.

Assessment:

1. Document indications for therapy, onset of symptoms, and any other agents used previously.

2. Ensure that appropriate lab studies, culture specimens, PPD skin testing, and CXR have been performed.

3. Determine if pregnant; drug may cause deafness in newborn.

Evaluate:

• Laboratory evidence of negative culture reports

• Resolution of infection and reports of symptomatic improvement

• Therapeutic serum drug levels (20–30 mcg/mL)

Succinylcholine chloride

(suck-sin-ill-**KOH**-leen)

Pregnancy Category: C

Anectine, Anectine Flo-Pack, Quelicin, Succinylcholine Chloride Min-I-Mix **(Rx)**

Classification: Depolarizing neuromuscular blocking agent

See also *Neuromuscular Blocking Agents.*

Action/Kinetics: Succinylcholine, an ultrashort-acting drug, initially excites skeletal muscle by combining with cholinergic receptors preferentially to acetylcholine. Subsequently, it prevents the muscle from contracting by prolonging the time during which the receptors at the neuromuscular junction cannot re-

spond to acetylcholine. The order of paralysis is levator muscles of the eyelid, mastication muscles, limb muscles, abdominal muscles, glottis muscles, the intercostals, the diaphragm, and all other skeletal muscles. Prolonged use may change from a depolarizing neuromuscular block (phase I block) to a block that resembles a nondepolarizing block (phase II block). This may be associated with prolonged respiratory depression and apnea. It has no effect on pain threshold, cerebration, or consciousness; thus, it should be used with sufficient anesthesia. Effects are not blocked by anticholinesterase drugs and may even be enhanced by them. Succinylcholine may cause a change in myocardial rhythm due to vagal stimulation due to surgical procedures (especially in children) and from potassium-mediated alterations in electrical conductivity (enhanced by cyclopropane and halogenated anesthetics). **IV: onset,** 30–60 sec; **duration:** 4–6 min; **recovery:** 8–10 min. **IM: Onset,** 2–3 min; **duration:** 10–30 min. Metabolized by plasma pseudocholinesterase to succinylmonocholine, which is a nondepolarizing muscle relaxant, and then to succinic acid and choline. About 10% succinylcholine is excreted unchanged in the urine.

Uses: Adjunct to general anesthesia to facilitate ET intubation and to induce relaxation of skeletal muscle during surgery or mechanical ventilation. *Investigational:* Reduce intensity of electrically induced seizures or seizures due to drugs.

Succinylcholine should be used only when facilities for ET intubation, artificial respiration, and oxygen administration are available immediately.

Contraindications: Use in those with genetically determined disorders of plasma pseudocholinesterase. Personal or family history of malignant hyperthermia. Myopathies associated with elevated CPK values.

---

bold italic = life threatening side effect

Acute narrow-angle glaucoma or penetrating eye injuries.

Special Concerns: Use with caution during lactation. Pediatric clients may be especially prone to myoglobinemia, myoglobinuria, and cardiac effects. Use of IV infusion is not recommended in children due to the risk of malignant hyperpyrexia. Use with caution in clients with severe liver disease, severe anemia, malnutrition, impaired cholinesterase activity, fractures. Also, use with caution in CV, pulmonary, renal, or metabolic diseases. Use with great caution in those with severe burns, electrolyte imbalance, hyperkalemia, those receiving quinidine, and those who are digitalized or recovering from severe trauma, as serious cardiac arrhythmias or cardiac arrest may result. Clients with myasthenia gravis may show resistance to succinylcholine. Those with fractures or muscle spasms may manifest additional trauma due to succinylcholine-induced muscle fasciculations.

Side Effects: *Skeletal muscle:* May cause **severe, persistent respiratory depression or apnea.** Muscle fasciculations, postoperative muscle pain. *CV:* Bradycardia or tachycardia, hypertension, hypotension, **arrhythmias, cardiac arrest.** *Respiratory:* **Apnea, respiratory depression.** *Other:* Fever, salivation, hyperkalemia, postoperative muscle pain, **anaphylaxis,** myoglobinemia, myoglobinuria, skin rashes, increased intraocular pressure, muscle fasciculation, myalgia, jaw rigidity, perioperative dreams in children, rhabdomyolysis with possible myoglobinuric acute renal failure. Repeated doses may cause tachyphylaxis.

Malignant hyperthermia: Muscle rigidity (especially of the jaw), tachycardia, tachypnea unresponsive to increased depth of anesthesia, increased oxygen requirement and carbon dioxide production, increased body temperature, metabolic acidosis.

OD **Overdose Management:** *Symptoms:* Skeletal muscle weakness, decreased respiratory reserve, low tidal volume, apnea. *Treatment:* Maintain a patent airway and respiratory support until normal respiration is ensured.

Drug Interactions:

Aminoglycoside antibiotics / Additive skeletal muscle blockade

Amphotericin B / ↑ Effect of succinylcholine due to induced electrolyte imbalance

Antibiotics, nonpenicillin / Additive skeletal muscle blockade

Beta-adrenergic blocking agents / Additive skeletal muscle blockade

Chloroquine / Additive skeletal muscle blockade

Cimetidine / Cimetidine inhibits pseudocholinesterase

Clindamycin / Additive skeletal muscle blockade

Cyclophosphamide / ↑ Effect of succinylcholine by ↓ breakdown of drug in plasma by pseudocholinesterase

Cyclopropane / ↑ Risk of bradycardia, arrhythmias, sinus arrest, apnea, and malignant hyperthermia

Diazepam / ↓ Effect of succinylcholine

Digitalis glycosides / ↑ Chance of cardiac arrhythmias, including ventricular fibrillation

Echothiophate iodide / ↑ Effect of succinylcholine by ↓ breakdown of drug in plasma by pseudocholinesterase

Furosemide / ↑ Skeletal muscle blockade

Halothane / ↑ Risk of bradycardia, arrhythmias, sinus arrest, apnea, and malignant hyperthermia

Isoflurane / Additive skeletal muscle blockade

Lidocaine / Additive skeletal muscle blockade

Lincomycin / Additive skeletal muscle blockade

Lithium carbonate / ↑ Skeletal muscle blockade

Magnesium salts / Additive skeletal muscle blockade

Narcotics / ↑ Risk of bradycardia and sinus arrest

Nitrous oxide / ↑ Risk of bradycardia, arrhythmias, sinus arrest, apnea, and malignant hyperthermia

Oxytocin / ↑ Effect of succinylcholine

Phenelzine / ↑ Effect of succinylcholine

Phenothiazines / ↑ Effect of succinylcholine

Polymyxin / Additive skeletal muscle blockade

Procainamide / ↑ Effect of succinylcholine

Procaine / ↑ Effect of succinylcholine by inhibiting plasma pseudocholinesterase activity

Promazine / ↑ Effect of succinylcholine

Quinidine / Additive skeletal muscle blockade

Quinine / Additive skeletal muscle blockade

Tacrine / ↑ Effect of succinylcholine

Thiazide diuretics / ↑ Effect of succinylcholine due to induced electrolyte imbalance

Thiotepa / ↑ Effect of succinylcholine by ↓ breakdown of drug in plasma by pseudocholinesterase

Trimethaphan / ↑ Effect of succinylcholine by inhibiting plasma pseudocholinesterase activity

Dosage
• **IM, IV**
Short or prolonged surgical procedures.
Adults, IV, initial: 0.3–1.1 mg/kg (average: 0.6 mg/kg); **then,** repeated doses can be given based on client response. **Adults, IM:** 3–4 mg/kg, not to exceed a total dose of 150 mg.
• **IV Infusion (Preferred)**
Prolonged surgical procedures.
Adults: Average rate ranges from 2.5 to 4.3 mg/min. Most commonly used are 0.1%–0.2% solutions in 5% dextrose, sodium chloride injection, or other diluent given at a rate of 0.5–10 mg/min depending on client response and degree of relaxation desired, for up to 1 hr.
• **Intermittent IV**
Prolonged muscle relaxation.
Initial: 0.3–1.1 mg/kg; **then,** 0.04–0.07 mg/kg at appropriate

intervals to maintain required level of relaxation.
• **IM, IV**
Electroshock therapy.
Adults, IV: 10–30 mg given 1 min prior to the shock (individualize dosage). **IM:** Up to 2.5 mg/kg, not to exceed a total dose of 150 mg.
ET intubation.
Pediatric, IV: 1–2 mg/kg; if necessary, dose can be repeated. **IM:** 3–4 mg/kg, not to exceed a total dose of 150 mg.

RESPIRATORY CARE CONSIDERATIONS

See also *Respiratory Care Considerations* for *Neuromuscular Blocking Agents.*
Administration/Storage:
1. An initial test dose of 0.1 mg/kg should be given to assess sensitivity and recovery time.
2. Review the drugs with which succinylcholine interacts.
3. Do not mix with anesthetic.
4. For IV infusion, use 1 or 2 mg/mL solution of drug in 5% dextrose injection, 0.9% sodium chloride, or other suitable IV solution. Succinylcholine is not compatible with alkaline solutions.
5. Alter the degree of relaxation by altering the rate of flow.
6. To reduce salivation, premedication with atropine or scopolamine is recommended.
7. A low dose of a nondepolarizing agent (such as tubocurarine) may be given to reduce the severity of muscle fasciculations.
8. Store the drug in the refrigerator at 2°C–8°C (36°F–46°F). Multidose vials are stable for 14 days or less at room temperature without significant loss of potency.
9. Have neostigmine or pyridostigmine available to reverse neuromuscular blockade.
Assessment:
1. List agents currently prescribed to ensure that none interact unfavorably. Note if the client is taking digitalis products or quinidine. These

clients are sensitive to the release of intracellular potassium.

2. Obtain baseline lab studies and VS. Assess clients with low plasma pseudocholinesterase levels. They are sensitive to the effects of succinylcholine and require lower doses.

3. Document any evidence of a history of MS, malignant hyperthermia, CPK myopathy, acute glaucoma, or eye injury, as drug is generally contraindicated.

Interventions:

1. A peripheral nerve stimulator should be used to assess the client's neuromuscular response and recovery. The order of paralysis is levator muscles of the eyelid, mastication muscles, limb muscles, abdominal muscles, glottis muscles, the intercostals, the diaphragm, and all other skeletal muscles. This is reversed with recovery.

2. Monitor VS and ECG. Succinylcholine can cause vagal stimulation resulting in bradycardia, hypotension, and cardiac arrhythmias, especially in children.

3. Observe for excessive, transient increase in intraocular pressure. Document and report as this can be dangerous to the eye.

4. Muscle fasciculations may cause the client to be sore and injured after recovery. Administer prescribed nondepolarizing agent (i.e., tubocurarine) and reassure that the soreness is likely caused by the unsynchronized contractions of adjacent muscle fibers just before the onset of paralysis.

5. Monitor closely for any evidence of malignant hyperthermia, unresponsive tachycardia, jaw spasm, or lack of laryngeal relaxation. Stop infusion and report. Temperature elevations are a late sign of this condition.

6. Document the length of time the client is taking the drug. It should be used only on a short-term basis and in a continuously monitored environment. Prolonged use may change from a depolarizing neuromuscular block (phase I block) to a block that resembles a nondepolarizing block (phase II block). This may be associated with prolonged respiratory depression and apnea.

7. Remember that client is fully conscious and aware of surroundings and conversations.

8. Drug does not affect pain or anxiety so administer analgesics and antianxiety agents as indicated.

9. When used for seizures, ensure that serum level of anticonvulsant agent is therapeutic, as succinylcholine does not cross the blood-brain barrier and will only suppress peripheral manifestations of seizures, not the central process.

Evaluate:
• Desired level of muscle relaxation/paralysis
• Suppression of the twitch response when tested with a peripheral nerve stimulator
• Facilitation of ET intubation and control of breathing during mechanical ventilation

Sufentanil

(soo-**FEN**-tah-nil)
Pregnancy Category: C
Sufenta **(Rx)**
Classification: Narcotic analgesic

See also *Narcotic Analgesics.*

Action/Kinetics: Onset, IV: 1.3–3 min. **Anesthetic blood concentration:** 8–30 mcg/kg. **t½:** 2.5 hr. Allows appropriate oxygenation of the heart and brain during prolonged surgical procedures. May be used in children.

Uses: Narcotic analgesic used as an adjunct to maintain balanced general anesthesia. To induce and maintain general anesthesia (with 100% oxygen), especially in neurosurgery or CV surgery.

Additional   Contraindications: Use during labor.

Special Concerns: Dosage must be decreased in the obese, elderly, or debilitated client.

Additional Side Effects: Erythema, chills, intraoperative muscle movement. *Extended postoperative respiratory depression.*

Dosage

- **IV**

Analgesia.

Adults, individualized, usual initial: 1–2 mcg/kg with oxygen and nitrous oxide; **maintenance:** 10–25 mcg as required.

For complicated surgery.

Adults: 2–8 mcg/kg with oxygen and nitrous oxide; **maintenance:** 10–50 mcg.

To induce and maintain general anesthesia.

Adults: 8–30 mcg/kg with 100% oxygen and a muscle relaxant; **maintenance:** 25–50 mcg. **Pediatric, less than 12 years:** 10–25 mcg/kg with 100% oxygen; **maintenance:** 25–50 mcg.

Induction and maintenance of general anesthesia in children less than 12 years of age undergoing CV surgery.

Initial: 10–25 mcg/kg with 100% oxygen; **maintenance:** 25–50 mcg.

RESPIRATORY CARE CONSIDERATIONS

See also *Respiratory Care Considerations* for *Narcotic Analgesics.*

Administration/Storage:

1. Dose should be reduced in the debilitated or elderly client.
2. The dose should be calculated based on lean body weight.

Evaluate: Desired level of analgesia

Sulfamethoxazole
(sul-fah-meth-**OX**-ah-zohl)

Pregnancy Category: C

Apo-Sulfamethoxazole ✚, Gantanol, Urobak **(Rx)**

Classification: Sulfonamide, intermediate-acting

See also *Sulfonamides.*

Action/Kinetics: t½: 8.6 hr. Sulfamethoxazole is also a component of Bactrim, Bactrim DS, Septra, and Septra DS.

Uses: Urinary and upper respiratory tract infections; lymphogranuloma venereum.

Special Concerns: May be an increased risk of severe side effects in elderly clients.

Dosage

- **Tablets**

Mild to moderate infections.

Adults, initially: 2 g; **then,** 1 g in morning and evening.

Severe infections.

Adults, initially: 2 g; **then,** 1 g t.i.d. **Infants over 2 months, initial:** 50–60 mg/kg; **then,** 25–30 mg/kg in morning and evening, not to exceed 75 mg/kg/day.

Lymphogranuloma venereum.

1 g b.i.d. for 2 weeks.

RESPIRATORY CARE CONSIDERATIONS

See also *General Respiratory Care Considerations for All Anti-Infectives.*

Evaluate:

- Resolution of infection
- Reports of symptomatic improvement

T

Terazosin
(ter-**AY**-zoh-sin)

Pregnancy Category: C

Hytrin **(Rx)**

Classification: Antihypertensive, alpha-1-adrenergic receptor blocking agent

Action/Kinetics: Terazosin blocks postsynaptic alpha-1-adrenergic receptors, leading to a dilation of both arterioles and veins, and ultimately, a reduction in BP. Both standing and supine BPs are lowered with no reflex tachycardia. The drug also relaxes smooth muscle of the prostate and bladder neck. Its usefulness in benign prostatic hypertrophy is due to alpha-1 receptor blockade, which relaxes the smooth muscle of the prostate and bladder neck and relieves pressure on the urethra. Bioavailability is not affected by food. **Onset:** 15 min. **Peak plasma levels:** 1–2 hr. t½: 9–12 hr. **Duration:** 24 hr. Terazosin is excreted as unchanged drug and inactive metabolites in both the urine and feces.

Uses: Alone or in combination with diuretics or beta-adrenergic blocking agents to treat hypertension. Treat symptoms of benign prostatic hyperplasia.

Special Concerns: Use with caution during lactation. Safety and efficacy have not been determined in children. Geriatric clients may be more sensitive to the hypotensive and hypothermic effects of terazosin.

Side Effects: *First-dose effect:* Marked postural hypotension and syncope. *CV:* Palpitations, tachycardia, postural hypotension, syncope, *arrhythmias,* chest pain, vasodilation. *CNS:* Dizziness, headache, somnolence, drowsiness, nervousness, paresthesia, depression, anxiety, insomnia, vertigo. *Respiratory:* Nasal congestion, dyspnea, sinusitis, epistaxis, bronchitis, *bronchospasm,* cold or flu symptoms, increased cough, pharyngitis, rhinitis. *GI:* Nausea, constipation, diarrhea, dyspepsia, dry mouth, vomiting, flatulence, abdominal discomfort or pain. *Musculoskeletal:* Asthenia, arthritis, arthralgia, myalgia, joint disorders, back pain, pain in extremities, neck and shoulder pain, muscle cramps. *Miscellaneous:* Peripheral edema, weight gain, blurred vision, impotence, chest pain, fever, gout, pruritus, rash, sweating, urinary frequency, UTI, tinnitus, conjunctivitis, abnormal vision, edema, facial edema.

OD **Overdose Management:** *Symptoms:* Hypotension, drowsiness, shock. *Treatment:* Restore BP and HR. Client should be kept supine; vasopressors may be indicated.

Volume expanders can be used to treat shock.
Laboratory Test Interferences: ↓ H&H, WBCs, albumin.

Dosage ⸺
• **Capsules**
Hypertension.
Individualized, initial: 1 mg at bedtime (this dose is not to be exceeded); **then,** increase dose slowly to obtain desired response. **Range:** 1–5 mg/day; doses as high as 20 mg may be required in some clients.
Benign prostatic hyperplasia.
Initial: 1 mg/day; dose should be increased to 2 mg, 5 mg, and then 10 mg once daily to improve symptoms and/or urinary flow rates.

RESPIRATORY CARE CONSIDERATIONS

See also *Respiratory Care Considerations* for *Antihypertensive Agents.*
Administration/Storage:
1. The initial dosing regimen must be carefully observed to minimize severe hypotension.
2. Monitor BP 2–3 hr after dosing as well as at the end of the dosing interval to ensure BP control has been maintained.
3. An increase in dose or b.i.d. dosing should be considered if BP control is not maintained at 24-hr interval.
4. To prevent dizziness or fainting due to a drop in BP, the initial dose should be taken at bedtime; the daily dose can be given in the morning.
5. If terazosin must be discontinued for more than a few days, the initial dosing regimen should be used if therapy is reinstituted.
6. Due to additive effects, caution must be exercised when terazosin is combined with other antihypertensive agents.
7. When treating BPH, a minimum of 4–6 weeks of 10 mg/day may be needed to determine if a beneficial effect has occurred.
Assessment
1. Document indications for therapy, noting onset, duration, and characteristics of symptoms.

2. Assess prostate gland, PSA level, and BPH score.

Interventions: A gradual increase in dose, i.e., 1 mg q day for 7 days, then 2 mg/day for 7 days, then 3 mg/day for 7 days, then 4 mg/day for 7 days, and then 5 mg /day, may assist to diminish adverse drug effects and client nonadherence, especially in the elderly.

Evaluate:
* Control of BP with hypertension
* Reports of improvement in symptoms R/T prostate enlargement

---

Terbutaline sulfate

(ter-**BYOU**-tah-leen)
Pregnancy Category: B
Brethaire, Brethine, Bricanyl **(Rx)**
Classification: Sympathomimetic, direct-acting; bronchodilator

---

See also *Sympathomimetic Drugs.*

Action/Kinetics: Terbutaline is specific for stimulating beta-2 receptors, resulting in bronchodilation and relaxation of peripheral vasculature. Minimum beta-1 activity. Drug action resembles that of isoproterenol. **PO: Onset:** 30 min; **maximum effect:** 2–3 hr; **duration:** 4–8 hr. **SC: Onset,** 5–15 min; **maximum effect:** 30 min–1 hr; **duration:** 1.5–4 hr. **Inhalation: Onset,** 5–30 min; **time to peak effect:** 1–2 hr; **duration:** 3–6 hr.

Uses: Bronchodilator in asthma, bronchitis, emphysema, bronchiectasis, pulmonary obstructive disease, and other conditions associated with reversible bronchospasms. *Investigational:* Inhibit premature labor.

Contraindications: Lactation.

Special Concerns: Safe use in children less than 12 years of age not established.

Additional Side Effects: *CV:* PVCs, ECG changes (e.g., atrial premature beats, AV block, sinus pause, ST-T wave depression, T-wave inversion, sinus bradycardia, atrial escape beat with aberrant conduction), tachycardia. *Respiratory:* Wheezing. *Miscellaneous:* Hypersensitivity reactions (including vasculitis), flushing, sweating, bad taste or taste change, muscle cramps, CNS stimulation, pain at injection site.

Laboratory Test Interferences: ↑ Liver enzymes.

Dosage ————————
* **Tablets**
  Bronchodilation.
  Adults and children over 15 years: 5 mg t.i.d. q 6 hr during waking hours, not to exceed 15 mg q 24 hr. If disturbing side effects are observed, dose can be reduced to 2.5 mg t.i.d. without loss of beneficial effects. Anticipate use of other therapeutic measures if client fails to respond after second dose. **Children 12–15 years:** 2.5 mg t.i.d., not to exceed 7.5 mg q 24 hr.
  Premature labor.
  2.5 mg q 4–6 hr until term.
* **SC**
  Bronchodilation.
  Adults: 0.25 mg. May be repeated 1 time after 15–30 min if no significant clinical improvement is noted. If client does not respond to the second dose, other measures should be undertaken. Dose should not exceed 0.5 mg over 4 hr.
* **IV Infusion**
  Premature labor.
  10 mcg/min initially; **then,** increase rate by 0.005 mg/min q 10 min until contractions cease or a maximum dose of 80 mcg/min is reached. The minimum effective dose should be continued for 4–8 hr after contractions cease. Terbutaline may also be given SC for preterm labor.
* **Metered Dose Inhaler**
  Bronchodilation.
  Adults and children over 12 years: 0.2–0.5 mg (1–2 inhalations) q 4–6 hr. Inhalations should be separated by 60-sec intervals. Dosage may be repeated q 4–6 hr.

RESPIRATORY CARE CONSIDERATIONS

See also *Respiratory Care Considerations* for *Sympathomimetic Drugs.*

Assessment:

1. Document indications for therapy, noting type, onset, duration, and characteristics of symptoms.

2. Auscultate and document baseline lung assessments with lung disorders and pulmonary function tests.

3. Document onset, frequency, and duration of contractions and fetal HR with preterm labor.

Interventions:

1. Observe respiratory client for evidence of drug tolerance and rebound bronchospasm.

2. Observe mother for evidence of headache, tremor, anxiety, palpitations, symptoms of pulmonary edema, and tachycardia. Monitor fetus for distress and report any increase in contractions.

3. Monitor mother and neonate for symptoms of hypoglycemia and mother for hypokalemia.

Client/Family Teaching:

1. Take oral medication with meals to minimize GI upset.

2. Report any persistent or bothersome side effects. The drug dose and administration times may need to be adjusted.

3. Do not increase dose or frequency if symptoms are not relieved. Report so dose can be reevaluated.

4. Advise to increase fluid intake to help liquefy secretions.

5. In clients with preterm labor, advise to notify provider immediately if labor resumes or unusual side effects are noted.

Evaluate:

• Improved pulmonary function

• Inhibition of premature labor

Terfenadine

(ter-**FEN**-ah-deen)
Pregnancy Category: C
Apo-Terfenadine ✦, Novo-Terfenadine ✦, Seldane **(Rx)**
Classification: Antihistamine, piperidine type

See also *Antihistamines*.

Action/Kinetics: Is said to manifest significantly less drowsiness and anticholinergic effects than other antihistamines. **Onset:** 1–2 hr; **peak effect:** 3–4 hr; **peak plasma levels:** 2 hr. **t½:** About 20 hr. **Duration:** Over 12 hr. Metabolized in the liver and excreted in the urine and feces.

Additional Use: *Investigational:* Histamine-induced bronchoconstriction in asthmatics; exercise and hyperventilation-induced bronchospasm.

Contraindications: Significant hepatic dysfunction. Use with drugs that prolong the QT interval, such as disopyramide, procainamide, quinidine, most antidepressants, and most neuroleptics. Consumption of grapefruit juice.

Special Concerns: Safety and efficacy in children less than 12 years of age have not been established. Hepatic insufficiency and any drug or food (e.g., grapefruit juice) that blocks the metabolism of terfenadine may cause serious CV effects (see *Side Effects* that follow).

Additional Side Effects: *Doses of 360 mg or more may cause serious CV effects, including death, cardiac arrest, torsades de pointes, and other ventricular arrhythmias (including QT interval prolongation).* Syncope may precede severe arrhythmias.

Drug Interactions:

Azole antifungal drugs / ↑ Risk of serious CV effects, including death, cardiac arrest, torsades de pointes, and other ventricular arrhythmias

Clarithromycin / ↑ Risk of serious CV effects, including death, cardiac arrest, torsades de pointes, and other ventricular arrhythmias

Diltiazem / Potential for ↑ risk of serious CV effects, including death, cardiac arrest, torsades de pointes, and other ventricular arrhythmias

Erythromycins / ↑ Risk of serious CV effects, including death, cardiac arrest, torsades de pointes, and other ventricular arrhythmias

Itraconazole / ↑ Risk of serious CV effects, including death, cardiac arrest, torsades de pointes, and other ventricular arrhythmias

Ketoconazole / ↑ Risk of serious CV effects, including death, cardiac ar-

rest, torsades de pointes, and other ventricular arrhythmias
Macrolide antibiotics / ↑ Risk of serious CV effects, including death, cardiac arrest, torsades de pointes, and other ventricular arrhythmias
Troleandomycin / ↑ Risk of serious CV effects, including death, cardiac arrest, torsades de pointes, and other ventricular arrhythmias

Dosage ⎯⎯⎯⎯⎯⎯⎯
• **Tablets**
Adults and children over 12 years: 60 mg q 12 hr as needed. **Children, 6 to 12 years of age:** 30–60 mg b.i.d.; **children, 3 to 6 years of age:** 15 mg b.i.d.

RESPIRATORY CARE CONSIDERATIONS

See also *Respiratory Care Considerations* for *Antihistamines*.
Administration/Storage: Clients should be advised not to consume grapefruit juice when taking terfenadine.
Assessment:
1. Document indications for therapy, noting onset, duration, and characteristics of symptoms.
2. List any other agents prescribed and the outcome. Note agents that should be avoided during this drug therapy.
3. Describe pulmonary and ENT assessment findings and note any sinus pressure.
Client/Family Teaching:
1. May take with food or milk to minimize GI upset. Do not consume grapefruit juice.
2. *Do not* exceed prescribed dosage or take with clarithomycin, macrolide antibiotics, azole antifungals, diltiazem, or troleandomycin because of the increased the risk of side effects, especially lethal arrhythmias. Review drug information or check with pharmacist and provider for any newly added adverse effects or contraindications.
3. Advise that with the H_1 antagonists, clinical effectiveness of one

group may diminish with continuous use. Changing to another group may restore drug effectiveness.
Evaluate: Improved airway exchange and relief of allergic manifestations

Tetracycline
(teh-trah-**SYE**-kleen)
Pregnancy Category: D
Achromycin Ophthalmic Ointment, Achromycin Ophthalmic Suspension, Actisite Periodontal Fiber **(Rx)**

Tetracycline hydrochloride
(teh-trah-**SYE** -kleen)
Pregnancy Category: D (topical solution is B)
Achromycin Topical Ointment, Achromycin V, Apo-Tetra ✸, Jaa Tetra ✸, Medicycline ✸, Nor-Tet, Novo-Tetra ✸, Nu-Tetra ✸, Panmycin, Robitet, Robicaps, Sumycin 250 and 500, Sumycin Syrup, Teline, Teline-500, Tetracap, Tetracyn ✸, Tetralan-250 and -500, Tetralan Syrup, Topicycline Topical Solution **(Rx)**
Classification: Antibiotic, tetracycline

See also *General Information* on *Tetracyclines*.
Action/Kinetics: t½: 7–11 hr. From 40% to 70% excreted unchanged in urine; 65% bound to serum proteins. Dosage is always expressed as the hydrochloride salt.
Additional   Use: Ophthalmic: Superficial ophthalmic infections due to *Staphylococcus aureus, Streptococcus, Streptococcus pneumoniae, Escherichia coli, Neisseria,* and *Bacteroides.* Prophylaxis of *Neisseria gonorrhoeae* in newborns. With oral therapy for treatment of *Chlamydia trachomatis.* **Topical:** Acne vulgaris, prophylaxis or treatment of infection following skin abrasions, minor cuts, wounds, or burns. **Tetracycline fiber:** Adult periodontitis. *Investigational:* Pleural sclerosing agent in malignant pleural effusions (administered by chest tube); in combination with gentamicin for *Vibrio vulnificus*

infections due to wound infection after trauma or by eating contaminated seafood. Mouthwash (use suspension) to treat nonspecific mouth ulcerations, canker sores, aphthous ulcers. Possible drug of choice for stage I Lyme disease.

Contraindications: The topical ointment should not be used in or around the eyes. Ophthalmic products should not be used to treat fungal diseases of the eye, dendritic keratitis, vaccinia, varicella, mycobacterial eye infections, or following removal of a corneal foreign body.

Special Concerns: The tetracycline fiber should be used with caution in clients with a history of oral candidiasis. Use of the fiber in chronic abscesses has not been evaluated. Safety and efficacy of the fiber have not been determined in children.

Additional Side Effects: Temporary blurring of vision or stinging following administration. Dermatitis and photosensitivity following ophthalmic use. *Use of the tetracycline fiber:* Oral candidiasis, glossitis, staining of the tongue, severe gingival hyperplasia, minor throat irritation, pain following placement in an abscessed area, throbbing pain, hypersensitivity reactions.

Dosage ————————————
• **Capsules, Syrup, Tablets**
   Mild to moderate infections.
Adults, usual: 500 mg b.i.d. or 250 mg q.i.d.
   Severe infections.
Adult: 500 mg q.i.d. **Children over 8 years:** 25–50 mg/kg/day in four equal doses.
   Brucellosis.
500 mg q.i.d. for 3 weeks with 1 g streptomycin IM b.i.d. for first week and once daily the second week.
   Syphilis.
Total of 30–40 g over 10–15 days.
   Gonorrhea.
Initially, 1.5 g; **then,** 500 mg q 6 hr until 9 g has been given.
   Gonorrhea sensitive to penicillin.
Initially, 1.5 g; **then,** 500 mg q 6 hr for 4 days (total: 9 g).
   GU or rectal Chlamydia trachomatis infections.

500 mg q.i.d. for minimum of 7 days.
   Severe acne.
Initially, 1 g/day; **then,** 125500 mg/day (long-term).
NOTE: The Centers for Disease Control have established treatment schedules for STDs.
Initially, 1 g/day; **then,** 125–500 mg/day (long-term).
• **Topical**
   Acne.
Apply topical solution to affected areas in the morning and at night, making sure that skin is completely wet after each application.
   Infections.
Apply OTC ointment (3%) to affected areas 1–4 times/day. A sterile bandage may be used.
• **Tetracycline Fiber**
   Adult periodontitis.
The fiber should be placed into the periodontal pocket until the pocket is filled (amount of fiber will vary with pocket depth and contour) ensuring that the fiber is in contact with the base of the pocket. The fiber should remain in place for 10 days, after which it is to be removed. The effectiveness of subsequent therapy with the fiber has not been assessed.

RESPIRATORY CARE CONSIDERATIONS

See also *Respiratory Care Considerations* for *Tetracyclines* and *General Respiratory Care Considerations for All Anti-Infectives.*

Administration/Storage:

1. To reconstitute solutions for IV use, vials containing 250 or 500 mg should be diluted with 5 or 10 mL, respectively, of sterile water for injection. Further dilution (100–1,000 mL) can be done with sodium chloride injection, 5% dextrose injection, 5% dextrose and sodium chloride, Ringer's injection, and lactated Ringer's injection.

2. Except for Ringer's and lactated Ringer's injections, calcium-containing solutions should not be used to dilute tetracycline HCl.

3. For IM administration, inject into a large muscle mass.

4. The tetracycline fiber product consists of a monofilament of ethylene/vinyl acetate copolymer evenly dispersed with tetracycline. The fiber provides for continuous release of tetracycline for 10 days. The fiber releases about 2 mcg/cm/hr of tetracycline.

5. Clients should avoid actions that may dislodge the fiber; i.e., they should not chew hard, crusty, or sticky foods; should not brush or floss near any treated areas; should not engage in hygienic practices that might dislodge the fiber; should not probe the treated area with tongue or fingers.

6. The dentist should be contacted immediately if the fiber is dislodged or falls out before the next scheduled visit or if pain or swelling occur.

Assessment:

1. Document indications for therapy and type, onset, characteristics, and duration of symptoms. Note any other agents or treatments prescribed.

2. Determine that appropriate cultures and/or diagnostic studies have been performed prior to starting therapy.

3. With long-term therapy, obtain baseline CBC and liver and renal function studies and monitor periodically.

Evaluate:

• Resolution of infection and reports of symptomatic improvement

• Evidence of ↓ acne lesions

• Radiologic evidence of resolution of effusion with desired pleural sclerosing

Theophylline

(thee-**OFF**-ih-lin)

Pregnancy Category: C

Immediate-release Capsules, Tablets, **Liquid Products:** Accurbron, Aquaphyllin, Asmalix, Bronkodyl, Elixomin, Elixophyllin, Lanophyllin, Lixolin, Pulmophylline ✿, Quibron-T/SR ✿, Quibron-T Dividose, Slo-Phyllin, Solu-Phyllin, Somnophyllin-T, Theo, Theoclear-80, Theolair, Theolixin ✿, Theomar, Theostat-80, Truxophyllin. **Timed-release Capsules and Tablets:**

Aerolate III, Aerolate Jr., Aerolate Sr., Apo-Theo LA ✿, Quibron-T/SR Dividose, Respid, Slo-Bid Gyrocaps, Slo-Phyllin Gyrocaps, Somophyllin-12 ✿, Somophyllin-CRT, Sustaire, Theo-24, Theo 250, Theobid Duracaps, Theobid Jr Duracaps, Theoclear L.A.-130 Cenules, Theoclear L.A.-260 Cenules, Theocot, Theochron, Theo-Dur, Theo-SR ✿, Theolair-SR, Theospan-SR, Theo-Time, Theophylline SR, Theovent Long-Acting, Uni-Dur, Uniphyl **(Rx)**

Classification: Antiasthmatic, bronchodilator

See also *Theophylline Derivatives*.

Action/Kinetics: Time to peak serum levels, oral solution: 1 hr; **uncoated tablets:** 2 hr; **chewable tablets:** 1–1.5 hr; **enteric-coated tablets:** 5 hr; **extended-release capsules and tablets:** 4–7 hr. In healthy adults, about 60% is bound to plasma protein whereas in neonates 36% is bound to plasma protein.

Additional Use: Oral liquid: Neonatal apnea as a respiratory stimulant. Theophylline and dextrose injection: Respiratory stimulant in neonatal apnea and Cheyne-Stokes respiration.

Dosage

• **Capsules, Tablets, Elixir, Oral Solution, Syrup**

See *Dosage* for *Oral Solution, Tablets,* under *Aminophylline*.

• **Extended-Release Capsules, Extended-Release Tablets**

See *Dosage* for *Extended-Release Tablets,* under *Aminophylline*.

• **Elixir, Oral Solution, Oral Suspension, Syrup**

Bronchodilator, chronic therapy.
9–12 years: 20 mg/kg/day; **6–9 years:** 24 mg/kg/day.
Neonatal apnea.
Loading dose: Using the equivalent of anhydrous theophylline administered by NGT, 5 mg/kg; **maintenance:** 2 mg/kg/day in two to three divided doses given by NGT.

RESPIRATORY CARE CONSIDERATIONS

See also *Respiratory Care Considerations* for *Theophylline Derivatives*.

Administration/Storage:
1. Dosage is individualized to maintain serum levels of 10–20 mcg/mL.
2. Dosage should be calculated based on lean body weight (theophylline does not distribute to body fat).
3. Serum theophylline levels should be monitored in chronic therapy, especially if the maximum maintenance doses are used or exceeded.
4. The extended-release tablets or capsules are not recommended for children less than 6 years of age. Dosage for once-a-day products has not been established in children less than 12 years of age.

Assessment:
1. Document indications for therapy, onset and duration of symptoms, and any other agents prescribed and the outcome.
2. Describe pulmonary assessment findings and note pulmonary function tests and ABG results if available.
3. If switching from IV therapy, wait 4 hr before administering intermediate-release forms; may administer extended-release form at time of discontinuation of IV.

Client/Family Teaching:
1. Take with food or milk to minimize GI upset.
2. Stress the importance of taking the drug only as prescribed; more is not better.
3. Do not crush or break slow-release forms of the drug.
4. Avoid cigarette smoking because it decreases drug's effectiveness.
5. Provide a printed list of side effects that require reporting if evident.
6. Caffeine- and xanthine-containing beverages and foods (chocolate, coffee, colas) and daily intake of charbroiled foods should be avoided because they tend to increase side effects of this drug.
7. Advise that fluid intake should be at least 2 L/day in order to decrease viscosity of secretions.
8. Do not take any OTC cough, cold, or breathing preparations without provider approval.

9. Report if symptoms do not improve or worsen with therapy.
10. Stress the importance of periodic tests for serum drug levels.

Evaluate:
• Improved pulmonary function
• Reports of ease in secretion removal and breathing
• Decreased apneic episodes in neonates
• Therapeutic serum drug levels (10–20 mcg/mL)

Ticarcillin disodium
(tie-kar-**SILL**-in)
Pregnancy Category: B
Ticar **(Rx)**
Classification: Antibiotic, penicillin

See also *Anti-Infectives* and *Penicillins.*

Action/Kinetics: This drug is a parenteral, semisynthetic antibiotic with an antibacterial spectrum of activity resembling that of carbenicillin. Primarily suitable for treatment of gram-negative organisms but also effective for mixed infections. Combined therapy with gentamicin or tobramycin is sometimes indicated for treatment of *Pseudomonas* infections. *The drugs should not be mixed during administration because of gradual mutual inactivation.* **Peak plasma levels:** IM, 25–35 mcg/mL after 1 hr; **IV,** 15 min. **t½:** 70 min. Elimination complete after 6 hr.

Uses: Bacterial septicemia, skin and soft tissue infections, acute and chronic respiratory tract infections caused by susceptible strains of *Pseudomonas aeruginosa, Proteus, Escherichia coli,* and other gram-negative organisms. GU tract infections caused by the above organisms and by *Enterobacter* and *Streptococcus faecalis.* Anaerobic bacteria causing empyema, anaerobic pneumonitis, lung abscess, bacterial septicemia, peritonitis, intra-abdominal abscess, skin and soft tissue infections, salpingitis, endometritis, pelvic inflammatory disease, pelvic abscess. Ticarcillin may be used in infections in which protective mechanisms are impaired such as during use of oncolytic or immunosuppressive drugs or in clients with acute leukemia. Clients seriously ill should receive higher doses such as in serious urinary tract and systemic infections.

Additional Contraindications: Pregnancy.

Special Concerns: Use with caution in presence of impaired renal function and for clients on restricted salt diets.

Additional Side Effects: Neurotoxicity and neuromuscular excitability, especially in clients with impaired renal function.

Additional Drug Interactions: Effect of carbenicillin may be enhanced when used in combination with gentamicin or tobramycin for *Pseudomonas* infections.

Laboratory Test Interferences: ↑ Alkaline phosphatase, AST, ALT.

Dosage —————————

- **IV Infusion, Direct IV, IM**
  Bacterial septicemia, intra-abdominal infections, skin and soft tissue infections, infections of the female genital system and pelvis, respiratory tract infections.
  Adults: 200–300 mg/kg/day by IV infusion in divided doses q 3, 4, or 6 hr, depending on the severity of the infection; **pediatric, less than 40 kg:** 200–300 mg/kg/day by IV infusion q 4 or 6 hr (daily dose should not exceed the adult dose).
  UTIs, uncomplicated.
  Adults: 1 g IM or direct IV q 6 hr; **pediatric, less than 40 kg:** 50–100 mg/kg/day IM or direct IV in divided doses q 6 or 8 hr.
  UTIs, complicated.
  Adults: 150–200 mg/kg/day by IV infusion in divided doses q 4 or 6 hr (usual dose is 3 g q.i.d. for a 70-kg client).
  Neonates with sepsis due to Pseudomonas, Proteus, *or* E. coli.
  Less than 7 days of age and less than 2 kg, 75 mg/kg q 12 hr; **more than 7 days of age and less than 2**

kg, 75 mg/kg q 8 hr; **less than 7 days of age and more than 2 kg,** 75 mg/kg q 8 hr; **more than 7 days of age and more than 2 kg,** 100 mg/kg q 8 hr. Can be given IM or by IV infusion over 10–20 min.

Clients with renal insufficiency should receive a loading dose of 3 g **IV,** and subsequent doses, as indicated by creatinine clearance.

RESPIRATORY CARE CONSIDERATIONS

See also *Respiratory Care Considerations* for *Penicillins.*

Administration/Storage:

1. Discard unused reconstituted solutions after 24 hr when stored at room temperature and after 72 hr when refrigerated.

2. For IM use, reconstitute each gram with 2 mL sterile water for injection, sodium chloride injection, or 1% lidocaine HCl (without epinephrine) to prevent pain and induration. The reconstituted solution should be used quickly and should be injected well into a large muscle.

3. For IV use, reconstitute each gram with 4 mL of the desired solution. Administer slowly to prevent vein irritation and phlebitis. A dilution of 1 g/20 mL (or more) will decrease the chance of vein irritation.

4. For an IV infusion, use 50 or 100 mL *ADD-Vantage* container of either 5% dextrose in water or sodium chloride injection and give by intermittent infusion over 30–120 min in equally divided doses.

5. Do not administer more than 2 g of the drug in each IM site.

6. Children weighing over 40 kg should receive the adult dose.

7. Ticarcillin should not be mixed together with amikacin, gentamicin, or tobramycin due to the gradual inactivation of these aminoglycosides .

8. Anticipate reduced dosage with liver or renal dysfunction.

Assessment:

1. Document indications for therapy and type and onset of symptoms.

2. Ensure that appropriate specimens have been sent for culture.

3. Obtain bleeding times and liver and renal function studies, and monitor during therapy.

Interventions:

1. Monitor client on high doses of drug for signs of electrolyte imbalance (especially sodium and potassium levels).

2. Note sodium content of drug (usually 4.75 mEq Na/g) and calculate accordingly for clients on strict sodium restrictions.

Evaluate:

• Laboratory evidence of negative culture reports

• Clinical evidence and reports of symptomatic improvement

Timolol maleate

(**TIE**-moh-lohl)
Pregnancy Category: C
Apo-Timol ✤, Apo-Timop ✤, Blocadren, Gen-Timolol ✤, Novo-Timol ✤, Nu-Timolol ✤, Timoptic, Timoptic in Acudose, Timoptic-XE **(Rx)**
Classification: Ophthalmic agent, beta-adrenergic blocking agent

---

See also *Beta-Adrenergic Blocking Agents.*

Action/Kinetics: Timolol exerts both beta-1- and beta-2-adrenergic blocking activity. Timolol has minimal sympathomimetic effects, direct myocardial depressant effects, and local anesthetic action. It does not cause pupillary constriction or night blindness. The mechanism of the protective effect in MI is not known. **Peak plasma levels:** 1–2 hr. **t½:** 4 hr. Metabolized in the liver. Metabolites and unchanged drug excreted through the kidney.

Timolol also reduces both elevated and normal intraocular pressure, whether or not glaucoma is present; it is thought to act by reducing aqueous humor formation and/or by slightly increasing outflow of aqueous humor. The drug does not affect pupil size or visual acuity. For use in eye: **Onset:** 30 min. **Maximum effect:** 1–2 hr. **Duration:** 24 hr.

Uses: Tablets: Hypertension (alone or in combination with other antihypertensives such as thiazide diuretics). Within 1–4 weeks of MI to reduce risk of reinfarction. Prophylaxis of migraine. *Investigational:* Ventricular arrhythmias and tachycardias, essential tremors.

Ophthalmic solution (Timoptic): Lower intraocular pressure in chronic open-angle glaucoma, selected cases of secondary glaucoma, ocular hypertension, aphakic (no lens) clients with glaucoma. *Ophthalmic gel forming solution (Timoptic-XE):* Reduce elevated intraocular pressure in glaucoma.

Contraindications: Hypersensitivity to drug. Bronchial asthma or bronchospasm including severe COPD.

Special Concerns: Use ophthalmic preparation with caution in clients for whom systemic beta-adrenergic blocking agents are contraindicated. Safe use in children not established.

Side Effects: *Systemic following use of tablets:* See *Beta-Adrenergic Blocking Agents.*

Following use of ophthalmic product: Few. Occasionally, ocular irritation, local hypersensitivity reactions, slight decrease in resting HR.

Drug Interactions: When used ophthalmically, possible potentiation with systemically administered beta-adrenergic blocking agents.

Laboratory Test Interferences: ↑ BUN, serum potassium, and uric acid. ↓ H&H.

Dosage —————————————

• **Tablets**

Hypertension.

Initial: 10 mg b.i.d. alone or with a diuretic; **maintenance:** 20–40 mg/day (up to 80 mg/day in two doses may be required), depending on BP and HR. If dosage increase is necessary, wait 7 days.

MI prophylaxis in clients who have survived the acute phase.
10 mg b.i.d.

Migraine prophylaxis.

Initially: 10 mg b.i.d. **Maintenance:** 20 mg/day given as a single dose; total daily dose may be increased to 30 mg in divided doses or decreased to 10 mg, depending on the response and client tolerance. If a satisfactory response for migraine prophylaxis is not obtained within 6–8 weeks using the maximum daily dose, the drug should be discontinued.

Essential tremor.
10 mg/day.
• **Ophthalmic Solution (Timoptic 0.25% or 0.5%)**
Glaucoma.
1 gtt of 0.25%–0.50% solution in each eye b.i.d. If the decrease in intraocular pressure is maintained, reduce dose to 1 gtt once a day.
• **Ophthalmic Gel-Forming Solution (Timoptic-XE 0.25% or 0.5%)**
Glaucoma.
1 gtt once daily.

RESPIRATORY CARE CONSIDERATIONS

See also *Respiratory Care Considerations* for *Beta-Adrenergic Blocking Agents* and *Antihypertensive Agents.*
Administration/Storage
Ophthalmic Solution
1. When client is transferred from another antiglaucoma agent, continue old medication on day 1 of timolol therapy (1 gtt of 0.25% solution). Thereafter, discontinue former therapy. Initiate with 0.25% solution. Increase to 0.50% solution if response is insufficient. Further increases in dosage are ineffective.
2. When client is transferred from several antiglaucoma agents, the dose must be individualized. If one of the agents is a beta-adrenergic blocking agent, it should be discontinued before starting timolol. Dosage adjustments should involve one drug at a time at 1-week intervals. The antiglaucoma drugs should be continued with the addition of timolol, 1 gtt of 0.25% solution b.i.d. (if response is inadequate, 1 gtt of 0.5% solution may be used b.i.d.). The following day, one of the other

antiglaucoma agents should be discontinued while the remaining agents should be continued or discontinued based on client response.
3. Before using the gel, invert the closed container and shake once before each use.
4. Other ophthalmics should be administered at least 10 min before the gel.
5. The ocular hypotensive effect has been maintained when switching clients from timolol solution given b.i.d. to the gel once daily.
Assessment
1. Document indications for therapy and onset, duration, and characteristics of symptoms.
2. Obtain baseline liver and renal function studies.
Evaluate:
• Control of hypertension with ↓ BP
• Prevention of myocardial reinfarction
• Migraine prophylaxis
• ↓ Intraocular pressures

Tobramycin sulfate
(toe-brah-**MY**-sin)
Pregnancy Category: D (B for ophthalmic use)
Parenteral: Nebcin, **Ophthalmic:** AK-Tob Ophthalmic Solution, Tobrex Ophthalmic Ointment, Tobrex Ophthalmic Solution **(Rx)**
Classification: Antibiotic, aminoglycoside

See also *Aminoglycosides.*
Action/Kinetics: This aminoglycoside is similar to gentamicin and can be used concurrently with carbenicillin. **Therapeutic serum levels: IM,** 4–8 mcg/mL. **t½:** 2–2.5 hr. Toxic serum levels: > 12 mcg/mL (peak) and > 2 mcg/mL (trough).
Uses: Systemic: Complicated and recurrent UTIs due to *Pseudomonas aeruginosa, Proteus, Escherichia coli, Klebsiella, Enterobacter, Serratia, Staphylococcus aureus, Citrobacter,* and *Providencia.* Lower respiratory tract infections due to *P. aeru-*

ginosa, Klebsiella, Enterobacter, E. coli, Serratia, and *S. aureus.* Intra-abdominal infections (including peritonitis) due to *E. coli, Klebsiella,* and *Enterobacter.* Septicemia in neonates, children, and adults due to *P. aeruginosa, E. coli,* and *Klebsiella.* Skin, bone, and skin structure infections due to *P. aeruginosa, Proteus, E. coli, Klebsiella, Enterobacter,* and *S. aureus.* Serious CNS infections, including meningitis. Can be used with penicillins or cephalosporins in serious infections when results of susceptibility testing are not yet known.

Ophthalmic: Treat superficial ocular infections due to *Staphylococcus, S. aureus, Streptococcus, S. pneumoniae,* beta-hemolytic streptococci, *Corynebacterium, E. coli, Haemophilus aegyptius, H. ducreyi, H. influenzae, H. parainfluenzae, Klebsiella pneumoniae, Neisseria, N. gonorrhoeae, Proteus, Acinetobacter calcoaceticus, Enterobacter, Enterobacter aerogenes, Serratia marcescens, Moraxella, Pseudomonas aeruginosa,* and *Vibrio.*

Contraindications: Ophthalmically to treat dendritic keratitis, vaccinia, varicella, fungal or mycobacterial eye infections, after removal of a corneal foreign body. Lactation.

Special Concerns: Use with caution in premature infants and neonates. Ophthalmic ointment may retard corneal epithelial healing.

Additional Side Effects: *Ophthalmic use:* Transient irritation, burning, stinging, itching, inflammation, angioneurotic edema, urticaria, vesicular and maculopapular dermatitis.

OD **Overdose Management:** *Symptoms (Ophthalmic Use):* Edema, lid itching, punctate keratitis, erythema, lacrimation.

Additional Drug Interactions: With carbenicillin or ticarcillin, tobramycin may have an increased effect when used for *Pseudomonas* infections.

Dosage —————————
• **IM, IV**

Non-life-threatening serious infections.
Adults: 3 mg/kg/day in three equally divided doses q 8 hr.
Life-threatening infections.
Up to 5 mg/kg/day in three or four equal doses. **Pediatric:** Either 2–2.5 mg/kg q 8 hr or 1.5–1.9 mg/kg q 6 hr; **neonates 1 week of age or less:** up to 4 mg/kg/day in two equal doses q 12 hr.
Impaired renal function.
Initially: 1 mg/kg; **then,** maintenance dose calculated according to information supplied by manufacturer.
• **Ophthalmic Ointment (0.3%)**
Acute infections.
0.5-in. ribbon q 3–4 hr until improvement is noted.
Mild to moderate infections.
0.5-in. ribbon b.i.d.–t.i.d.
• **Ophthalmic Solution (0.3%)**
Acute infections.
Initial: 1–2 gtt q 15–30 min until improvement noted; **then,** reduce dosage gradually.
Moderate infections.
1–2 gtt 2–6 times/day.

RESPIRATORY CARE CONSIDERATIONS

See also *Respiratory Care Considerations* for *Aminoglycosides.*
Administration/Storage:
1. Prepare IV solution by diluting calculated dose of tobramycin with 50–100 mL of dextrose or saline solution and infuse over 30–60 min.
2. Use proportionately less diluent for children than for adults.
3. Do not mix with other drugs for parenteral administration.
4. Store drug at room temperature no longer than 2 years.
5. Discard solution of drug containing up to 1 mg/mL after 24 hr at room temperature.
Evaluate:
• Laboratory evidence of negative culture reports
• Resolution of ophthalmic infection
• Therapeutic serum drug levels (4–8 mcg/mL) with systemic therapy

Tocainide hydrochloride
(toe-**KAY**-nyd)
Pregnancy Category: C
Tonocard **(Rx)**
Classification: Antiarrhythmic, class IB

See also *Antiarrhythmic Agents.*
Action/Kinetics: Tocainide, which is similar to lidocaine, decreases the excitability of cells in the myocardium by decreasing sodium and potassium conductance. Tocainide increases pulmonary and aortic arterial pressure and slightly increases peripheral resistance. Is effective in both digitalized and nondigitalized clients. **Peak plasma levels:** 0.5–2 hr. **t½:** 11–15 hr. **Therapeutic serum levels:** 4–10 mcg/mL. **Duration:** 8 hr. Approximately 10% is bound to plasma protein. From 28% to 55% is excreted unchanged in the urine. Alkalinization decreases the excretion of the drug although acidification does not produce any changes in excretion.
Uses: Life-threatening ventricular arrhythmias, including ventricular tachycardia. Has not been shown to improve survival in clients with ventricular arrhythmias. *Investigational:* Myotonic dystrophy, trigeminal neuralgia.
Contraindications: Allergy to amide-type local anesthetics, second- or third-degree AV block in the absence of artificial ventricular pacemaker. Lactation.
Special Concerns: There is an increased risk of death when used in those with non-life-threatening cardiac arrhythmias. Safety and efficacy have not been established in children. Use with caution in clients with impaired renal or hepatic function (dose may have to be decreased). Geriatric clients may have an increased risk of dizziness and hypotension; the dose may have to be reduced in these clients due to age-related impaired renal function.
Side Effects: *CV: Increased arrhythmias,* increased ventricular rate (when given for atrial flutter or fibrillation), CHF, tachycardia, hypotension, *con-*duction disturbances,* bradycardia, chest pain, LV failure, palpitations. *CNS:* Dizziness, vertigo, headache, tremors, confusion, disorientation, hallucinations, ataxia, paresthesias, numbness, nervousness, altered mood, anxiety, incoordination, walking disturbances. *GI:* N&V, anorexia, diarrhea. *Respiratory: Pulmonary fibrosis, fibrosing alveolitis,* interstitial pneumonitis, *pulmonary edema,* pneumonia. *Hematologic:* Leukopenia, *agranulocytosis,* hypoplastic anemia, *aplastic anemia,* bone marrow depression, neutropenia, *thrombocytopenia and sequelae as septicemia and septic shock. Musculoskeletal:* Arthritis, arthralgia, myalgia. *Dermatologic:* Rash, skin lesion, diaphoresis. *Other:* Blurred vision, visual disturbances, nystagmus, tinnitus, hearing loss, lupus-like syndrome.
OD **Overdose Management:** *Symptoms:* Initially are CNS symptoms including tremor (see above). GI symptoms may follow (see above). *Treatment:* Gastric lavage and activated charcoal may be useful. In the event of respiratory depression or arrest or seizures, maintain airway and provide artificial ventilation. An IV anticonvulsant (e.g., diazepam, thiopental, thiamylal, pentobarbital, secobarbital) may be required if seizures are persistent.
Drug Interactions:
Cimetidine / ↓ Bioavailability of tocainide
Metoprolol / Additive effects on wedge pressure and cardiac index
Rifampin / ↓ Bioavailability of tocainide
Laboratory Test Interferences: Abnormal liver function tests (especially in early therapy). ↑ ANA.

Dosage
• **Tablets**
Antiarrhythmic.
Adults, individualized, initial: 400 mg q 8 hr, up to a maximum of 2,400 mg/day; **maintenance:** 1,200–1,800 mg/day in divided doses. Total daily dose of 1,200 mg may be

adequate in clients with liver or kidney disease.

Myotonic dystrophy.
800–1,200 mg/day.

Trigeminal neuralgia.
20 mg/kg/day in three divided doses.

RESPIRATORY CARE CONSIDERATIONS

See also *Respiratory Care Considerations* for *Antiarrhythmic Agents*.

Assessment:
1. Document indications for therapy and type, onset, and duration of symptoms.
2. Obtain baseline ECG, CBC, electrolytes, and liver and renal function studies. Potassium deficits should be corrected before initiating tocainide therapy.
3. Assess and document cardiac and pulmonary assessment findings.

Evaluate:
• Control of lethal ventricular arrhythmias
• ↓ Muscle spasm and pain
• Therapeutic serum drug levels (4–10 mcg/mL)

Torsemide
(**TOR**-seh-myd)
Pregnancy Category: B
Demadex **(Rx)**
Classification: Loop diuretic

See also *Diuretics, Loop*.
Action/Kinetics: Onset, IV: Within 10 min; **PO:** within 60 min. **Peak effect, IV:** Within 60 min; **PO:** 60–120 min. **Duration:** 6–8 hr. **t½:** 210 min. Metabolized by the liver and excreted through the urine. Food intake delays the time to peak effect by about 30 min, but the overall bioavailability and the diuretic activity are not affected.
Uses: Congestive heart failure, chronic renal failure, hepatic cirrhosis, hypertension.
Contraindications: Lactation.
Special Concerns: Clients sensitive to sulfonamides may show allergic reactions to torsemide. Safety and efficacy in children have not been determined.

Side Effects: *CNS:* Headache, dizziness, asthenia, insomnia, nervousness, syncope. *GI:* Diarrhea, constipation, nausea, dyspepsia, edema, *GI hemorrhage,* rectal bleeding. *CV:* ECG abnormality, chest pain, atrial fibrillation, hypotension, ventricular tachycardia, shunt thrombosis. *Respiratory:* Rhinitis, increase in cough. *Musculoskeletal:* Arthralgia, myalgia. *Miscellaneous:* Sore throat, excessive urination, rash.
Laboratory Test Interferences: Hyperglycemia, hyperuricemia, hypokalemia, hypovolemia.

Dosage ————————————
• **Tablets, IV**
  Congestive heart failure.
Adults, initial: 10 or 20 mg once daily.
  Chronic renal failure.
Adults, initial: 20 mg once daily.
  Hepatic cirrhosis.
Adults, initial: 5 or 10 mg once daily given with an aldosterone antagonist or a potassium-sparing diuretic.
  Hypertension.
Adults, initial: 5 mg once daily. If this dose does not lead to an adequate decrease in BP within 4–6 weeks, the dose may be increased to 10 mg once daily. If the 10-mg dose is not adequate, an additional antihypertensive agent is added to the treatment regimen.

RESPIRATORY CARE CONSIDERATIONS

See also *Respiratory Care Considerations* for *Diuretics, Loop*.

Administration/Storage:
1. Oral and IV doses are therapeutically equivalent, and clients may be switched to and from the IV form with no change in dose.
2. If the response is inadequate for the initial dose used for CHF, chronic renal failure, or hepatic cirrhosis, the dose can be doubled until the desired diuretic response is obtained. Doses greater than 200 mg for CHF or chronic renal failure and greater than 40 mg for hepatic cirrhosis have not been adequately studied.

3. Torsemide may be given at any time in relation to a meal.

4. The IV dose is given slowly over a period of 2 min.

5. The dose does not need to be adjusted for geriatric clients.

Assessment:

1. Document indications for therapy and type and onset of symptoms.

2. List other agents prescribed and the outcome.

3. Query client and note any sensitivity to sulfonamides.

4. List drugs currently prescribed to ensure none interact unfavorably.

5. Obtain baseline VS, serum blood sugar, uric acid, and potassium levels and monitor periodically. Drug may increase blood sugar and uric acid levels.

6. Assess and document baseline pulmonary, renal, and CV data.

7. Initially monitor VS, daily weight, and I&O.

Evaluate:

• Promotion of diuresis

• Reduction of edema in furosemide refractory clients

• ↓ BP

• Reduction of interdialysis weight gain and promotion of Na, Cl, and water excretion

Triamcinolone
(try-am-**SIN**-oh-lohn)
Dental Paste: Kenalog in Orabase, Oracort, Oralone **(Rx)**. **Tablets:** Aristocort, Atolone, Kenacort **(Rx)**

Triamcinolone acetonide
(try-am-**SIN**-oh-lohn)
Dental Paste: Oracort ✦. **Inhalation Aerosol:** Azmacort, Nasacort, Nasacort AQ **(Rx)**. **Parenteral:** Kenaject-40, Kenalog-10 and -40, Tac-3 and -40, Triam-A, Triamonide 40, Trilog **(Rx)**. **Topical Aerosol:** Kenalog **(Rx)**. **Topical Cream:** Aristocort, Aristocort A, Delta-Tritex, Flutex, Kenac, Kenalog, Kenalog-H, Kenonel, Triac-et, Triaderm ✦, Trianide Mild, Trianide Regular, Triderm, Trymex **(Rx)**. **Topical Lotion:** Kenalog, Kenonel **(Rx)**. **Topical Ointment:** Aristocort, Aristocort A, Kenac, Kenalog, Kenonel, Triaderm ✦, Trymex **(Rx)**

Triamcinolone diacetate
(try-am-**SIN**-oh-lohn)
Parenteral: Amcort, Aristocort Forte, Aristocort Intralesional, Aristocort Parenteral ✦, Articulose L.A., Kenacort Diacetate, Triam-Forte, Triamolone 40, Trilone, Tristoject. **Syrup:** Aristocort Syrup ✦ **(Rx)**

Triamcinolone hexacetonide
(try-am-**SIN**-oh-lohn)
Aristospan Intra-Articular, Aristospan Intralesional **(Rx)**
Classification: Corticosteroid, synthetic

See also *Corticosteroids*.

Action/Kinetics: More potent than prednisone.   Intermediate-acting. Has no mineralocorticoid activity. **Onset:** Several hours. **Duration:** One or more weeks. **t½:** Over 200 min.

Additional Use: Pulmonary emphysema accompanied by bronchospasm or bronchial edema. Diffuse interstitial pulmonary fibrosis. With diuretics to treat refractory CHF or cirrhosis of the liver with ascites. Multiple sclerosis. Inflammation following dental procedures. Triamcinolone acetonide for PO inhalation is used for maintenance treatment of asthma. Triamcinolone hexacetonide is restricted to intra-articular or intralesional treatment of rheumatoid arthritis and osteoarthritis.

Special Concerns: Use during pregnancy only if benefits clearly outweigh risks. Use with special caution in clients who have decreased renal function or renal disease. Dose must be highly individualized.

Additional Side Effects: Intra-articular, intrasynovial, or intrabursal administration may cause transient flushing, dizziness, local depigmentation, and rarely, local irritation. Exacerbation of symptoms has also been reported. A marked increase in

T

---

bold italic = life threatening side effect

swelling and pain and further restricted joint movement may indicate septic arthritis. Intradermal injection may cause local vesicular ulceration and persistent scarring.

Syncope and anaphylactoid reactions have been reported with triamcinolone regardless of route of administration.

Dosage

Triamcinolone

- **Tablets**

Adrenocortical insufficiency (with mineralocorticoid therapy).
4–12 mg/day.

Acute leukemias (children).
1–2 mg/kg.

Acute leukemia or lymphoma (adults).
16–40 mg/day (up to 100 mg/day may be necessary for leukemia).

Edema.
16–20 mg (up to 48 mg may be required until diuresis occurs).

Tuberculosis meningitis.
32–48 mg/day.

Rheumatic disease, dermatologic disorders, bronchial asthma.
8–16 mg/day.

SLE.
20–32 mg/day.

Allergies.
8–12 mg/day.

Hematologic disorders.
16–60 mg/day.

Ophthalmologic diseases.
12–40 mg daily.

Respiratory diseases.
16–48 mg/day.

Triamcinolone acetonide

- **IM Only (Not for IV Use)**
2.5–60 mg/day, depending on the disease and its severity.

- **Intra-articular,   Intrabursal, Tendon Sheaths**
2.5–5 mg for smaller joints and 5–15 mg for larger joints, although up to 40 mg has been used.

- **Intradermal**
1 mg/injection site (use 3 mg/mL or 10 mg/mL suspension only).

- **Topical: 0.025%, 0.1%, 0.5% Ointment or Cream; 0.025%, 0.1% Lotion; Paste: 0.1%; Aerosol—to deliver 0.2 mg)**

Apply sparingly to affected area b.i.d.–q.i.d. and rub in lightly.

- **Metered Dose Inhaler**

Adults, usual: 2 inhalations (about 200 mcg) t.i.d.–q.i.d., not to exceed 1,600 mcg/day. High initial doses (1,200–1,600 mcg/day) may be needed in some clients with severe asthma. **Pediatric, 6–12 years:** 1–2 inhalations   (100–200   mcg) t.i.d.–q.i.d., not to exceed 1,200 mcg/day. Use in children less than 6 years of age has not been determined.

- **Intranasal Spray (Nasacort)**

Seasonal and perennial allergic rhinitis.

Adults and children over 12 years of age: 2 sprays (110 mcg) into each nostril once a day (i.e., for a total dose of 220 mcg/day). The dose may be increased to 440 mcg/day given either once daily or q.i.d. (1 spray/nostril).

Triamcinolone diacetate

- **IM Only**
40 mg/week.

- **Intra-articular, Intrasynovial**
5–40 mg.

- **Intralesional, Sublesional**
5–48 mg (no more than 12.5 mg/injection site and 25 mg/lesion).

Triamcinolone hexacetonide **Not for IV use.**

- **Intra-articular**
2–6 mg for small joints and 10–20 mg for large joints.

- **Intralesional/Sublesional**
Up to 0.5 mg/sq. in. of affected area.–

RESPIRATORY CARE CONSIDERATIONS

See also *Respiratory Care Considerations* for *Corticosteroids.*
Administration/Storage:
1. Initially the aerosol should be used concomitantly with systemic steroid. After 1 week, a gradual withdrawal of systemic steroid should be initiated. The next reduction should be made after 1–2 weeks, depending on the response. If symptoms of insufficiency occur, the dose of systemic steroid can be in-

creased temporarily. Also, the dose of systemic steroid may need to be increased in times of stress or a severe asthmatic attack.

2. The acetonide products should not be used if they clump due to exposure to freezing temperatures.

3. A single IM dose of the diacetate provides control from 4–7 days up to 3–4 weeks.

4. Triamcinolone acetonide nasal spray for allergic rhinitis may be effective as soon as 12 hr after initiation of therapy. If improvement is not seen within 2–3 weeks, the client should be reevaluated.

Assessment:

1. Document indications for therapy and type, onset, and characteristics of symptoms.

2. Assess area requiring treatment and describe findings.

3. Obtain blood sugar, CBC, electrolytes, and serum cortisol level with long-term use.

Client/Family Teaching:

1. Take at the same time each morning.

2. Ingest a liberal amount of protein because with regular use of this drug, clients may experience gradual weight loss, associated with anorexia, muscle wasting, and weakness. Refer to dietitian for assistance in meal planning and preparation.

3. Remind client to lie down if feeling faint. Report if syncopal episodes persist and interfere with daily activities.

4. Report any evidence of abnormal bruising, bleeding, weight gain, edema, or dyspnea.

5. Advise that drug may suppress reactions to skin allergy testing.

6. With topical application, apply to clean, slightly moist skin. Report if area does not improve with therapy or if symptoms worsen.

7. With nasal spray or inhaler, review appropriate method of administration, watch client self-administer, and stress proper care and storage of equipment.

8. Report immediately any new onset

of depression as well as aggravation of existing depressive symptoms.

Evaluate:

• ↓ Immune and inflammatory responses in autoimmune disorders and allergic reactions

• Improved airway exchange

• Restoration of skin integrity

• Relief of pain and inflammation with improved joint mobility

---

Triamterene

(try-**AM**-ter-een)

Pregnancy Category: B

Dyrenium **(Rx)**

Classification: Diuretic, potassium-sparing

See also *Diuretics.*

Action/Kinetics: Triamterene is a mild diuretic that acts directly on the distal tubule. It promotes the excretion of sodium—which is exchanged for potassium or hydrogen ions—bicarbonate, chloride, and fluid. The drug increases urinary pH. It is also a weak folic acid antagonist. **Onset:** 2–4 hr. **Peak effect:** 6–8 hr. **Duration:** 7–9 hr. **t½:** 3 hr. From one-half to two-thirds of the drug is bound to plasma protein. Triamterene is metabolized to hydroxytriamterene sulfate, which is also active. About 20% is excreted unchanged through the urine. Triamterene is also found in Dyazide.

Uses: Edema due to CHF, hepatic cirrhosis, nephrotic syndrome, steroid therapy, secondary hyperaldosteronism, and idiopathic edema. May be used alone or with other diuretics. *Investigational:* Prophylaxis and treatment of hypokalemia, adjunct in the treatment of hypertension.

Contraindications: Hypersensitivity to drug, severe or progressive renal insufficiency, severe hepatic disease, anuria, hyperkalemia, hyperuricemia, gout, history of nephrolithiasis. Lactation.

Special Concerns: Safety and efficacy have not been determined in children.

Side Effects: *Electrolyte:* Hyperkalemia, electrolyte imbalance. *GI:* Nausea, vomiting (may also be indicative of electrolyte imbalance), diarrhea, dry mouth. *CNS:* Dizziness, drowsiness, fatigue, weakness, headache. *Hematologic:* Megaloblastic anemia, thrombocytopenia. *Renal:* Azotemia, interstitial nephritis. *Miscellaneous:* **Anaphylaxis,** photosensitivity, hypokalemia, jaundice, muscle cramps, rash.

OD **Overdose Management:** *Symptoms:* Electrolyte imbalance, especially hyperkalemia. Also, nausea, vomiting, other GI disturbances, weakness, hypotension, reversible acute renal failure. *Treatment:* Immediately induce vomiting or perform gastric lavage. Electrolyte levels and fluid balance should be evaluated and treated if necessary. Dialysis may be beneficial.

Drug Interactions:
Amantadine / ↑ Toxic effects of amantadine due to ↓ renal excretion
Angiotensin-converting enzyme inhibitors / Significant hyperkalemia
Antihypertensives / Potentiated by triamterene
Captopril / ↑ Risk of significant hyperkalemia
Cimetidine / ↑ Bioavailability and ↓ clearance of triamterene
Digitalis / Inhibited by triamterene
Indomethacin / ↑ Risk of nephrotoxicity and acute renal failure
Lithium / ↑ Chance of lithium toxicity due to ↓ renal clearance
Potassium salts / Additive hyperkalemia
Spironolactone / Additive hyperkalemia

Laboratory Test Interferences: Triamterene may impart blue fluorescence to urine, interfering with fluorometric assays (e.g., lactic dehydrogenase, quinidine). ↑ BUN, creatinine. ↑ Serum uric acid in clients predisposed to gouty arthritis.

Dosage ————
Capsules.
Diuretic. **Adults, initial:** 100 mg

b.i.d. after meals; **maximum daily dose:** 300 mg.

RESPIRATORY CARE CONSIDERATIONS

See also *Respiratory Care Considerations* for *Diuretics.*
Administration/Storage:
1. Minimize nausea by giving the drug after meals.
2. Triamterene dosage is usually reduced by one-half when another diuretic is added to the regimen.
Assessment:
1. Take a complete drug history, noting drugs with which triamterene interacts.
2. Obtain baseline serum electrolytes, renal function studies, and uric acid levels before administering the drug.
3. Determine that a CBC and an ECG have been performed prior to initiating therapy.
Interventions:
1. Monitor serum electrolytes, BUN, uric acid, and CBC and report any variations.
2. If the client has any history of CAD, obtain an ECG and be alert to the development of cardiac arrhythmias.
3. If the client has a history of alcoholism, megaloblastic anemia may occur because triamterene is a weak antagonist of folic acid. Monitor the CBC and WBC differential periodically.
4. Observe for hyperkalemia; this is an indication to withdraw the drug because cardiac irregularities may result.
Evaluate:
• ↓ Edema
• Reports of ↑ diuresis
• ↓ BP

————COMBINATION DRUG————
Trimethoprim and Sulfamethoxazole
(sul-fah-meh-**THOX**-ah-zohl, try-**METH**-oh-prim)
Pregnancy Category: C
Apo-Sulfatrim ✦, Bactrim, Bactrim DS, Bactrim IV, Bactrim Pediatric, Bactrim

Roche ✦, Cotrim, Cotrim D.S., Cotrim Pediatric, Novo-Trimel ✦, Novo-Trimel DS ✦, Nu-Cotrimix ✦, Pro-Trin ✦, Roubac ✦, Septra, Septra DS, Septra IV, Sulfatrim, Trisulfa ✦, Trisulfa S ✦ **(Rx)**
Classification: Antibacterial

See also *Sulfonamides.*
Content: These products contain the antibacterial agents sulfamethoxazole and trimethoprim. See also *Sulfamethoxazole.*

Oral Suspension: Sulfamethoxazole, 200 mg and trimethoprim, 40 mg/5 mL.

Tablets: Sulfamethoxazole, 400 mg and trimethoprim, 80 mg/tablet.

Double Strength (DS) Tablets: Sulfamethoxazole, 800 mg and trimethoprim, 160 mg/tablet.

Concentrate for injection: Sulfamethoxazole, 80 mg and trimethoprim, 16 mg/mL.

Uses: PO, Parenteral: UTIs due to *Escherichia coli, Klebsiella, Enterobacter, Pseudomonas mirabilis* and *vulgaris,* and *Morganella morganii.* Enteritis due to *Shigella flexneri* or *S. sonnei. Pneumocystis carinii* pneumonitis in children and adults. **PO:** Acute otitis media in children due to *Haemophilus influenzae* or *Streptococcus pneumoniae.* Traveler's diarrhea in adults due to *E. coli.* Prophylaxis of *P. carinii* pneumonia in immunocompromised clients (including those with AIDS). Acute exacerbations of chronic bronchitis in adults due to *H. influenzae* or *S. pneumoniae. Investigational:* Cholera, salmonella, nocardiosis, prophylaxis of recurrent UTIs in women, prophylaxis of neutropenic clients with *P. carinii* infections or leukemia clients to decrease incidence of gram-negative rod bacteremia. Treatment of acute and chronic prostatitis. Decrease chance of urinary and blood bacterial infections in renal transplant clients.

Additional Contraindications: Infants under 2 months of age. During pregnancy at term. Megaloblastic anemia due to folate deficiency. Lactation.

Special Concerns: Use with caution in impaired liver or kidney function. AIDS clients may not tolerate or respond to this product. Use with caution in clients with possible folate deficiency.

Additional Drug Interactions:
Cyclosporine / ↓ Effect of cyclosporine; ↑ risk of nephrotoxicity
Dapsone / ↑ Effect of both dapsone and trimethoprim
Methotrexate / ↑ Risk of methotrexate toxicity due to displacement from plasma protein binding sites
Phenytoin / ↑ Effect of phenytoin due to ↓ hepatic clearance
Sulfonylureas / ↑ Hypoglycemic effect of sulfonylureas
Thiazide diuretics / ↑ Risk of thrombocytopenia with purpura in geriatric clients
Warfarin / ↑ PT
Zidovudine / ↑ Serum levels of AZT due to ↓ renal clearance

Laboratory Test Interferences: Jaffe alkaline picrate reaction overestimation of creatinine by 10%.

Dosage
• **Oral Suspension, Double-Strength Tablets, Tablets**
  UTIs, shigellosis, bronchitis, acute otitis media.
Adults: 1 DS tablet, 2 tablets, or 4 teaspoonfuls of suspension q 12 hr for 10–14 days. **Pediatric:** Total daily dose of 8 mg/kg trimethoprim and 40 mg/kg sulfamethoxazole divided equally and given q 12 hr for 10–14 days. (*NOTE:* For shigellosis, give adult or pediatric dose for 5 days.) For clients with impaired renal function the following dosage is recommended: creatinine clearance of 15–30 mL/min: one-half the usual regimen and for creatinine clearance less than 15 mL/min: use is not recommended.
  Chancroid.
1 DS tablet b.i.d. for at least 7 days (alternate therapy: 4 DS tablets in a single dose).
  Pharyngeal gonococcal infection

T

due to penicillinase-producing Neisseria gonorrhoeae.

720 mg trimethoprim and 3,600 mg sulfamethoxazole once daily for 5 days.

Prophylaxis of P. carinii pneumonia.

Adults: 160 mg trimethoprim and 800 mg sulfamethoxazole q 24 hr.
Children: 150 mg/m² of trimethoprim and 750 mg/m² sulfamethoxazole daily in equally divided doses b.i.d. on three consecutive days per week. The total daily dose should not exceed 320 mg trimethoprim and 1,600 mg sulamethoxazole.

Treatment of P. carinii pneumonia.

Adults and children: Total daily dose of 15–20 mg/kg trimethoprim and 100 mg/kg sulfamethoxazole divided equally and given q 6 hr for 14–21 days.

Prophylaxis of P. carinii pneumonia in immunocompromised clients.

1 DS tablet daily.

Traveler's diarrhea.

Adults, 1 DS tablet q 12 hr for 5 days.

Prostatitis, acute bacterial.

1 DS tablet b.i.d. until client is afebrile for 48 hr; treatment may be required for up to 30 days.

Prostatitis, chronic bacterial.

1 DS tablet b.i.d. for 4–6 weeks.

• **IV**

UTIs, shigellosis, acute otitis media.

Adults and children: 8–10 mg/kg/day (based on trimethoprim) in two to four divided doses q 6, 8, or 12 hr for up to 14 days for severe UTIs or 5 days for shigellosis.

Treatment of P. carinii pneumonia

Adults and children: 15–20 mg/kg/day (based on trimethoprim) in 3–4 divided doses q 6–8 hr for up to 14 days.

RESPIRATORY CARE CONSIDERATIONS

See also *General Respiratory Care Considerations for All Anti-Infectives.*

Administration/Storage:

1. The IV infusion must be administered over a period of 60–90 min.

2. Each 5-mL vial must be diluted to 125 mL with D5W and used within 6 hr. If the amount of fluid should be restricted, each 5 mL can be diluted up to 75 mL with D5W and used within 2 hr. The diluted solution should not be refrigerated.

3. The IV infusion should not be mixed with any other drugs or solutions.

4. If the diluted IV infusion is cloudy or precipitates after mixing, it should be discarded and a new solution prepared.

Assessment:

1. Obtain baseline lab data to evaluate cultures and liver and renal functions. Anticipate reduced dose with renal dysfunction.

2. Assess for anemia (leukopenia and granulocytopenia) because megaloblastic anemia due to folate deficiency is a contraindication as drug inhibits ability to produce folinic acid.

3. Simultaneous administration of folinic acid (6–8 mg/day) may prevent antifolate drug effects.

4. Document, when known, in clients infected with AIDS virus as they may be intolerant to this product.

5. List all drugs currently prescribed to ensure none interact unfavorably.

Evaluate:

• Resolution of infection
• Negative culture results
• Prophylaxis of *P. carinii* pneumonia.

Trimetrexate glucuronate

(**try**-meh-**TREX**-ayt gloo-**KYOU**-roh-nayt)
Pregnancy Category: D
NeuTrexin **(Rx)**
Classification: Miscellaneous anti-infective

See also *Anti-Infectives.*

Action/Kinetics: Trimetrexate inhibits the enzyme dihydrofolate reductase that results in interference with thymidylate biosynthesis and inhibition of folate-dependent formyl-transferases. This leads to inhibition of purine synthesis and disruption of DNA, RNA, and protein synthesis and ultimately cell death. Trimetrexate must be given together with leucovorin to prevent serious or life-threatening complications, including bone marrow suppression, oral and GI mucosal ulceration, and renal and hepatic dysfunction. **t½:** 11 hr. The drug is highly bound to plasma protein and is metabolized by the liver. The metabolites also appear to have an inhibitory effect on dihydrofolate reductase.

Uses: As alternative therapy with concurrent leucovorin for the treatment of moderate to severe *Pneumocystis carinii* pneumonia in immunocompromised clients. Treatment is indicated in clients with AIDS who are intolerant of or refractory to trimethoprim-sulfamethoxazole (TMP/SMZ) therapy or in whom this combination is contraindicated. *Investigational:* Treatment of non-small-cell lung, prostate, or colorectal cancer.

Contraindications: Hypersensitivity to trimetrexate, leucovorin, or methotrexate. Use during lactation.

Special Concerns: Use with caution in clients with impaired hematologic, renal, or hepatic function. Safety and efficacy have not been determined for clients less than 18 years of age for use in treating histologically confirmed PCP.

Side Effects: *GI:* N&V. *Hematologic:* Neutropenia, thrombocytopenia, anemia. *Hepatic:* Hepatic toxicity manifested by increased ALT, AST, alkaline phosphatase, and bilirubin. *Renal:* Increased serum creatinine. *Electrolytes:* Hyponatremia, hypocalcemia.

OD **Overdose Management:** *Symptoms:* Primarily hematologic. *Treatment:* Discontinue trimetrexate and administer leucovorin at a dose of 40 mg/m² q 6 hr for 3 days.

Drug Interactions: Since trimetrexate is metabolized by the P-450 enzyme system in the liver, drugs that stimulate or inhibit this enzyme system may cause drug interactions that may alter plasma levels of trimetrexate (e.g., erythromycin, rifabutin, rifampin).

Acetaminophen / May alter the levels of trimetrexate metabolites
Cimetidine / May ↓ metabolism of trimetrexate
Clotrimazole / ↓ Metabolism of trimetrexate
Ketoconazole / ↓ Metabolism of trimetrexate
Miconazole / ↓ Metabolism of trimetrexate

Dosage ⎯⎯⎯⎯⎯⎯⎯⎯
• **IV Infusion**
Pneumocystis carinii *pneumonia.*
Adults: 45 mg/m² once daily by IV infusion over 60–90 min. Leucovorin is given IV at a dose of 20 mg/m² over 5–10 min q 6 hr for a total daily dose of 80 mg/m². Leucovorin may also be given orally in four doses of 20 mg/m² spaced equally throughout the day (the oral dose should be rounded up to the next higher 25-mg increment). Doses of trimetrexate and leucovorin are modified depending on hematologic toxicity. If neutrophils are between 750 and 1,000/mm³ and platelets between 50,000 and 75,000/mm³, the dose of trimetrexate remains at 45 mg/m² once daily but the dose of leucovorin is increased to 40 mg/m² q 6 hr. If neutrophils are between 500 and 749/mm³ and platelets between 25,000 and 49,999, the dose of trimetrexate is reduced to 22 mg/m² once daily and the dose of leucovorin is 40 mg/m² q 6 hr. If neutrophils are less than 500/mm³ and platelets are less than 25,000/mm³, trimetrexate is discontinued for 9 days with leucovorin still given at a dose of 40 mg/m² q 6 hr; from days 10 to 21, trimetrexate should be interrupted up to 96 hr.

RESPIRATORY CARE CONSIDERATIONS

See also *General Respiratory Care*

Considerations for All Anti-Infectives.

Administration/Storage:

1. Leucovorin therapy must be given for 72 hr after the last dose of trimetrexate.

2. The recommended course of therapy is 21 days for trimetrexate and 24 days for leucovorin.

3. The lyophilized powder is reconstituted with 2 mL of 5% dextrose injection or sterile water for injection to yield a concentration of 12.5 mg/mL. The reconstituted product appears as a pale greenish-yellow solution. The solution should not be used if it is cloudy or a precipitate is observed. The solution should be filtered before dilution.

4. The powder should not be reconstituted with solutions containing either chloride ion or leucovorin as precipitation occurs immediately.

5. The reconstituted solution may be further diluted with 5% dextrose injection to yield a final concentration of from 0.25 to 2 mg/mL.

6. Before and after administering trimetrexate, the IV line must be flushed thoroughly with at least 10 mL of 5% dextrose injection.

7. Trimetrexate and leucovorin solutions must be given separately.

8. If trimetrexate comes in contact with the skin or mucosa, the areas should be immediately and thoroughly washed with soap and water.

9. After reconstitution, the solution is stable under refrigeration or at room temperature for at least 24 hr. The reconstituted solution should not be frozen. Any unused portion should be discarded after 24 hr.

Assessment:

1. Document indications for therapy, any other agents prescribed, and the outcome.

2. Note if client is intolerant or refractory to trimethoprim-sulfamethoxazole.

3. List drugs currently prescribed to ensure none interact unfavorably.

4. Determine any hypersensitivity to leucovorin, methotrexate, or trimetrexate.

5. Obtain baseline hematologic profile and liver and renal function studies. During therapy, obtain these values twice a week to assess hematologic, renal, and hepatic functions.

Interventions:

1. Drug is to be administered concurrently with leucovorin to avoid its hematologic, hepatic, renal, and GI toxicities.

2. Clients who require concomitant therapy with myelosuppressive, nephrotoxic, or hepatotoxic drugs should be carefully monitored.

3. To allow for use of full therapeutic doses of trimetrexate, anticipate that zidovudine therapy should be discontinued during trimetrexate therapy.

4. Observe client carefully and report any changes. It may be difficult to distinguish side effects caused by trimetrexate from symptoms due to underlying medical conditions.

5. Trimetrexate should be discontinued for the following:

• Serum transaminase or alkaline phosphatase increases to more than 5 times the upper limit of the normal range

• Serum creatinine increases to 2.5 mg/dL

• Mucosal toxicity becomes so severe it interferes with oral intake

• Body temperature increases to more than 40.5°C (105°F) when taken orally

Evaluate: Resolution of PCP in immunocompromised clients

Tripelennamine hydrochloride

(try-pell-**EN**-ah-meen)
PBZ, PBZ-SR, Pelamine, Pyribenzamine
✢ **(Rx)**
Classification: Antihistamine, ethylenediamine derivative

See also *Antihistamines.*

Action/Kinetics: GI effects more pronounced than other antihistamines. **Duration:** 4–6 hr.

Special Concerns: Safe use during pregnancy has not been established. Use is not recommended in neonates. Geriatric clients may be more sensitive to the usual adult dose.

Side Effects: Low incidence. Moderate sedation, mild GI distress, paradoxical excitation, hyperirritability.

Dosage ————————————
• **Tablets**
Adults, usual: 25–50 mg q 4–6 hr; **pediatric:** 1.25 mg/kg (37.5 mg/m²) q 6 hr as needed, not to exceed 300 mg/day.
• **Extended-Release Tablets**
Adults: 100 mg q 8–12 hr as needed, up to a maximum of 600 mg/day. Do not use sustained-release form in children.

RESPIRATORY CARE CONSIDERATIONS

See also *Respiratory Care Considerations* for *Antihistamines*.
Evaluate: Reports of ↓ allergic manifestations

Tromethamine
(troh-**METH**-ah-meen)
Pregnancy Category: C
Tham, Tham-E **(Rx)**
Classification: Systemic alkalizing agent

Action/Kinetics: Tromethamine, an organic amine, is a buffering and systemic alkalizing agent. It actively binds hydrogen ions, thereby decreasing and correcting acidosis. It promotes the excretion of acids, carbon dioxide, and electrolytes and is thought to be able to neutralize some intracellular acid. It acts as an osmotic diuretic, increasing urine flow. Seventy-five percent of the drug is eliminated within 8 hr, the remainder within 3 days.
Uses: Prevention and correction of systemic acidosis, especially that accompanying cardiac bypass surgery, correction of acidity of acid citrate dextrose (ACD) blood in cardiac bypass surgery, and cardiac arrest.
Contraindications: Uremia and anuria.

Special Concerns: Use with caution in newborns and infants. Administer with caution to clients with renal disorders.
Side Effects: *Respiratory:* Respiratory depression, especially in those with chronic hypoventilation or getting drugs that depress respiration. *Other:* Fever, hypervolemia, transient decrease of blood glucose. *At injection site:* Extravasation may cause inflammation, vascular spasms, and tissue damage (e.g., chemical phlebitis, thrombosis, necrosis, sloughing). *In newborn:* **Hemorrhagic liver necrosis when given by umbilical vein.**
OD **Overdose Management:** *Symptoms:* Alkalosis, overhydration, hypoglycemia (severe and prolonged), solute overload. *Treatment:* Discontinue the infusion and treat symptoms.

Dosage ————————————
Minimum amount to correct acid-base imbalance. The amount of tromethamine can be estimated using the buffer base deficit of the extracellular fluid: mL of 0.3 M tromethamine solution required = body weight (kg) × base deficit (mEq/L) × 1.1
• **Slow IV Infusion**
Acidosis in cardiac bypass surgery.
Adults: 500 mL (150 mEq or 18 g) as a single dose. Severe cases may require 1,000 mL. The dose should not exceed 500 mg/kg over a period of not less than 1 hr.
• **Injection into Ventricular Cavity or Large Peripheral Vein**
Acidosis in cardiac arrest (given at the same time as other standard procedures are being applied).
If chest is open. Adults: 62–185 mL (2–6 g) into the ventricular cavity (not into the cardiac muscle). **If chest closed. Adults:** 111–333 mL (3.6–10.8 g) into a large peripheral vein.
• **Addition to Pump Oxygenator Acid Citrate Dextrose Blood**
For acidity in ACD blood.

15–77 mL (0.5–2.5 g) added to each 500 mL of ACD blood. Usually 62 mL (2 g) added to 500 mL of ACD blood is adequate.

RESPIRATORY CARE CONSIDERATIONS

Administration/Storage:

1. Tests on blood pH, pCO_2, bicarbonate, glucose, and electrolytes should be determined before, during, and after administration of tromethamine.

2. Concentration of solution administered *must not* exceed 0.3 M.

3. Prepare a 0.3-M solution of tromethamine by adding 1,000 mL of sterile water for injection to 36 g of lyophilized tromethamine.

4. Infuse slowly.

5. Administer into the largest antecubital vein through a large needle or indwelling catheter and elevate limb.

6. For treatment of cardiac arrest, the drug may be injected into the ventricular cavity if the chest is open. If the chest is not open, the drug may be injected into a large peripheral vein.

7. Do not administer longer than 1 day unless acute life-threatening situation exists.

8. Discontinue administration *immediately,* if extravasation occurs:

• Administer 1% procaine hydrochloride with hyaluronidase to reduce venospasm and to dilute the drug in the tissues.

• Phentolamine mesylate (Regitine) has been used for local infiltration for its adrenergic blocking properties.

• If necessary, a nerve block of the autonomic fibers may be done.

Assessment:

1. Note if the client has any history of urinary or bladder problems.

2. Obtain baseline renal and hepatic function studies.

3. Determine that pH, pCO_2, bicarbonate, glucose, and electrolytes have been analyzed before administering drug.

4. If the client is female and of childbearing age, check to determine if pregnant.

Interventions:

1. Observe for respiratory depression and have mechanical ventilation equipment readily available.

2. Document and report any complaints of weakness, presence of moist pale skin, tremors, and a full bounding pulse. These are symptoms of hypoglycemia, which can occur after a rapid or high dose of the drug has been administered.

3. Maintain an accurate record of I&O.

4. Assess for nausea, diarrhea, tachycardia, oliguria, weakness, numbness, or tingling sensations. These are symptoms of hyperkalemia and are more likely to occur in clients with impaired renal function.

5. Monitor serum electrolytes, blood glucose levels, pH, and hepatic and renal function studies periodically throughout drug therapy. Report any abnormal findings.

6. Observe closely for extravasation, as the drug is extremely irritating to the vein.

Evaluate:

• Neutralization of ACD blood in pump oxygenator

• Correction of systemic acidosis, with serum pH within desired range

---

Tubocurarine chloride

(too-boh-kyour-**AR**-een)

Pregnancy Category: C

(Rx)

Classification: Nondepolarizing neuromuscular blocking agent

See also *Neuromuscular Blocking Agents.*

Action/Kinetics: Cumulative effects may occur. Most likely of the nondepolarizing drugs to cause histamine release. Narrow margin between therapeutic dose and toxic dose. Overdosage chiefly treated by artificial respiration, although neostigmine, atropine, and edrophonium chloride should also be on hand.

Onset, IV: 1 min; **IM:** 15–25 min.

Time to peak effect, IV: 2–5 min.

Duration, IV: 20–40 min. **t½:** 1–3 hr. About 43% excreted unchanged in urine.

Uses: Muscle relaxant during surgery or setting of fractures and dislocations; spasticity caused by injury to or disease of CNS. Treat seizures electrically induced or induced by drugs. Diagnosis of myasthenia gravis. **Additional Contraindications:** Drug may cause excessive secretion and circulatory collapse. Clients in whom release of histamine is hazardous.

Special Concerns: Use with caution during pregnancy and lactation and in children. If repeated doses are used before delivery, the newborn may manifest decreased skeletal muscle activity. Children up to 1 month of age may be more sensitive to the effects of tubocurarine. Use with extreme caution in clients with renal dysfunction, liver disease, or obstructive states.

Additional Side Effects: *Allergic reactions.*

Additional Drug Interactions:

Acetylcholine / Acetylcholine antagonizes effect of tubocurarine

Anticholinesterases / Anticholinesterases antagonize effect of tubocurarine

Calcium salts / ↑ Effect of tubocurarine

Diazepam / Diazepam may cause malignant hyperthermia with tubocurarine

Potassium / Antagonizes effect of tubocurarine

Propranolol / ↑ Effect of tubocurarine

Quinine / ↑ Effect of tubocurarine

Succinylcholine chloride / ↑ Relaxant effect of both drugs

Dosage ─────────────

• **IV, IM**

Adjunct to surgical anesthesia.

Adults, IM, IV, initial: 6–9 mg (40–60 units); **then,** 3–4.5 mg (20–30 units) in 3–5 min if needed. Supplemental doses of 3 mg (20 units) can be given for prolonged

procedures. Dosage can be calculated on the basis of 1.1 units/kg. **Pediatric, up to 4 weeks of age, IV, initial:** 0.3 mg/kg; **then,** give subsequent doses in increments of ⅕–⅙ the initial dose. **Infants and children, IV:** 0.6 mg/kg.

Electroshock therapy.

Adults, IV: 0.165 mg/kg (1.1 units/kg) given over 30–90 sec. It is recommended that the initial dose be 3 mg less than the calculated total dose.

Diagnosis of myasthenia gravis.

Adults, IV: 0.004–0.033 mg/kg. A test dose should be given within 2–3 min with IV neostigmine, 1.5 mg, to minimize prolonged respiratory paralysis.

RESPIRATORY CARE CONSIDERATIONS

See also *Respiratory Care Considerations* for *Neuromuscular Blocking Agents.*

Administration/Storage:

1. The drug should be given IV as a sustained injection over 1–1.5 min. It may also be given IM.

2. Tubocurarine should be given in incremental doses until relaxation is reached.

3. The initial dose should be decreased if the inhalation anesthetic used enhances the action of curariform drugs or if the client has compromised renal function.

4. Review the drugs with which tubocurarine interacts.

5. Tubocurarine is incompatible with alkaline solutions and may form a precipitate when mixed with them (e.g., methohexital sodium or thiopental sodium).

6. After IV administration, expect the peak action to occur in 2–5 min and the effect to last 25–90 min.

7. Have neostigmine methylsulfate available as an antidote.

Assessment

1. Document indications for therapy and onset, duration, and characteristics of symptoms.

2. Utilize a peripheral nerve stimula-

T

tor to assess neuromuscular response and recovery.

3. Obtain baseline ECG, VS, and lab studies.

Interventions:

1. Monitor VS and ECG. Drug can cause vagal stimulation resulting in bradycardia, hypotension, and cardiac arrhythmias.

2. Document length of time client is receiving the drug. It should be used only on a short-term basis and in a continuously monitored environment.

3. Remember that client may be fully conscious and aware of surroundings and conversations.

4. Drug does not affect pain or anxiety so administer analgesics and antianxiety agents as indicated.

Evaluate:

• Desired level of skeletal muscle relaxation

• Control of drug or electrically induced seizures

• Diagnosis of myasthenia gravis

V

Vancomycin hydrochloride

(van-koh-**MY**-sin)
Pregnancy Category: C
Lyphocine, Vancocin, Vancocin CP
★, Vancoled **(Rx)**
Classification: Antibiotic, miscellaneous

See also *Anti-Infectives*.

Action/Kinetics: This antibiotic, derived from *Streptomyces orientalis*, diffuses in pleural, pericardial, ascitic, and synovial fluids after parenteral administration. It appears to bind to bacterial cell wall, arresting its synthesis and lysing the cytoplasmic membrane by a mechanism that is different from that of penicillins and cephalosporins. Vancomycin may also change the permeability of the cytoplasmic membranes of bacteria, thus inhibiting RNA synthesis. The drug is bactericidal for most organisms and bacteriostatic for enterococci. It is poorly absorbed from the GI tract. **Peak plasma levels, IV:** 33 mcg/mL 5 min after 0.5-g dosage. **t½, after PO:** 4–8 hr for adults and 2–3 hr for children; **t½, after IV:** 4–11 hr for adults and ranging from 2–3 hr in children to 6–10 hr for newborns. The half-life is increased markedly in the presence of renal impairment (240 hr has been not-

ed). Primarily excreted in urine unchanged. Auditory and renal function tests are indicated before and during therapy.

Uses: PO. Antibiotic-induced pseudomembranous colitis due to *Clostridium difficile*. Staphylococcal enterocolitis. Severe or progressive antibiotic-induced diarrhea caused by *C. difficile* that is not responsive to the causative antibiotic being discontinued; also for debilitated clients.

IV. Severe staphylococcal infections in clients who have not responded to penicillins or cephalosporins, who cannot receive these drugs, or who have resistant infections. Infections include lower respiratory tract infections, bone infections, endocarditis, septicemia, and skin and skin structure infections. Alone or in combination with aminoglycosides to treat endocarditis caused by *Streptococcus viridans* or *S. bovis*. Must combine with an aminoglycoside to treat endocarditis due to *Streptococcus faecalis*. Used with rifampin, an aminoglycoside (or both) to treat early onset prosthetic valve endocarditis caused by *Staphylococcus epidermidis* or other diphtheroids. Prophylaxis of bacterial endocarditis in pencillin-allergic clients who have congenital heart disease or rheumatic or other acquired or valvular heart disease if such clients are undergoing dental or surgical procedures of the upper respiratory tract. The parenteral dosage form may be given PO to treat pseudomembranous colitis or staphylococcal enterocolitis due to *C. difficile*.

Contraindications: Hypersensitivity to drug. Minor infections. Lactation.

Special Concerns: Use with extreme caution in the presence of impaired renal function or previous hearing loss. Geriatric clients are at a greater risk of developing ototoxicity.

Side Effects: Ototoxicity (may lead to deafness), nephrotoxicity (may lead to uremia). *Red-neck syndrome:* Chills, erythema of neck and back, fever, paresthesias. *Dermatologic:* Urticaria, macular rashes. *Allergic:* Drug fever, hypersensitivity, **anaphylaxis.** *Miscellaneous:* Nausea, tinnitus, eosinophilia, neutropenia (reversible), hypotension (due to rapid administration). Thrombophlebitis at site of injection. Deafness mayprogress after drug is discontinued.

Drug Interactions
Aminoglycosides / ↑ Risk of nephrotoxicity
Anesthetics / Risk of erythema and histamine-like flushing in children
Muscle relaxants, nondepolarizing / ↑ Neuromuscular blockade

Dosage ——————————
• **Capsules, Oral Solution**
Adults: 0.5–2 g/day in three to four divided doses for 7–10 days. Alternatively, 125 mg t.i.d.–q.i.d. for *C. difficile* may be as effective as the 500-mg dosage. **Children:** 40 mg/kg/day in three to four divided doses for 7–10 days, not to exceed 2 g/day. **Neonates:** 10 mg/kg/day in divided doses.
• **IV**
Severe staphylococcal infections.
Adults: 500 mg q 6 hr or 1 g q 12 hr. **Children:** 10 mg/kg/6 hr. **Infants and neonates, initial:** 15 mg/kg for one dose; **then,** 10 mg/kg q 12 hr for neonates in the first week of life and q 8 hr thereafter up to 1 month of age.

Prophylaxis of bacterial endocarditis in dental, oral, or upper respiratory tract procedures in penicillin-allergic clients.
Adults: 1 g vancomycin over 1 hr plus 1.5 mg/kg gentamicin (IV or IM), not to exceed 80 mg, 1 hr before the procedure. May repeat once, 8 hr after the initial dose. **Children:** 20 mg/kg vancomycin plus 2 mg/kg gentamicin (IV or IM), not to exceed 80 mg, 1 hr before the procedure. May repeat once, 8 hr after the initial dose.

RESPIRATORY CARE CONSIDERATIONS

See also *General Respiratory Care Considerations for All Anti-Infectives.*

Administration/Storage:
1. Dosage must be reduced in clients with renal disease; see package insert for procedure.
2. The oral solution is prepared by adding 115 mL distilled water to the 10-g container. The appropriate dose of oral solution may be mixed with 1 oz of water or flavored syrup to improve the taste. The diluted drug may also be given by NGT.
3. The parenteral form may be administered PO by diluting the 1-g vial with 20 mL distilled or deionized water (each 5 mL contains about 250 mg vancomycin).
4. For IV use, dilute each 500-mg vial with 10 mL of sterile water. This may be further diluted in 200 mL of dextrose or saline solution and infused over 60 min.
5. Intermittent infusion is the preferred route, but continuous IV drip may be used.
6. Avoid rapid IV administration because this may result in hypotension, nausea, warmth, and generalized tingling. Administer over 1 hr in at least 200 mL of NSS or D5W.
7. Avoid extravasation during injections as this may cause tissue necrosis.
8. Reduce risk of thrombophlebitis

by rotating injection sites or adding additional diluent.

9. Aqueous solution is stable for 2 weeks.

10. Once rubber stopper is punctured, ampule should be refrigerated to maintain stability.

Assessment:

1. Document indications for therapy and type, onset, and duration of symptoms.

2. Determine that baseline renal and auditory functions (including 8th cranial nerve function) have been assessed.

3. Anticipate reduced dose with renal dysfunction.

4. Ensure that baseline CBC and cultures have been performed.

Interventions:

1. Monitor and record weight, VS, and I&O; ensure adequate hydration.

2. Assess and report any evidence of adverse drug effects, such as:

• Ototoxicity, demonstrated by tinnitus, progressive hearing loss, dizziness, and/or nystagmus

• Nephrotoxicity, demonstrated by albuminuria, hematuria, anuria, casts, edema, and uremia

3. During IV drug administration ensure that peak and trough drug levels are performed at the prescribed dosing interval, usually 30 min prior to scheduled IV dose (trough) and 1 hr following IV dose (peak) to accurately assess serum levels.

Evaluate:

• Laboratory evidence of negative culture reports

• Relief of S&S R/T infection

• Serum drug levels within therapeutic range (trough 1–5 mcg/mL; peak 20–50 mcg/mL)

Vecuronium bromide

(vh-kyour-**OH**-nee-um)

Pregnancy Category: C

Norcuron **(Rx)**

Classification: Nondepolarizing neuromuscular blocking agent

See also *Neuromuscular Blocking Agents.*

Action/Kinetics: Less likely than other agents to cause histamine release. Effects can be antagonized by anticholinesterase drugs. **Onset:** 2.5–3 min; **peak effect:** 3–5 min; **duration:** 25–40 min using balanced anesthesia. It is about one-third more potent than pancuronium, but its duration of action is shorter at initial equipotent doses. No cumulative effects noted after repeated administration. **t½, elimination:** 65–75 min; a shortened half-life (35–40 min) has been noted in late pregnancy. Metabolized in liver and excreted through the kidney and bile. Is bound to plasma protein. Recovery may be doubled in clients with cirrhosis or cholestasis; renal failure does not affect recovery time.

Uses: To induce skeletal muscle relaxation during surgery or mechanical ventilation. To facilitate ET intubation. As an adjunct to general anesthesia. *Investigational:* To treat electrically induced seizures or seizures induced by drugs.

Additional Contraindications: Use in neonates, obesity. Sensitivity to bromides.

Special Concerns: Pediatric clients from 7 weeks to 1 year of age are more sensitive to the effects of vecuronium leading to a recovery time up to 1½ times that for adults. The dose for children aged 1–10 years of age must be individualized and may, in fact, require a somewhat higher initial dose and a slightly more frequent supplemental dosing schedule than adults. Clients with myasthenia gravis or Eaton-Lambert syndrome may experience profound effects with small doses of vecuronium. Cardiovascular disease, old age, and edematous states result in increased volume of distribution and thus a delay in onset time—the dose should *not* be increased.

Additional Side Effects: Moderate to severe skeletal muscle weakness, which may require artificial respiration. *Malignant hyperthermia.*

Additional Drug Interactions

Bacitracin / ↑ Muscle relaxation

following high IV or IP doses of ba-citracin

Sodium colistimethate / ↑ Muscle relaxation following high IV or IP doses of sodium colistimethate

Tetracyclines / ↑ Muscle relaxation following high IV or IP doses of tet-racyclines

Succinylcholine ↑ Effect of vecuro-nium.

Dosage

• **IV Only**

Intubation.

Adults and children over 10 years of age. 0.08–0.1 mg/kg.

For use after succinylcholine-as-sisted ET intubation.

0.04–0.06 mg/kg for inhalation anes-thesia and 0.05–0.06 mg/kg using balanced anesthesia. (*NOTE:* For hal-othane anesthesia, doses of 0.15–0.28 mg/kg may be given with-out adverse effects.)

For use during anesthesia with enflurane or isoflurane after steady state established.

0.06–0.085 mg/kg (about 15% less than the usual initial dose).

Supplemental use.

IV only: 0.01–0.015 mg/kg given 25–40 min following the initial dose; **then,** given q 12–15 min as needed. **IV infusion:** Initiated after recovery from effects of initial IV dose of 0.08–0.1 mg/kg has started. **Initial:** 0.001 mcg (1 mg)/kg; **then** adjust according to client response and re-quirements. Average infusion rate: 0.0008–0.0012 mg/kg/min (0.8–1.2 mcg/kg/min). After steady-state enflu-rane, isoflurane, and possibly halo-thane anesthesia has been estab-lished: IV infusion should be re-duced by 25%–60%.

RESPIRATORY CARE CONSIDERATIONS

See also *Respiratory Care Considera-tions* for *Neuromuscular Blocking Agents.*

Administration/Storage:

1. Dosage must be individualized and depends on prior or concomitant use of anesthetics or succinylcho-line.

2. Vecuronium may be mixed with saline, 5% dextrose alone or with sa-line, lactated Ringer's solution, and sterile water for injection.

3. Vecuronium should be used within 8 hr of reconstitution.

4. Anticipate the onset of action to oc-cur within 1–5 min and the effect to last 20–40 min.

5. The drug should be refrigerated after reconstitution.

6. Have neostigmine, pyridostig-mine, or edrophonium available to reverse vecuronium; atropine helps counteract muscarinic effects.

Assessment

1. Document indications for therapy and anticipated time frame for utiliza-tion.

2. Obtain baseline ECG, VS, CBC, electrolytes, and liver and renal function studies.

Interventions:

1. A peripheral nerve stimulator should be used to assess the client's neuromuscular response and recov-ery.

2. Monitor VS and ECG. Drug can cause vagal stimulation resulting in bradycardia, hypotension, and car-diac arrhythmias.

3. Muscle fasciculations may cause the client to be sore or injured after re-covery. Administer prescribed non-depolarizing agent and reassure that the soreness is likely caused by the unsynchronized contractions of ad-jacent muscle fibers just before the on-set of paralysis.

4. Monitor closely for any evidence of malignant hyperthermia, unrespon-sive tachycardia, jaw spasm, or lack of laryngeal relaxation. Stop infusion and report. Temperature elevations are a late sign of this condition.

5. Document length of time client is receiving the drug. It should be used only on a short-term basis and in a continuously monitored environ-ment.

6. Remember client is fully con-

V

scious and aware of surroundings and conversations.

7. Drug does not affect pain or anxiety so administer analgesics and antianxiety agents as indicated.

8. Prolonged use, as in an ICU setting, may lead to skeletal muscle weakness and symptoms consistent with muscle disuse atrophy. This may complicate ventilator weaning and some clients may require extensive physical therapy.

Evaluate:

• Desired level of skeletal muscle relaxation

• Facilitation of intubation and tolerance of mechanical ventilation

• Suppression of the twitch response when tested with a peripheral nerve stimulator

---

Verapamil
(ver-**AP**-ah-mil)
Pregnancy Category: C
Apo-Verap ✹, Calan, Calan SR, Covera HS, Isoptin, Isoptin I.V. ✹, Isoptin SR, Novo-Veramil ✹, Nu-Verap ✹, Verelan **(Rx)**
Classification: Calcium channel blocking agent

See also *Calcium Channel Blocking Agents.*

Action/Kinetics: Slows AV conduction and prolongs effective refractory period. IV doses may slightly increase LV filling pressure. The drug moderately decreases myocardial contractility and peripheral vascular resistance. Worsening of heart failure may result if verapamil is given to clients with moderate to severe cardiac dysfunction. **Onset: PO,** 30 min; **IV,** 3–5 min. **Time to peak plasma levels (PO):** 1–2 hr (5–7 hr for extended-release). **t½, PO:** 4.5–12 hr with repetitive dosing; **IV, initial:** 4 min; **final:** 2–5 hr. **Therapeutic serum levels:** 0.08–0.3 mcg/mL. **Duration, PO:** 8–10 hr (24 hr for extended-release); **IV:** 10–20 min for hemodynamic effect and 2 hr for antiarrhythmic effect. Verapamil is metabolized to norverapamil, which possesses 20% of the activity of verapamil.

NOTE: Covera HS is designed to deliver verapamil in concert with the 24-hr circadian variations in BP.

Uses: PO: Angina pectoris due to coronary artery spasm (Prinzmetal's variant), chronic stable angina including angina due to increased effort, unstable angina (preinfarction, crescendo). With digitalis to control rapid ventricular rate at rest and during stress in chronic atrial flutter or atrial fibrillation. Prophylaxis of repetitive paroxysmal supraventricular tachycardia. Essential hypertension. Sustained-release tablets are used to treat essential hypertension (Step I therapy). **IV:** Supraventricular tachyarrhythmias. Atrial flutter or fibrillation *Investigational:* PO for prophylaxis of migraine, manic depression (alternate therapy), exercise-induced asthma, recumbent nocturnal leg cramps, hypertrophic cardiomyopathy, cluster headaches.

Contraindications: Severe hypotension, second- or third-degree AV block, cardiogenic shock, severe CHF, sick sinus syndrome (unless client has artificial pacemaker), severe LV dysfunction. Cardiogenic shock and severe CHF unless secondary to SVT that can be treated with verapamil. Lactation. Use of verapamil, IV, with beta-adrenergic blocking agents (as both depress myocardial contractility and AV conduction). Ventricular tachycardia.

Special Concerns: Infants less than 6 months of age may not respond to verapamil. Use with caution in hypertrophic cardiomyopathy, impaired hepatic and renal function, and in the elderly.

Side Effects: *CV:* CHF, bradycardia, ***AV block, asystole,*** premature ventricular contractions and tachycardia (after IV use), peripheral and pulmonary edema, hypotension, syncope, palpitations, AV dissociation, ***MI, CVA.*** *GI:* Nausea, constipation, abdominal discomfort or cramps, dyspepsia, diarrhea, dry mouth. *CNS:* Dizziness, headache, sleep disturbances, depression, amnesia, paranoia, psychoses, hallucinations, jitteriness, confusion, drowsiness, vertigo.

V

IV verapamil may increase intracranial pressure in clients with supratentorial tumors at the time of induction of anesthesia. *Dermatologic:* Rash, dermatitis, alopecia, urticaria, pruritus, erythema multiforme, **Stevens-Johnson syndrome.** *Respiratory:* Nasal or chest congestion, dyspnea, SOB, wheezing. *Musculoskeletal:* Paresthesia, asthenia, muscle cramps or inflammation, decreased neuromuscular transmission in Duchenne's muscular dystrophy. *Other:* Blurred vision, equilibrium disturbances, sexual difficulties, spotty menstruation, sweating, rotary nystagmus, flushing, gingival hyperplasia, polyuria, nocturia, gynecomastia, claudication, hyperkeratosis, purpura, petechiae, bruising, hematomas, tachyphylaxis.

OD **Overdose Management:** *Symptoms:* Extension of side effects. *Treatment:* Beta-adrenergics, IV calcium, vasopressors, pacing, and resuscitation.

Additional Drug Interactions:
Antihypertensive agents / Additive hypotensive effects
Barbiturates / ↓ Bioavailability of verapamil
Calcium salts / ↓ Effect of verapamil
Carbamazepine / ↑ Effect of carbamazepine due to ↓ breakdown by liver
Cimetidine / ↑ Bioavailability of verapamil
Cyclosporine / ↑ Plasma levels of cyclosporine possibly leading to renal toxicity
Digoxin / ↑ Risk of digoxin toxicity due to ↑ plasma levels
Disopyramide / Additive depressant effects on myocardial contractility and AV conduction
Etomidate / Anesthetic effect of etomidate may be ↑ with prolonged respiratory depression and apnea
Lithium / ↓ Lithium plasma levels; lithium toxicity also observed
Muscle relaxants, nondepolarizing / ↑ Neuromuscular blockade due to effect of verapamil on calcium channels
Prazosin / Acute hypotensive effect
Quinidine / Possibility of bradycardia, hypotension, AV block, ventricular tachycardia, and pulmonary edema
Ranitidine / ↑ Bioavailability of verapamil
Rifampin / ↓ Effect of verapamil
Sulfinpyrazone / ↑ Clearance of verapamil
Theophyllines / ↑ Effect of theophyllines
Vitamin D / ↓ Effect of verapamil
Warfarin / Possible ↑ effect of either drug due to ↓ plasma protein binding
NOTE: Since verapamil is significantly bound to plasma proteins, interaction with other drugs bound to plasma proteins may occur.↓

Laboratory Test Interferences: ↑ Alkaline phosphatase, transaminase.

Dosage —————————
• **Tablets**
Angina at rest and chronic stable angina.
Individualized. Adults, initial: 80–120 mg t.i.d. (40 mg t.i.d. if client is sensitive to verapamil); **then,** increase dose to total of 240–480 mg/day. Covera HS is given once daily at bedtime in doses of either 180 or 240 mg.
Arrhythmias.
Dosage range in digitalized clients with chronic atrial fibrillation: 240–320 mg/day in divided doses t.i.d.–q.i.d. For prophylaxis of nondigitalized clients: 240–480 mg/day in divided doses t.i.d.–q.i.d. Maximum effects are seen within 48 hr.
Essential hypertension.
Initial, when used alone: 80 mg t.i.d. Doses up to 360 mg daily may be used. Effects are seen in the first week of therapy. In the elderly or in people of small stature, initial dose should be 40 mg t.i.d.
• **Extended-Release   Capsules and Tablets**
Essential hypertension.

Initial: 240 mg/day in the a.m (120 mg/day in the elderly or people of small stature). If response is inadequate, increase dose to 240 mg in the a.m. and 120 mg in the evening and then 240 mg q 12 hr. Covera HS is given once daily at bedtime in doses of either 180 or 240 mg.

- **IV, Slow**
  Supraventricular tachyarrhythmias.

Adults, initial: 5–10 mg (0.075–0.15 mg/kg) given over 2 min (over 3 min in older clients); **then,** 10 mg (0.15 mg/kg) 30 min later if response is not adequate. **Infants, up to 1 year:** 0.1–0.2 mg/kg (0.75–2 mg) given as an IV bolus over 2 min; **1–15 years:** 0.1–0.3 mg/kg (2–5 mg, not to exceed 5 mg total dose) over 2 min. If response to initial dose is inadequate, it may be repeated after 30 min, but not more than a total of 10 mg should be given to clients from 1 to 15 years of age.

RESPIRATORY CARE CONSIDERATIONS

See also *Respiratory Care Considerations* for *Calcium Channel Blocking Agents.*

Administration/Storage:

1. Before administration, ampules should be inspected for particulate matter or discoloration.

2. IV dosage should be administered under continuous ECG monitoring with resuscitation equipment readily available.

3. Give as a slow IV bolus (5–10 mg) over 2 min (3 min to elderly clients) to minimize toxic effects.

4. Ampules should be stored at 15°C–30°C (59°F–86°F) and protected from light.

5. Do not give verapamil in an infusion line containing 0.45% sodium chloride with sodium bicarbonate because a crystalline precipitate will form.

6. Do not give verapamil by IV push in the same line used for nafcillin infusion because a milky white precipitate will form.

7. Verapamil should not be mixed with albumin, amphotericin B, hydralazine, trimethoprim/sulfamethoxazole, or diluted with sodium lactate in polyvinyl chloride bags.

8. Verapamil will precipitate in any solution with a pH greater than 6.

9. Dosage of verapamil in the elderly should always be individualized because the pharmacologic effects are more pronounced and more prolonged.

10. The SR tablets (120 mg) may be useful for small stature and elderly clients who require less medication.

11. The sustained release tablets should be taken with food.

12. Verelan pellet filled capsules may be carefully opened and the contents sprinkled on a spoonful of applesauce. The applesauce should be swallowed immediately without chewing and is followed with a glass of cool water to ensure complete swallowing of the pellets. Subdividing the contents of a capsule is not recommended.

Assessment:

1. Document indications for therapy and onset and duration of symptoms.

2. List other agents prescribed and the outcome.

3. Review list of prescribed medications to ensure that none interact unfavorably.

4. Obtain baseline ECG, CBC, and liver and renal function studies. Anticipate reduced dosage for clients with hepatic or renal impairment.

Interventions:

1. Monitor VS and assess for bradycardia and hypotension, symptoms that may indicate overdosage. Verapamil may lower BP to dangerously low levels if the client already has a low BP.

2. *Do not* administer concurrently with IV beta-adrenergic blocking agents.

3. Unless treating verapamil overdosage, withhold any medication that elevates serum calcium levels and check with provider.

4. Clients receiving concurrent digoxin therapy should be assessed

for symptoms of toxicity and have digoxin levels checked periodically.

5. If disopyramide is to be used, do not administer for at least 48 hr before verapamil to 24 hr after verapamil administration.

6. Administer extended-release tablets with food to minimize fluctuations in serum levels.

Evaluate:
• ↓ Frequency and severity of anginal attacks
• Control of BP
• Restoration of normal sinus rhythm (usually 10 min after IV administration)
• Therapeutic serum drug levels (0.08–0.3 mcg/mL)

Z

Zafirlukast
(zah-**FIR**-loo-kast)
Pregnancy Category: B
Accolate **(Rx)**
Classification: Antiasthmatic

Action/Kinetics: Zafirlukast is a selective and competitive antagonist of leukotriene receptors D_4 and E_4, which are components of slow-reacting substance of anaphylaxis. It is believed that cysteinyl leukotriene occupation of receptors causes asthma, including airway edema, smooth muscle constriction, and altered cellular activity associated with the inflammatory process. Zafirlukast inhibits bronchoconstriction caused by sulfur dioxide and cold air in clients with asthma. The drug also attenuates the early- and late-phase reaction in asthmatics caused by inhalation of antigens such as grass, cat dander, ragweed, and mixed antigens. Zafirlukast is rapidly absorbed after PO use. However, the bioavailabilty may be decreased when taken with food. **Peak plasma levels:** 3 hr. **t½, terminal:** About 10 hr. The drug is over 99% bound to plasma proteins. It is extensively metabolized in the liver, with about 90% excreted in the feces and 10% in the urine. Zafirlukast inhibits certain cytochrome P450 isoenzymes.

Uses: Prophylaxis and chronic treatment of asthma in adults and children 12 years of age and older.

Contraindications: Use to terminate an acute asthma attack, including status asthmaticus. Lactation.

Special Concerns: The clearance is reduced in clients 65 years of age and older. Safety and efficacy have not been determined in children less than 12 years of age.

Side Effects: *GI:* N&V, diarrhea, abdominal pain, dyspepsia. *CNS:* Headache, dizziness. *Miscellaneous:* Infection, generalized pain, asthenia, accidental injury, myalgia, fever, back pain.

Drug Interactions
Aspirin / ↑ Plasma levels of zafirlukast
Erythromycin / ↓ Plasma levels of zafirlukast
Terfenadine / ↓ Plasma levels of zafirlukast
Theophylline / ↓ Plasma levels of zafirlukast
Warfarin / Significant ↑ PT
Laboratory Test Interferences: ALT.

Dosage

• **Tablets**
Asthma.
Adults and children aged 12 and older: 20 mg b.i.d.

RESPIRATORY CARE CONSIDERATIONS
Administration/Storage
1. The drug is to be taken 1 hr before or 2 hr after meals.

bold italic = life threatening side effect   **Z**

2. The drug is to be protected from light and moisture and stored at controlled room temperatures of 20°C–25°C (68°F–77°F).

Assessment

1. Document indications for therapy and onset, duration, and characteristics of symptoms. List other agents trialed with the outcome.
2. Note cardiopulmonary assessment findings.
3. Obtain baseline labs and pulmonary function studies.

Client/Family Teaching

1. Advise to take 1 hr before or 2 hr after meals to prevent loss of bioavailability.
2. Drug should be taken regularly and during symptom-free periods. Do not increase or decrease dose without provider approval.
3. Reinforce that drug is not appropriate for acute episodes of asthma. Continue all other antiasthma medications as prescribed.
4. Review peak flow meter use and set targets for intervention or additional therapy.
5. Instruct to avoid triggers, i.e., dust, chemicals, cigarette smoke, pollutants, pets, and perfumes.
6. Advise to practice reliable birth control during therapy and not to breast feed.

Evaluate: Inhibition of bronchoconstriction with asthma

Zileuton
(zye-**LOO**-ton)
Pregnancy Category: C
Zyflo **(Rx)**
Classification: Antiasthmatic, leukotriene receptor inhibitor

Action/Kinetics: As a specific inhibitor of 5-lipoxygenase, zileuton inhibits the formation of leukotrienes. Leukotrienes are substances that induce various biological effects including aggregation of neutrophils and monocytes, leukocyte adhesion, increase of neutrophil and eosinophil migration, increased capillary permeability, and contraction of smooth muscle. These effects of leukotrienes contribute to edema, secretion of mucus, inflammation, and bronchoconstriction in asthmatic clients. By inhibiting leukotriene formation, zileuton reduces bronchoconstriction due to cold air challenge in asthmatics. The drug is rapidly absorbed from the GI tract; **peak plasma levels:** 1.7 hr. Zileuton is metabolized in liver and mainly excreted through the urine. **t½:** 2.5 hr.

Uses: Prophylaxis and chronic treatment of asthma in adults and children over 12 years of age.

Contraindications: Active liver disease or transaminase elevations greater than or equal to three times the upper limit of normal. Hypersenstivity to zileuton. Treatment of bronchoconstriction in acute asthma attacks, including status asthmaticus. Lactation.

Special Concerns: Use with caution in clients who ingest large quantities of alcohol or who have a past history of liver disease. Safety and efficacy have not been determined in children less than 12 years of age.

Side Effects: *GI:* Dyspepsia, nausea, constipation, flatulence, vomiting. *CNS:* Headache, dizziness, insomnia, malaise, nervousnes, somnolence. *Body as a whole:* Unspecified pain, abdominal pain, chest pain, asthenia, accidental injury, fever. *Musculoskeletal:* Myalgia, arthralgia, neck pain/rigidity. *GU:* Urinary tract infection, vaginitis. *Miscellaneous:* Conjunctivitis, hypertonia, lymphadenopathy, pruritus.

Laboratory Test Alteration: ↑ ALT. Low white blood cell count.

Drug Interactions
Propranolol / ↑ Effect of propranolol
Terfenadine / ↑ Effect of terfenadine due to ↓ clearance
Theophylline / Doubling of serum theophylline levels → ↑ effect
Warfarin / ↑ Prothrombin time

Dosage ————
• **Tablets**
   Symptomatic treatment of asthma.
Adults and children over 12 years of age: 600 mg q.i.d.

Z

RESPIRATORY CARE CONSIDERATIONS

Administration/Storage

1. Zileuton may be taken with meals and at bedtime.

2. Clients should not decrease the dose or stop taking any other antiasthmatics when taking zileuton.

Assessment

1. Document onset, characteristics, and severity of disease. Note triggers and list currently prescribed medications.

2. Obtain baseline CBC, PFT's and LFT's and monitor during therapy.

3. Screen for excessive alcohol use and any evidence of liver disease.

Client/Family Teaching

1. Take regularly as directed (may take with meals and at bedtime) and continue other antiasthmatic medications as prescribed.

2. Drug will not reverse bronchospasm during acute asthma attack; use bronchodilators and seek medical attention if symptoms are severe or peak flow readings indicate need.

3. Instruct that drug inhibits formation of those substances that cause bronchoconstrictive symptoms in asthmatics.

4. Review use of peak flow meter and teach client how to monitor airway effectiveness, when to increase medications, and when to seek immediate medical attention based on peak flow readings.

5. Advise to notify provider immediately if experiencing RUQ pain, lethargy pruritus, jaundice, fatigue, or flu-like symptoms (S&S of liver toxicity).

6. Report for CBC, regularly scheduled LFT's and evaluation of pulmonary status. Bring record of peak flow readings.

7. Review triggers (i.e., smoke, cold air, and exercise) that may cause increased hyperresponsiveness which can last up to a week. Advise that if more than the usual or maximum number of inhalations of short-acting bronchodilator treatment in a 24 hr period are required, they should notify the provider.

Evaluate: Asthma prophylaxis with improved airway exchange.

(Page 528 is Blank)

APPENDIX ONE
Controlled Substances in the United States and Canada

Controlled Substances Act—United States

The U.S. Federal Controlled Substances Act of 1970 placed drugs controlled by the Act into five categories or schedules based on their potential to cause psychologic and/or physical dependence as well as on their potential for abuse. The schedules are defined as follows:

Schedule (C-I): Includes substances for which there is a high abuse potential and no current approved medical use (e.g., heroin, marijuana, LSD, other hallucinogens, certain opiates and opium derivatives).

Schedule (C-II): Includes drugs that have a high abuse potential and a high ability to produce physical and/or psychologic dependence and for which there is a current approved or acceptable medical use.

Schedule (C-III): Includes drugs for which there is less potential for abuse than drugs in Schedule II and for which there is a current approved medical use. Certain drugs in this category are preparations containing limited quantities of codeine. Also, anabolic steroids are classified in Schedule III.

Schedule (C-IV): Includes drugs for which there is a relatively low abuse potential and for which there is a current approved medical use.

Schedule (C-V): Drugs in this category consist mainly of preparations containing limited amounts of certain narcotic drugs for use as antitussives and antidiarrheals. Federal law provides that limited quantities of these drugs (e.g., codeine) may be bought without a prescription by an individual at least 18 years of age. The product must be purchased from a pharmacist who must keep appropriate records. However, state laws vary, and in many states such products require a prescription.

Controlled Substances—Canada

In Canada, narcotics are governed by the Narcotics Control regulations and are designated by the letter N. Drugs that are considered subject to abuse, have an approved medical use, and are not narcotics are designated by the letter C.

Generally prescriptions for Schedule II (high-abuse-potential) drugs cannot be transmitted over the phone and they cannot be refilled. Prescriptions for Schedule III, IV, and V drugs may be refilled up to five times within 6 months. Schedule II drugs are not necessarily "stronger" than drugs in Schedules III, IV, or V; Schedule II drugs are classified as such due to their high abuse potential.

	Drug Schedule	
Drug	United States	Canada
Alfentanil	II	N
Alprazolam	IV	*
Amobarbital	II	C
Amphetamine	II	Not available
Aprobarbital	III	*
Benzphetamine	III	Not available
Buprenorphine	V	*
Butabarbital	III	C
Butorphanol	*	C
Chloral hydrate	IV	*
Chlordiazepoxide	IV	*
Clonazepam	IV	*
Clorazepate	IV	*
Codeine	II	N
Dextroamphetamine	II	C
Diazepam	IV	*
Diethylpropion	IV	C
Estazolam	IV	*
Ethchlorvynol	IV	*
Fenfluramine	IV	*
Fentanyl	II	N
Fluoxymesterone	III	*
Flurazepam	IV	*
Glutethimide	III	*
Halazepam	IV	Not available
Hydrocodone	Not available	N
Hydromorphone	II	N
Levomethadyl acetate HCl	II	Not available
Levorphanol	II	N
Lorazepam	IV	*
Mazindol	IV	*
Meperidine	II	N
Mephobarbital	IV	C
Meprobamate	IV	*
Methadone	II	N
Methamphetamine	II	Not available
Metharbital	III	C
Methylphenidate	II	C
Methyltestosterone	III	*
Methyprylon	III	*
Midazolam	IV	*
Morphine	II	N
Nalbuphine	*	C

Nandrolone decanote	III	*
Nandrolone phenpropionate	III	*
Opium	II	N
Oxandrolone	III	*
Oxazepam	IV	*
Oxycodone	II	N
Oxymetholone	III	*
Oxymorphone	II	N
Paraldehyde	IV	*
Paregoric	III	N
Pemoline	IV	*
Pentazocine	IV	N
Pentobarbital		
PO, parenteral	II	C
Rectal	III	C
Phendimetrazine	III	Not available
Phenmetrazine	II	Not available
Phenobarbital	IV	C
Phentermine	IV	C
Prazepam	IV	Not available
Propoxyphene	IV	N
Quazepam	IV	Not available
Secobarbital		
PO	II	C
Parenteral	II	*
Rectal	III	*
Stanozolol	III	*
Sulfentanil	II	N
Talbutal	III	*
Temazepam	IV	*
Testosterone cypionate in oil	III	*
Testosterone enanthante in oil	III	*
Testosterone in aqueous suspension	III	*
Testosterone propionate in oil	III	*
Testosterone transdermal system	III	*
Triazolam	IV	*
Zolpidem tartrate	IV	*

*Not controlled

APPENDIX TWO
Elements of a Prescription

In order to safely communicate the exact elements desired on a prescription, the following items should be addressed:

A. The prescriber: Name, address, and phone number and associated practice/speciality

B. The client: Name and address and telephone number

C. The prescription itself: Name of the medication (generic or trade); quantity to be dispensed (e.g., number of tablets or capsules, 1 vial, 1 tube, volume of liquid); the strength of the medication (e.g., 125-mg tablets, 250 mg/5 mL, 80 mg/1 mL, 10%); and directions for use (e.g., 1 tablet t.i.d.; 2 gtt to each eye q.i.d.; 1 teaspoonful q 8 hr for 10 days; apply a thin film to lesions b.i.d. for 14 days)

D. Other elements: Date prescription is written, signature of the provider, number of refills; provider number: state license number and Drug Enforcement Agency (DEA) number (when applicable); and brand-product-only indication (when applicable)

A typical prescription is depicted as follows:

A. **Julia Bryan, MSN, RN, CPNP**
Pediatric Associates
1611 Kirkwood Highway
Wilmington, DE 19805
302-645-8261

Date: July 10, 1997

B. **For: Kathryn Woods, Age 8**
27 East Parkway
Lewes, DE 19958
123-555-1234

C.

Rx **Amoxicillin   250 mg/5 mL**
Disp. 150 mL
Sig: 1 teaspoon PO q 8 hr x 10 days

D.
Refills: 0

Provider signature
Provider/State license number

Interpretation of prescription: The above prescription is written by Pediatric Nurse Practitioner Julia Bryan for Kathryn Woods and is for amoxicillin suspension. The concentration desired is 250 mg/5 mL (i.e., 250 mg per teaspoonful). The directions for taking the medication are 1 teaspoon (i.e., 5 mL) by mouth every 8 hr for 10 days. The prescriber wants 150 mL dispensed and there are no refills allowed.

APPENDIX THREE
Pregnancy Categories: FDA Assigned

A: Adequate and well-controlled studies have failed to demonstrate a risk to the fetus in the first trimester of pregnancy (and there is no evidence of risk in later trimesters).

B: Animal reproduction studies have failed to demonstrate a risk to the fetus and there are no adequate and well-controlled studies in pregnant women.

C: Animal reproduction studies have shown an adverse effect on the fetus and there are no adequate and well-controlled studies in humans, but potential benefits may warrant use of the drug in pregnant women despite potential risks.

D. There is positive evidence of human fetal risk based on adverse reaction data from investigational or marketing experience or studies in humans, but potential benefits may warrant use of the drug in pregnant women despite potential risks.

X: Studies in animals or humans have demonstrated fetal abnormalities and/or there is positive evidence of human fetal risk based on adverse reaction data from investigational or marketing experience, and the risks involved in use of the drug in pregnant women clearly outweigh potential benefits.

The use of drugs during pregnancy should be avoided unless the benefits of therapy far outweigh the risk of fetal malformation. This also applies to any OTC drugs, cigarettes, alcohol, excessive caffeine consumption, and street or recreational drugs.

The stages of fetal development include:

1. Days 0–14: Fertilization to implantation
2. Days 18–60: Organogenesis
3. Eight weeks to birth: Organ maturation

APPENDIX FOUR

Commonly Used Laboratory Test Values

Identified normal values will vary depending on the laboratory, quality controls utilized, and methods used for assay. For clarification, check with the laboratory that performed the analysis.

Serum, Plasma, and Blood

Test	Range	Units	SI Range	Units
Acetone, serum	0.3–2.0	mg/dL	51.6–344.0	µmol/L
Acid phosphatase	0.1–5.0	U/L	2.7–10.7	IU/L
Alanine aminotransferase [ALT] (SGPT)	8–20	U/L	8–20	U/L
Albumin, serum	3.5–5.0	g/dL	35–50	g/L
Alcohol (serum levels)				
No significant influence	< 0.05% or 50	mg/dL	10.8	mmol/L
Alcohol influence present	0.05–0.10% or 50–100	mg/dL	10.8–21.6	mmol/L
Reaction time affected	0.10–0.15% or 100–150	mg/dL	21.6–32.5	mmol/L
Indicative of alcohol intoxication	0.15% or 150	mg/dL	32.5	mmol/L
Severe alcohol intoxication	> 0.25% or 250	mg/dL	54.2	mmol/L
Coma	0.30% or 300	mg/dL	65.1	mmol/L

Test	Conventional value	Conventional unit	SI value	SI unit
Aldosterone	<16	ng/dL (fasting)	<0.45	nmol/L
	4–30	ng/dL (sitting)	0.11–0.84	nmol/L
Alkaline phosphatase	30–120	U/L	0.5–2	μkat/L
Alpha-1-antitrypsin	80–260	mg/dL	0.8–2.6	g/L
Ammonia [NH_4^+]	15–45	μg/dL	11–35	μmol/L
Amylase, serum	60–160	Somogyi U/dL	30–170	U/L
Anion gap	10–17	mEq/L	10–17	mmol/L
Antinuclear antibodies (ANA)	Negative at 1:20 dilution			
Aspartate aminotransferase [AST] (SGOT)	8–33	U/L	8–33	U/L
B_{12}	130–770	pg/mL		
Bilirubin, total (serum)	0.1–1	mg/dL	2–18	μmol/L
Bilirubin, conjugated (direct)	0.1–0.3	mg/dL	1.7–5.1	μmol/L
Blood urea nitrogen/creatinine ratio	10.1–20:1		Average 15:1	
Calcium, serum	8.8–10.4	mg/dL	2.2–2.58	mmol/L
Calcium, ionized	4.4–5.0	mg/dL	1.1–1.24	mmol/L
Carcinoembryonic antigen (CEA)	<2.5	ng/mL (nonsmoker)	<2.5	μg/L
	<5.0	ng/mL (smoker)	<5.0	μg/L
Ceruloplasmin	18–45	mg/dL	180–450	mg/L
Chloride, serum	95–105	mEq/L	95–105	mmol/L
Cholesterol				
Desirable level	<200	mg/dL	<5.20	mmol/L
Moderate risk	200–240	mg/dL	5.2–6.3	mmol/L
High risk	>240	mg/dL	>6.3	mmol/L
Cold agglutinins	1:8 antibody titer			
Copper	70–140	μg/dL	11–22	μmol/L
Cortisol, serum				
0800 hours	4–19	μg/L	110–520	nmol/L
1600 hours	2–15	μg/L	50–410	nmol/L
2400 hours	5		140	nmol/L

Test	Range	Units	SI Range	Units
Creatine kinase (CK)				
Isoenzymes	0–130	U/L	0–2.167	μkat/L
MB fraction	>5 in MI	%	>0.05	1
MB (mass assay)	normal 1.2–3.0	ng/mL		
AMI	>5	ng/mL	>0.05	1
Creatine phosphokinase				
Male	5–35	μg/mL	55–170	U/L
Female	5–25	μg/mL	30–135	U/L
CPK-MB (heart)	0–6%			
Creatinine, serum	0.6–1.2	mg/dL	50–110	μmol/L
Creatinine clearance	75–125	mL/min	1.24–2.08	mL/sec
Erythrocyte count (RBC)				
Male	4.3–5.9	$10^6/mm^3$	4.3–5.9	10^{12}/L
Female	3.5–5	$10^6/mm^3$	3.5–5	10^{12}/L
Erythrocyte sedimentation rate (ESR)				
Male	0–20	mm/hr	0–20	mm/hr
Female	0–30	mm/hr	0–30	mm/hr
Ferritin				
Male	46–637	ng/mL		
Female	10–260	ng/mL	Not available	Not available
Fibrinogen split products	2–10	μg/mL		
Folate	1.5–20.6	pg/mL		
Free thyroxine index (FTI)	1.1–4.7	mcg/dL		
Gamma-glutamyl transferase (GGT)				
Male	4–23	IU/L	9–69	U/L
Female	3–13	IU/L	4–33	U/L
Gases, arterial blood				
pO_2	75–105	mm Hg	10–14	kPa
pCO_2	35–45	mm Hg	4.7–6	kPa

Test	Conventional	Units	SI	Units
Glucose, plasma (fasting)	70–110	mg/dL	3.9–6.1	mmol/L
Glucose, postprandial (fasting)	<140	mg/dL/2 hr	<7.77	mmol/L
Glycosylated HbA1-C	<7.5	%		
Immunoglobulins (Ig)				
Total	900–2,200	mg/dL	9.0–22.0	g/L
IgG	600–1,900	mg/dL	6.0–19.0	g/L
IgA	60–330	mg/dL	0.6–3.3	g/L
IgM	45–145	mg/dL	0.45–1.45	g/L
IgD	0.5–3.0	mg/dL	0.005–0.03	g/L
IgE	10–506	U/mL	0.1–5.06	U/L
Iron, serum				
Male	80–180	µg/dL	14–32	µmol/L
Female	60–160	µg/dL	11–29	µmol/L
Iron binding capacity	250–460	µg/dL	45–82	µmol/L
Iron saturation	15–55	%		
Lactic acid				
Arterial	0.5–1.6	mEq/L	0.5–1.6	mmol/L
Venous	0.5–2.2	mEq/L	0.5–2.2	mmol/L
Lactic dehydrogenase (LDH)	70–250	U/L	70–250	U/L
Lead				
Normal	10–20	µg/dL	<0.9	µmol/L
Acceptable	20–40	µg/dL	<1.9	µmol/L
Lipase	14–280	mU/mL	14–280	U/L
	20–180	IU/L		
Lipoproteins				
Low density (LDL)	50–190	mg/dL	1.3–4.9	mmol/L
High density (HDL)				
Male	30–70	mg/dL	0.8–1.8	mmol/L
Female	30–85	mg/dL	0.8–2.2	mmol/L

Test	Range	Units	SI Range	Units
Leukocyte count (WBC)	4,500–10,000	mm³	4.5–10	10⁹/L
Magnesium, serum	1.8–3	mg/dL	0.8–1.2	mmol/L
	1.6–2.4	mEq/L	0.8–1.2	mmol/L
Myoglobin				
Positive elevation (with AMI)	14–53	ng/mL	Not available	Not available
5' Nucleotidase	<17	U/L	<17	U/L
Osmolality, plasma	280–300	mOsm/kg	280–300	mmol/kg
Phosphate, serum	2.5–5	mg/dL	0.8–1.6	mmol/L
Potassium, serum	3.5–5	mEq/L	3.5–5	mmol/L
Prolactin	<20	ng/mL	<20	mcg/L
Prostate-specific antigen (PSA)				
Normal	0–4	ng/mL	Not available	Not available
BPH	4–19	ng/mL	Not available	Not available
Prostate CA	10–120	ng/mL	Not available	Not available
Protein				
Total	6–8	g/dl	60–80	g/L
Albumin	3.5–5.0	g/dl	35–50	g/L
Fibrinogen	0.2–0.4	g/dl	2–4	g/L
Globulin	1.5–3.0	g/dl	15–30	g/L
Renin				
Supine	0.2–2.3	ng/mL	0.2–2.3	μg/L
Upright	1.6–4.3	ng/mL	1.6–4.3	μg/L
Reticulocyte count				
Male	0.5–1.5%		0.005–0.015 X 10³	
Female	0.5–2.5%		0.005–0.025 X 10³	
Rheumatoid factor	<1:20 titer			
Sodium, serum	135–147	mEq/L	135–147	mmol/L

Test		Conventional		SI value	SI unit
Testosterone					
	Female	<60	mcg/mL		
	Male	300–900	mcg/mL		
Thyroid binding globulin (TBG)		12–28	µg/dL	150–360	nmol/L
Thyroid stimulating hormone (TSH)		2–11	µU/mL	2–11	mU/L
Thyroxine (T₄)		5–12	µg/dL	51–142	nmol/L
Thyroxine, free serum		0.8–2.8	ng/dL	10–36	pmol/L
Transferrin		170–370	mg/dL	1.7–3.7	g/L
Triglycerides		<160	mg/dL	<1.8	mmol/L
Triiodothyronine (T₃)		0.075–0.2	mg/dL	1.2–3.4	nmol/L
Troponin I		<0.5	ng/mL		
	Diagnostic AMI	>2	ng/mL		
T₃ uptake		25–35	%	0.25–0.35	1
T₄ uptake		0.8–1.1		1	
Urea nitrogen		5–20	mg/dL	1.8–7.1	mmol/L
Uric acid					
	Male	3.5–7.0	mg/dL	202–416	µmol/L
	Female	2.4–6.0	mg/dL	143–357	µmol/L
Vitamin B₁₂		130–770	pg/mL		
Zinc protoporphyrin		15–77	µg/dL	0.24–1.23	µmol/L
Zinc, serum		75–150	µg/dL	11.5–23	µmol/L

"SI units" is the abbreviation of *Système International d'Unités*. It is a uniform system of reporting numerical values, permitting interchangeability of information among nations and between disciplines.

Chernecky, C. C., Krech, R. L., and Berger, B. J. (1993). Laboratory Tests and Diagnostic Procedures. *Philadelphia, PA: W. B. Saunders.*
Jacobs, D. S., Kaster, B. L., Demott, W. R., and Wolfson, W. L. (1988). Laboratory Test Handbook, 2nd ed. *St. Louis, MO: Mosby/Lexi-Comp.*
Kee, J. L. (1995). Laboratory and Diagnostic Tests with Nursing Implications, *4th ed. Norwalk, CT: Appleton & Lange.*
Young, D. S. Implementation of SI Units for Clinical Laboratory Data. Annals of Internal Medicine 106:114–129, 1987. *(Courtesy American College of Physicians.)*

ADDITIONAL PHYSIOLOGIC VALUES

HEMATOLOGY

Red blood cell (RBC) count

Male: $4.3–5.9 \times 10^6/mm^3$, $4.3–5.9 \times 10^{12}/L$ (SI units)

Female: $3.5–5 \times 10^6/mm^3$, $3.5–5.0 \times 10^{12}/L$ (SI units)

RBC indices

Mean corpuscular hemoglobin (MCH), 27–33 pg (standard and SI)

Mean corpuscular hemoglobin concentration (MCH), 33–37 g/dL, 330–370, g/L (SI units)

Mean corpuscular volume (MCV) 76–100 μm^3, 76–100 fL

Hemoglobin

Male: 13.5–18 g/dL, 135–180 g/L (SI units)

Female: 11.5–15.5 g/dL, 115–155 g/L (SI units)

Glycosylated (HbA1-C), <7.5%, 5–6% (desired)

Hematocrit

Male: 40–52% (0.40–0.52)

Female: 35–46% (0.35–0.46)

Platelets	$130–400 \times 10^3/mm^3$
White blood cells (leukocytes)	5,000–10,000/mm³
Neutrophils	50–70%
Segments	50–65%
Bands	0–5%
Basophils	0.25–0.5%
Eosinophils	1–3%
Monocytes	2–6%
Lymphocytes	25–40%
T-lymphocytes	60–80% of lymphocytes
B-lymphocytes	10–20% of lymphocytes
Bleeding time	1–3 min (Duke)
	1–5 min (Ivy)
Coagulation time (Lee White)	5–15 min
Prothrombin time	10–15 sec (same as control)
Partial thromboplastin time (PTT)	60–70 sec
Thrombin time	Within 5 sec of control
INR recommended range	
Standard therapy	2.0–3.0
High-dose therapy	2.5–3.5
Activated partial thromboplastin time (APTT)	30–45 sec

BLOOD GASES

Whole blood oxygen, capacity	17–24 vol %
Arterial	
Saturation	96–100% of capacity
pCO_2	35–45 mm Hg
pO_2	75–100 mm Hg
pH	7.38–7.44
Bicarbonate, normal range	24–28 mEq/L
Base excess (BE)	+2 to –2 (±2 mEq/L)
Venous	
Saturation	60–85% capacity
pCO_2	40–54 mm Hg
pO_2	20–50 mm Hg

| pH | 7.36–7.41 |
| Bicarbonate, normal range | 22–28 mEq/L |

CEREBROSPINAL FLUID (CSF)

Cell count	0–8/mm³
Chloride	118–132 mEq/L
Culture	No organisms
Glucose	40–80 mg/dL
Pressure	75–175 cm water
Protein	15–45 mg/dL
Sodium	145–150 mg/dL

URINALYSIS (ROUTINE)

Reference Values (Adult)

Color	Light straw to dark amber
Appearance	Clear
Odor	Aromatic
Foam	White (small amount)
pH	4.5–8.0 (average is 6)
Specific gravity (SG)	1.005–1.030 (1.015–1.024, normal fluid intake)
Protein	2–8 mg/dL (negative reagent strip test)
Glucose	Negative
Ketones	Negative
Microscopic examination	
RBC	1–2 per low-power field
WBC	3–4
Casts	Occasional hyaline

URINE CHEMISTRY

Aldosterone	2–26 μ/24 hr, 5.6–73 nmol/24 hr (SI units)
Amylase	4–37 U/L/2 hr
Bilirubin and bile	Negative to 0.02 mg/dL
Electrolytes	
Calcium	7.4 mEq/24 hr
Chloride	70–250 mEq/24 hr
Magnesium	15–300 mg/24 hr
Phosphorus, inorganic	0.9–1.3 g/24 hr
Potassium	25–120 mEq/24 hr
Sodium	40–220 mEq/24 hr
Glucose	0
5-Hydroxyindoleacetic acid (HIAA)	2–10 mg/24 hr
Ketones	0
Nitrogenous constituents	
Ammonia	30–50 mEq/24 hr
Creatinine clearance	100–200 mL/min
Creatinine	Males: 20–26 mg/kg/24 hr Females: 14–22 mg/kg/24 hr
Protein	0–5 mg/dL/24 hr
Urea	6–17 g/24 hr
Uric acid	0.25–0.75 g/24 hr
Osmolality	200–1,200 mOsm/L
Porphobilinogen	0.2 mg/24 hr

Steroids
  17-Hydroxycorticosteroids   Males: 5–15 mg/24 hr
                                     Females: 3–13 mg/24 hr
  17-Ketosteroids   Males: 8–25 mg/24 hr
                                     Females: 5–15 mg/24 hr
Urobilinogen   0–4 mg/24 hr
Vanillylmandelic acid (VMA)   1.5–7.5 mg/24 hr

APPENDIX FIVE
Nomogram for Estimating Body Surface Area

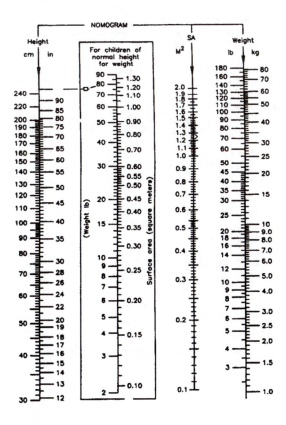

Directions for use: (1) Determine client height. (2) Determine client weight. (3) Draw a straight line to connect the height and weight. Where the line intersects on the surface area line is the derived body surface area (M²).

Reprinted with permission from Behrman, R. E., Kliegman, R., and Arvin, A. M., eds. *Nelson Textbook of Pediatrics,* 15th ed. (Philadelphia: W. B. Saunders Company, 1996).

APPENDIX SIX
Easy Formulas for IV Rate Calculation

In order to calculate the continuous drip rate for an IV infusion, the following information is necessary:

    a. amount of solution to be infused
    b. time for infusion to be administered
    c. *drop factor (found in the tubing package)

$$\frac{\text{Total volume to be infused}}{\text{Total hours for infusion}} \times \frac{\text{*drop factor}}{60 \text{ min/hr}} = \text{gtt/min or cc/hr or mL/hr}$$

*If drop factor is: 60 gtt/min, then use 1 in the formula
                         10 gtt/min, then use ⅙ in the formula
                         15 gtt/min, then use ¼ in the formula
                         20 gtt/min, then use ⅓ in the formula

Example: Infuse 1,000 cc over 8 hr using tubing with a drop factor of 10 gtt/min.

$$\frac{1,000 \text{ cc}}{8 \text{ hr}} \times \frac{1}{6} = 20.8 \text{ or } 21 \text{ cc/hr}$$

When administering intermittent infusions, as with antibiotic therapy, use the following formula:

$$\text{Total volume to be infused} \div \frac{\text{minutes to administer}}{60 \text{ min/hr}} = \frac{\text{mL}}{\text{hr}}$$

Example: Administer 3 g Zosyn in 100 cc of D5W over 45 min

$$100 \div \frac{45}{60} \quad \text{(invert to multiply)}$$

or

$$100 \times \frac{60}{45} = 133.3 \text{ or } 134 \frac{\text{mL}}{\text{hr}}$$

APPENDIX SEVEN
Commonly Accepted Therapeutic Drug Levels

Drug	Peak	Trough
Amikacin	20–30 mcg/mL	1–5 mcg/mL
Gentamicin	5–10 mcg/mL	1–2 mcg/mL
Netilmicin	4–10 mcg/mL	1–2 mcg/mL
Streptomycin	25 mcg/mL	–
Tobramycin	4–10 mcg/mL	1–2 mcg/mL
Vancomycin	20–50 mcg/mL	1–5 mcg/mL

Drug	Therapeutic Range
Amiodarone	0.5–2.5 mcg/mL
Amitriptyline	50–200 ng/mL
Bepridil HCl	1–2 ng/mL
Carbamazepine	4–10 mcg/mL
Desipramine	50–200 ng/mL
Digoxin	0.5–2.2 ng/mL
Disopyramide	2–8 mcg/mL
Doxepin	50–200 ng/mL
Flecainide acetate	0.2–1.0 mcg/mL
Haloperidol	3–10 ng/mL
Heparin	1.5–3 times normal clotting time
Lidocaine	1.5–5 mcg/mL
Lithium	0.4–1.0 mEq/L (maintenance)
Mezlocillin sodium	35–45 mcg/mL
Mexiletine HCl	0.5 mcg/mL
Milrinone	150–250 ng/mL
Nicardipine	0.028–0.05 mcg/mL
Nifedipine	0.025–0.1 mcg/mL
Phenobarbital	15–40 mcg/mL (as anticonvulsant)
Phenytoin	10–20 mcg/mL
Primidone	5–12 mcg/mL
Procainamide	4–8 mcg/mL
Propafenone	0.5–3 mcg/mL
Propranolol	50–200 ng/mL

Drug	Therapeutic Range
Quinidine	2–6 mcg/mL
Salicylic acid	150–300 mcg/mL (as anti-inflammatory)
Theophylline	10–20 mcg/mL
Tocainide HCl	4–10 mcg/mL
Valproic acid	50–100 mcg/mL
Verapamil	0.08–0.3 mcg/mL

APPENDIX EIGHT
Table of Weights and Measures

Weights	Exact Equivalents	Approximate Equivalents
1 ounce (oz)	28.35 g	30 g
1 pound (lb)	453.6 g	454 g
1 gram (g)	0.0353 oz	0.035 oz
1 kilogram (kg)	2.205 lb	2.2 lb
Fluid Measures		
1 teaspoon (t)		5 mL
1 tablespoon (T)	3 tsp	15 mL (½ fl oz)
1 fluid ounce (fl oz)	29.57 mL	30 mL
1 pint (16 fl oz)	473.0 mL	473 mL
1 quart(32 fl oz)	946 mL	945 mL
1 gallon (128 fl oz)	3.785 L	3.8 L
1 milliliter (mL)	0.0352 fl oz (Imperial)	0.0345 fl oz
1 liter (L)	2.11 pt	2 pt
Lengths		
1 inch (in)	2.54 cm	2.5 cm
1 foot (ft)	30.48 cm	30.0 cm
1 yard (yd)	0.914 m	0.9 m
1 centimeter (cm)	0.3937 in	
1 meter (m)	39.4 in	

Approximate Conversions to Metric Measures

To Convert	To	Multiply By
Inches	Centimeters	2.54
Feet	Centimeters	30.48
Grains	Grams	0.065
Ounces	Grams	28.35
Pounds	Kilograms	0.45
Teaspoons, Medical	Milliliters	5.0
Tablespoons	Milliliters	15.0
Fluid ounces	Milliliters	29.57
Cups	Liters	0.24
Pints	Liters	0.47
Quarts	Liters	0.95
Gallons	Liters	3.8

Approximate Conversions to Metric Measures

To Convert	To	Multiply By
Millimeters	Inches	0.039
Centimeters	Inches	0.39
Grams	Grains	15.432
Kilograms	Pounds	2.2
Milliliters	Fluid ounces	0.034
Liters	Pints	2.1
Liters	Quarts	1.06
Liters	Gallons	0.26
Deg. Fahrenheit	Deg. Celsius	5/9 (after subtracting 32)
Deg. Celsius	Deg. Fahrenheit	9/5 (then add 32)

Index

Boldface = generic drug name
italics = therapeutic drug class

Regular type = trade names
CAPITALS = combination drugs

Boldface = generic drug name
Italics = therapeutic drug class

Regular type = trade names
CAPITALS = combination drugs

Boldface = generic drug name
italics = therapeutic drug class

Regular type = trade names
CAPITALS = combination drugs

Boldface = generic drug name
italics = therapeutic drug class

Regular type = trade names
CAPITALS = combination drugs

Boldface = generic drug name
italics = therapeutic drug class

Regular type = trade names
CAPITALS = combination drugs

Boldface = generic drug name
italics = therapeutic drug class

Regular type = trade names
CAPITALS = combination drugs

Boldface = generic drug name   Regular type = trade names
italics = therapeutic drug class   CAPITALS = combination drugs

Boldface = generic drug name
italics = therapeutic drug class
Regular type = trade names
CAPITALS = combination drugs

Boldface = generic drug name
italics = therapeutic drug class

Regular type = trade names
CAPITALS = combination drugs

Boldface = generic drug name
italics = therapeutic drug class

Regular type = trade names
CAPITALS = combination drugs

Boldface = generic drug name
italics = therapeutic drug class

Regular type = trade names
CAPITALS = combination drugs

Boldface = generic drug name
italics = therapeutic drug class

Regular type = trade names
CAPITALS = combination drugs

Boldface = generic drug name   Regular type = trade names
italics = therapeutic drug class   CAPITALS = combination drugs